PHARMACOLOGICAL APPROACHES TO THE TREATMENT OF BRAIN AND SPINAL CORD INJURY

W0227319

PHARMACOLOGICAL APPROACHES TO THE TREATMENT OF BRAIN AND SPINAL CORD INJURY

EDITED BY

DONALD G. STEIN
Clark University
Worcester, Massachusetts

AND

BERNHARD A. SABEL
University of Munich
Munich, Federal Republic of Germany

PLENUM PRESS • NEW YORK AND LONDON

Library of Congress Cataloging in Publication Data

Luxembourg Conference on Recovery from Brain and Spinal Cord Injury (2nd: 1986:
  Walferdange, Luxembourg)
  Pharmacological approaches to the treatment of brain and spinal cord injury.
  "Based on the Second Luxembourg Conference on Recovery from Brain and Spinal
Cord Injury, held July 7-11, 1986, in Walferdange, Luxembourg"—T.p. verso.
  Includes bibliographies and index.
  1. Brain damage—Chemotherapy—Evaluation—Congresses. 2. Spinal cord—
Wounds and injuries—Chemotherapy—Evaluation—Congresses. I. Stein, Donald G.
II. Sabel, Bernhard A. III. Title. [DNLM: 1. Brain Injuries—drug therapy—congresses.
2. Spinal Cord Injuries—drug therapy—congresses. WL 354 L977 1986p]
  RC387.5.L89 1986   617′.481061   88-5942
  ISBN-13: 978-1-4612-8249-5   e-ISBN-13: 978-1-4613-0927-7
  DOI: 10.1007/978-1-4613-0927-7

Based on the Second Luxembourg Conference on Recovery from Brain and Spinal
Cord Injury, held July 7-11, 1986, in Walferdange, Luxembourg

© 1988 Plenum Press, New York
Softcover reprint of the hardcover 1st edition 1988

A Division of Plenum Publishing Corporation
233 Spring Street, New York, N.Y. 10013

To Darel and Liz

CONTRIBUTORS

YOSEF BAWNIK • Department of Neurobiology, The Weizmann Institute of Science, Rehovot, Israel 76100

MICHAEL S. BEATTIE • Departments of Surgery (Neurologic Surgery) and Anatomy, and Spinal Cord Injury Research Center, The Ohio State University, Columbus, Ohio 43210

MICHAEL BELKIN • Goldschleger Eye Institute, Tel Aviv University, Tel Hashomer, Israel

SIMÓN BRAILOWSKY • National Institute of Sciences and Technology, D.I.F., Mexico 14000 D.F., Mexico. *Present address:* Laboratory of Neurophysiology, C.N.R.S., 91190 Gif sur Yvette, France

JACQUELINE C. BRESNAHAN • Departments of Surgery (Neurologic Surgery) and Anatomy, and Spinal Cord Injury Research Center, The Ohio State University, Columbus, Ohio 43210

R. DAL TOSO • Fidia Research Laboratories, 35031 Abano Terme, Italy

PAUL DE KONING • Division of Molecular Neurobiology, Rudolf Magnus Institute for Pharmacology, and Institute of Molecular Biology and Medical Biotechnology, University of Utrecht, 3584 CH Utrecht, The Netherlands

PAUL DELREE • Department of Human Physiology and Physiopathology, University of Liège, Institute L. Frédéricq, B-4020 Liège, Belgium

PAUL DEMEDIUK • Department of Neurology, University of California, San Francisco, and Center for Neural Injury, Veterans Administration Medical Center, San Francisco, California 94121

GARY L. DUNBAR • Brain Research Laboratory, Department of Psychology, Clark University, Worcester, Massachusetts 01610. *Present address:* Department of Psychology, Central Michigan University, Mt. Pleasant, Michigan 48852

ALAN I. FADEN • Department of Neurology, University of California, San Francisco, and Center for Neural Injury, Veterans Administration Medical Center, San Francisco, California 94121

DENNIS M. FEENEY • Departments of Psychology and Physiology, The University of New Mexico, Albuquerque, New Mexico 87131

G. FERRARI • Fidia Research Laboratories, 35031 Abano Terme, Italy

WILLEM HENDRIK GISPEN • Division of Molecular Neurobiology, Rudolf Magnus Institute for Pharmacology, and Institute for Molecular Biology and Medical Biotechnology, University of Utrecht, 3584 CH Utrecht, The Netherlands

ADRIAN HAREL • Department of Neurobiology, The Weizmann Institute of Science, Rehovot, Israel 76100

FRANZ HEFTI • Department of Neurology, University of Miami School of Medicine, Miami, Florida 33101

STEPHEN E. KARPIAK • Division of Neuroscience, New York State Psychiatric Institute, and Departments of Psychiatry and Biochemistry and Molecular Biophysics, College of Physicians and Surgeons, Columbia University, New York, New York 10032

ANDREW KERTESZ • Research Institute, St. Joseph's Hospital, University of Western Ontario, London, Ontario N6A 4V2, Canada

VERED LAVIE • Department of Neurobiology, The Weizmann Institute of Science, Rehovot, Israel 76100

PHILIPPE P. LEFEBVRE • Department of Human Physiology and Physiopathology, University of Liège, Institute L. Frédéricq, B-4020 Liège, Belgium

A. LEON • Fidia Research Laboratories, 35031 Abano Terme, Italy

PIERRE LEPRINCE • Department of Human Physiology and Pathophysiology, University of Liège, Institute L. Frédéricq, B-4020 Liège, Belgium

YU S. LI • Division of Neuroscience, New York State Psychiatric Institute, and Departments of Psychiatry and Biochemistry and Molecular Biophysics, College of Physicians and Surgeons, Columbia University, New York, New York 10032

SAHEBARAO P. MAHADIK • Division of Neuroscience, New York State Psychiatric Institute, and Departments of Psychiatry and Biochemistry and Molecular Biophysics, College of Physicians and Surgeons, Columbia University, New York, New York 10032

TRACY K. MCINTOSH • Department of Neurology, University of California, San Francisco, and Center for Neural Injury, Veterans Administration Medical Center, San Francisco, California 94121. *Present address:* Laboratory for Neuroscience Research, Department of Surgery, University of Connecticut Health Center, Farmington, Connecticut 06032

GUSTAVE MOONEN • Department of Human Physiology and Physiopathology, University of Liège, Institute L. Frédéricq, B-4020 Liège, Belgium

MANUEL NIETO-SAMPEDRO • Department of Psychobiology, University of California at Irvine, Irvine, California 92717

VIVIANE PALLAGE • Department of Neurophysiology and Biology of Behavior, Center of Neurochemistry, C.N.R.S., 67084 Strasbourg, France

JEAN-MICHEL RIGO • Department of Human Physiology and Pathophysiology, University of Liège, Institute L. Frédéricq, B-4020 Liège, Belgium

BERNARD ROGISTER • Department of Human Physiology and Pathophysiology, University of Liège, Institute L. Frédéricq, B-4020 Liège, Belgium

BERNHARD A. SABEL • Institute of Medical Psychology, University of Munich, School of Medicine, 8000 Munich 2, Federal Republic of Germany

MICHAL SCHWARTZ • Department of Neurobiology, The Weizmann Institute of Science, Rehovot, Israel 76100

S. D. SKAPER • Fidia Research Laboratories, 35031 Abano Terme, Italy, and Department of Biology and School of Medicine, University of California at San Diego, La Jolla, California 92093

ARIE SOLOMON • Goldschleger Eye Institute, Tel Aviv University, Tel Hashomer, Israel

DONALD G. STEIN • Departments of Psychology and Biology, Clark University, Worcester, Massachusetts 01610. *Present address:* Dean of the Graduate School and Associate Provost for Research, Rutgers University at Newark, Newark, New Jersey 07102

CATHY STEIN-IZSAK • Department of Neurobiology, The Weizmann Institute of Science, Rehovot, Israel 76100

BRADFORD T. STOKES • Departments of Surgery (Neurologic Surgery) and Anatomy, and Spinal Cord Injury Research Center, The Ohio State University, Columbus, Ohio 43210

RICHARD L. SUTTON • Departments of Psychology and Physiology, The University of New Mexico, Albuquerque, New Mexico 87131

G. TOFFANO • Fidia Research Laboratories, 35031 Abano Terme, Italy

GUY TONIOLO • Department of Neurophysiology and Biology of Behavior, Center of Neurochemistry, C.N.R.S., 67084 Strasbourg, France

G. VANTINI • Fidia Research Laboratories, 35031 Abano Terme, Italy

WILLIAM J. WEINER • Department of Neurology, University of Miami School of Medicine, Miami, Florida 33101

BRUNO WILL • Department of Neurophysiology and Biology of Behavior, Center of Neurochemistry, C.N.R.S., 67084 Strasbourg, France

JUSTIN A. ZIVIN • Department of Neurology, San Diego Veterans Administration Medical Center, and Department of Neurosciences, University of California, San Diego, La Jolla, California 92093

PREFACE

Although there are over 400,000 people each year in the United States alone who suffer from traumatic injury to the central nervous system (CNS), no pharmacological treatment is currently available. Considering the enormity of the problem in terms of human tragedy as well as the economic burden to families and societies alike, it is surprising that so little effort is being made to develop treatments for these disorders. Although no one can become inured to the victims of brain or spinal cord injuries, one reason that insufficient time and effort have been devoted to research on recovery is that it is a generally held medical belief that nervous system injuries are simply not amenable to treatment. At best, current therapies are aimed at providing symptomatic relief or focus on rehabilitative measures and the teaching of alternative behavioral strategies to help patients cope with their impairments, with only marginal results in many cases.

Only within the last decade have neuroscientists begun to make serious inroads into understanding and examining the inherent "plasticity" found in the adult CNS. Ten years or so ago, very few researchers or clinicians would have thought that damaged central neurons could sprout new terminals or that intact nerve fibers in a damaged pathway could proliferate to replace inputs from neurons that died as a result of injury.

It would have been even more radical to propose that specific pharmacological agents might serve to salvage or spare brain or spinal neurons from the devastating effects of traumatic injury. Anyone who proposed that injured brains produce special proteins that enhance neuronal survival and promote new axonal growth, or that glial cells may play a pivotal role in the enhancement of functional recovery from CNS trauma, would have found his scientific credibility at stake.

Today, neuroscience is in the midst of a scientific revolution. Long-held beliefs and research paradigms are being seriously reevaluated in the face of new discoveries about the nature of neuronal and glial plasticity in the central nervous system. These discoveries are dramatically altering the way we think about recovery and are permitting, for the first time, some optimism that brain injury might be treated with pharmacological agents.

Both of us have studied various ways of promoting recovery from severe brain injuries, and in the course of our research, we realized that there was no current overview of this important field. In July, 1986, an international conference on experimental approaches to the treatment of brain and spinal cord injuries was held in Walferdange, Luxembourg. A number of American and European colleagues who have been deeply concerned with finding the means to promote functional recovery from brain and spinal injuries were invited to discuss and share their research findings in an informal, collegial setting.

The present volume summarizes the contemporary research in this area, ranging from clinical neuropsychology to the possible role of oncogenes in neuroplasticity. Each of the participants brought a special expertise to discuss. Some investigators were primarily concerned with neurotransmitter biochemistry in the brain or spinal cord and the alterations that occurred after injury; others discussed the question of how endogenous or exogenous "trophic" substances might work to promote survival of damaged neurons or new axonal growth. We also invited colleagues who sought to determine how some of the secondary damage that accompanies CNS injury could be characterized and prevented. Finally, there were others with behavioral concerns who were interested in determining whether new, experimental substances could be used to enhance cognitive and functional recovery after traumatic brain injury.

As with previous Clark University/Luxembourg meetings, this one, too, was made possible through the generosity of Mr. Henry J. Leir, a Clark University benefactor who has long been interested in fostering international cooperation in the sciences and the humanities. We were also fortunate to receive generous grants from the following pharmaceutical companies that enabled us to bring colleagues to Luxembourg from ten countries. We wish to thank Fidia Research Laboratories of Italy; P.F. Medicament, France; American Cyanamid, U.S.A.; Schering, AG, Fed. Rep. Germany; Abbott Laboratories, U.S.A.; Cybila, GmBH, Fed. Rep. Germany; Travenol Laboratories, U.S.A.; Eli Lilly & Company, U.S.A.; and E.I. DuPont Pharmaceuticals, U.S.A., for their support, interest, and encouragement of this meeting.

As was the case in the past, we were very happy to have the continued support of Dr. Gaston Schaber, Luxembourg Ministry of Education, as well as the kindness and hospitality of the Mayor of Walferdange and the excellent staff of the Institute Pedagogique, who did everything in their power to ensure a successful and pleasant meeting; we eagerly look forward to future collaborations with them.

Finally, we owe a warm and grateful "thank you" to our respective spouses, Darel Stein and Elizabeth Sabel, for their unswerving support and patience through the good and the bad times.

D.G.S., B.S.

Worcester, Massachusetts

CONTENTS

1. THERAPEUTIC APPROACHES IN SUBJECTS WITH BRAIN
LESIONS 1

SIMÓN BRAILOWSKY

1. Introduction 1
2. Developmental, Degenerative, and Regenerative Factors
   Related to Brain Plasticity 3
3. Mechanisms of Cell Damage Linked to Ischemia 5
4. Drugs Used to Treat Ischemic Cell Damage 9
5. Management of Medical and Neurological Complications .. 10
6. Requirements in the Design of a Clinical Trial 12
7. Individualization of Drug Therapy 13
8. The GABA Technique of Reversible Brain Dysfunction ... 14
   References 18

2. ARACHIDONIC ACID METABOLITES AND MEMBRANE LIPID
CHANGES IN CENTRAL NERVOUS SYSTEM INJURY 23

PAUL DEMEDIUK AND ALAN I. FADEN

1. Introduction 24
2. Membrane Lipid Changes in CNS Injury 24
   2.1. Direct Membrane Effects 24
   2.2. Eicosanoid Production 29
3. Pharmacological Intervention 32
   3.1. Direct Membrane Protection 32
   3.2. Eicosanoid Blockade 33
4. Research in Progress 35
5. Conclusion 35
   References 36

3. EXPERIMENTAL SPINAL CORD INJURY: STRATEGIES FOR ACUTE
   AND CHRONIC INTERVENTION BASED ON ANATOMIC,
   PHYSIOLOGICAL, AND BEHAVIORAL STUDIES 43

MICHAEL S. BEATTIE, BRADFORD T. STOKES, AND JACQUELINE C.
BRESNAHAN

1. Introduction and a Brief History of Spinal Cord Injury
   Research 43
2. Current Methods for Lesion Production 44
   2.1. Impact Injuries 44
   2.2. Slow(er) Compression Injuries 45
3. The Time Course of Events following Injury 45
   3.1. The Acute Phase and the Concept of a Progressive
        Lesion 46
   3.2. The Chronic Phase: Potential Reorganization and
        Rehabilitation 47
4. The Features of the Lesion 47
   4.1. At the Impact Site 47
   4.2. The Distributed Nature of the Lesion 51
5. Assessing Behavioral and Neurological Recovery 51
6. Examples of Attempts at Pharmacological Intervention ... 52
   6.1. In the Acute Phase 53
   6.2. In the Chronic Phase 54
   6.3. Adjuncts to Pharmacological Treatment 55
7. Studies Using the Ohio State Impaction Device 56
   7.1. The Ohio State Feedback-Controlled Impactor 56
   7.2. Production of Lesions with Predictable Outcomes ... 56
   7.3. The Role of Ionic Ca^{2+} in the Acute Phase ... 61
8. Future Strategies for Pharmacological Intervention ... 65
   8.1. In the Acute Phase 65
   8.2. In the Chronic Phase 66
9. Summary and Conclusions 68
   References 68

4. SEROTONIN ANTAGONISTS REDUCE CENTRAL NERVOUS
   SYSTEM ISCHEMIC DAMAGE.............................. 75

JUSTIN A. ZIVIN

1. Introduction 75
2. Review of the Effects of Serotonin in Stroke 76
3. New Methods for the Study of CNS Ischemia 78

3.1. Rabbit Spinal Cord Ischemia Model 78
3.2. Microsphere Embolic Stroke Model 80
4. Biochemical Studies of the Effects of Serotonin in CNS
   Ischemia 82
5. Pharmacological Studies of the Effects of Serotonin
   Antagonists and Agonists in CNS Ischemia 83
6. Microsphere Studies of the Effects of Serotonin Antagonists
   on Stroke 86
   References 87

5. OPIATE ANTAGONISTS IN CNS INJURY 89

TRACY K. MCINTOSH AND ALAN I. FADEN

1. Introduction 89
2. Opiate Antagonists 90
3. Rationale for Use of Opiate Antagonists in CNS Injury ... 91
   3.1. Opiate Antagonists in the Treatment of Spinal Cord
        Injury 92
   3.2. Opiate Antagonists and Traumatic Brain Injury 95
4. Role of Specific Opioids and Opiate Receptors in CNS
   Injury 95
5. Opiate Antagonists in CNS Injury: Clinical Studies 98
6. Future Directions 98
   References 99

6. ADAPTIVE CHANGES IN CENTRAL DOPAMINERGIC NEURONS
   AFTER INJURY: EFFECTS OF DRUGS 103

FRANZ HEFTI AND WILLIAM J. WEINER

1. Introduction 103
2. Anatomy and Function of Mesencephalic Dopaminergic
   Neurons 104
3. Compensatory Changes in Transmitter Release 107
4. Pharmacological Stimulation of DA Synthesis and Release
   in Dopaminergic Neurons Surviving Partial Nigrostriatal
   Lesions 109
5. Compensatory Changes in Postsynaptic Receptor
   Sensitivity 114
   References 116

7. Catecholamines and Recovery of Function after Brain
   Damage 121

Dennis M. Feeney and Richard L. Sutton

1. Historical Background 121
   1.1. Tactile Placing 121
   1.2. Visual Cliff 122
   1.3. Hemiplegic Rat Model 122
   1.4. Norepinephrine and the Importance of Experience .. 123
   1.5. Hemiplegic Cat Model 125
   1.6. Binocular Vision 125
2. Theoretical Bases 126
   2.1. Morphological Changes 126
   2.2. Vicariation 127
   2.3. Behavioral Substitution 127
   2.4. Cerebral Blood Flow and Cholinergic System 127
   2.5. Diaschisis, RFD, and Metabolic Studies 128
3. Recent Data 132
   3.1. Cytochrome Oxidase 132
   3.2. Idazoxan 132
   3.3. Locus Coeruleus and Cerebellum 133
   3.4. Phentermine and Phenylpropanolamine 134
   3.5. Transplants 135
   3.6. Cortical Contusion 135
   3.7. Clinical Data 136
   3.8. Drug Contraindications 138
4. Future Directions 138
   4.1. Mechanisms 138
   4.2. Optimizing Therapy 139
   References 139

8. Ganglioside Involvement in Membrane-Mediated
   Transfer of Trophic Information: Relationship to G_{M1}
   Effects following CNS Injury 143

R. Dal Toso, S. D. Skaper, G. Ferrari, G. Vantini, G. Toffano,
and A. Leon

1. Introduction 144
   1.1. Neuronotrophic Activity after Injury 144
   1.2. Trophic Effects and Exogenous Factors 144
   1.3. Trophic Effects and Membrane Constituents 145
2. Evidence for Ganglioside Involvement in the
   Biotransduction of Membrane-Mediated Information 146
   2.1. Chemical Diversity of the Gangliosides 146

2.2. Tissue Distribution and Cellular Localization 148
2.3. Membrane Organization 149
3. Evidence for Ganglioside Involvement in Neuronal Cell
Responsiveness to Neuronotrophic Factors 151
3.1. Studies in Normal Neuronal Development and
"Accidents of Nature" 152
3.2. Studies Utilizing Neuroblastoma Cells 153
3.3. Studies Utilizing Primary PNS Neurons and
PC_{12} Cells 154
3.4. Studies Utilizing Primary CNS Neurons 157
4. G_{M1} Effects *in Vivo:* Possible Relationship with
Neuronotrophic Factors 158
References 159

9. ANATOMIC MECHANISMS WHEREBY GANGLIOSIDE TREATMENT
INDUCES BRAIN REPAIR: WHAT DO WE REALLY KNOW? 167

BERNHARD A. SABEL

1. Introduction 168
2. Regeneration and Sprouting after Brain Injury 170
2.1. Gangliosides in Development and Peripheral Nerve
Regeneration 170
2.2. Sprouting in Adulthood 171
2.3. Sprouting in Development 176
2.4. Conclusions on Sprouting 180
3. Preventing Secondary Degeneration after Brain Injury 181
3.1. Degeneration in Adulthood 181
3.2. Degeneration in Development 185
4. Other Mechanisms 187
4.1. Denervation Supersensitivity 187
4.2. Synaptic Efficiency 188
5. Discussion 188
6. Recommendations for Future Research 190
References 191

10. GANGLIOSIDES AND FUNCTIONAL RECOVERY FROM BRAIN
INJURY 195

GARY L. DUNBAR AND DONALD G. STEIN

1. Introduction 196
2. Behavioral Recovery following Damage to the
Septohippocampal System 196

3. Behavioral Recovery following Damage or Denervation of
   Cortical Structures 197
   3.1. Recovery after Lesions to the Cholinergic Forebrain
        Nuclei 197
   3.2. Recovery after Cortical Lesions 198
   3.3. Recovery after Ischemia 200
4. Behavioral Recovery following Nigrostriatal Damage 201
   4.1. Early Studies on Recovery following Nigrostriatal
        Damage 201
   4.2. Later Studies on Recovery after Nigrostriatal Damage 202
   4.3. Recent Data on Recovery after Nigrostriatal Damage   204
   4.4. Recent Data on Recovery after Bilateral Lesions of the
        Caudate Nucleus 204
5. General Discussion and Conclusions 210
   References 215

11. ACUTE GANGLIOSIDE EFFECTS LIMIT CNS INJURY:
    FUNCTIONAL AND BIOCHEMICAL CONSEQUENCES 219

STEPHEN E. KARPIAK, YU S. LI, AND SAHEBARAO P. MAHADIK

1. Long-Term Ganglioside Effects: Increased Plasticity 219
2. Acute Ganglioside Effects 220
   2.1. Unilateral Entorhinal Cortical Lesions 220
   2.2. Bilateral Entorhinal Cortical Lesions 221
   2.3. Nigrostriatal Transection: Reduced Asymmetry 222
3. G_{M1} Ganglioside Reduces Edema: Protection of Membrane
   Na^+,K^+-ATPase 223
   3.1. Membrane Na^+,K^+-ATPase 224
   3.2. Protection of Striatal Na^+,K^+-ATPase after
        Hemitransection 224
4. Ganglioside Treatment Reduces Mortality from Ischemia .. 226
   4.1. Global Ischemia Model 226
   4.2. Reduced Mortality following Ganglioside Injections ... 227
5. Mechanism: Membrane Protection 228
   References 229

12. A RATIONALE FOR THE USE OF MELANOCORTINS IN NEURAL
    INJURY 233

PAUL DE KONING AND WILLEM HENDRIK GISPEN

1. Introduction 233
2. Trophic Influences of Melanocortins in Development 235

3. Melanocortins and CNS Plasticity 236
4. Regeneration in the Peripheral Nervous System 239
5. Melanocortins and PNS Plasticity 240
    5.1. Recovery of Function following a Crush Lesion 240
    5.2. Route of Administration 243
    5.3. Electrophysiology 243
    5.4. Histology 246
6. Neurotrophic Effect and Pathophysiological Mechanism ... 247
7. Local Application of α-MSH and the Repair of Transected
    Rat Sciatic Nerve 249
8. Clinical Perspectives 251
    References 253

13. Developmental Neurobiology and Physiopathology of
Brain Injury 259

Gustave Moonen, Paul Delree, Pierre Leprince, Jean-Michel
Rigo, Bernard Rogister, and Philippe P. Lefebvre

1. Introduction 260
2. Neuronal Proliferation 260
3. Neuronal Migration 262
    3.1. Plasminogen Activators 262
    3.2. Cell Adhesion Molecules 263
    3.3. Extracellular Matrix Components 263
4. Neuronal Stabilization 265
    4.1. Neuronotrophic Factors 266
    4.2. Neuronotoxic Factors 268
    4.3. Interference between Neuronotrophic and
         Neuronotoxic Activities 270
5. Growth (Mitogenic) Factors 270
6. Conclusion 274
    References 275

14. Growth-Associated Triggering Factors and Central
Nervous System Response to Injury 281

Michal Schwartz, Adrian Harel, Cathy Stein-Izsak, Arie
Solomon, Vered Lavie, Yosef Bawnik, and Michael Belkin

1. Introduction 282
2. Background and Literature Survey 283

2.1. Regeneration-Associated Events in the Neuron 283
2.2. Neuronal–Microenvironment Reciprocal Relationship 285
3. Results Obtained in the Visual System 286
3.1. Modifications of Neuronal Environment and
     Regeneration 287
3.2. Messenger RNA Derived from Nonneuronal Cells and
     Regeneration 294
References 296

15. GROWTH FACTOR INDUCTION AND ORDER OF EVENTS IN CNS REPAIR

15. GROWTH FACTOR INDUCTION AND ORDER OF EVENTS IN CNS
REPAIR 301

MANUEL NIETO-SAMPEDRO

1. Introduction 302
2. Cellular Events That Follow CNS Injury 302
3. Neuronal Survival after CNS Injury 303
3.1. Central Neuronotrophic Factors and Secondary
     Neuronal Death 304
3.2. Excitotoxicity and Secondary Neuronal Death 305
3.3. Preventing Secondary Neuronal Death 307
3.4. Replacing Lost Neurons: Injury-Induced
     Neuronotrophic Factors and Transplant Survival 308
4. Reactive and Regenerative Growth after CNS Injury 310
4.1. Reactive Synaptogenesis 312
4.2. Functional Significance of Reactive Synaptogenesis ... 312
4.3. Neurite-Promoting Factors and Axonal Sprouting 313
4.4. Regenerative Synaptogenesis and Transplant–Host
     Integration 315
5. Multiple Roles of Astroglia 318
5.1. The "Glial Scar" or Neo-Glia Limitans 318
5.2. The Control of Glial Populations in Adult CNS:
     Mitogens, Morphogens, and Inhibitors 320
5.3. Astrocytes Accumulate and Detoxify Glutamate 321
5.4. Astrocytes Produce Factors That Promote Neuronal
     Survival, Sprouting, and Substrate Attachment 323
5.5. Transplants of Purified Astrocytes Promote Functional
     Recovery 324
5.6. Control of the Neural Environment by Astrocytes: A
     Neuron–Astrocyte Unit of Function 326
6. Cellular Sources of Trophic Factors 326
7. Timing of the Intervention in CNS Repair 328

8. Conclusion 331
   References 332

16. NERVE GROWTH FACTOR: EFFECTS ON CNS NEURONS AND ON
    BEHAVIORAL RECOVERY FROM BRAIN DAMAGE 339
    BRUNO WILL, FRANZ HEFTI, VIVIANE PALLAGE, AND GUY TONIOLO

    1. Introduction 339
    2. The Nerve Growth Factor and Its Effects
       on PNS Neurons 340
    3. Effects of NGF on CNS Neurons 341
    4. Effects of NGF on Behavior 347
    5. Discussion 353
       References 356

17. RECOVERY FROM STROKE 361
    ANDREW KERTESZ

    1. Introduction 361
    2. Pharmacological Intervention and First-Stage Recovery 363
    3. Pharmacological Treatment in Second-Stage Recovery 366
    4. Factors in Second-Stage Recovery 367
    5. The Measurements of Deficit 368
    6. Recovery Rates and Time Intervals 369
    7. Lesion Size and Recovery 369
    8. Lesion Location and Recovery 370
    9. Cerebral Asymmetry 371
   10. Functional Reorganization 371
   11. Implications for Pharmacological Trials in Patients 373
       References 373

INDEX. 377

1

THERAPEUTIC APPROACHES IN SUBJECTS WITH BRAIN LESIONS

SIMÓN BRAILOWSKY

ABSTRACT. The pharmacological treatment of subjects who sustain a brain lesion, either accidentally (trauma, stroke) or surgically (tumor excision, stereotactic lesions, etc.) is generally aimed at preventing further damage from pathology such as edema, hemorrhage, infection, seizures, or renal or cardiopulmonary failure. The efficacy of these treatments can be observed in the period immediately following the insult. However, the long-term effects, if any, of these treatments, or any interactions between the drugs used and mechanisms involved in functional recovery, have often been ignored.

A brief review of some basic aspects of the response of neural and nonneural cells to injury is offered, with some comments on events occurring during histogenesis and in the initiation and regulation of inflammatory and immune responses that might be relevant to the problem of brain plasticity. I then discuss some of the mechanisms of cell damage common to different forms of injury (e.g., trauma, hemorrhage, thrombosis) such as membrane permeability changes, intracellular calcium alterations, and the role of certain neurotransmitters in the genesis of acute neuronal loss. Special emphasis on ischemia is made, with a review of the pharmacological treatment of stroke and comments on the importance of the management of the medical and neurological complications of a brain lesion. I conclude with a discussion of the requirements in the design of clinical trials oriented towards the individualization of drug therapy.

Finally, I summarize our own investigations with a pharmacological model of reversible brain dysfunction using GABA, an endogenous inhibitory neurotransmitter, in both rats and monkeys.

1. INTRODUCTION

In a previous paper,[7] we referred to the common attitude of clinicians dealing with brain-injured patients. These cases often generate a mixed feeling of pessimism not only among medical personnel but also in the patient's family. The limited availability of specific drugs to treat brain lesions has, however, stimulated efforts both to understand the mechanisms involved in the pathophysiology of neural

SIMÓN BRAILOWSKY • National Institute of Sciences and Technology, D.I.F., Mexico 14000 D.F., Mexico. *Present address:* Laboratory of Neurophysiology, C.N.R.S., 91190 Gif sur Yvette, France.

injury and to find new remedial interventions to help these patients. In Table I we have assembled some of the theories and mechanisms invoked to explain the recovery processes found clinically and experimentally. Far from being exhaustive, this list demonstrates that (1) many changes occur after a brain lesion, as most of the mechanisms proposed are not mutually exclusive, (2) that there are many possible levels of pharmacological intervention to alter the course of a brain lesion, and (3) that some confusion exists among researchers when naming a phenomenon related to the already vague term of "plasticity." For example, what is the difference between "redundancy" and "multiple control"?

Generally speaking, the main objective in the medical treatment of patients with brain injury is to reduce neurological deficits and prevent the progression of neural damage. In spite of undeniable progress in the neurosciences and the increasing power of new electrophysiological and brain-imaging techniques (PET scanning, nuclear magnetic resonance, etc.), we are still unable to distinguish between reversible and irreversible damage in the period immediately following brain injury. Nevertheless, every clinician recognizes that some patients will show spontaneous recovery. This fact, in conjunction with the awareness of the dynamic character of brain lesions, should provide the basis for investigation of therapies aimed at favoring the recovery process.

As Norman Geschwind stated[23]:

> It is a salient principle that one can probably never speak of a fixed neurological lesion. Damage in every location is followed by a sequence of changes, both local and distant, some instantaneous and others proceeding over years. . . . It is possible that many [of these] changes, perhaps the majority, are unfavorable, serving to prevent the expression of latent restorative processes. Study of these unfavorable mechanisms may be even more important than investigations of spontaneous recovery in leading to improved methods of therapy.

Geschwind's insight will serve to establish our framework for the discussion of some of the factors to be considered in the medical treatment of patients with brain injury.

TABLE I. Brain Plasticity after Injury:
Proposed Theories and Mechanisms

Theories	Mechanisms
Sparing	Reactive synaptogenesis
Redundancy	Regenerative sprouting
Multiple control	Postsynaptic supersensitivity
Substitution	Presynaptic hyperactivity
Compensation	Silent afferents ("unmasking")
Diaschisis ("neural shock")	Sustained collaterals
Restoration (restitution)	Remote disinhibition
Vicariation	Release of occlusion
	Release or reactivation of developmental processes

Stroke is one of the main causes of neurological disability. For this reason, many attempts have been made to alter its progression toward stabilization or reversal of neurological impairment. The epidemiologic importance of this syndrome warrants a brief review of the rationales employed by clinicians in the pharmacological treatment of these patients. We use this pathological condition to examplify current efforts to influence functional recovery after CNS damage. Information on drug treatment of other types of neural injury is more limited, although promising (for review, see ref. 19). It should be stressed that progress in the pharmacological treatment of patients with brain injuries should be based on our understanding of normal brain mechanisms: from receptors to behavior, from environmental influences to genetics, all levels should be considered.

I review briefly some basic aspects of the response of neural and nonneural cells to injury with some comments on events occurring during histogenesis that we consider relevant to the problem of brain plasticity; Dr. Moonen and co-workers (Chapter 13) and Dr. Nieto-Sampedro (Chapter 15) refer to some of them in more detail. A short discussion of some of the reactions and mechanisms of cell damage linked to ischemia with special emphasis on those changes that may be common to other forms of injury follows. I then examine some of the more specific pharmacological aspects of stroke with comments on some of the drugs used to treat ischemic damage; the importance of the management of medical and neurological complications of a brain lesion is emphasized with a discussion of the requirements for the design of clinical trials aimed at the final goal, individualization of drug therapy. Finally, I summarize our own investigations with a pharmacological model of reversible brain dysfunction using GABA, an endogenous inhibitory neurotransmitter, in both rats and monkeys.

2. DEVELOPMENTAL, DEGENERATIVE, AND REGENERATIVE FACTORS RELATED TO BRAIN PLASTICITY

When a nerve fiber is cut, a complex sequence of events is triggered inside the neuron and in neighboring cells (see Fig. 1). The detailed mechanisms of many of these events are still to be clarified; for example, the character of the signal produced by the severed axon to induce the well-known chromatolytic changes in the cell soma is still unknown,[28] and the processes by which an injured neuron loses all incoming terminals after axotomy and recovers them if the axon reestablishes contact with its target[55] are also obscure. We know that many trophic factors exist between neurons and between neurons and glia and that these must play a role in plastic phenomena. The identification of macromolecules implicated in cell recognition, cell adhesion, axonal guidance, and regulation of gene expression offers new possibilities of intervention in the healing process after injury.

The increased resolution of separation and immunologic techniques has permitted the isolation of molecular markers of many of the nonneural cells that

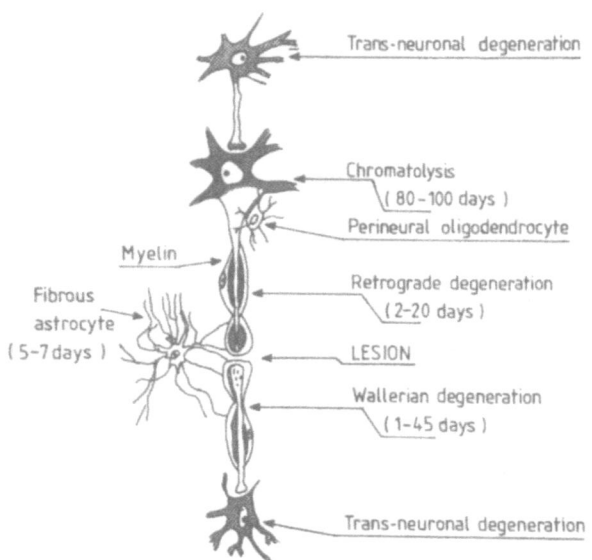

FIGURE 1. Schematic view of neuronal and glial responses to nerve injury. An approximate time course of these events is included to illustrate the dynamic character of the process. The participation of glia (astrocytes and oligodendrocytes) at the central level and of Schwann cells in the periphery should be considered an integral element of both positive and negative reactions of the nervous system to noxious influences (for details, see text).

participate in developmental, degenerative, and regenerative processes. Use of antibodies to these markers has made it possible to identify which cells react in response to a lesion or in an eventual recovery response. The interactions between neurons and glia are now better understood. We know, for example, that extracts of Schwann cell cultures promote regeneration of cholinergic processes *in vivo*,[33] that adult oligodendrocytes proliferate only in presence of neurons and not when neurons are absent,[60] and that mitogenic activity of regrowing axons has been observed in Schwann cells during Wallerian degeneration (see ref. 11). We know also that nonneural cells secrete molecules that promote neurite extension in culture by formation of substrate adhesion molecules (SAM) such as laminin, fibronectin, and heparan sulfate proteoglycan[12]; SAMs are major components of the basal lamina, a structure thought to determine which areas of the nervous system will remain intrinsic (i.e., inside the brain–blood barrier) rather than peripheral after an injury.[59] The laminin-induced promotion of neurite outgrowth is much higher in developing tissues, whereas in the adult nervous system its immunoreactivity is limited to basement membranes.[12,13] After axotomy, Schwann cells proliferate and provide laminin-rich pathways that may guide and stimulate axonal regrowth.[33,48]

Characterization of cell adhesion molecules (CAM) can help understand how neural and nonneural cells establish contact. Specific CAMs exist in neuron-to-neuron communication (N-CAM), in neuron-to-astrocyte adhesion (Ng-CAM), in neuronal migration (Ng-CAM and L-1), and in myelination (MAG). Failure of axonal regrowth after injury might be caused by abortive expression of these guiding and promoting signals.

Finally, astrocytes appear to play a major role in the initiation and regulation of intracerebral inflammatory and immune responses.[57] In the brain, and more specifically, in the vicinity of blood vessels, astrocytes can behave as specialized antigen-presenter cells (APC). T lymphocytes recognize antigen only when it is presented on the membrane of an APC. Astrocytes and other APCs (monocytes, macrophages) release interleukin-1 (IL-1), which stimulates T cells to produce IL-2, an essential factor for the full expression of the T-cell cycle, and γ-interferon, which stimulates further APC expression, IL-1 release, and secretion of prostaglandin E (PGE). Recently, IL-2 has been shown to induce proliferation and differentiation of oligodendrocytes, suggesting a role in the inflammatory lesions of multiple sclerosis and in gliosis consecutive to brain injury.[4]

The glial proliferation in which all types of nonneural cells participate[34] may impede reorganization through displacement of synaptic terminals[6] or interfere with growing axon sprouts. Raisman[45] considers the latter to be the main limiting factor in recovery through reinnervation. Recently, Wells and Bernstein[59] reviewed the data on the influence of scar formation and neuronal regeneration after trauma. They concluded that the failure of the axon to reestablish synaptic connections results from a combination of both inadequate neuronal growth properties and the scar formation processes rather than either alone (see also ref. 21). Nevertheless, as Nieto-Sampedro discusses (Chapter 15), astrocytes may also play a beneficial role after neural injury.

3. MECHANISMS OF CELL DAMAGE LINKED TO ISCHEMIA

The neurodegenerative changes observed after a brain lesion depend on the characteristics of the etiopathogenic agent. For example, neurological disorders such as epilepsy, Huntington's chorea, parkinsonism, and olivopontocerebellar atrophy show neuronal losses localized to different structures, suggesting different causative factors, whereas common mechanisms have been proposed for brain damage induced by excitotoxins and by anoxic/ischemic accidents.[47,49]

I consider briefly some of the mechanisms of cell damage linked to ischemia from the clinical point of view and then examine, in some detail, how disturbances in intracellular calcium occupy a center position in the sequence of events leading to neuronal death. I finally refer to some recent evidence on the role of neurotransmitters in the genesis of acute neuronal loss.

The possible causes of reduction in cerebral blood flow (CBF) are many. They can occur either acutely, i.e., circulatory arrest, cerebral embolism, trauma with hemorrhage, rupture of an aneurism, etc., or they may evolve progressively as in asphyxia, transient focal ischemic attacks, progressing stroke, etc. The latter category is sometimes difficult to define, particularly in cases of acute carotid system infarction (see ref. 29). It is of paramount importance to establish, as soon as possible, the etiology of the ischemic accident, particularly in cases of intracranial bleeding or evolving hypertensive encephalopathy. The physician must take into account this time window when choosing a medical treatment for his patient, as neuronal damage increases proportionally with progressing ischemia.

Concerning the acute progressing stroke, the general impression is that 18 to 24 hr without progression, in cases where the site of focal ischemia is in the carotid system, is sufficient to categorize the stroke as "completed." If the lesion is in the vertebrobasilar territory, a longer period of time (up to 72 hr) is necessary. Completed stroke then refers to a condition in which the focal neurological deficit is stable.

A focus of ischemia usually presents three zones: (1) a central ischemic zone where the blood flow is under 10 ml/100 g per min and that eventually will progress to infarction, (2) a bordering zone, now called "ischemic penumbra,"[1] where blood flow is between 10 and 15 ml/100 g per min, and (3) a collateral zone, frequently hyperemic.[58]

There are many factors that can influence the outcome of an ischemic attack: completness of ischemia (incomplete ischemia appears to be more hazardous than complete ischemia), collateral circulation, duration of ischemia, presence of edema (see ref. 58), pH, and serum glucose concentration. The latter has been shown to be a critical factor: the level of carbohydrate in the brain will determine whether the ischemic zone will cause cerebral infarction or will result in more limited damage. Plum's[44] hypothesis is that hyperglycemia induces a chain of events: high tissue lactoacidosis → neuronal death, astrocyte swelling, endothelial leakage, and disintegration → infarction → severe extracellular edema. Therefore, special care should be taken in patients at risk for hyperglycemia.

The pathophysiology of neural injury from ischemia is shown in Fig. 2. Independently of the origin, local ischemia will eventually produce an increase in intracellular calcium, triggering what has been called "the calcium cascade."

The Ca^{2+} cascade refers to the chain of events produced by an abnormal increase in cytosolic calcium. The disruption of membranal Ca^{2+}-ATPase pump activity can be the consequence of energy failure (depletion of high-energy phosphates) or prolonged depolarization. The increased intracellular Ca^{2+} will activate two subclasses of protein kinases: the calcium and calmodulin-dependent protein kinase and the calcium and phosphatidylserine-dependent kinase or protein kinase C[39]; these kinases will trigger different mechanisms normally tightly controlled, including neurotransmitter release (via stimulation of inositol triphosphate and diacylglycerol formation) and hydrolysis of arachidonic acid

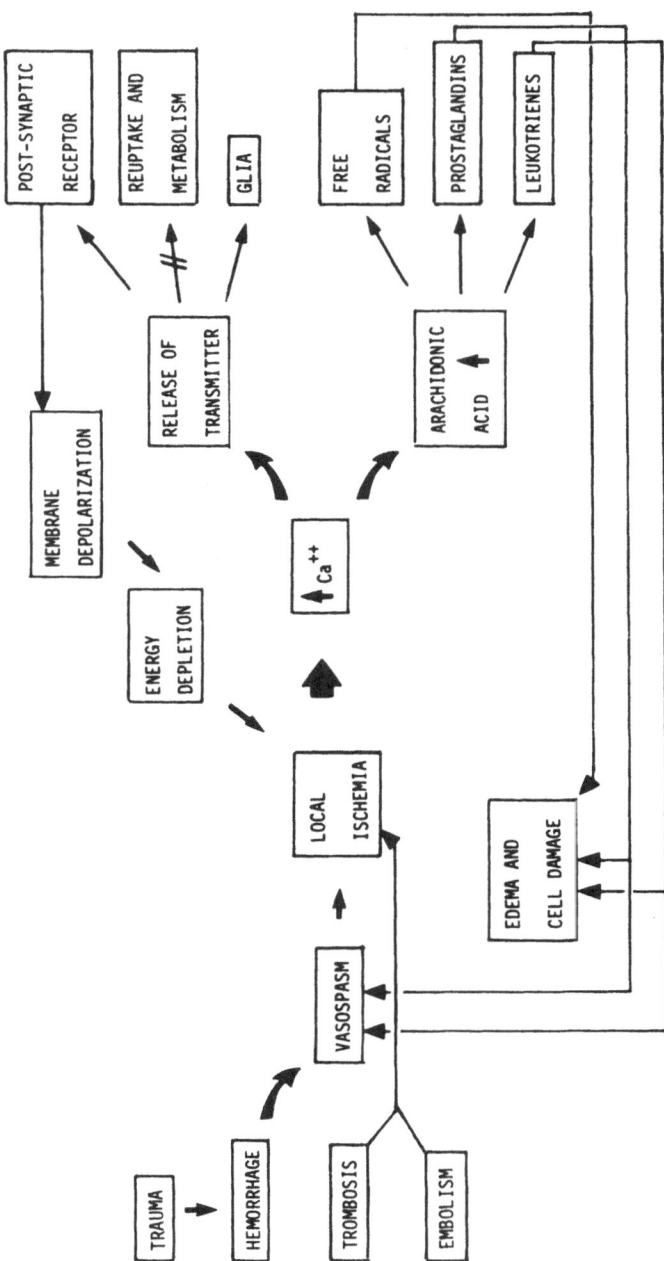

FIGURE 2. Pathophysiology of neural injury. Sequence of events consecutive to traumatic or ischemic/anoxic insults that can lead to an eventual increase in intracellular calcium concentrations. Further details of the "calcium cascade" in the text.

(AA) via phospholipase A_2. Increased neurotransmitter release will induce inositol phospholipid (IP) turnover; in general, this turnover is associated with an increase in the intracellular concentration of calcium. In this way, occupation of both neuronal and glial receptors by the released molecules will induce degradation of IP to produce diacylglycerol (DAG) and inositol triphosphate (IP_3). The former, operating within the plane of the membrane, will activate protein kinase C (PKC), whereas IP_3 will be released into the cytoplasm to mobilize Ca^{2+} stores.[5] The PKC can phosphorylate several target proteins to induce physiological responses. Interestingly, PKC can be selectively activated by tumor-promoting phorbol esters (see ref. 40) substituting for DAG. Recently, phorbol esters have been shown to potentiate synaptic transmission in the hippocampus,[37] a structure in which plastic phenomena such as long-term potentiation (LTP) have been well characterized. Moreover, glutamate, an excitatory amino acid that participates in hypoxic cell damage (*vide infra*), has been shown to be involved in the generation of LTP and in stimulation of IP in the brain.[50]

The enzymatic reactions associated with stimulation of PKC and with mobilization of intracellular Ca^{2+} through IP_3 have been proposed to be the site of action of certain oncogenes (see ref. 5) known to stimulate cell proliferation. Dr. Schwartz and co-workers (Chapter 14) presents evidence on the possible role of oncogenes in regeneration and nerve repair.

The increased formation of arachidonic acid, a precursor of vasoactive substances (prostaglandins and leukotrienes), will further worsen blood flow and, as a substrate for xanthine oxidase and cytochrome P450, will give rise to free radicals, which will cause peroxidation of lipid membranes of neurons and endothelial cells affecting their selective permeability. The release of AA will also stimulate several cyclases with the formation of cyclic nucleotides and the resulting activation of various protein kinases. This will result in further alteration of neurotransmitter release and inactivation mechanisms.[20] Drs. Demediuk and Faden (Chapter 2) elaborate further on this ''AA cascade.''

Increased synaptic activity, probably mediated by release of excitatory neurotransmitters, will eventually produce cell death.[46] The cell death observed after treatment with agonists of excitatory amino acid receptors such as kainic acid or N-methyl-D-aspartate (NMDA) is also a calcium-dependent phenomenon.[22] Interestingly, these authors found that as early as 1 min after incubation of cerebellar slices with kainate (100 μM), Golgi cells started showing signs of degeneration, and a 4-min exposure to this drug was enough to cause irreversible damage.[25] These authors suggest that massive release of excitatory neurotransmitters is responsible for acute neuronal necrosis, a hypothesis put forward by Olney[44] and supported by the protective effects of excitatory amino acid receptor blockers in a rat model of forebrain ischemia.[49] The deleterious effects of agonists like NMDA seem to be mediated by an intracellular increase in calcium concentration.[36]

If excitotoxic influences may explain ischemia-induced infarction, we are still unable to understand the mechanisms involved in the temporary depression of the surviving systems that mediate functional recovery. This point is discussed further in Section 8 of this chapter.

4. DRUGS USED TO TREAT ISCHEMIC CELL DAMAGE

As we have seen, the abnormally elevated intracellular concentration of calcium is both the consequence of several mechanisms and the origin of a number of reactions that can lead to cell damage. All these levels of calcium's action may be modified by drugs (see ref. 56).

1. Chelating agents. Drugs such as EDTA have the ability to bind extra-cellular Ca^{2+}. However, to our knowledge, there are no clinical studies with these agents in stroke patients.
2. Calcium channel blockers: nifedipine, nimodipine, flunarizine, verapamil. Most of these drugs have shown mainly a vasodilator activity. However, their action on ischemic tissue is different from that observed in normal cells: they may prevent vasospasm in the absence of ischemia and increase edema formation when the latter is present.[58] Recently, calcium antagonist receptors have been localized to specific synaptic regions in the brain,[24] but their functional significance remains to be elucidated.
3. Inactivators of the Ca^{2+}–calmodulin complex: phenothiazines. Intracellular calcium accumulation can be prevented by pretreatment with chlorpromazine. However, in hypoxic or ischemic conditions, promethazine had lethal effects on 75 to 80% of the animals.
4. Arachidonic acid antagonists. To date, there are no agents that can specifically inhibit AA hypermetabolism. However, a number of drugs have been used against the negative effects of some of its byproducts. Reducing agents such as α-tocopherol, ascorbic acid, glutathione, etc. may protect cells from hydroxyl radicals (OH·). Xanthine oxidase inhibitors such as allopurinol may decrease production of superoxide anions and hydrogen peroxide. Inhibitors of prostaglandin synthesis such as indomethacin reduce thromboxane levels when given before ischemia and protect adenylate cyclase from ischemic changes[53] in gerbils. However, in ischemic baboons, it significantly increases edema. Prostacyclin (PGI_2), a vasodilator and inhibitor of platelet aggregation, has been administered to stroke patients with controversial results. More tests are needed before any conclusion can be reached about this agent.
5. Pharmacological protection: barbiturates. Properties such as stabilization of neuronal membranes, decreased calcium influx, lowering of intracranial pressure, diminished release of AA, and overall decrease of

cellular metabolism have made these drugs interesting candidates for protection against brain ischemia. However, the experimental and clinical evidence of their efficacy is not resolved. For instance, the dosages used are much larger than those ordinarily employed, and treatment, when effective, had to be given within the first 60 min of the onset of ischemia. Moreover, removal of barbiturates may be followed by fatal elevation of intracranial pressure.[61] More data are needed from carefully controlled randomized clinical trials with long-term follow-up to validate the usefulness of barbiturate protection.

6. Opioids. Endogenous morphinelike substances have been suggested to participate in the pathophysiology of both ischemic and traumatic injuries.[3,15] Naloxone, the commonly used antagonist for opiate toxicity, has been tested in stroke patients with controversial results.[17] Animal experiments also show conflicting results; for example, Baskin et al.[3] report beneficial effects of an opiate agonist, dynorphin(1–13), in cats with occlusion of the right middle cerebral artery, whereas Tang[52] did not find this protective effect in gerbils with bilateral carotid occlusion. Moreover, this author reports protective effects of a specific κ opioid receptor agonist (U-50,488E) in his gerbil model, and Faden and Jacobs,[16] using a selective antagonist for the same receptor, find improvement in neurological recovery after ischemic spinal cord injury in rabbits. Finally, use of drugs with mixed agonist–antagonist actions on the opiate receptor (in this case, levallorphan) has been reported to reverse neurological deficits in patients with acute ischemic stroke.[26] Perhaps the differences in animal models or in drugs used may account for these discrepancies. Meanwhile, naloxone continues to be used in many clinical settings.[61]

To summarize, Table II illustrates some therapeutic measures and their rationale in patients with completed stroke.

5. Management of Medical and Neurological Complications

The management of medical and neurological complications of a brain lesion is as important as the treatment of the lesion itself. Special attention should be paid to cardiac and pulmonary functions, the nutritional and metabolic status, excretory functions, dermatological and vascular risks arising from bed rest and immobility, and neurological complications such as seizures or alterations of consciousness. It is also crucial to control underlying pathological conditions such as ischemic heart disease, diabetes, or hypertension.[27,61]

TABLE II. Therapy of Completed Strokes[a]

Microcirculation
  Rationale: To improve blood flow to the "ischemic penumbra" (ischemically impaired but viable brain tissue)
  Drugs
    Prostacyclin or its stable prostaglandin analogues: Unproven value
    Naloxone: May be used acutely (0.4 to 0.8 mg)
    Aminophylline: Without benefit in controlled studies
    Vasopressors: May be beneficial during angiography, but of unproven efficacy (and may be hazardous) in thromboembolic strokes
    Hypotensors: Acutely may aggravate the ischemic stroke

Platelet antiaggregation drugs
  Rationale: To prevent platelet hyperaggregability associated with stroke
  Drugs
    Aspirin: Reduces stroke recurrences
    Dipyridamole: Dubious synergistic activity with aspirin
    Sulfinpyrazone: No more effective than aspirin
    Clofibrate and flurbiprofen: More clinical trials are needed

Anticoagulation
  Rationale: To prevent possible coagulation and a thromboembolic stroke syndrome
  Drugs
    Anticoagulants: Of little use in completed strokes; heparin may be used if recovery is in progress or the deficit is small
    Fibrinolysins (streptokinase, urokinase, and tissue plasminogen activators): Of theoretical value from studies in coronary artery disease

Biorheologic factors
  Rationale: To reduce blood viscosity and improve blood flow to the "ischemic penumbra"
  Drugs
    Dextran or albumin infusion: May improve neurological status
    Perfluorocarbons (fluosol): Carry oxygen; may be useful by exchange transfusion
    Pentoxyfilline: Reduces red blood cell deformability and therefore blood viscosity
    Ancrod (snake venom): To reduce fibrinogen (experimental)

Antiedema agents
  Rationale: To improve "vasogenic" edema associated with brain tumors but rarely with stroke
  Drugs
    Steroids (dexamethasone, methylprednisolone): Have not been shown to be of any benefit in acute ischemic strokes; their use should be abandoned
    Dehydrating agents (mannitol, glycerol): As a temporary measure to prevent herniation syndromes

Pharmacological protection
  Rationale: To decrease cerebral metabolic rate until circulation is restored, to reduce intracranial pressure, to block the "calcium cascade," and to decrease free radical generation
  Drugs
    Barbiturates: No carefully controlled, randomized clinical trials support their use in man

(continued)

12 SIMÓN BRAILOWSKY

TABLE II. (*Continued*)

Calcium channel blockers (nifedipine, nimodipine, etc.): Of theoretical value from studies in
myocardial infarction; potential of side effects (vasodilatation and increased edema)
Allopurinol: To block xanthine oxidase, which generates free radicals; effects on human
brain ischemia not yet known
Other agents: Piracetam, prexilene, imidazole derivates, etc.; more information is needed

aFrom: Kistler *et al.*,[31] Fishman,[20] and Yatsu *et al.*[61]

6. REQUIREMENTS IN THE DESIGN OF A CLINICAL TRIAL

It is unfortunate to realize that part of our inability to reach valid conclusions concerning the efficacy of a given medical treatment in patients with brain lesions arises from incorrect design of clinical trials.[51] The alarming frequency of improperly applied statistical tests is one of the reasons, but not the only one. The difficulty of establishing a group of patients with comparable degree of pathology, and in sufficient number, should not prevent the proper evaluation of potentially useful treatments.

Many designs for clinical trials have been proposed (for example, see refs. 42 and 43), and the importance of having a statistical consultant has been repeatedly underlined.[51] In this chapter, we can only make a few recommendations worth considering by both clinicians and experimentalists concerned with clinical trials:

1. Specific outcomes of therapy must be measured.
2. The accuracy of diagnosis and the severity of the disease must be comparable.
3. Dosage should be individualized in order to be able to compare relative efficacy at equivalent toxicity or relative toxicity at equivalent efficacy.
4. Placebo effects must be controlled (evaluation of subjective effects).
5. Compliance should be assessed before assignment of experimental regimen.
6. Sample size should be estimated before the beginning of a clinical trial.
7. Sufficient follow-up duration must be established.
8. Ethical considerations may determine the choice of control groups.

Finally, I should mention the fact that the acceptance of a medical treatment for a defined population is also based on national policies. For example, drug approval regulations in the United States have been considered too long (an average for a new drug, from initial studies in normal volunteers to the conditional approval by FDA, is from 8 to 10 years). A better design for clinical trials may abbreviate this duration.

7. INDIVIDUALIZATION OF DRUG THERAPY

I should make a short comment on some of the possible sources of variability in response to drug treatment (see Table III), as they are variables that have to be taken into account before conclusions can be reached on the beneficial or deleterious effects of any substance.

A detailed analysis of these factors and others not mentioned here, such as gender, psychological variables (emotional state, motivation, familial support, etc.), pre- and postlesion exposure to drugs, and socially determined variables, has been dealt with elsewhere.[7] The age factor is considered below.

Pharmacokinetic and pharmacodynamic parameters are quantifiable variables that can be manipulated experimentally, but other sources of variability are more difficult to control. Patient compliance is one of them. In this context, the interaction between the physician and the patient may determine the success or failure of a medical treatment. We believe that compliance can be facilitated when both parties, physician and patient, share information concerning the disease, the treatment, and the expectancies of this treatment. Unfortunately, this information is frequently confined to the patient's medical record.

Finally, we should add that the context in which a drug is administered can significantly alter drug response. Both the family environment and the social

TABLE III. Individualization of Drug Therapy:
Sources of Variability in Response to
Drug Treatment

Patient compliance
Medication errors
Pharmacokinetic parameters
    Availability
    Urinary excreation
    Binding to plasma proteins
    Clearence
    Volume of distribution
    Half-life
    Effective and toxic concentrations
    Physiological variables
    Pathological variables
    Genetic variables
    Drug interactions
    Tolerance
Pharmacodynamic parameters
    Drug–receptor interactions
    Functional state
    Placebo effects

---

setting in which the patient lives have to be considered in the optimization of medical treatment. Drugs are not the only solution for brain-injured patients. Rehabilitation measures have to include social support, for a patient with a positive mood has a much better opportunity to develop fully the potentials offered by the plasticity of the brain.

8. THE GABA TECHNIQUE OF REVERSIBLE BRAIN DYSFUNCTION

It is conceivable that both functional deficits and behavioral recovery following a brain lesion are the result of alterations in neurotransmitter regulation. In an already classic book on restoration of function after brain injury, Luria[35] pointed to this fact and proposed that pharmacological modification of neurotransmitter levels could be a valid form of intervention. Based on his experiments with inhibitors of cholinesterase in man, he stated:

> There is reason to suppose that the mediator metabolism does not remain undisturbed in a synapse which is affected by edema as a result of trauma. Long before the terminal filaments and their endings show signs of gross fragmentation and destruction, the mediator metabolism is probably deranged, which would explain the inactive state of synapses in which no gross structural damage is apparent. If this hypothesis is correct, it may also be postulated that modification of the mediator metabolism (the chemical mechanism of transmission at the synapse) by activation of acetylcholine will help to restore normal synaptic transmission and to revive temporarily inhibited functions.

Drs. Feeney and Sutton (Chapter 7) and Zivin (Chapter 4) describe this approach employing catecholaminergic agonists and serotonin antagonists, respectively, to influence the outcome of brain injury.

We have been interested in the GABA system both to elucidate its participation in the lesion and recovery processes and as a pharmacological tool to reproduce the phenomenology of a brain deficit. This inhibitory neurotransmitter is particularly sensitive to changes in cerebral blood flow (see references in ref. 9), and significant increases in its extracellular concentrations have been detected after ischemia and/or hypoxia.

Using chronic, localized perfusion of GABA into the motor cortex of freely moving animals, we have been able to induce a reversible hemiplegia in the rat.[9] Focal administration has several advantages including a reduction in intra- and interanimal variability in cerebral drug concentration and a reduction in collateral drug effects on other organs. Moreover, this technique permits us to overcome variations related to blood–brain barrier permeability or effects on other distant structures.

The technique consists of the chronic delivery of minute quantities of GABA directly into the structure of interest through osmotic minipumps. These devices are implanted subcutaneously and connected through a plastic catheter to an intracerebral cannula. We have infused the rat motor cortex with GABA (100 $\mu g/\mu l$) or saline for 7 days (1 $\mu l/hr$) and studied the temporal evolution of the clinical deficit, as evaluated with a motor test of coordinated walking on an elevated narrow wooden beam. In this test, trained rats maintain all four paws on the upper surface of the beam while walking towards their home cage, located at the opposite end of the bar, whereas animals with motor deficits are either unable to run (maximal deficit score), drag the limb contralateral to the operated side, or show slips, falls, or defects in paw placing (for a full description of the scoring system, see ref. 9). A dose of 100 $\mu g/\mu l$ was chosen based on previous experiments in which the effects of the amino acid were evaluated using the evoked potential technique.

The GABA-infused group showed significant differences (higher deficits) in 4 of the 7 days of treatment. The motor deficit found in the saline-treated animals was similar to the one produced by motor cortex aspiration, even in those cases in which the excision of cortical tissue included bigger areas. From these experiments we conclude that the GABA-induced deficit lasted longer than that produced by the trauma of the cannula itself or by deficits provoked by aspiration of large cortical areas.

After our findings of significant differences in motor deficit between GABA-treated and saline-infused animals (both groups having the same extent of structural lesion), we compared the deficit induced by the inhibitory neurotransmitter in young adult (6–9 months) and aged (24 months) rats. The latter group showed longer and more pronounced deficits after GABA infusion than the young rats (see Fig. 3).

Originally, we proposed[9] the usefulness of this rat model of reversible hemiplegia for screening pharmacological agents used in patients with brain lesions or to study substances that might facilitate recovery processes. Because we were interested in possible interactions between GABA and drugs claimed to interact with this amino acid, we studied the effect of phenytoin (a widely used anticonvulsant both in neurology and neurosurgery) in our rat model.[10] Administration of phenytoin concurrently with chronic GABA infusion resulted in a significant increase in the severity of the hemiplegic syndrome. The drug had no deleterious effects on motor function when administered either before GABA (always in trained animals) or after GABA, when the animals had already recovered from the motor deficit (14 days after intracortical implantation of the cannulas used to deliver the amino acid).

We have also employed this method to evaluate the effects of dopaminergic manipulation in both young adult and aged hemiplegic animals.[32] Haloperidol, a dopaminergic antagonist widely used in humans, has been reported to induce a reappearance of the motor disturbances produced by cortical lesions in recovered animals[54] and to antagonize the facilitation of recovery produced by amphetamine in motor-cortex-lesioned rats[18] (see also Chapter 7). For these reasons, we

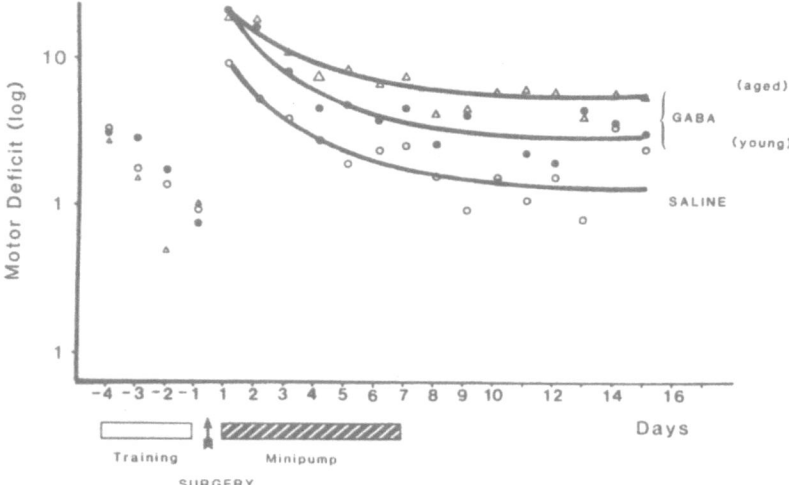

FIGURE 3. Comparison of motor performance of young adult (filled circles) and aged (triangles) GABA-treated animals and saline-infused young rats (open circles). The solutions (1 μl/hr for 7 days) were administered to the left somatosensory cortex via osmotic minipumps. Implantations are indicated by the arrow ("surgery"). All groups showed a trend towards better performance in the training period. The GABA-treated animals had greater deficits than the saline-treated animals. Note that the aged group slowly recovered after the end of drug treatment, although they never attained presurgery performance levels (represented on a log scale). Further details and references in the text.

studied the effects of the neuroleptic on young and aged animals who had recovered from GABA-induced motor dysfunction (15 to 45 days after minipump implantation). After confirming stability in motor performance on the beam test for at least 3 days, 0.1 mg/kg i.p. of the drug was given. All the animals, including the controls (unoperated), showed some degree of deficit under the effects of the drug (see Fig. 4), consisting mainly of hesitation and a wider hindlimb base while walking but without any evidence of lateralized defects. The GABA-treated animals showed a deficit contralateral to the lesion that was identical to the one produced during the GABA infusion period and much more severe than the dysfunction seen in the control group.

An interesting trend was observed between the young and the aged groups: the aged subjects showed, as in the GABA infusion period, a slower and less complete recovery (see Fig. 4). These data indicate differential sensitivity of aged and young animals to both GABAergic and dopaminergic manipulation.

These experiments with phenytoin and haloperidol suggest that GABAergic mechanisms are involved in the initial stages of functional deficit after a brain lesion and that phenytoin administration in brain-damaged individuals in the initial postlesion stage may be deleterious, whereas dopaminergic neurotransmission is implicated in the late stages of functional recovery after motor cortex lesions. Moreover, aged animals appear to be more sensitive to dopaminergic

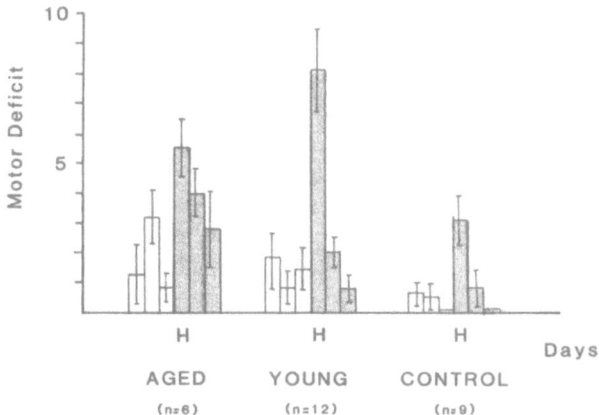

FIGURE 4. Effects of haloperidol (0.1 mg/kg) on motor performance of young adult and aged rats studied for six consecutive days. The drug was administered on day "H," and its effects were studied 30 min after injection and on the next 2 days. Each bar represents the day's mean ± S.E.M. The control group (unoperated animals) showed nonspecific impairment in motor performance without any evidence of lateralization. The "aged" and "young" animals received the drug after recovery or stabilization from the GABA-mediated potentiation of cortical hemiplegia. Haloperidol induced the reappearance of the unilateral motor deficit in these animals. The aged group showed significantly slower recovery after the drug, whereas the young animals returned to predrug motor scores on the day after administration. For details, see text.

blockade once the recovery process has begun. The clinical implications of the latter observation are that aged patients can also recover from brain lesions but that this recovery is slower and more easily disruptable than that in younger subjects. Definite strategies for rehabilitation can thus be suggested: aged, brain-damaged patients require longer training, and more attention should be exercised when administering drugs that influence the dopaminergic system. Conversely, pharmacological manipulation of this system may be attempted to enhance recovery. The findings of Feeney and Sutton (Chapter 7) with amphetamine in stroke patients represent a good example.

Functional deficits may result not only from processes that decrease brain excitability, such as the ones considered above, but also after epileptic processes, that is, consequent to increased neuronal activity. An irritative focus may disrupt normal function of the implicated structure and of all those areas to which the affected area projects. In the case of epilepsy, there is a clear correlation between the affected area and the resulting functional abnormality. Moreover, we have proposed a possible relationship between the motor syndrome observed after GABA infusion and Todd's phenomenon, also called postepileptic paralysis.[9] This "paralysis" can affect any area of the cortex, depending on where the epileptic focus is located, and is reversible. The clinical deficits reported can be motor (from hemiparesis to aphasia) or sensory (paresthesias), but it is also possible that cognitive dysfunctions exist and pass undetected. The generality of the phenomenon suggests a common inhibitory mechanism.[14]

We are presently applying the technique of chronic intracortical GABA infusion in the photosensitive baboon, *Papio papio*. This animal has been considered one of the best animal models of human epilepsy because the only manipulation necessary to induce clinical manifestations of epilepsy in this monkey is intermittent light stimulation.[38] Electrophysiological experiments have shown that there is a discrete area in the frontorolandic cortex from which epileptic discharges triggered by light stimulation that precedes myoclonic activity are generated. We infused GABA into this region in a manner similar to that described for the rat, producing a complete blockade of the photosensitivity. No other clinical deficit was observed. As in the case of hemiplegia, these effects were reversible, as the animals returned to their previous state of photosensitivity in the week following GABA application.

However, at the end of the GABA infusion period (7 days), we observed the appearance of spontaneous epileptic discharges originating in the GABA-treated areas. This "GABA withdrawal syndrome" lasted for 3 to 4 days, with return to normal electrical activity afterwards. The spontaneous hyperactivity of this cortical region after GABA infusion seems to be a rebound in excitability after chronically elevated inhibitory neurotransmission. It is possible that this rebound represents a local disinhibition after chronic enhancement of GABA levels or facilitatory activity from other structures projecting to this cortical area. If the latter is the case (remote effects), we should be able to demonstrate some "diaschisislike" phenomenon such as the compensatory excitability changes that may be common to lesion experiments in which recovery processes are also implicated.

Further experiments are necessary to explore the applicability of this technique to reversible inactivation of other structures and the mechanisms involved. The temporal evolution of both the deficit and the recovery process after GABA inactivation offers a good time window through which we can examine brain plasticity.

ACKNOWLEDGMENTS. I would like to thank Dr. R. Naquet for helpful comments on the manuscript and Drs. Menini and Silva-Barrat for their assistance in the preparation of this chapter.

REFERENCES

1. Astrup, J., Siesjo, B. K., and Symon, L., 1981, Threshholds in cerebral ischemia—the ischemic penumbra, *Stroke* **12**:723–725.
2. Baskin, D. S., and Hosobuchi, Y., 1981, Naloxone reversal of ischemic neurological deficits in man, *Lancet* **2**:272–275.

3. Baskin, D. S., Hosobuchi, Y., Loh, H. H., and Lee, N. M., 1984, Dynorphin(1–13) improves survival in cats with focal cerebral ischemia, *Nature* **312:**551–552

4. Benveniste, E. N., and Merrill, J. E., 1986, Stimulation of oligodendroglial proliferation and maturation by interleukin-2, *Nature* **321:**610–613.

5. Berridge, M. J., and Irvine, R. F., 1984, Inositol trisphosphate, a novel second messenger in cellular signal transduction, *Nature* **312:**315–321.

6. Blinzinger, K., and Kreutzberg, G. W., 1968, Displacement of synaptic terminals from regenerating motorneurons by microglial cells, *Z. Zellforsch.* **85:**145–157.

7. Brailowsky, S., 1980, Neuropharmacological aspects of brain plasticity, in: *Recovery of Function: Theoretic Considerations for Brain Injury Rehabilitation* (P. Bach-y-Rita, ed.), H. Huber, Bern, pp. 187–215.

8. Brailowsky, S., and Knight, R. T., 1984, Inhibitory modulation of cat somatosensory cortex: A pharmacological study, *Brain Res.* **322:**310–315.

9. Brailowsky, S., Knight, R. T., Blood, K., and Scabini, D., 1986, GABA-induced potentiation of cortical hemiplegia, *Brain Res.* **362:**322–330.

10. Brailowsky, S., Knight, R. T., and Efron, R., 1986, Phenytoin increases the severity of cortical hemiplegia in rats, *Brain Res.* **376:**71–77.

11. Bunge, R. P., and Waksman, B. H., 1985, Glial development and interactions, *Trends Neurosci.* **8:**424–427.

12. Davis, G. E., Varon, S., Engvall, E., and Manthorpe, M., 1985, Substratum-binding neurite-promoting factors: Relationships to laminin, *Trends Neurosci.* **8:**528–532.

13. Edelman, G. M., 1986, Cell adhesion molecules in neural histogenesis, *Annu. Rev. Physiol.* **48:**417–430.

14. Efron, R., 1961, Post-epileptic paralysis: Theoretical critique and report of a case, *Brain* **84:**381–394.

15. Faden, A. I., 1983, Neuropeptides and stroke: Current status and potential applications, *Stroke* **14:**169–172.

16. Faden, A. I., and Jacobs, T. P., 1985, Opiate antagonist WIN44,441-3 stereospecifically improves neurologic recovery after ischemic spinal injury, *Neurology (N.Y.)* **35:**1311–1315.

17. Fallis, R. J., Fisher, M., and Lobo, R. A., 1984, A double blind trial of naloxone in the treatment of acute stroke, *Stroke* **15:**627–629.

18. Feeney, D. M., Gonzalez, A., and Law, W. A., 1982, Amphetamine, haloperidol and experience interact to affect rate of recovery after motor cortex injury, *Science* **217:**855–857.

19. Feeney, D. M., and Sutton, R. L., 1987, Pharmacotherapy for recovery of function after brain injury, *CRC Crit. Rev. Clin. Neurobiol.* **3:**135–197.

20. Fishman, R. A., 1986, Brain edema, in: *Stroke*, Volume 1 (H. J. M. Barnett, J. P. Mohr, B. M. Stein, and F. M. Yatsu, eds.), Churchill Livingstone, New York, pp. 119–126.

21. Freed, W. J., Medinaceli, L. de, and Wyatt, R. J., 1985, Promoting functional plasticity in the damaged nervous system, *Science* **227:**1544–1552.

22. Garthwaite, G., Hajos, F., and Garthwaite, J., 1986, Ionic requirements for neurotoxic effects of excitatory amino acid analogues in rat cerebellar slices, *Neuroscience* **18:**437–447.

23. Geschwind, N., 1985, Mechanisms of change after brain lesions, *Ann. N.Y. Acad. Sci.* **457:**1–12.

24. Gould, R., Murphy, K. M. M., and Snyder, S. H., 1985, Autoradiographic localization of calcium channel antagonist receptors in rat brain with [³H]nitrendipine, *Brain Res.* **330:**217–223.

25. Hajos, F., Garthwaite, G., and Garthwaite, J., 1986, Reversible and irreversible neuronal damage caused by excitatory amino acid analogues in rat cerebellar slices, *Neuroscience* **18:**417–436.

26. Handa, N., Matsumoto, M., Nakamura, M., Yoneda, S., Kimura, K., Sugitani, Y., Tanaka, K., Takano, T., and Kamada, T., 1985, Reversal of neurological deficits by levallorphan in patients with acute ischemic stroke, *J. Cereb. Blood Flow Metab.* **5:**469–472.

27. Isaacs, B., 1978, Stroke, in: *Textbook of Geriatric Medicine and Gerontology*, 2nd ed. (J. C. Brocklehurst, ed.), Churchill Livingstone, Edinburgh, pp. 201–220.
28. Jacobson, M., 1978, *Developmental Neurobiology*, 2nd ed., Plenum Press, New York, pp. 271–279.
29. Jones, H. R., and Millikan, C. H., 1976, Temporal profile (clinical course) of acute carotid system cerebral infarction, *Stroke* 7:64–71.
30. Katzman, R., Clasen, R., Klatzo, I., Meyer, J. S., Pappius, H. M., and Waltz, A. G., 1977, Brain edema in stroke, *Stroke* 8:512–540.
31. Kistler, J. P., Ropper, A. H., and Heros, R. C., 1984, Theory of ischemic cerebral vascular disease due to atherothrombosis, *N. Engl. J. Med.* 311:100–105.
32. Knight, R. T., and Brailowsky, S., 1984, Possible role of dopamine in the functional recovery from hemiplegia in aged rats, *Soc. Neurosci. Abstr.* 10:448.
33. Kromer, L. F., and Conrbrooks, C. J., 1985, Transplants of Schwann cell cultures promote axonal regeneration in the adult mammalian brain, *Proc. Natl. Acad. Sci. U.S.A.* 82:6330–6334.
34. Ludwin, S. K., 1984, Proliferation of mature oligodendrocytes after trauma to the central nervous system, *Nature* 308:274–275.
35. Luria, A. R., 1948, *Restoration of Function after Brain Injury*, Macmillan, New York, p. 10 (reprinted 1963).
36. MacDermott, A. B., Mayer, M. L., Westbrook, G. L., Smith, S. J., and Barker, J. L., 1986, NMDA-receptor activation increases cytoplasmic calcium concentration in cultured spinal cord neurons, *Nature* 321:519–522.
37. Malenka, R. C., Madison, D. V., and Nicoll, R. A., 1986, Potentiation of synaptic transmission in the hippocampus by phorbol esters, *Nature* 321:175–177.
38. Menini, C., and Naquet, R., 1986, Les myoclonies, *Rev. Neurol.* 142:3–28.
39. Nestler, E. J., Walaas, S. I., and Greengard, P., 1984, Neuronal phosphoproteins: Physiological and clinical implications, *Science* 225:1357–1364.
40. Nishizuka, Y., 1984, Turnover of inositol phospholipids and signal transduction, *Science* 225:1365–1370.
41. Olney, J. W., 1978, Neurotoxicity of excitatory amino acids, in: *Kainic Acid as a Tool in Neurobiology* (E. G. McGeer, J. W. Olney, and P. L. McGeer, eds.), Raven Press, New York, pp. 95–121.
42. Peto, R., Pike, M. C., Armitage, P., Breslow, N. E., Cox, D. R., Howard, S. V., Mantel, N., McPherson, K., Peto, J., and Smith, P. G., 1976, Design and analysis of randomized clinical trials requiring prolonged observation of each patient, *Br. J. Cancer* 34:585–612.
43. Peto, R., Pike, M. C., Armitage, P., Breslow, N. E., Cox, D. R., Howard, S. V., Mantel, N., McPherson, K., Peto, J., and Smith, P. G., 1977, Design and analysis of randomized clinical trials requiring prolonged observation of each patient, *Br. J. Cancer* 35:1–39.
44. Plum, F., 1983, What causes infarction in ischemic brain?, *Neurology (N.Y.)* 33:222–233.
45. Raisman, G., 1978, What hope for repair of the brain? *Ann. Neurol.* 3:101–106.
46. Rothman, S. M., 1983, Synaptic activity mediates death of hypoxic neurons, *Science* 220:536–537.
47. Rothman, S., 1984, Synaptic release of excitatory amino acid neurotransmitter mediates anoxic neuronal death, *J. Neurosci.* 4:1884–1891.
48. Sanes, J. R., and Covault, J., 1985, Axon guidance during reinnervation of skeletal muscle, *Trends Neurosci.* 8:523–528.
49. Simon, R. P., Swan, J. H., Griffiths, T., and Meldrum, B. S., 1984, Blockade of N-methyl-D-aspartate receptors may protect agains ischemic damage in the brain, *Science* 226:850–852.
50. Sladeczek, F., Pin, J. P., Recasens, M., Bockaert, J., and Weiss, S., 1985, Glutamate stimulates inositol phosphate formation in striatal neurones, *Nature* 317:717–719.
51. Spence, J. D., and Donner, A., 1982, Problems in design of stroke treatment trials, *Stroke* 13:94–99.

52. Tang, A. H., 1985, Protection from cerebral ischemia by U-50,488E, a specific kappa opioid analgesic agent, *Life Sci.* **37:**1475–1482.
53. Taylor, M. D., Palmer, G. C., and Callahan, A. S., 1984, Protective action by methylprednisolone, allopurinol and indomethacin against stroke-induced damage to adenylate cyclase in gerbil cerebral cortex, *Stroke* **15:**329–335.
54. van Hasselt, P., 1973, Effects of butyrophenones on motor function in rats after recovery from brain damage, *Neuropharmacology* **12:**245–249.
55. Watson, W. E., 1974, Physiology of neuroglia, *Physiol. Rev.* **54:**245–271.
56. Weir, B., 1984, Calcium antagonists, cerebral ischemia and vasospasm, *Can. J. Neurol. Sci.* **11:**239–246.
57. Wekerle, H., Linington, C., Lassman, H., and Meyermann, R., 1986, Cellular immune reactivity within the CNS, *Trends Neurosci.* **9:**271–277.
58. Welch, K. M. A., and Barkley, G. L., 1986, Biochemistry and pharmacology of cerebral ischemia, in: *Stroke*, Volume 1. (H. J. M. Barnett, J. P. Mohr, B. M. Stein, and F. M. Yatsu, eds.), Churchill Livingstone, New York, pp. 75–90.
59. Wells, M. R., and Bernstein, J. J., 1985, Scar formation and the barrier hypothesis in failure of mammalian central nervous system regeneration, in: *Trauma of the Central Nervous System* (R. G. Dacey, Jr., H. R. Winn, R. W. Rimel, and J. A. Jane, eds.), Raven Press, New York, pp. 245–257.
60. Wood, P. M., and Bunge, R. P., 1986, Evidence that axons are mitogenic for oligodendrocytes isolated from adult animals. *Nature* **320:**756–758.
61. Yatsu, F. M., Pettigrew, L. C., Jr., and Grotta, J. C., 1986, Medical therapy of ischemic strokes, in: *Stroke*, Volume 2 (H. J. M. Barnett, J. P. Mohr, B. M. Stein, and F. M. Yatsu, eds.), Churchill Livingstone, New York, pp. 1069–1083.

2

ARACHIDONIC ACID METABOLITES AND MEMBRANE LIPID CHANGES IN CENTRAL NERVOUS SYSTEM INJURY

PAUL DEMEDIUK AND ALAN I. FADEN

ABSTRACT. Following various forms of trauma to the brain and spinal cord, a series of membrane lipid changes occur that include large increases in free fatty acids and diacylglycerols and decreases in selected phospholipids and cholesterol. Occurrence of peroxidative damage is also indicated by decreased levels of membrane antioxidants and increased levels of peroxidation products. Among the free fatty acids, arachidonate shows the largest relative increase. A consequence of arachidonate release is its metabolism through the cyclooxygenase and lipoxygenase pathways to produce prostaglandins, leukotrienes, and other eicosanoids, compounds with very potent physiological effects. The potential consequences of the membrane lipid alterations include changes in membrane permeability, edema induction, and reductions in activities of membrane-bound enzymes such as Na^+,K^+-ATPase. The production of the eicosanoids may be related to the platelet aggregation, reduction in blood flow, and capillary damage seen following central nervous system trauma.

Using two different animals (cat, rat) and two different models of mechanical spinal cord injury (compression, weight drop), we have demonstrated a biphasic response in membrane lipid metabolism. Very early changes (1 min to 1 hr) are characterized by increases in free fatty acids and eicosanoids, which peak at 30 min and are declining by 1 hr post-injury. There is also a more delayed secondary increase in free fatty acid levels with associated decreases in selected phospholipids; these changes appear to peak at 24 hr post-injury.

By using specific drugs as pharmacological probes to inhibit release or effects of the lipid changes, we are currently studying the role of arachidonic acid metabolites on secondary CNS injury following trauma or ischemia.

PAUL DEMEDIUK AND ALAN I. FADEN • Department of Neurology, University of California, San Francisco, and Center for Neural Injury, Veterans Administration Medical Center, San Francisco, California 94121.

23

1. INTRODUCTION

Delayed, progressive injury may follow a variety of insults to the central nervous system (CNS), including hypoglycemia, hypoxia, seizures, ischemia, and mechanical trauma. There is increasing evidence to indicate that a major component of this delayed injury is the release or production of endogenous pathophysiological factors in response to the initial insult. It is believed that these factors may contribute to the propagation of the injury through a variety of mechanisms including reductions in blood flow, alterations in the local metabolic environment, and cell membrane damage with effects on membrane-dependent enzymes. In addition to the postulated role of direct membrane damage in the trauma process, glycerophospholipid components of the cell membrane may also act as a source of release of potentially injurious molecules including free fatty acids (FFA), platelet-activating factor, prostaglandins, and leukotrienes.

2. MEMBRANE LIPID CHANGES IN CNS INJURY

2.1. DIRECT MEMBRANE EFFECTS

2.1.1. LIPID HYDROLYSIS

The delayed, self-propagating cell death that is characteristic of certain types of CNS injury appears to be related to biochemical changes. One very early target of biochemical changes that cause cellular damage appears to be the cell membrane via activation of lipid hydrolytic enzymes (lipases). Experiments by Bazan and co-workers[5] demonstrated that global ischemia and epileptic seizures are accompanied by a rapid increase in brain FFA levels, with the largest relative change being observed in arachidonic acid. Similar increases in FFA concentration have since been observed in brain during hypoxia,[38] hypoglycemia,[2] cold-induced injury,[13] and severe focal ischemia[85] and in spinal cord following mechanical trauma[22] (Table I). Diacylglycerols (DG) have also been documented to accumulate following CNS trauma.

In normal brain and spinal cord, the concentrations of FFA and DG are very low. The lowest reported FFA values for brain are those of Yoshida et al.,[116] who measured a concentration of 64 nmol/g wet weight for rat brain frozen in situ with liquid nitrogen. However, the range of brain FFA concentrations typically found in the literature varies from 140 to 170 nmol/g wet weight, including more recent results from Yoshida et al.[115] Control FFA levels of feline spinal cord in situ average 95 nmol/g wet weight.[23] Rat spinal cord has been found to have control FFA levels of 150 nmol/g wet weight (A. I. Faden, P. H. Chan, and S. Longar, unpublished results). In all cases, the polyunsaturated arachidonate and docosahexaenoate species represent extremely small proportions of the total

TABLE I. Changes in Eicosanoid Levels following Traumatic Injury

Injury type	PGE$_2$	PGF$_{2\alpha}$	TXA$_2$	PGI$_2$	LTs	References
Cold injury (brain)	↑	↑	Not measured	Not measured	Not measured	80
Brain ischemia	↑	↑	↑	↑	↑	15, 74
Concussive brain trauma	↑	↑	Not measured	↓	Not measured	28
Seizures (brain)	↑	↑	↑	Not measured	Not measured	6
Spinal cord trauma	↑	↑	↑	No change	↑	22, 55

FFA fraction. Control DG concentrations in brain and spinal cord have been measured at 100–170 nmol/g and 65 nmol/g wet weight, respectively.[22,23,60,99]

Traumatic insults to the brain or spinal cord produce marked increases in total FFA and DG levels (Fig. 1). Regional variability and gray/white matter differences in lipid hydrolysis have been demonstrated.[9,22,87] Observable differences occur very rapidly (as early as 30 sec) after initiation of trauma. Insults that cause no apparent permanent functional loss (i.e., induced seizures) are subject to a relatively modest increase in FFA levels to approximately 450 nmol/g wet weight. More severe injury states (i.e., complete brain ischemia) that result in permanent measurable losses of CNS function elevate FFA and DG levels to 800–1200 nmol/g and 450–520 nmol/g wet weight. In most cases, these changes are monophasic over the experimental time period with a pronounced maximum and then a decline within 60–180 min. Unfortunately, only relatively short time periods have been studied (<3 hr), and very little is known regarding the fate of membrane lipids at longer times following injury. Recent

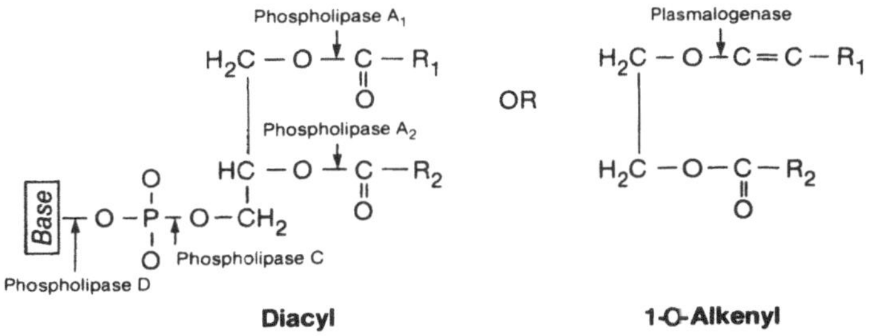

FIGURE 1. Typical phospholipid structures and points of enzymatic hydrolysis by various lipases. In the CNS, approximately 15–20% of the total phospholipid is in the 1-O-alkenyl or plasmalogen form, primarily as plasmenylethanolamine.

preliminary data indicated that more delayed time-dependent changes also occur, with peak effects at 24 hr (Table II).

Theoretically, the released FFA could arise by hydrolytic activity acting on a number of different lipid pools that are known to be rich in fatty acids. Cholesterol esters, mono-, di-, and triacylglycerols, and the glycerophospholipids all contain esterified fatty acyl groups. The sphingolipids contain a fatty acyl group in an amide linkage, which is very resistant to hydrolysis. In the CNS the most abundant and easily liberated fatty acids are those attached through ester linkages to the glycerolipids.[19] Within the glycerolipid fraction, the phosphoglycerides greatly predominate in the CNS and have thus received the greatest attention. The increase in DG levels is also most probably related to altered glycerophospholipid metabolism.

Phosphoglycerides can be conveniently depicted as consisting of a glycerol backbone with various functional groups attached to the glyceryl alcohols by ester or ether linkages (Fig. 2). The 2 position is generally much higher in polyunsaturated acyl content than the 1 position. As seen in Fig. 2, (1,2)-diacyl- or 1-O-alkenyl,2-acylphospholipids are subject to hydrolytic attack by five classes of lipases.[19,102]

Phospholipases of the A type produce a FFA and lysophospholipid; phospholipases C and D produce a DG and phosphatidic acid, respectively. Alkenyl phospholipids (plasmalogens) may undergo hydrolysis at the 1 position via a plasmalogenase. The remaining fatty acyl group in a lysophospholipid produced by the action of phospholipase A_1, A_2, or plasmalogenase is then susceptible to hydrolysis by lysophospholipases, which are very active in brain.[97] Free fatty acids may also be liberated by the sequential action of diacylglycerol lipase and monoacylglycerol lipase. Diacylglycerols can be formed nonhydrolytically from glycerophospholipids by reversal of the synthetic enzyme 1,2-diacylglycerol:

TABLE II. Changes in Biochemical Parameters following Impact Trauma to the Rat Spinal Cord[a]

Variable	Control	2 hr	24 hr	1 week
Total FFA (nmol/mg wet weight)	265.8	329.7	502.6	321.2
20:4 (nmol/mg wet weight)	19.6 ± 4.9	17.9 ± 6.2	58.2 ± 20.1	16.7 ± 6.2
Total lipid P (nmol/mg wet weight)	74.1 ± 8.8	67.7 ± 7.9	46.2 ± 6.7	67.9 ± 9.3
Na^+, K^+-ATPase (μmol Pi/mg protein/hr)	7.5 ± 2.1	15.9 ± 2.6	1.7 ± 1.2	1.7 ± 0.9
H_2O (%)	68.2 ± 0.3	69.7 ± 0.5	72.2 ± 0.5	70.0 ± 0.6

[a]Data expressed as mean $\pm$ S.D., $n = 6$.

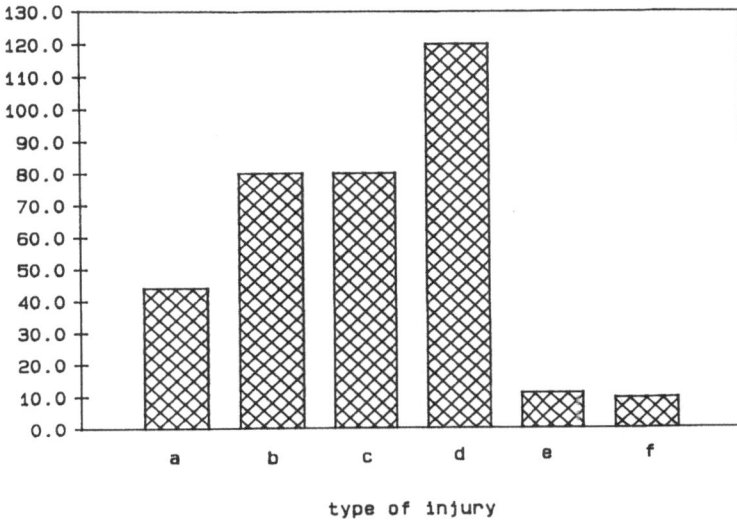

FIGURE 2. Maximal total free fatty acid levels resulting from the following types of trauma to the CNS: (a) induced brain seizures, (b) brain hypoglycemia, (c) brain ischemia, (d) spinal cord compression. Data for e and f are control brain and spinal cord values, respectively. (Taken from references 2, 5, 22, 23, 115, 116.)

CDP-choline cholinephosphostranferase, which catalyzes the reaction of CMP with phosphatidylcholine to produce CDP-choline and DG.[26]

Based on current data, it is not possible to pinpoint either the particular phospholipid source(s) of trauma-induced FFA and DG or the specific lipases that are activated following CNS injury. However, it seems likely that multiple phospholipid classes and lipases are involved. Increases in the activities of phospholipase A_1 and A_2 (acting on phosphatidylcholine and phosphatidylethanolamine) and lysophospholipase have been seen in ischemic dog and gerbil brains.[22,27,52] Phospholipase C activity has been found to increase in cat brain after experimental concussive injury.[106] Phospholipid degradation has been demonstrated following brain ischemia[7] and cold injury to the brain.[13] The specific phospholipid species that are hydrolyzed vary with type of injury and with time after initiation of injury, further indicating activation of multiple lipases.

The mechanisms leading to the disruption of normal metabolism of membrane lipids after CNS injury are poorly understood. Both cAMP and Ca^{2+} have been postulated to be involved. An elevation of cAMP (possibly via trauma-related release of neurotransmitters) may trigger activation of phospholipases through phosphorylation of lipomodulin (lipocortin, macrocortin), a protein that inhibits phospholipases by binding to the enzyme.[51] When phosphorylated, lipomodulin dissociates from phospholipases, and the enzymes become active. Increases in intracellular free Ca^{2+} are also associated with alterations in lipid metabolism both through direct activation of phospholipases of the A and C types and through calcium-dependent binding of calmodulin to phospholipase A_2.[75] There is strong, albeit indirect, evidence for early elevation of intracellular free Ca^{2+} after CNS trauma.[96,117] Phospholipids are normally recycled through a series of energy-dependent reactions. As a result, the steady-state phospholipid content of cellular membranes is not depleted, and the intracellular concentrations of FFA are maintained at low levels. In CNS injury, however, requisite energy stores are depleted. As a result, the reacylation of liberated fatty acids into phospholipids may be impeded and thus contribute to the injury-induced rise of FFA.[8,97]

Elevations in FFA and DG following CNS trauma may damage cells and affect physiological processes by altering membrane structure and fluidity. At low concentrations, FFA and DG readily intercalate into membranes, producing significant changes in the packing and acyl group motion of the constituent lipid molecules. Typical control values of both FFA and DG are approximately 0.4 mol% of the pool of total phospholipids. In severe CNS trauma these values increase to as high as 8 mol%, levels at which fatty acids have been shown to perturb both model and biological membranes.[50,57,61,101] In addition, DG, which can undergo rapid transmembrane flip-flop (unlike phospholipids), may affect membrane curvature.[3,93]

Physiologically, a number of membrane-related effects of FFA and DG have been observed. In erythrocytes, low levels of FFA stabilize cells against osmotic fragility, whereas higher concentrations facilitate osmotic hemolysis in hypotonic medium.[84] Free fatty acids have also been shown to inhibit calcium uptake by sarcoplasmic reticulum vesicles from rabbit skeletal muscle.[58] In addition, FFA inhibit the Na^+-dependent synaptosomal uptake of proline, aspartate, glutamate, and γ-aminobutyric acid and reduce synaptosomal Na^+,K^+-ATPase activity.[13,84,86] Intracerebral injections of arachidonic acid in rats selectively destroy the outer leaflet of capillary plasma membranes in white matter.[105] Diglycerides stimulate transepithelial sodium transport in frog skin epithelium[114] and the Ca^{2+}-activated, phospholipid-dependent protein kinase C from rat brain.[72] Diglycerides also markedly increase phospholipase-catalyzed hydrolysis of phospholipid bilayers.[20]

Because proper membrane structure is essential for function, perturbations of cell membranes may result in functional deficits that contribute to cell death. An often-cited indicator of membrane damage is the change in activity of the enzyme Na^+,K^+-ATPase. This enzyme is membrane bound and phospholipid dependent, with its activity requiring an intact membrane structure.[35,40,107] Membrane damage would be expected to alter the structural configuration of the Na^+,K^+-ATPase, with resultant reduction in enzymatic activity. The Na^+,K^+-

ATPase has shown rapid and persistent declines in activity after reversible brain ischemia,[39] spinal cord injury,[16] and cold injury to the brain.[13]

2.1.2. PEROXIDATION

The univalent reduction of molecular oxygen in living tissues produces free radicals such as superoxide anions, hydrogen peroxide, and hydroxyl radicals.[37] These activated oxygen species can initiate a chain peroxidation process with polyunsaturated fatty acyl side chains of membrane lipids.[68] Glycerophospholipids of the CNS are very rich in polyunsaturates. The first step in lipid peroxidation is the abstraction of a hydrogen atom from a fatty side chain by an oxygen-derived free radical, resulting in a lipid radical that undergoes molecular rearrangement to form a conjugated diene. The radical diene then undergoes reaction with molecular oxygen to give a peroxy radical, which can abstract a hydrogen from an adjacent polyunsaturate to form a hydroperoxide and new lipid radical, which propagates the chain reaction. Additional reactions of hydroperoxides lead to a variety of products, including aldehydes and alkyl radical fragments that can form cross links with similar products as adjacent acyl chains. The resultant change in the chemical nature of the affected fatty side chains should be accompanied by physical changes in the membrane structure and function.[18,56,103] There is strong indirect evidence to indicate that peroxidative damage to membrane lipids of the CNS contributes to the progressive pathophysiology of CNS injury.[14,24,64,100,116] A more thorough discussion of lipid peroxidation and CNS injury is beyond the scope of this text. However, several excellent reviews have recently been published.[46,47]

2.2. EICOSCANOID PRODUCTION

The eicosanoids are biologically active metabolites of free arachidonic acid that have been implicated in the response of the CNS to injury. Eicosanoids include prostaglandins (PGs), leukotrienes (LTs), thromboxane A_2 (TXA_2), prostacyclin (PGI_2), and hydroperoxy- and hydroxyeicosatetraenoic acids (HPETEs, HETEs). The PGs and LTs are designated by letters and numbers (e.g., PGF_2, LTC_4), with the letters referring to ring substituents and amino acid substituents, respectively (see Fig. 3). The numbers indicate the number of double bonds. All 2 and 4 series PGs and LTs are biologically active. The normal levels of these compounds in brain and spinal cord are very low but rise markedly in response to injury. Eicosanoids have been shown to rise in animals following drug-induced and electroshock convulsions,[6] ischemia,[15,74] cold injury,[80] and fluid concussive injury.[28] Compression trauma and impact trauma to spinal cord have also recently been shown to cause eicosanoid increases.[22,55]

Most mammalian cells generate eicosanoids in response to a wide variety of

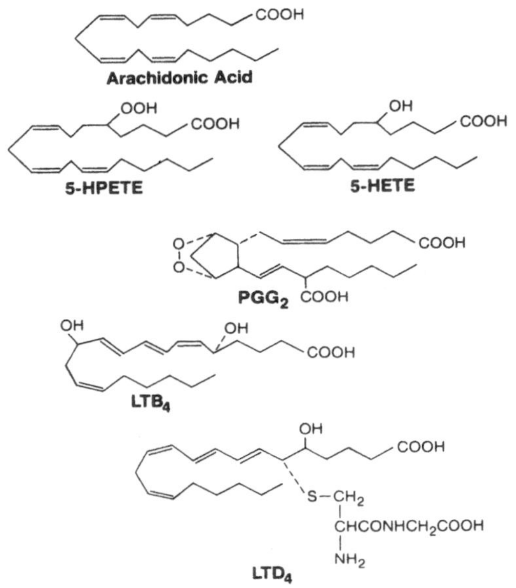

FIGURE 3. Arachidonic acid and some representative cyclooxygenase and lipoxygenase metabolites.

stimuli.[111] Because these compounds are not stored in cells, synthesis immediately precedes release. The overall rate-limiting step of eicosanoid biosynthesis is the hydrolytic production of free arachidonate. Arachidonic acid may be metabolized through two different multienzyme systems, cyclooxygenase and/or lipoxygenase. The cyclooxygenase pathway catalyzes the formation of biologically active PGs and TXA_2 through the unstable endoperoxides PGG_2 and PGH_2. Conversion of PGG_2 to PGH_2 is accompanied by generation of oxygen free radicals. Prostaglandin H_2 acts as precursor for PGD_2, PGE_2, PGF_2, PGI_2, and TXA_2. Lipoxygenases act on arachidonate to generate HPETEs with hydroperoxy groups at differing carbon atoms. 5-Lipoxygenase produces 5-HPETEs, which are the precursors for the biologically active LTB_2, LTC_4, LTD_4, and LTE_4. A new group of lipoxygenase derivatives, the lipoxins, have recently been demonstrated to be synthesized via the 15-lipoxygenase product 15-HPETE.[92]

Because a variety of different denominators (milligrams protein, grams wet weight, nanomoles lipid P) have been used for normalizing tissue eicosanoid levels, it is difficult to compare literature values directly among various studies. Qualitative comparisons, however, show that although many forms of CNS trauma are characterized by eicosanoid increases, the particular pattern, magnitude, and time scale of these increases differ depending on the type of injury and the species used. For example, compression trauma of feline spinal cord and impact trauma of rabbit spinal cord result in 2.5- and fivefold increases in PGI_2, and five- and 14-fold increases in TXB_2; in contrast, impact trauma to dog spinal cord caused no measurable increase in PGI_2 and a 16-fold increase in TXB_2.[22,23,55] In cat, rabbit, and dog spinal cord, postinjury TXB_2 levels were three- to tenfold higher than PGI_2 levels. Reversible cerebral ischemia in the gerbil has been found to increase PGI_2 and TXB_2 two- and fourfold. In contrast to spinal cord, though, the postinjury levels of gerbil brain PGI_2 were 20- to 40-fold higher than those of TXB_2. Significant increases in PGE_2 and PGI_2 have been found in several trauma states. Cold injury to rat brain causes large increases in $PGF_{2\alpha}$.[80] Compression of feline spinal cord and impact injury to canin spinal cord results in significant elevations of PGE_2 and $PGF_{2\alpha}$.[22] Substances with leukotrienelike immunoreactivity have been found to increase following brain ischemia in gerbils[74] and after compression of the feline spinal cord.[4] See Table I for a summary of eicosanoid changes in CNS trauma.

Because of the variety of biological and pathophysiological actions attributed to the eicosanoids,[73,90,111] these metabolites of arachidonic acid have been proposed to contribute to the progression of CNS injury. In addition to their role in cellular inflammation, eicosanoids have effects on CNS vascular homeostasis.[108] Thromboxane A_2 is the most potent naturally occurring vasoconstrictor and promoter of platelet aggregation, whereas PGI_2 is a strong opposing vasodilator and antiaggregant. Prostaglandin F_2 is a vasoconstrictor and platelet aggregator. Leukotrienes C_4, D_4, and E_4 have been shown to have potent vasoconstrictor activity.[29,88,98] In the CNS, these compounds (with the exception of PGI_2) may therefore contribute to postischemic and postconcussive hypoperfusion, formation of platelet microthrombi, and impairment of microcirculation.[21,83] The oxygen free radicals released during eicosanoid biosynthesis may also produce membrane damage, as previously discussed. Leukotrienes B_4, C_4, and D_4 also may act to increase permability of vascular tissue, resulting in extravasation of blood elements into surrounding tissue.[81,112] Finally, LTB_4 is a potent chemoattractant, which may be a factor in the accumulation of leukocytes that has been observed following brain ischemia and spinal cord compression.[45,69] The specific cell types from which eicosanoids are released following CNS trauma have not yet been clearly delineated. Neurons and astrocytes in culture have both been reported to synthesize PGF_2, PGE_2, and TXB_2,[59,76] whereas astrocytes have also been demonstrated to have a very low PGI_2-synthesizing capacity. Cerebral blood vessels have a significant biosynthetic capacity for PGI_2 but lack the ability to synthesize TXA_2.[1,41] Platelets, which accumulate in injured CNS tissue, may also act as a source of eicosanoids.

The particular phospholipid precursor(s) from which arachidonate is released for eicosanoid production is also not known. Only 1–2% of the total arachidonate released by brain or spinal cord following injury is converted to eicosanoids. This observation may indicate that only those arachidonate molecules that are released in close proximity to the cyclooxygenase and lipoxygenase systems are metabolized.

3. PHARMACOLOGICAL INTERVENTION

3.1. DIRECT MEMBRANE PROTECTION

3.1.1. INHIBITION OF HYDROLYSIS

Following CNS trauma, lipid hydrolysis products may lead to direct membrane perturbation. Lipid hydrolysis products may also be metabolized to biologically active factors that may exacerbate the injury state. Therefore, inhibitors of lipase activity are of potential interest, both as pharmacological probes and as possible therapeutic agents. Unfortunately, at the present time there are few and relatively nonspecific lipase inhibitors. A further drawback to many of these compounds is that they may have diverse systemic effects unrelated to lipid metabolism. Compounds that have been shown to inhibit phospholipases or acylglycerol lipases generally work either by binding to the enzyme or by associating with the substrate so as to alter interaction with the enzyme. An example of a binding inhibitor is the previously discussed protein lipomodulin,[34,51] which can be induced by glucocorticoids. Lipomodulin inhibits both phospholipase A_2 and phospholipase C. Lipase inhibitors that interact with the substrate encompass a wide range of chemical types. Cationic amphiphilic drugs such as the antimalarial quinacrine (mepacrine) and chlorpromazine inhibit phospholipases A_2 and C,[54,66,67] as do the polyamines spermidine and putrescine.[91] Some anesthetics also appear to inhibit lipase activity.[94,104] RHC 80267 [6-di(O-carbamolyl)cyclohexanone oxime)hexane], which was originally developed as a diacylglycerol lipase inhibitor, has recently been shown to also inhibit phospholipases A_2 and C.[78] Vitamin E (α-tocopherol), a naturally occurring antioxidant, has been suggested to retard the action of phospholipases by interactions with unsaturated phospholipids.[65]

In the context of CNS injury, lipase inhibitors other than corticosteroids have received little attention. Synthetic corticoids such as dexamethasone and methylprednisolone, which induce lipomodulin, have been used clinically and experimentally for treatment of ischemic stroke, head injury, and spinal cord injury with conflicting claims of efficacy.[11,31,42,77]

3.1.2. ANTIOXIDANTS

The strong indirect evidence for the role of lipid peroxidation in cellular damage following CNS trauma suggests that antioxidant compounds may be of therapeutic importance. A number of substances have been proposed as possible pharmacological antioxidant agents. These include such diverse molecules as dimethylsulfoxide (DMSO), ascorbic acid, selenium, desferrioxamine, vitamin E, superoxide dismutase, methylprednisolone, and disulfiram.[25,46,71,110,115] However, only a few have been tested in CNS injury states, with vitamin E (α-tocopherol) receiving the most attention. Yoshida and co-workers[12,115] have shown that vitamin E supplementation in the rat diminishes compression-induced brain edema and increases blood flow, whereas vitamin E deficiency enhances edema and blood flow reduction in the same model. Yamamoto et al.[113] have reported improvement in brain energy metabolism and neurological function as a result of pretreating rats with vitamin E prior to reversible cerebral ischemia. Pretreatment of rats with vitamin E has also been reported to lessen FeC12-induced focal brain edema.[109]

3.2. EICOSANOID BLOCKADE

3.2.1. INTRODUCTION

In addition to blocking lipolytic arachidonic acid release, there are numerous points at which the synthesis of cyclooxygenase and lipoxygenase metabolites of arachidonate may potentially be inhibited (Fig. 4). In recent years, the pharmaceutical industry has been active in synthesizing and testing a wide variety of cyclooxygenase and lipoxygenase cascade inhibitors as well as eicosanoid receptor antagonists.

3.2.2. CYCLOOXYGENASE CASCADE INHIBITORS

The initial step in the cyclooxygenase pathway is the conversion of arachidonate to PGG_2 by prostaglandin endoperoxide synthase. This reaction is inhibited by a wide variety of substances, thereby preventing production of further biologically active metabolites.[33] These types of inhibitors, which include fatty acid analogues and ibuprofen, bind to the active site of the enzyme but are not themselves metabolized. Irreversible inhibitors include aspirin and act by covalently modifying the active site. Reversible noncompetitive inhibitors are represented by indomethacin, which is thought to work via a free-radical-trapping process. Another set of drugs that have been of interest are the imidazole

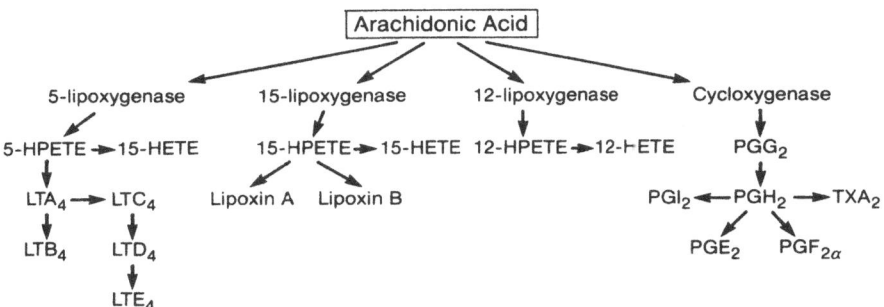

FIGURE 4. Biosynthetic pathways of eicosanoid production.

and pyridine derivatives, which selectively inhibit TXA_2 synthesis,[17] presumably by coordinating with a heme unit that is necessary for activity of thromboxane synthetase. Prostacyclin, which acts as a vasodilator and antiaggregator of platelets, has also been postulated to be of potential use in cerebrovascular disease.

Cyclooxygenase and thromboxane synthetase inhibitors have been used in both clinical and experimental settings, including human stroke and animal models of ischemia and spinal cord injury. Both positive and negative trials of aspirin in human stroke have been reported. Certain of the negative reports may have reflected inadequate sample size. There is also a question as to whether optimal doses have been used.[53] The cyclooxygenase inhibitors ibuprofen and meclofenamate have recently been shown to preserve posttraumatic spinal cord blood flow in contusion-injured cat.[43] Indomethacin administration has given inconsistent results in both experimental and clinical brain ischemia.[44,48] One suggestion for these inconsistencies is that inhibition of cyclooxygenase may increase substrate availability to the lipoxygenase system, thereby increasing leukotriene levels. The pyridine-based thromboxane synthetase inhibitor has been shown to prevent loss of energy metabolites and elimination of electrophysiological response in arachidonate-induced cerebral platelet thromboembolism in rats.[36] To date, only a very small number of multidisciplinary studies have been performed that correlate cyclooxygenase metabolite inhibitors with improvements in biochemistry, physiology, and neurological function following any CNS injury.

3.2.3. LIPOXYGENASE AND MIXED CYCLOOXYGENASE–LIPOXYGENASE INHIBITION

As with cyclooxygenase, the lipoxygenases are inhibited by a number of different compounds including nordihydroguaiaretic acid (NDGA), acetylenic fatty acids, and pyrazoline derivatives.[10,49,82] Acetylenic fatty acids and NDGA are reversible competitive inhibitors that bind to the enzyme active site and have differential inhibitory potencies toward the three major forms of lipoxygenase.[89] The pyrazoline derivatives such as nafazatrom [2,4-dihydro-5-methyl-2-(naphthyloxy)ethyl-3H-pyrazol-3-one] and BW755C [3-amino-1-(m-[trifluoromethyl]-phenyl)-2-pyrazoline] can also inhibit cyclooxygenase activity, with BW755C being a much more potent cyclooxygenase inhibitor than nafazatrom.[82] To date, there are no published reports of the use of these drugs in studies of CNS injury.

3.2.4. RECEPTOR ANTAGONISTS

There are a few drugs available that may block the physiological effects of certain cyclooxygenase and lipoxygenase metabolites of arachidonic acid through their actions as specific receptor antagonists. Antagonists have been developed for TXA_2 and for LTD_4.[62,79] However, no antagonists are currently available for any of the prostaglandins or for the other leukotrienes. As yet there are no reports evaluating the effects of TXA_2 or LTD_4 receptor antagonists in CNS injury.

4. RESEARCH IN PROGRESS

Our laboratories have been actively involved in a multidisciplinary study of the role of membrane lipid changes and arachidonic acid metabolites in the progression of experimental spinal cord injury. Quantified changes in lipid metabolites and membrane function following impact trauma are being correlated with pharmacological intervention and behavioral outcome. Studies to date have used two different species (cat and rat) and two different injury models (compression and impact) to examine early (<1 hr) and delayed (2 hr to 1 week) changes in membrane lipids (Table II). Compression of feline spinal cord with a 170-g weight for 5 min caused rapid increases in FFA and eicosanoid levels. Thirty minutes of recovery after removal of the compression resulted in a 35% decline in total FFA, with the largest decrease occurring in arachidonate. Eicosanoid levels continued to rise at this time. No significant change was observed in total phospholipid levels in spite of a statistically significant decline in the ethanolamine glycerophospholipid fraction. Studies using impact trauma in the rat[32] have extended the time periods at which lipid alterations have been determined to 1 week, with additional sampling points at 2 and 24 hr. As seen in Table II, traumatic spinal cord injury in rats caused a delayed time-dependent increase in free fatty acids (FFA) and concomitant decreases in total phospholipids. The largest percentage increases were found for polyunsaturated fatty acids, including arachidonic and docosahexaenoic acid. Associated with these changes were a reduction in the activity of Na^+,K^+-ATPase and the development of spinal cord edema (data not shown). Quantitation of eicosanoid levels is in progress. All future experiments will utilize this rat model of spinal injury.

5. CONCLUSION

It has been proposed that the progressive tissue necrosis observed following a traumatic injury to the CNS is mediated through the release of endogenous factors that exert deleterious physicochemical or physiological effects. Factors that are postulated to play a role in the progression of CNS injury include, among others, endogenous opioids,[30] excitatory amino acids,[70] and metabolites of membrane glycerophospholipids. This chapter has focused on the potential effects of changes in membrane lipid metabolism.

Lefer[63] has recently set forth several criteria that should be met in order to demonstrate the involvement of a putative mediator in an injury state. First, the potential mediator(s) must be demonstrated to increase either at the injury site or in the blood. Second, the pathophysiological action(s) of the putative mediator(s) should be such that it induces or contributes to the injury state. Finally, pharmacological intervention that inhibits formation or antagonizes the action of the putative mediator(s) should significantly attenuate the degree of injury and improve functional outcome. In this chapter, evidence has been presented that glycerophospholipid hydrolysis products and arachidonic acid metabolites of the cyclooxygenase and lipoxygenase enzymic pathways meet the first two criteria for CNS trauma and ischemia. Pharmacological studies are currently being performed to determine if the third criterion will also be met. It is hoped that studies of this type will lead to the identification of pathophysiological factors that are of major importance in secondary CNS injury following trauma or ischemia. It may then be possible to design clinically relevant therapies for treating patients relatively early after CNS injury, which may prevent or greatly attenuate functional deficits.

ACKNOWLEDGMENTS. The authors would like to thank Ms. Jane Vink for her patience in the typing of this manuscript and Ms. Ingeborg Sacksen for technical support. Supported by NIH research grant NS-14543.

REFERENCES

1. Abdel-Halim, M. S., Lunden, I., Cseh, Q., and Anggard, E., 1980, Prostaglandin profiles in nervous tissue and blood vessels of brain of various animals, *Prostaglandins* **19**:249–258.
2. Agardh, C. D., Chapman, A. G., Nilsson, B., and Siesjo, B. K, 1981, Endogenous substrates utilized by rat brain in severe insulin-induced hypoglycemia, *J. Neurochem.* **36**:490–500.
3. Allan, D., Thomas, P., and Michell, R. H., 1978, Rapid transbilayer diffusion of 1,2-diacylglycerol and its relevance to control of membrane curvature, *Nature* **276**:289–290.
4. Anderson, D. K., Saunders, R. D., Demediuk, P., Dugan, L. L., Braughler, J. M., Hall, E. D., Means, E. D., and Horrocks, L. A., 1985, Lipid hydrolysis and peroxidation in injured spinal cord: Partial protection with methylprednisolone or vitamin E and selenium, *CNS Trauma* **2**:257–267.
5. Bazan, N. G., 1970, Effect of ischemia and electroconvulsive shock on free fatty acid pool in the brain, *Biochim. Biophys. Acta* **218**:1–10.
6. Bazan, N. G., 1976, Free arachidonic acid and other lipids in the nervous system during early ischemia and after electroshock, *Adv. Exp. Med. Biol.* **72**:317–335.
7. Bazan, N. G., and Rodriguez de Turco, E. B, 1980, Membrane lipids in the pathogenesis of brain edema: Phospholipids and arachidonic acid, the earliest membrane components changed at the onset of ischemia, *Adv. Neurol.* **28**:197–205.
8. Bazan, N. G., Bazan, H. E. P., Kennedy, W. G., and Joel, C. D., 1971, Regional distribution and rate of production of free fatty acids in rat brain, *J. Neurochem.* **18**:1387–1394.
9. Bhakoo, K. K., Crockard, H. A., and Ascelles, P. T., 1984, Regional studies of changes in brain fatty acids following experimental ischemia and reperfusion in the gerbil, *J. Neurochem.* **43**:1025–1031.
10. Bokoch, G. M., and Reed, P. W., 1982, Evidence for inhibition of leukotriene A_4 synthesis by

5,8,11,14-eicosatetraynoic acid in guinea pig polymorphonuclear leukocytes, *J. Biol. Chem.* **256:**4156–4163.

11. Bracken, M. G., Collins, W. F., Freeman, D. F., Shepard, M. J. Wagner, F. W., Silten, R. M., Hellenbrand, K. G., Ransohoff, J., Hunt, W. E., Perot, P. L., Grossman, R. G., Green, B. A., Eisenberg, H. M., Rifkinson, O. N., Goodman, J. H., Meagher, J. N., Fischer, B., Clifton, G. L., Flamm, E. S., and Rawe, S. E., 1984, Efficacy of methlprednisolene in acute spinal cord injury, *J.A.M.A.* **251:**45–52.

12. Busto, R., Yoshida, S., Ginsberg, M. D., Alanso, O., Smith, D W., and Goldberg, W. J., 1984, Regional blood flow in compression-induced brain edema in rats: Effect of dietary vitamin E, *Ann. Neurol.* **15:**441–448.

13. Chan, P. H., Longar, S., and Fishman, R. A., 1983, Phospholipid degradation and edema development in cold-injured rat brain, *Brain Res.* **277:**329–337.

14. Chan, P. H., Fishman, R. A., Schmidley, J. W., and Chen, S. F., 1984, Release of polyunsaturated fatty acids from phospholipids and alteration of brain membrane integrity by oxygen-derived free radicals, *J. Neurosci. Res.* **12:**595–605.

15. Chen, S. T., Hsu, C. Y., Hogan, E. L., Halushka, P. V., Linet, O. I., and Yatsu, P. M., 1986, Thromboxane, prostacyclin, and leukotrienes in cerebral ischemia, *Neurology (N.Y.)* **36:**466–470.

16. Clendenon, N. R., Allen, N., Gordon, W. A., and Bingham, W. G., 1978, Inhibition of Na^+,K^+-activated ATPase activity following experimental spinal cord trauma, *J. Neurosurg.* **49:**563–568.

17. Cross, P. E., Dickinson, R. P., Parry, M. J., and Randall, M. J., 1985, Selective thromboxane synthetase inhibitors, *J. Med. Chem.* **28:**1427–1432.

18. Curtis, M. T., Gilfor, D., and Farber, J. L., 1984, Lipid peroxidation increases the molecular order of microsomal membranes, *Arch. Biochem. Biophys.* **235:**644–649.

19. Dawson, R. M. C., 1973, *Form and Function of Phospholipids,* Elsevier/North Holland, Amsterdam.

20. Dawson, R. M. C., Hemington, N. L., and Irvine, R. F., 1983, Diacylglycerol potentiates phospholipase attack upon phospholipid bilayers: Possible connection with cell stimulation, *Biochem. Biophys. Res. Commun.* **117:**196–210.

21. De La Torre, J. S., 1982, Spinal cord injury. Review of basic and applied research, *Spine* **6:**315–335.

22. Demediuk, P., Saunders, R. D., Anderson, D. K., Means, E. D., and Horrocks, L. A., 1985, Membrane lipid changes in laminectomized and traumatized cat spinal cord, *Proc. Natl. Acad. Sci. U.S.A.* **82:**7071–7075.

23. Demediuk, P., Saunders, R. D., Clendenan, N. R., Anderson, D. K., Means, E. D., and Horrocks, L. A., 1985, Changes in lipid metabolism in traumatized spinal cord, *Prog. Brain. Res.* **63:**211–226.

24. Demopoulos, H. B., Flamm, E. S., Pietronigro, D. D., and Seligman, M. L., 1980, The free radical pathology and the microcirculation in the major central nervous system disorders, *Acta Physiol. Scand. [Suppl.]* **492:**91–118.

25. Demopoulos, H. B., Flamm, E. S., Seligman, M. L., Pietronigro, D. D., Tomasula, J., and DeCrescito, V., 1982, Further studies on free radical pathology in the major central nervous system disorders: Effect of very high doses of methylprednisolone on the functional outcome, morphology, and chemistry of experimental spinal cord impact injury, *Can. J. Physiol. Pharmacol.* **60:**1415–1424.

26. Dorman, R. V., Dabrowiecki, Z., and Horrocks, L. A., 1983, Effects of CDPcholine and CDPethanolamine on the alterations in rat brain lipid metabolism induced by global ischemia, *J. Neurochem.* **40:**276–279.

27. Edgar, A. D., Strosznajder, J., and Horrocks, L. A, 1982, Activation of ethanolamine phospholipase A_2 in brain during ischemia, *J. Neurochem.* **39:**1111–1116.

Inhibition of lipid peroxidation in spinal cord homogenates by various drugs, *Exp. Neurol.* **81**:714–721.

72. Mori, T., Takai, Y., Yu, B., Takahashi, J., Nishizuka, Y., and Fujikara, T., 1982, Specificity of the fatty acyl moieties of diacylglycerol for the activation of calcium-activated phospholipid-dependent protein kinase, *J. Biochem.* **91**:427–431.

73. Moskowitz, M. A., and Coughlin, S. R., 1981, Basic properties of the prostaglandins, *Stroke* **12**:696–701.

74. Moskowitz, M. A., Kiwak, K. J., Hekimian, K., and Levine, L., 1984, Synthesis of compounds with the properties of leukotrienes C_4 and D_4 in gerbil brains after ischemia and reperfusion, *Science* **224**:886–889.

75. Moskowitz, N., Andres, A., Silva, W., Shapira, L., Schook, W., and Puszkin, S., 1985, Calcium-dependent binding of calmodulin to phospholipase A_2 subunits induces enzyme activation, *Arch. Biochem. Biophys.* **241**:413–417.

76. Murphy, S., Jeremy, J., Pearce, B., and Dandona, P., 1985, Eicosanoid synthesis and release from primary cultures of rat central nervous system astrocytes and meningeal cells, *Neurosci. Lett.* **61**:61–65.

77. Norris, J. W., and Hachinski, V. C., 1985, Megadose steroid therapy in ischemic stroke, *Stroke* **16**:150–157.

78. Oglesby, T. D., and Gorman, R. R., 1984, The inhibition of arachidonic acid metabolism in human platelets by RHC 80267, a diacylglycerol lipase inhibitor, *Biochim. Biophys. Acta* **793**:269–277.

79. Olanoff, L. S., Cook, J. A., Eller, T., Knapp, D. R., and Halushka, P. V., 1985, Protective effects of trans-13-ATP, a thromboxane receptor antogenist, in endotoxemia, *J. Cardiovasc. Pharmacol.* **7**:114–120.

80. Pappius, H. M., Wolfe, L. S., 1983, Functional disturbances in brain following injury: Search for underlying mechanisms, *Neurochem. Res.* **8**:63–72.

81. Peck, M. J., Piper, P. J., and Williams, T. J., 1981, The effect of leukotrienes C_4 and D_4 on the microvasculture of guinea pig skin, *Prostaglandins* **21**:315–320.

82. Radmark, O., Malmsten, C., and Samuelsson, B., 1980, The inhibitory effects of BW775c on arachidonic acid metabolism in human polymorphonuclear leukocytes, *FEBS Lett.* **110**:213–215.

83. Raichle, M. E., 1983, The pathophysiology of brain ischemia, *Ann. Neurol.* **13**:2–10.

84. Raz, A., and Livne, A., 1973, Differential effects of lipids on the osmotic fragility of erythrocytes, *Biochim. Biophys. Acta* **311**:222–229.

85. Rehncrona, S., Westerberg, E., Akesson, B., and Siesjo, B. K, 1982, Brain cortical fatty acids and phospholipids during and following complete and severe incomplete ischemia, *J. Neurochem.* **38**:84–93.

86. Rhoads, D. E., Kaplan, M. A., Petersen, N. A., and Raghupathy, E., 1982, Effects of free fatty acids on synaptosomal amino acid uptake systems, *J. Neurochem.* **38**:1255–1260.

87. Rodriguez de Turco, E. B., Morelli de Liberti, S., and Bazan, N. G., 1983, Stimulation of free fatty acid and diacylglycerol accumulation in cerebrum and cerebellum during bicuculline-induced status epilepticus. Effect of pretreatment with *o*-methyl-*p*-tyrosine and *p*-chlorophenylalanine, *J. Neurochem.* **40**:252–259.

88. Rosenblum, W. I., 1985, Constricting effect of leukotrienes on cerebral arterioles of mice, *Stroke* **16**:262–263.

89. Salari, H., Braguet, P., and Borgeat, P., 1984, Comparative effects of indomethacin, acetylenic acids, 15-HETE, nordihydroguaiaretic acid, and BW755c on the metabolism of arachidonic acid in human leukocytes and platelets, *Prostaglandins Leukotrienes Med.* **13**:53–60.

90. Samuelsson, B., 1983, Leukotrienes: Mediators of immediate hypersensitivity reactions and inflammation, *Science* **220**:568–575.

91. Sechi, A. M., Cubrini, L., Landi, L., Pasguali, P., and Lenax, G., 1978, Inhibition of

50. Hill, D. J., Dawidowicz, E. A., Andrews, M. L., and Karnovsky, M. J., 1983, Modulation of microsomal glucose-6-phosphatase translocase activity by free fatty acids: Implications for lipid domain structure in microsomal membranes, *J. Cell Physiol.* **115**:1–8.

51. Hirata, F., 1981, The regulation of lipomodulin, a phospholipase inhibitory protein, in rabbit neutrophils by phosphorylation, *J. Biol. Chem.* **256**:7730–7733.

52. Hirashima, Y., Koshu, K., Kamiyama, K., Nishijima, M., Endo, S., and Takaku, A., 1984, Activities of phospholipase A_1, A_2, lysophospholipase, and acyl CoA: Lysophospholipid acyl transferase, in: *Recent Progress in the Study and Therapy of Brain Edema* (K. G. Go and A. Baethman, eds.), Plenum Press, New York, pp. 213–221.

53. Hirsh, J., 1985, Progress review: The relationship between dose of aspirin, side-effects, and antithrombotic effectiveness, *Stroke* **16**:5–9.

54. Hostetler, K. Y., and Matsuzawa, Y., 1981, Studies on the mechanism of drug-induced lipidosis. Cationic amphiphilic drug inhibition of lysosonal phospholipases A and C, *Biochem. Pharmacol.* **30**:1121–1126.

55. Hsu, C. Y., Halushka, P. V., Hogan, E. L., Banik, N. L., Lee, W. A., and Perot, P. L., 1985, Alteration of thromboxane and prostacyclin levels in experimental spinal cord injury, *Neurology (N.Y.)* **35**:1003–1009.

56. Jain, S. K., 1984, The accumulation of malondialdehyde, a product of lipid peroxidation, can disturb aminophospholipid organization in the membrane bilayer of human erythrocytes, *J. Biol. Chem.* **259**:3391–3394.

57. Karnovsky, M. J., Kleinfeld, A. M., Hoover, R. L., and Klausner, R. D., 1982, The concept of lipid domains in membranes, *J. Cell Biol.* **94**:1–6.

58. Katz, A. M., Nash-Adler, P., Watras, J., Messine, F. C., and Takenaka, H., and Louis, C. F., 1982, Fatty acid effects on calcium influx and efflux in sarcoplasmic reticulum vesicles from rabbit skeletal muscle, *Biochim. Biophys. Acta* **687**:17–26.

59. Keller, M., Jakisch, R., Seregi, A., and Hertting, G., 1985, Comparison of prostanoid forming capacity of neuronal and astroglial cells in primary cultures, *Neurochem. Int.* **7**:655–665.

60. Keough, K. M. W., MacDonald, G., and Thompson, W., 1972, A possible relation between phosphoinositides and the diglyceride pool in rat brain, *Biochem. Biophys. Acta* **270**:337–347.

61. Klausner, R. D., Kleinfeld, A. M., Hoover, R. L., and Karnovsky, M. J., 1980, Lipid domains in membranes. Evidence derived from structural perturbations induced by free fatty acids and lifetime heterogeneity analysis, *J. Biol. Chem.* **255**:1286–1295.

62. Ku, T. W., McCarthy, M. E., Weichman, B. M., and Gleason, J. G., 1985, Synthesis and LTD_4 antagonist activity of 2-norleukotriene analogues, *J. Med. Chem.* **28**:1847–1853.

63. Lefer, A. M., 1985, Eicosanoids as mediators of ischemia and shock, *Fed. Proc.* **44**:275–280.

64. Lo, W. D., and Betz, A. L., 1986, Oxygen free-radical reduction of brain capillary rubidium uptake, *J. Neurochem.* **46**:394–398.

65. Lucy, J. A., 1972, Functional and structural aspects of biological membranes: A suggested role for vitamin E in the control of membrane permeability and stability, *Ann. N.Y. Acad. Sci.* **16**:4–11.

66. Lullmann, H., and Wehling, M., 1979, The binding of drugs to different polar lipids *in vitro*, *Biochem. Pharmacol.* **28**:3409–3415.

67. Marcus, H. B., and Bull, E. G., 1969, Inhibition of lipolytic processes in rat adipose tissue by antimalarial drugs, *Biochim. Biophys. Acta* **187**:486–491.

68. Mead, J. F., 1976, Free radical mechanisms of lipid damage and consequences for cellular membranes, in: *Free Radicals in Biology*, Volume 1 (W. A. Pryor, ed.), Academic Press, New York, pp. 51–68.

69. Means, E. D., and Anderson, D. K., 1983, Neuronophagia by leukocytes in experimental spinal cord injury, *J. Neuropathol. Exp. Neurol.* **42**:707–719.

70. Meldrum, B., 1985, Excitatory amino acids and anoxic/ischemic brain damage, *Trends Biochem. Sci.* **10**:47–48.

71. Misiorowski, R. L., Chvapil, M., Snider, B. J., Weinstein, P. R., and Vostal, J. J., 1983,

28. Ellis, E. F., Wright, J. F., Wei, E. P., and Kontos, H. A., 1981, Cyclooxygenase products of arachidonic acid metabolism in cat cerebral cortex after experimental concussive brain injury, *J. Neurochem.* **37**:892–896.
29. Ezra, D., Boyd, L. M., Feuerstein, B., and Goldstein, R. E., 1983, Coronary constriction by leukotriene C_4, D_4, and E_4 in the intact pig heart, *Am. J. Cardiol.* **51**:1451–1454.
30. Faden, A. I., Jacobs, T. P., and Holaday, J. W., 1981, Opiate antagonist improves neurological recovery after spinal injury, *Science* **211**:493–494.
31. Faden, A. I., Jacobs, T. P., and Patrick, D. H., 1984, Megadose corticosteroid therapy following experimental spinal cord injury, *J. Neurosurg.* **60**:712–717.
32. Faden, A. I., Molineaux, C. J., Rosenberger, J. G., Jacobs, T. P., and Cox, C. M., 1985, Endogenous opioid immunoreactivity in rat spinal cord following traumatic injury, *Ann. Neurol.* **17**:386–390.
33. Flower, R. J., and Vane, J. R., 1974, Some pharmacological and biochemical aspects of prostaglandin biosynthesis and its inhibition, in: *Prostaglandin Synthase Inhibitors* (H. J. Robinson and J. R. Vane, eds.), Raven Press, New York, pp. 9–18.
34. Flower, R. J., and Blackwell, G. J., 1979, Antiinflammatory steroids induce biosynthesis of a phospholipase A_2 inhibitor which prevents prostaglandin generation, *Nature* **278**:456–459.
35. Fourcans, B., and Jain, M. K., 1974, Role of phospholipids in transport and enzymatic reactions, *Adv. Lipid Res.* **12**:146–166.
36. Fredriksson, K., Rosen, I., Johansson, B. B., and Wieloch, T., 1985, Cerebral platelet thromboembolism and thromboxane synthetase inhibition, *Stroke* **16**:800–805.
37. Fridovich, I., 1978, The biology of oxygen radicals, *Science* **201**:875–888.
38. Gardiner, M., Nilsson, B., Rehncrona, S., and Siesjo, B. K, 1981, Free fatty acids in moderate and severe hypoxia, *J. Neurochem.* **36**:1500–1505.
39. Goldberg, W. J., Watson, B. D., Busto, R., Kurchner, H., Santiso, M., and Ginsberg, M. D., 1984, Concurrent measurement of Na^+,K^+-ATPase activity and lipid peroxides in rat brain following reversible global ischemia, *Neurochem. Res.* **9**:1737–1747.
40. Goldman, S. S., and Albers, R. W., 1973, Sodium-potassium activated adenosine triphosphatase. IX. The role of phospholipids, *J. Biol. Chem.* **248**:876–874.
41. Hagen, A. A., White, R. P., Terragno, N. A., and Robertson, J. T., 1978, Synthesis of prostaglandins by bovine cerebral arteries, *Fed. Proc.* **37**:384–390.
42. Hall, E. D., and Braughler, J. M., 1982, Glucocorticoid mechanisms in acute spinal cord injury: A review and therapeutic rationale, *Surg. Neurol.* **18**:320–327.
43. Hall, E. D., and Wolf, D. F., 1986, A pharmacological analysis of the pathophysiological mechanisms of posttraumatic spinal cord ischemia, *J. Neurosurg.* **64**:951–961.
44. Hallenbeck, J. M., Leitch, D. R., Dutka, A. J., Greenbaum, L. J., and McKee, A. E., 1982, Prostacyclin I_2, indomethacin, and heparin promote postischemic neuronal recovery in dogs, *Ann. Neurol.* **12**:145–156.
45. Hallenbeck, J. M., Dutka, A. J., Tanishima, T., Kochanek, P. M., Kumaroo, K. K., Thompson, C. B., Obrenovitch, T. P., and Cantreras, T. J., 1986, Polymorphonuclear leukocyte accumulation in brain regions with low blood flow during the early postischemic period, *Stroke* **17**:246–253.
46. Halliwell, B., and Gutteridge, J. M. C., 1985, Oxygen radicals and the nervous system, *Trends Biochem. Sci.* **10**:22–26.
47. Hammond, B., Kontos, H. A., and Hess, M. L., 1985, Oxygen radicals in the adult respiratory distress syndrome, in myocardial ischemia and reperfusion injury, and in cerebral vascular damage, *Can. J. Physiol. Pharmacol.* **63**:173–187.
48. Harris, R., Bayhan, M., Branston, N. M., Watson, A., and Syman, L., 1982, Modulation of the pathophysiology of primate focal cerebral ischemia by indomethacin, *Stroke* **13**:17–24.
49. Higgs, G. A., and Flower, R. J., 1981, Anti-inflammatory drugs and the inhibition of arachidonate lipoxygenase, in: *SRS-A and Leukotrienes* (P. J. Piper, ed.), John Wiley & Sons, New York, pp. 197–207.

phospholipase A_2 and pholpholipase C by polyamines, *Arch. Biochem. Biophys.* **186**:248–254.

92. Serhan, C. N., Hamberg, M., and Samuelsson, B., 1984, Lipoxins: Novel series of biologically active compounds formed from arachidonic acid in human leukocytes, *Proc. Natl. Acad. Sci. U.S.A.* **81**:5335–5339.

93. Sheetz, M. P., and Singer, S. J., 1974, Biological membranes as bilayer couples. A molecular mechanism of drug–erythrocyte interactions, *Proc. Natl. Acad. Sci. U.S.A.* **71**:4457–4461.

94. Shiu, G. K., Nemoto, E. M., and Alexander, H. L., 1981, Brain free fatty acid changes during global ischemia with barbiturate anesthesia and hypothermia, *Br. J. Anaesth.* **53**:304–310.

95. Siesjo, B. K., Ingvar, M., and Westerberg, E., 1982, The influence of bicuculline-induced seizures on free fatty acid concentrations in cerebral cortex, hippocampus, and cerebellum, *J. Neurochem.* **39**:796–803.

96. Stokes, B. T., Fox, P., and Hollinden, G., 1983, Extracellular calcium activity in the injured spinal cord, *Exp. Neurol.* **85**:561–572.

97. Sun, G. Y., Su, K. L., Der, O. M., and Tang, W., 1979, Enzymic regulation of arachidonate metabolism in brain membrane phosphoglycerides, *Lipids* **14**:229–235.

98. Tagari, P., DuBoulay, G. H., Aitken, V., and Boullin, P. J., 1983, Leukotriene D_4 and the cerebral vasculature *in vivo* and *in vitro*, *Prostaglandins Leukotrienes Med.* **11**:281–297.

99. Tang, W., and Sun, G. Y., 1985, Effects of ischemia on free fatty acids and diacylglycerols in developing rat brain, *Int. J. Dev. Neurosci.* **3**:51–56.

100. Triggs, W. J., and Willmore, L. J., 1984, *In vivo* lipid peroxidation in rat brain following intracortical Fe^{2+} injection, *J. Neurochem.* **42**:976–980.

101. Usher, J. R., Epand, R. M., and Papahadjopoulos, D., 1978, The effect of free fatty acids on the thermotropic phase transition of dimyristroyl glycerophosphocholine, *Chem. Phys. Lipids* **22**:245–253.

102. Van den Bosch, H., 1980, Intracellular phospholipases A, *Biochim. Biophys. Acta* **604**:191–246.

103. van Dugin, G., Verkleij, A. J., and de Kruijff, B., 1984, Influence of phospholipid peroxidation on the phase behavior of phosphatidylcholine and phosphatidylethanolamine in aqueous dispersions, *Biochemistry* **23**:4969–4977.

104. Vigo, C., Lewis, G. P., and Piper, P. J., 1980, Mechanisms of inhibition of phospholipase A_2, *Biochem. Pharmacol.* **29**:623–627.

105. Wakai, S., Aritake, K., Asano, T., and Takakura, K., 1982, Selective destruction of the outer leaflet of the capillary endothelial membrane after intra-cerebral injection of arachidonic acid, *Acta Neuropathol. (Berl.)* **58**:303–306.

106. Wei, E. P., Lamb, R. G., and Kontos, H. A., 1982, Increased phospholipase C activity after experimental brain injury, *J. Neurosurg.* **56**:695–698.

107. Wheeler, K. P., Walker, J. A., and Barker, D. M., 1975, Lipid requirement of the membrane sodium-plus-potassium ion-dependent adenosine triphosphatase system, *Biochem. J.* **146**:713–722.

108. White, R. P., and Hagan, A. A., 1982, Cerebrovascular actions of prostaglandins, *Pharmacol. Ther.* **18**:313–331.

109. Willmore, L. J., and Rubin, J. J., 1984, Effects of antiperoxidants on $FeCl_2$-induced lipid peroxidation and focal edema in rat brain, *Exp. Neurol.* **83**:62–70.

110. Willmore, L. J., and Rubin, J. J., 1984, The effect of tocopherol and dimethyl sulfoxide on focal edema and lipid peroxidation induced by isocortical injection of ferrous chloride, *Brain Res.* **296**:389–392.

111. Wolfe, L. S., 1982, Eicosanoids: Prostaglandins, thromboxanes, leukotrienes, and other derivatives of carbon-20 unsaturated fatty acids, *J. Neurochem.* **38**:1–14.

112. Woodward, D. F., and Ledgard, S. E., 1985, Effect of LTD_4 on conjuctival vasopermeability and blood–aqueous barrier integrity, *Invest. Ophthalmol. Vis. Sci.* **26**:481–485.

113. Yamamoto, M., Shima, T., Uozumi, T., Sogabe, T., Yamada, K., and Kawasaki, T., 1983, A possible role of lipid peroxidation in cellular damages caused by cerebral ischemia and the protective effect of vitamin E, *Stroke* **14**:977–982.
114. Yorio, T., Torres, S., and Tarapoom, N., 1980, Alterations in membrane permeability by diacylglycerol and phosphatidylcholine containing arachidonic acid, *Lipids* **18**:96–99.
115. Yoshida, S., Busto, R., and Ginsborg, M. D., 1983, Compression-induced brain edema: Modification by prior depletion and supplementation of vitamin E, *Neurology (N.Y.)* **33**:166–172.
116. Yoshida, S., Abe, K., Busto, R., Watson, B. O., Kogure, K., and Ginsberg, M. D., 1982, Influence of transient ischemia on lipid-soluble antioxidants, free fatty acids, and energy metabolites in rat brain, *Brain Res.* **245**:307–316.
117. Young, W., Yen, V., and Blight, A., 1982, Extracellular calcium ion activity in experimental spinal cord contusion, *Brain Res.* **253**:105–113.

3

Experimental Spinal Cord Injury

Strategies for Acute and Chronic Intervention Based on Anatomic, Physiological, and Behavioral Studies

Michael S. Beattie, Bradford T. Stokes, and Jacqueline C. Bresnahan

ABSTRACT. Much of the current research on mechanisms and treatments of injury to the spinal cord employs techniques for controlled impaction of the cord after laminectomy. The resultant injury and its sequelae are often conceived in terms of an acute phase, when progressive degradation occurs, and a chronic phase, when whatever compensatory mechanisms available must act. This chapter reviews previous attempts to affect the outcome of spinal cord contusion injuries using pharmacological approaches aimed at both the acute and chronic phases, attempts to relate studies of contusion injuries to studies of recovery of function after spinal transections and funiculotomies, and suggests future strategies for intervention that recognize the widely distributed effects of spinal lesions on the central nervous system. The use of a new, feedback-controlled impaction device in such studies is discussed, and the importance of careful, longitudinal assessments of motor function in animal models is stressed. Advances in the treatment of spinal cord injury will depend on the creative application of advances in basic neurobiology to controlled laboratory models incorporating behavioral, physiological, and morphological criteria of recovery.

1. Introduction and a Brief History of Spinal Cord Injury Research

In 1911, Allen introduced a technique for the production of experimental spinal cord contusion in dogs that has remained one of the most widely used methods

MICHAEL S. BEATTIE, BRADFORD T. STOKES, AND JACQUELINE C. BRESNAHAN • Departments of Surgery (Neurologic Surgery), Anatomy, and Physiology, and Spinal Cord Injury Research Center, The Ohio State University, Columbus, Ohio 43210.

43

for the laboratory simulation of human spinal cord injury. Since then, a large number of studies have been conducted to determine the nature of the lesion resulting from various kinds of trauma to the cord and the potential for pharmacological intervention to ameliorate its deleterious consequences. Several substantive reviews of this literature have appeared.[8,30,38,99,126] Much of the work done to date has focused on the acute effects of trauma, i.e., on the events and mechanisms responsible for the degradation of neural tissue subsequent to an injury that does not primarily sever axons or destroy neurons. The concept of a progressive lesion has been central to much of spinal cord injury research, with the thought that ameliorating progressive destruction might be an effective strategy for treatment soon after injury.[4,126] This emphasis on the early posttrauma events in spinal cord injury is, at least in part, in contrast to neuropsychological studies of recovery from damage to telencephalic structures (see refs. 44,81,108), which have emphasized the mechanisms of long-term recoveries from CNS damage. In this chapter, we review methods for the experimental production of spinal cord injury and strategies for pharmacological intervention, touching both on treatments aimed at stopping the progression of the lesion and on treatments and behavioral strategies that might serve to enhance long-term recovery. We discuss in some detail the features of experimental spinal cord lesions with emphasis on the relationship of these features to interventive strategies, including those aimed at both short-term and long-term reduction of deficits.

2. CURRENT METHODS FOR LESION PRODUCTION

In research on spinal cord regeneration, the traditional approach has been complete surgical transection (see review by Windle[122]), and particular attention has been paid to the documentation of transection completeness.[61] The goal of injury models, on the other hand, has been to produce tissue damage like that seen in fracture–dislocation injuries, penetrating injuries, or progressive compression such as that which occurs with spinal metastatic tumors.

2.1. IMPACT INJURIES

Models of fracture–dislocation injuries have been based primarily on Allen's[2] method; a weight of known mass is dropped through a vented tube onto the exposed dorsal surface of the spinal cord from varying heights. The magnitude of the resultant impact has often been expressed as the product of the mass times the distance dropped, i.e., "g-cm," although it is widely recognized that this unit is not very meaningful in any physical sense (e.g., the force imparted to the cord by a 5-g weight dropped 20 cm does not equal that produced by a 10-g weight dropped 10 cm). Since the physical properties of the impact itself are not readily measured, however, the convenience of this measure has encouraged its continued use in the literature, usually with careful attention to reporting both the weight and surface area of the impactor and the distance dropped. Although the lack of interlaboratory reliability of the method is by now notorious,[125] recent careful applications of the method have indeed shown that different levels of injury can be produced by varying the distance or mass.[12,46,123] An attempt to reduce variability use has been made of a curved "anvil" to provide support for the spinal cord *in situ*.[46] This approach seems to have promise, but even with this technique, it is clear that the production of an intermediate lesion is difficult. Rather, there was a sharp transition zone (in terms of "g-cm" of impact) between animals showing rapid and complete recovery and those showing persistent paralysis.

Some attempts have been made to measure the physical parameters of impact injuries using the weight-drop method (see ref. 30 for a review). These studies provided the background for the development of the feedback-controlled impactor developed at Ohio State and described below.

2.2. SLOW(ER) COMPRESSION INJURIES

Tarlov[115] and Rivlin and Tator[95,96] have used an epidural balloon and aneurysm clip to compress the spinal cord, respectively. Slow compression of the spinal cord has also been accomplished by static loading of the surface of the spinal cord for varying lengths of time[35,78] or by slowing compressing the cord with a vicelike apparatus.[101]

3. THE TIME COURSE OF EVENTS FOLLOWING INJURY

It is convenient to divide the effects of impact (especially) or compression injury into "acute" and "chronic" stages. Acute effects are those that are the immediate effects of the lesion or a direct consequence of it (e.g., shearing forces that disrupt axons and cellular components). Chronic effects might be classified as those that persist after the effects of edema or swelling have subsided and must include the possible effects of reorganization and neural and behavioral plasticity, which may be both positive and negative.

The categorization of the putative progressive events following injury is difficult, since the delineation of degenerative and reparative processes is not always obvious. In addition, the roles of blood flow changes, edema, ischemia, autolytic enzymes, etc. are difficult to categorize as "acute" or "chronic," since they may develop and persist over time courses overlapping those in which reparative processes may be taking place. It is clear, however, that the long-term consequences of the lesion must be evaluated only after a considerable length of time. Periods of 3 to 4 weeks or longer have often been considered adequate for stabilization of the anatomic and neurological consequences of impact injuries. Less attention has been focused on the very-long-term outcome of experimental injuries. This is in some degree because of the time-consuming nature of such studies, but it may well be that most studies of partial lesions fail to describe adequately the residual capacities of the subjects involved. This may be particularly important in evaluating the effects of pharmacological agents; multiple measures over the full time course of potential recovery may be needed to evaluate adequately the effects of any particular agent. Attention to whether a drug effect represents actions on initial destructive events or on the residual capacities of organisms with chronic lesions may have theoretical importance for planning treatment strategies aimed at different aspects of spinal trauma.

3.1. THE ACUTE PHASE AND THE CONCEPT OF A PROGRESSIVE LESION

One of the most striking features of spinal cord impact injuries is the lack of obvious damage immediately following the impact; spinal cords removed rapidly after an impact injury appear surprisingly intact. In contrast, functional deficits are apparent immediately, even in the absence of gross pathology. For example, after a "400 g-cm" impact injury to the cat thoracic spinal cord, somatosensory evoked potentials (SEPs) are completely abolished just after impact.[126] These may then return transiently, only to disappear again at times coincident with the development of obvious white matter pathology.

Young[126] has pointed out that the lack of obvious pathology at early postimpact times does not necessarily mean that cells and axons remain intact; the manifestations of even immediate cell death take time. Functional or biochemical studies may reveal alterations not observable with standard anatomic techniques. For example, studies by LaMotte and colleagues[74,109] showed enhanced permeability to horseradish peroxidase (HRP) in axons, even at the periphery of the white matter, between 15 min and 3 hr post-impact, suggesting that axonal membranes are altered even though electron microscopy shows little or no evidence of membrane breakdown.[23] In addition, there is clear evidence for a rapid depression in Na^+,K^+-ATPase,[28] a membrane-bound enzyme, and the rapid appearance of arachidonate metabolites as soon as a few minutes after injury[5] (see P. Demediuk and A. I. Faden, Chapter 2). The release of these metabolites is paralleled by rapid increases in lipoxygenase activities, suggesting that the injury initiates a progressive cascade of membrane-related biochemical events that may be irreversible. Such observations suggest that the destructive effects of the trauma are initiated almost immediately.

The evidence for a truly progressive lesion, then, comes from additional observations (e.g., ref. 126). First, the transient return of SEPs noted above suggests that there is an initial conduction block in white matter axons, followed by recovery. The secondary loss of the transient SEP recovery might then reflect the spread of the destructive events initiated by membrane alterations, ischemia, etc. Second, spinal white matter blood flow probably remains stable for 2 to 3 hr following impact,[126] although recent data dispute this claim.[69] A third line of evidence for lesion progression comes from studies that have purported to show protective effects of early interventions, e.g., naloxone, spinal cord hypothermia, high-dose corticosteroids, and opiate antagonists.

3.2. THE CHRONIC PHASE: POTENTIAL REORGANIZATION AND REHABILITATION

After these destructive events have subsided and the lesion is established, i.e., the irreversibly damaged neurons have died and the remaining affected neurons have recovered either from direct damage or from denervation, a new steady state is reached. This new organization reflects direct and indirect alterations produced by the lesion and is the product of such dynamic processes as regeneration, collateral sprouting, denervation supersensitivity, and transsynaptic changes. It is this reorganized system that must be used to reestablish functional integrity, and understanding the reorganization should help in the appropriate design of treatment strategies.

4. THE FEATURES OF THE LESION

Although considerable attention has been paid to the site of impact itself and to the resulting tissue degradation, axonal destruction, glial changes, etc., it is clear that an impact lesion to the spinal cord results, in the long term, in a highly distributed lesion. This is illustrated schematically in Fig. 1A, where an impact site in the rat spinal cord is shown in relation to the whole CNS. The distributed nature of the lesion results, of course, from the fact that disruption of axons passing through the impact site has both anterograde and retrograde effects on diverse and distant neuronal cell groups in both the distal spinal segments and rostral spinal cord, brainstem, and forebrain centers.

4.1. AT THE IMPACT SITE

The first macroscopic signs following impact injury are petechial hemorrhages in the gray matter followed by central hemmorrhagic necrosis. Destruction of axons is first evident in the region close to the gray matter and progresses in a central-to-peripheral direction.[12,23] The rate of this progression depends on the degree of severity of the injury.[6,23] Axonal disruption is characterized by the damming of the products of axoplasmic transport in the stumps of transected axons and, later, Wallerian degeneration of the isolated distal segments (see Fig. 2). Axons surviving the injury are characteristically located at the periphery of

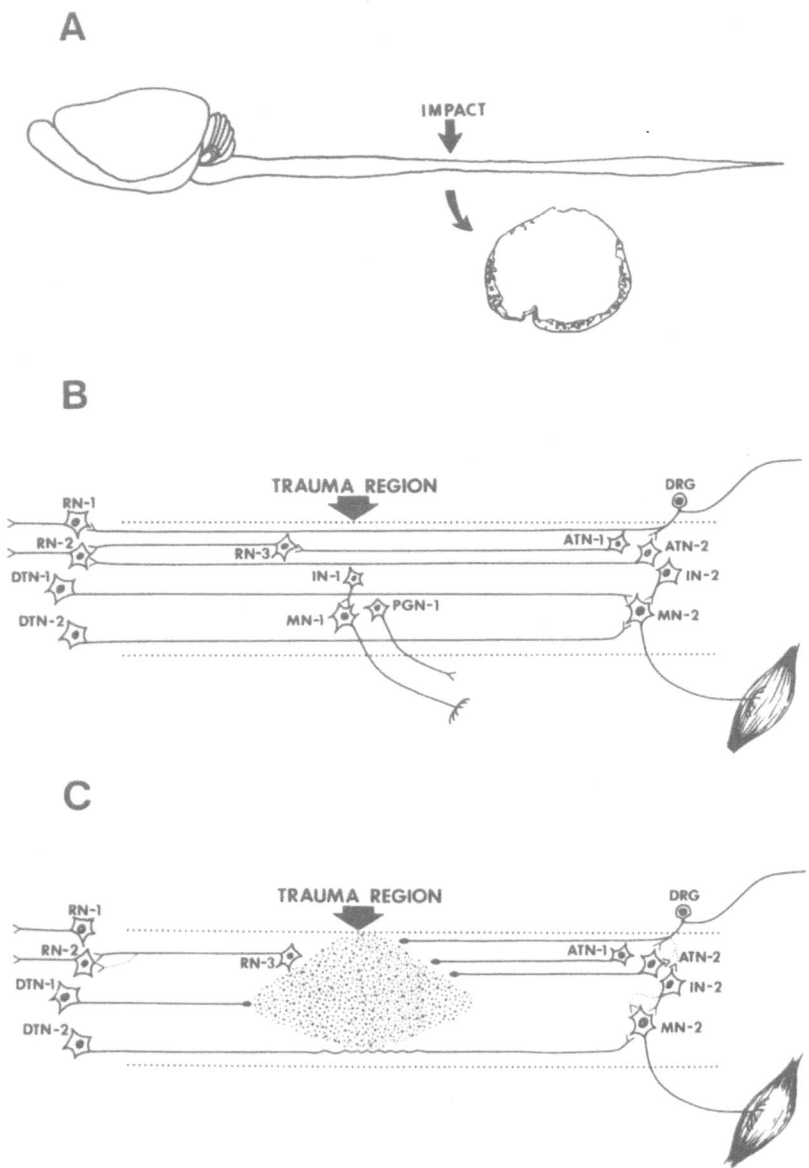

FIGURE 1. A schematic diagram of a lesion in the thoracic spinal cord. A: The spinal cord and brain of a rat with an indication of the impact site. The histological appearance of the spinal cord at the impact site is shown in cross section below. B: The normal spinal cord with several neurons indicated. The sensory input from dorsal root ganglion neurons (DRG) to the caudal portion of the spinal cord as well as their branches to the brainstem sensory relay neurons (RN-1) are indicated.

the cord,[12,13,23] tend to be smaller in diameter,[13] and tend to have reduced myelin sheaths.[12] Dying back of the severed axons[27,70] occurs for a few millimeters on either side of the injury impact site, and it is possible that some of these axons attempt regeneration.[27,75,122] The degenerative debris at the lesion epicenter is phagocytosed by macrophages, which constitute 30% of the volume of the lesion site by 1 week after an impact injury.[12] Degenerating axons away from the lesion site are also phagocytosed by macrophages, which have been observed to enter still intact myelin sheaths to gain access to the degenerating debris.[23] By 2 to 3 weeks post-lesion, cystic cavities are beginning to be formed by fibroblasts, which separate the cavities from the remaining neural and glial tissue,[7] and by several weeks later, well-developed scars with collagen fibrils can be observed.[23] Remyelination of axons at the lesion site is accomplished by both oligodendroglia and Schwann cells.[12,23]

4.1.1. THE PARTIAL LESION

As discussed above, spinal cord contusion rarely results in complete destruction of all spinal axons. A peripheral rim of fibers typically remains.[12,13,23−25,33] These fibers may have abnormal physiological properties with reduced conduction velocities and increased refractory periods and temperature sensitivity.[126] However, less than 10% of the white matter is sufficient to subserve locomotor function in animal experiments.[1,12,24,36,121] Those in the ventral funiculus are of particular importance.[1,36]

4.1.2. FACTORS LIMITING POTENTIAL RECOVERY

Factors limiting potential recovery include the extent of gray matter loss, which determines the degree of segmental and autonomic denervation of the periphery, as well as the loss of second-order neurons relaying somatosensory

---

Ascending tract neurons (ATN-1 and -2), spinal interneurons (IN-1 and -2), motor neurons (MN-1 and -2), and autonomic preganglionic neurons (PGN-1) in the spinal cord are also shown. Additional relay neurons in the rostral spinal cord (RN-3) and brainstem (RN-2) are indicated as well. Descending tract neurons (DTN-1 and -2) are shown projecting from rostral sites to the spinal cord. After a spinal cord injury at the site indicated as the trauma region, axotomy, denervation, and compensatory processes ensue. The final status of some of the processes is indicated in C. The ascending tract neurons (ATN-1 and -2) are axotomized, and the rostrally projecting collaterals of DRG neurons (DRG) are pruned. The interneurons (IN-1), motor neurons (MN-1), and preganglionic neurons (PGN-1) at the impact site are destroyed by the lesion. Axons passing through the lesion are also mostly destroyed, although some at the periphery (axon of DTN-2) survive, but with some alterations of conduction properties. The degeneration of the isolated distal segments of the axons produces denervation of neurons both rostrally and caudally. Vacated postsynaptic sites may induce collateral axonal sprouting of intact neurons (e.g., IN-1 and RN-3) or of neurons that have had their axonal arbors pruned (e.g., DRG). Other functional alterations produced by the lesion include denervation supersensitivity and unmasking of previously ineffective synapses (see text for further explanation).

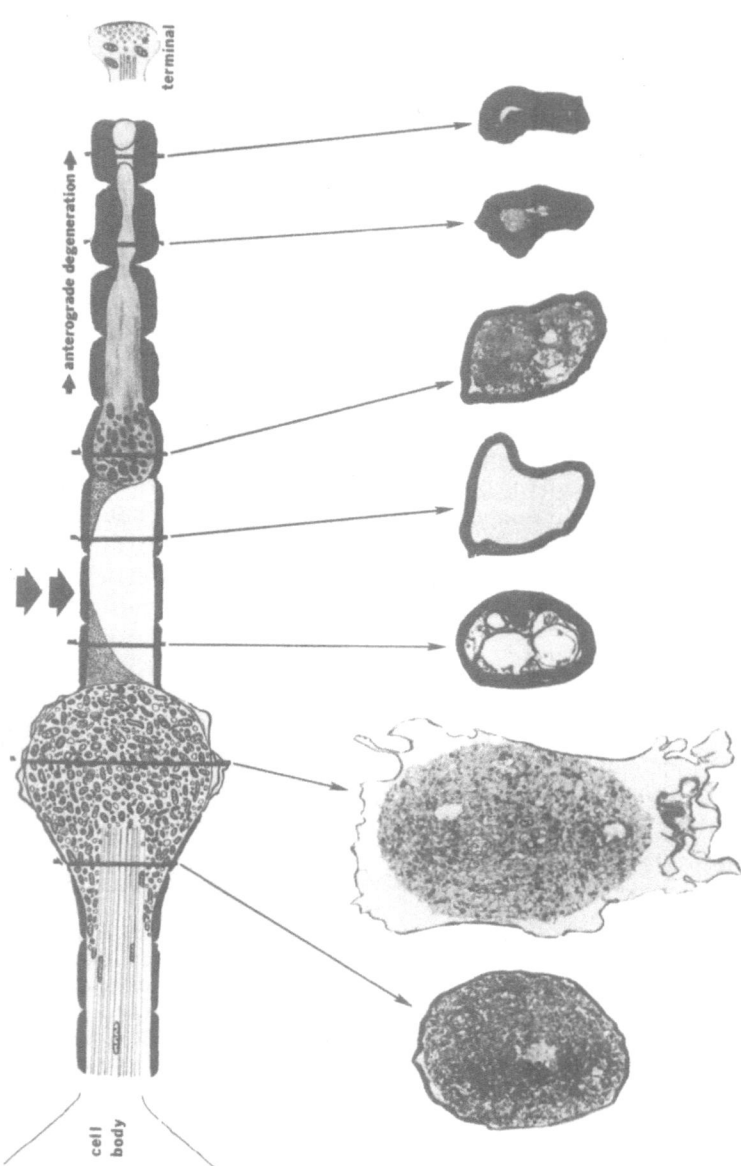

FIGURE 2. Alterations of an individual axon that result from traumatic injury. On the top is a schematic representation of an axon that has been interrupted at a lesion site, and below are actual electron micrographs that represent cross sections through axons at the level indicated on the schematic. The proximal segment (on the left) is still connected to the cell body, and the damming of the products of axoplasmic flow produces swelling of the proximal stump. It is from this region that regenerative sprouts will be produced. The distal segment of the axon (on the right) is separated from the cell body and undergoes Wallerian degeneration including the terminal portions of the axonal tree. (From Bresnahan.[23])

and proprioceptive input to rostral and caudal centers. The limiting factors for sensory and locomotor recovery in models using thoracic cord impacts are the extent to which long ascending and descending fibers are functionally spared and the extent to which distributed lesion effects can be overcome. It is especially relevant here that a rim of fibers be spared. Their functional status, the role they play in sensorimotor function in the normal animals, and their potential capacity to interfere with or mediate recovery are important in understanding how pharmacological agents might better the outcomes of actual traumatic injuries.

4.2. THE DISTRIBUTED NATURE OF THE LESION

The wide distribution of axonal degeneration in the CNS seen following impact injuries in macaques[25] serves to illustrate the considerable extent of denervation both rostral and caudal to the lesion proper, including brainstem and thalamic structures. Such widespread denervation might be expected to contribute to widespread and diverse functional effects.

As shown schematically in Fig. 1, denervation of systems rostral and caudal to the lesion results from the anterograde degeneration of damaged axons. Retrograde changes also occur in surviving neurons whose axons have been disrupted. In addition to chromatolysis, dendritic alterations,[52] synaptic stripping,[11] and expansion of remaining collaterals have been reported.[84] Some neurons escape direct damage to both their cell bodies and axons but still can be affected by the lesion through denervation and whatever compensatory responses occur to that denervation. In the acute phase, this takes the form of spinal shock[102] or diaschisis,[83] phenomena that may be important in the initial lack of function and the mechanisms of which are still unknown. Other functional changes in the acute phase may be produced by unmasking of previously ineffective synapses.[119] Some responses to denervation develop over time as spinal shock subsides and include denervation supersensitivity,[53,106] collateral axonal sprouting or reactive synaptogenesis,[29,54] and behavioral compensation, which includes learning. Denervation has also been invoked as a possible cause of the central pain states frequently experienced by spinal cord injury patients.[79] Indeed, collateral axonal sprouting has been suggested as a cause of spasticity and hyperreflexia in caudal spinal reflexes after injury (e.g., ref. 54); perhaps sensory systems can exhibit "spasticity" in response to denervation as well.

5. ASSESSING BEHAVIORAL AND NEUROLOGICAL RECOVERY

The somatosensory evoked potential has been one of the most frequently employed methods of assessing neural transmission in the spinal cord.[125,126] Typically, hindlimb sensory nerves are stimulated, and evoked potentials are recorded over the rostral spinal cord, the brainstem, and (most frequently) the somatosensory cortex. Measures of sensory function in awake, behaving animals after spinal lesions have been less frequently used, but most require extensive training and testing of the animals.[118] The hot plate test, in which the subject is placed on a hot plate and the latency to lick the hindpaw is measured, has been used as an assessment of pain perception in animals with spinal cord lesions.[50] This latter test, however, requires a complex motor response, which might be affected by the lesion as well, so it is not a purely "sensory" task. With the exception of the SEP, however, no task is purely "sensory," as all require some motor output to affirm reception of the sensory event.

The most commonly used measure of motor function following spinal cord damage is simple rating of general locomotor ability, e.g., the Tarlov scale.[115] More refined assessments of locomotor function include evaluation of treadmill walking[37,57,58,98] and walking on narrow beams[54] or wire grids.[24,104] A gross measure of postural adjustment to body displacement was developed by Rivlin and Tator[95]; this test measures an animal's ability to maintain its position on an inclined plane, the angle of which is gradually increased. A physiological measure of the integrity of pathways descending from the brainstem that influence postural reflexes is muscle activity produced by free fall.[59] The vestibular freefall responses have quantifiable components that are differentially affected by spinal cord lesions, and the residual responses correlate with locomotor ability.[59] Motor evoked potentials[76] have also been used to assess the integrity of descending motor pathways.

6. EXAMPLES OF ATTEMPTS AT PHARMACOLOGICAL INTERVENTION

The multifaceted nature of the spinal lesion after injury has precipitated a wide range of hypotheses on the nature of both the acute and chronic lesion. These have been matched by a search for the combination of pharmaceutical agents that is best able to arrest or reverse the developing pathology. Since little agreement exists on the mechanisms by which such changes take place, there continues to be much confusion about which agents to use and when to give them. The development of clear cause-and-effect hypotheses has also been impeded by a lack of biomechanically defined models and well-controlled behavioral studies to evaluate the most important criterion of their efficacy, the recovery of function. Most investigators would agree, however, that any therapeutic approach to the pharmacology of spinal injury must take into account the biphasic temporal nature of lesion development. Because the acute and chronic phases of these sequelae may be quite different mechanistically, we discuss them here in separate sections. As noted above, however, this distinction does not always imply that separate mechanisms are involved.

6.1. IN THE ACUTE PHASE

Historically, treatment modalities in experimental spinal cord injury have attempted to deal with the immediate sequelae of the injury itself. Certain approaches such as the use of osmotic diuretics,[31] hypothermia,[63,73,117] antiadrenergic compounds,[66,88,91] hyperbaric oxygenation,[51,67,124] enzyme therapy,[60] and local anesthetics[47] have all had their proponents but only limited success in reversing or arresting the damage. Two of these (hypothermia and hyperbaric oxygenation) have been used in a series of clinical trials that have been difficult to interpret because of their lack of double-blind methodology and the inconclusive nature of the results.[125] The remainder have found little support elsewhere.

Steroids have traditionally been used to treat human spinal cord injury. Such clinical approaches were based on a wide range of dosages in experimental animal work that appear to improve neurological function[5,34,78] or prevent changes in neural tissue normally associated with spinal trauma.[17,18] Others have found little effect with similar protocols.[41,66] Higher-dosage paradigms have been suggested[19,78,129] but have not always been clearly effective.[40] Issues of an increase in experimental complications and potential mortality problems have been raised.[40,56] In spite of recent improvements,[5,123] there is still a need for double-blind experimental protocols in established animal models using such high dosages. Until then, controversy about mechanisms of action and potential therapeutic use of these agents will continue.[14,20]

The endogenous opioids may play a role in the spinal injury process. Evidence suggests that naloxone, an opiate antagonist, leads to neurological improvement when administered just after injury (see T. K. McIntosh and A. I. Faden, Chapter 5). Although not clearly established, its mechanisms of action were thought to be mediated through a prevention or improvement of the spinal ischemia known to accompany severe injury[128]; more recent evidence disputes this finding.[69,120] In addition, drugs that are known to increase blood flow dramatically (calcium channel blockers such as nimodipine) are without effect on the production of spinal lesions.[42,48] Further evidence also suggests that naloxone, at the high dosages used, may exert its effects by nonopioid effects. These include its capacity to inhibit lipid peroxidation[72] and reverse the decrease of extracellular calcium activity.[112] High doses of naloxone and the more effective thyrotropin-releasing hormone (TRH) therapy (see ref. 39, for example), as discussed by McIntosh and Faden (Chapter 5), could also have their effects through alternate classes of opioid receptors. A hypothesis that the κ opioid receptor, which binds TRH and naloxone less well, is involved in these sequelae to injury has been presented and supported by recent evidence.[38] Agents that seem to perturb this putative dynorphin receptor axis beneficially may therefore replace TRH and naloxone for the treatment of spinal trauma.[38]

Others have proposed that the generation of free radical reactions in traumatized tissue[32] induces lipid peroxidation and hydrolysis in cellular membranes. The consequent release of free fatty acids (arachidonate), activation of certain phospholipases, and destruction of ionic homeostasis that ensue have all been targets of recent attempts to reverse the pathology.[4] Such attempts have included a variety of antioxidants such as vitamin E,[5] selenium,[5] coenzyme Q,[114] megadose corticosteroids,[17] and high-dose opiate antagonists[72]; TRH, mentioned above, may also work through such mechanisms.[77] Recent studies that have provided a clearer picture of the additive interaction between calcium and lipid peroxidation during spinal injury have resulted in newer models to test functional efficacy.[16] Evidence for functional recovery using such interventions is so far lacking, but future trials in experimental populations are likely.

6.2. IN THE CHRONIC PHASE

A recent study by Robinson and Goldberger[97] has shown that some of the long-term consequences of complete spinal transection on hindlimb locomotor performance can be ameliorated by pharmacological interventions. These authors studied treadmill locomotor performance in adult cats that had received spinal transections at least 3 months prior to testing and found that bicuculline (400–600 μg/kg) significantly enhanced treadmill performance and positive supporting reactions. Hindlimb proprioceptive placing was unaffected. Naloxone (100 μg/kg) had no effect on locomotor tests but induced micturition in some animals, as previously reported by Thor et al.[116]

Recently, it has been suggested that clonidine, an α_2-adrenergic receptor agonist, can improve functional recovery in cats with long-term paralysis and sensory loss following impact–contusion injuries.[85] However, the interpretation of this study has been questioned.[38] The results remain interesting in light of earlier work in acute spinal cats showing that clonidine and other adrenergic agonists can enhance the activity of isolated spinal locomotor generating circuits.[49,58,98]

Drug treatments have more often been used to attempt to ameliorate the chronic effects of lesions to the brain. For example, amphetamine treatments reinstate visual placing responses in cats with chronic, extensive posterior cortical lesions.[82] Similarly, Amassian et al.[3] showed return of contact placing after lesions to the ventral anterior thalamus with amphetamine, and Braun et al.[21,22] used amphetamine to restore visual placing and brightness discrimination in rats. Beattie et al.[10] showed that amphetamine administration greatly improved the performance of a conditioned avoidance response (CAR) in rats with nearly complete neocortical ablations. Further, this effect was highly drug dependent: animals performed at normal levels under the drug but performed miserably the next day if saline vehicle injections were substituted for amphetamine.[80] Performance could be maintained, however, if a course of gradual drug withdrawal was employed.[80]

The significance of these studies in the present context is that drug treatment allowed the expression of residual capacities not evident without treatment. Thus, the apparent neurological status following injury is not necessarily a good index of the actual capability of the animal, and the possibility remains that pharmacological or other adjunctive therapies can increase recovery in the chronic stages after CNS trauma. Such enhancements after spinal cord injury might reflect actions of agents on regions remote from the lesion, actions enhancing conduction through the rim of spared fibers,[125] or actions that promote the ability of spared systems to compensate for both local and remote alterations caused by the injury. Strategies aimed at promoting the ability of the organism to use spared systems after spinal injury have not, to our knowledge, been attempted. Such experiments, using amphetamine and other agents, have recently been initiated in our laboratories.

6.3. Adjuncts to Pharmacological Treatment

Adjuncts to pharmacological therapies are exemplified by the studies of Feeney and colleagues[43] (D. M. Feeney and R. L. Sutton, Chapter 7). These authors showed that positive amphetamine effects in chronic decorticated cats depended on practice of locomotion; i.e., there was a significant drug–practice interaction.

Using cats with complete spinal transections, Smith and colleagues[103] showed that exercise can affect treadmill locomotion mediated by the isolated lumbosacral spinal cord. Cats had their spinal cords transected as adults and were then maintained either without exercise or on a regimen of repeated treadmill locomotion tests. Animals with exercise exhibited significantly better hindlimb treadmill locomotion in that they were able to maintain alternate stepping at higher treadmill speeds. It is not clear whether this result arises from central properties of the isolated segments or from the ability of the hindlimb musculature to respond to central output. Perhaps both are involved. In any event, the performance of the function in question during the recovery period results in an enhancement of its expression in the long term. Although this might seem obvious from the perspective of rehabilitation medicine, such factors have rarely been studied systematically in recovery from experimental spinal cord trauma. The use of direct muscle stimulation as an adjunct to rehabilitation therapy in humans has, however, been reported[90]; it is clear that maintenance of muscle tone, bone density, and limb mobility are important for the expression of any central recovery that might occur or that might be enhanced by pharmacological approaches.

7. STUDIES USING THE OHIO STATE IMPACTION DEVICE

Our extensive past experience with the Allen weight-drop method confirmed other reports of unacceptable variability and led to the development in our center of a feedback-dependent, computer-controlled injury device. Details of the construction of the device and anatomic, behavioral, and physiological analyses of the consequences of the lesions produced by it are found elsewhere.[24,86,87,104,113] The major features of these studies and their potential use in pharmacological trials of the future are described below.

7.1. THE OHIO STATE FEEDBACK-CONTROLLED IMPACTOR

Since previous trials with injury devices indicated that the mobility of spinal tissues could vary by as much as 50% under the same injury conditions, we sought to construct a device that could normalize or account for these differences in individual variability and deliver predictable and reliable contusion injuries by negative feedback control. By controlling either the displacement or the force of the impact head of the device, we have been able to create such a range of predictable spinal injuries.

A schematic of the device is shown in Fig. 3. The use of wide-bandwidth displacement and force transducers allows voltage signals to be generated over a wide range of injury protocols. These are provided to the hybrid computer, where they are compared with the preset impact signal selected by the investigator. The difference between the actual impact and the desired impact signal is used to correct, on a millisecond basis, the actual output of the impact power amplifier.

The waveform produced by the pattern generator is selected by the investigator and consists of eight independently controlled time periods during which displacement or force can be programmed. The probe attached to the power amplifier is driven into the spinal substance during the extension phase, remains at that position during a plateau component, and is rapidly withdrawn to a position well above the spinal surface to avoid the multiple contacts encountered using standard injury devices. The total timing sequence rarely exceeds 20 msec in duration. Force and displacement information from the controller is arithmetically manipulated by the Apple II+ to calculate and store the six biomechanical parameters of interest.

7.2. PRODUCTION OF LESIONS WITH PREDICTABLE OUTCOMES

7.2.1. BEHAVIORAL OUTCOMES AND RELIABILITY

An initial study[24] used the new device to produce lesions that had a variety of behavioral outcomes. Parameters that produced an intermediate lesion with a recoverable but persisting behavioral deficit were then used to analyze the relia-

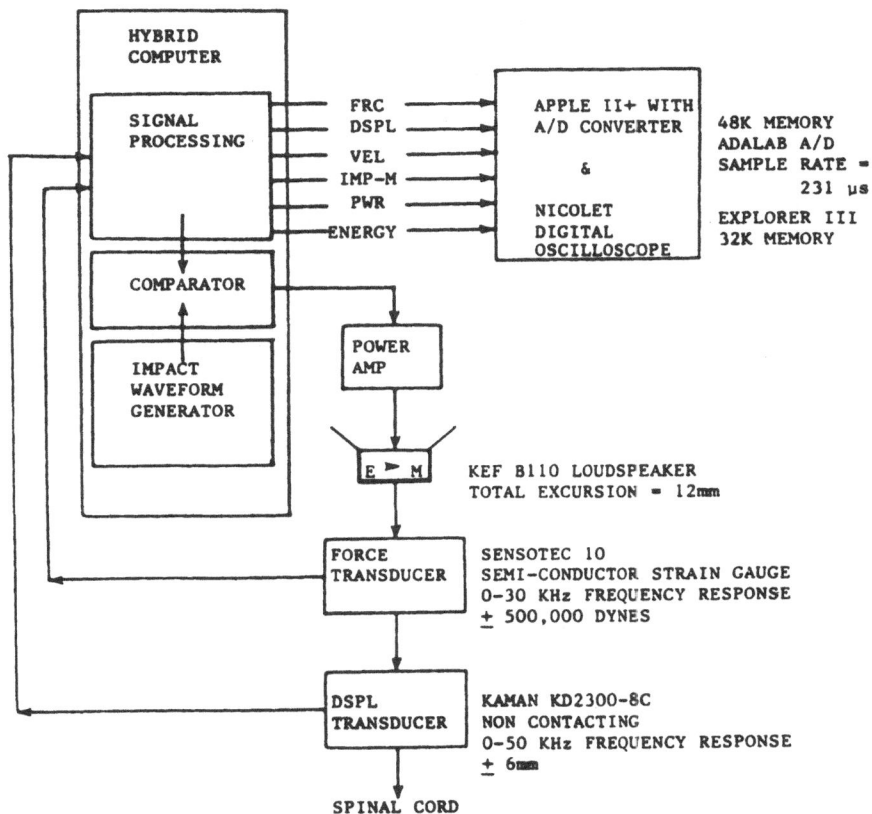

FIGURE 3. Block diagram of the Ohio State impaction device. The injury assembly is comprised of a loudspeaker (electromechanical transducer) with the injury shaft and head attached to the speaker cone. The power amplifier drives the speaker, and sensitive force and displacement transducers provide feedback signals to the hybrid computer controller. These signals are used to control the intended output signal (from the impact waveform generator) to the injury assembly. Force and displacement signals are also sent to the data acquisition system (Apple II+, Nicolet digital oscilloscope) for signal processing and subsequent display of the biomechanical parameters of the injury.

bility of the device for producing consistent lesions and behavioral outcomes. We selected a battery of behavioral tests to assess neurological function, which included a general measure of locomotor ability, walking in an open field[115]; a test of fine locomotor skill requiring hindlimb placement using tactile and proprioceptive cues, walking on a widely spaced wire grid; and a test of postural compensation for body displacement, the inclined plane test.[95] Subjects were tested for 21 days postoperatively.

Varying the force of the impact produced a variety of lesions that resulted in a range of behavioral deficits from very mild transient deficits to total paraplegia. The physical descriptors of the impacts (force, displacement, impulse momentum, velocity, power, and energy) all correlated very highly with the behavioral results; performance in the open field and on the inclined plane were most highly correlated during the first week of the recovery period, and performance on the grid was most highly correlated during the second and third weeks postoperatively. A second group of animals that sustained consistent impacts (displacement was preset and feedback controlled and varied only ±3%) showed very consistent patterns of behavioral deficits and recovery (see Fig. 4).

In a second experiment,[104] cord displacement was held constant, and the duration of the displacement was varied in three groups of animals. The behavioral performance of these subjects fell on either side of that of the animals described above (see Fig. 5), with the shorter duration of displacement (light injury group) producing lesions that resulted in a smaller deficit on all behavioral measures and the two longer-displacement groups (the intermediate- and heavy-injury groups) showing a larger deficit. In fact, these latter two groups showed very little behavioral recovery even after 3 weeks; a longer period of testing might have revealed further recovery.

The three behavioral tests appeared to be sensitive to different aspects of spinal cord function following lesions. The open field and the inclined plane were most sensitive early in the recovery period, particularly in those animals with mild deficits, whereas the grid-walking task appeared to be sensitive to residual deficits, even when performance on the other tasks was normal or near normal. In severely debilitated animals, however, the grid-walking task cannot be performed.

7.2.2. ANATOMIC PATHOLOGY

The anatomic results from the first experiment[24] correlated very highly with the physical descriptors of the impact. The lesion volume and the maximal cross-sectional area of the cord occupied by the lesion both showed significant correlations with all of the impact parameters. The anatomic results also correlated well with the behavioral results; performance in the open field and on the inclined plane during the early part of the recovery period was significantly correlated to the lesion measures, as was performance on the grid during the later part of the recovery period.

7.2.3. BIOMECHANICAL CONSIDERATIONS

A thorough knowledge of the time history of the biomechanics of injury to each experimental animal is important for predicting the functional outcome. Our injury protocols and device allow accurate placement of the impact probe on the spinal surface prior to injury by force feedback from the corresponding trans-

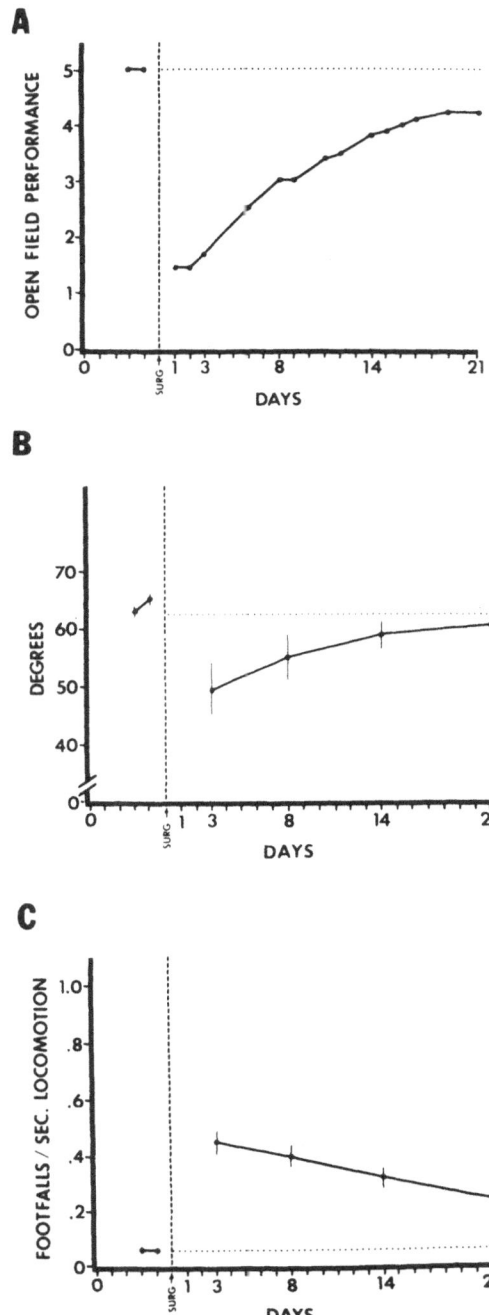

FIGURE 4. Performance of a group of animals with consistent impactions of the spinal cord on the three behavioral measures (A, open field walking; B, inclined plane; C, walking on wire grid; see text for explanation) used to evaluate recovery following spinal cord injury. (From Bresnahan *et al.*[24])

MICHAEL S. BEATTIE *ET AL.*

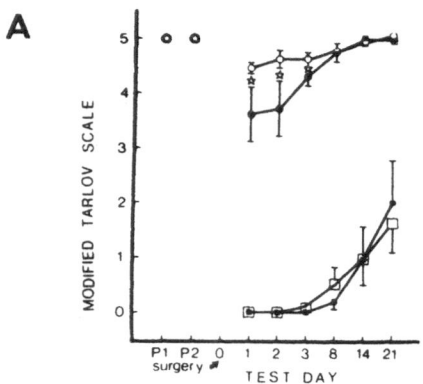

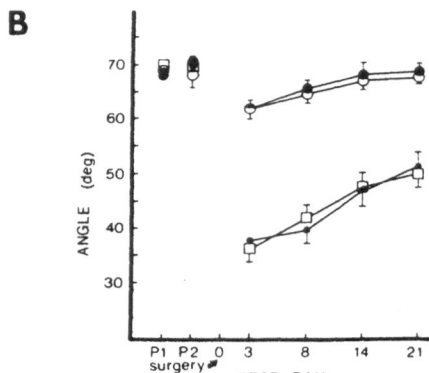

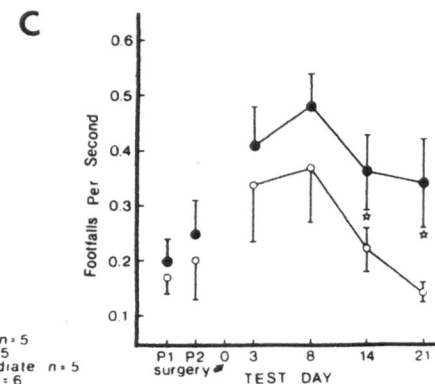

FIGURE 5. Behavioral evaluation of
open-field walking (A), inclined
plane tests (B), and grid walking (C)
for control and light-, intermediate-,
and heavy-injury groups. All animals
were tested for a minimum of 2 days
preoperatively and at least on days 3,
8, 14, and 21 postoperatively. Stars
indicate significant differences between the normal group and the light-
injury group at the 0.05 level at least.

ducer and immediate knowledge of the individual variability of mechanical characteristics of the spinal compartment. Highly reliable injury paradigms can be achieved, particularly in the displacement mode.[87] Both of these criteria allow the separation of experimental groups at the time of injury, a distinct advantage over those paradigms that must take days and sometimes weeks to produce results. The advantages to those interested in the therapeutic pharmacology of spinal injury is obvious. The capacity to control the anatomic extent of the lesion is constantly improving[105]; this will allow us to define further the number of fibers required for functional recovery.[12]

7.3. The Role of Ionic Ca^{2+} in the Acute Phase

Numerous observations now support the general hypothesis that calcium entry into the intracellular environment is a major factor in cell death after spinal trauma.[127] Several studies have provided the direct evidence supporting this conclusion. First, intraaxonal calcification has been shown to occur in spinal injury.[6] Second, atomic absorption spectrometry of injured cords has revealed marked calcium elevations (fivefold by 8 hr) at the injury site.[64] Third, calcium chloride superfusion of the normal spinal cord induces changes similar to those induced by spinal injury.[9] Fourth, extracellular calcium in injured spinal cords falls to <0.01 mM at the injury site (compared to an average 1.2 mM normally).[110,131] Thus, major shifts in the ionic balance occur as immediate sequelae to severe injuries that probably precipitate intracellular toxicity. Calcium influx under these conditions begins those processes that degrade structural proteins[89,100] and activate the enzymatic tools that eventually destroy the integrity of neural and glial elements.[68]

Although the magnitude of the depression in extracellular calcium seems consistent in the studies above, the actual time course and recovery patterns are quite different.[111,131] Although one study emphasized the depression of calcium in gray matter at the impact site to less than 0.1 mM for up to 4 hr,[131] another presented evidence for a spontaneous recovery to 0.6 mM over the first 3 hr independent of electrode location.[111] In addition, the former study described an initial depression of extracellular calcium followed by partial recovery in white matter, with a later fall at 2–3 hr post-injury. Such a biphasic response has considerable importance for pharmacological manipulations of extracellular recovery curves after injury. For instance, the same authors[129] conclude that the prevention of the late fall in extracellular calcium by high-dose corticosteroid therapy is of potential benefit. Recovery curves produced by naloxone intervention restore calcium to normal levels within 2 hr of administration.[112] In the absence of data supporting the importance of extracellular calcium recovery, this controversy is of little consequence. Recent evidence does, however, support the hypothesis that recovery of calcium in the extracellular space may be of considerable importance to the eventual neurological outcome.[104,112] We review these findings here along with preliminary evidence that inappropriate recovery patterns may exacerbate the problem of calcium entry into toxic cells and therefore interrupt or worsen the recovery process.

7.3.1. Correlation with Behavioral Outcome

As discussed above, the characteristics of our new spinal injury device allow us to test the hypothesis that indices of acute trauma can be correlated with behavioral or neuropathological outcome. We have recently examined[104,113] the extracellular calcium recovery curves from three populations of animals injured with known biomechanical predictors.[24,86] Figure 6 is a summary of the results of this work. Here, we show that recovery of calcium in the extracellular space follows different rates depending on the magnitude of impact injury. Note that the "light-injury" group shows complete spontaneous recovery within 3 hr after injury. Mechanical descriptors of the injury paradigm for this group are well below those in the intermediate and heavy groups.[87] In order to evaluate neurological recovery in these groups, we have used the behavioral indices discussed above. As an illustration of the differences in the groups, we have included a figure from this published work (Fig. 5). In the modified Tarlov comparison, the light-injury group is the only one to recover completely. Further experiments are in progress to characterize the behavioral indices of such injuries more completely and couple them to anatomic losses of the spinal neuropil.[105] Although not showing a causal relationship, we have provided evidence that recovery of extracellular calcium can be associated with neurological recovery processes. If spontaneous recovery of extracellular calcium can be associated with behavioral recovery, can pharmacological intervention have a similar effect? Two attempts to investigate that question are discussed below.

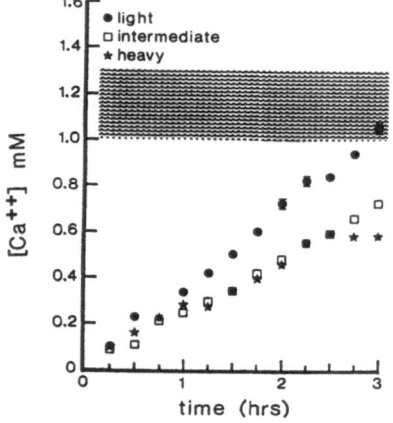

FIGURE 6. Extracellular calcium activities in the injured rat spinal cord. The recordings are averaged over 15-min periods, and the recording electrodes are placed in the center of the lesion site at a depth of approximately 1500 μm. The light-injury group shows recovery to normal levels (1.08 mM) by the end of the recording period.

7.3.2. EFFECTS OF NALOXONE

Our previous work has confirmed that high-dose naloxone, if given just after injury, can completely reverse the tissue extracellular hypocalcia.[112] The dose–response relationship of these findings is illustrated here. At the high doses[45,128] that invoke neurological improvement (10 mg/kg), calcium is restored within 3 hr; smaller dosages (1.0 mg/kg) lead to incomplete restoration (Fig. 7). Early experiments that indicated a prevention of ischemia by these high-dose protocols[128] have recently been questioned.[69,120] It is likely that the effects are principally mediated by other mechanisms such as prevention of membrane destruction by antioxidant properties.[72]

7.3.3. EFFECTS OF NIMODIPINE

In contrast to naloxone, the calcium channel blocker nimodipine has little effect on recovery from spinal injury.[48] This is perhaps at least superficially surprising, since it could potentially block calcium entry and dramatically reverse spinal ischemia.[71,107] Our preliminary data suggest the potential reason for this failure (Fig. 8). In this series of experiments, nimodipine administered as a bolus at the same time as naloxone induces a quicker recovery of calcium in the extracellular space (<1.0 hr). The slope of the recovery curve is also much steeper than that of naloxone recovery. Recovery to normal levels is, however, short lived, since a reversal of normal values takes place at 2 hr. We speculate that during this reversal phase further calcium entry is taking place in marginally injured neurons. This entry, under conditions in which blood flow is rapidly being normalized, may be the spinal cord equivalent of the calcium paradox phenomenon that occurs during myocardial reperfusion damage.[26]

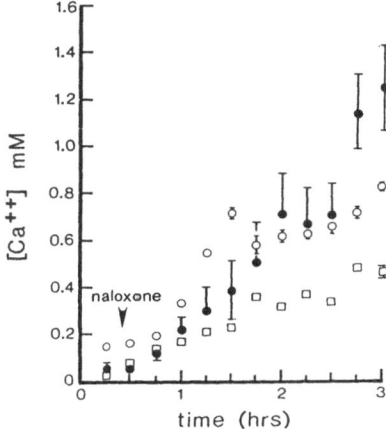

FIGURE 7. Extracellular calcium activity as affected by naloxone after spinal cord injury in the dog. In three groups of animals ($n > 6$ for each; control, open squares; 1.0 mg/kg naloxone, open circles; 10 mg/kg naloxone, closed circles), recovery curves are plotted for free calcium in the interstitial space after spinal cord injury (400 g-cm). Naloxone hydrochloride was administered as an i.v. bolus at 20 min post-injury for both drug groups; an equivalent bolus of vehicle was administered for the control group. Note the partial recovery in the 1.0 mg/kg group with complete recovery in the 10 mg/kg group.

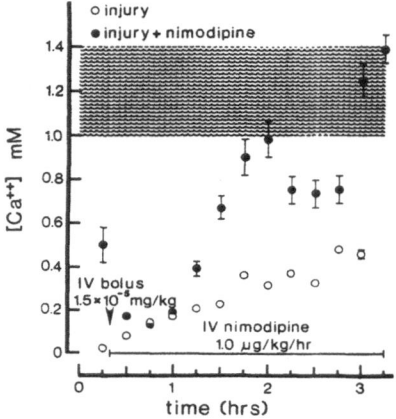

FIGURE 8. Nimodipine restitiution of extracellular calcium activity after spinal cord injury in the dog. The spinal cord was injured with a 400 g-cm impact, and extracellular calcium concentration was monitored and summed for 15-min intervals after injury at time 0. Nimodipine (closed circles ± S.E.M.) injected as a bolus at 20 min post-injury and continuously infused (1.0 μg/kg per hr) thereafter resulted in a rapid (<1.0 hr) restoration of free calcium to normal levels. Control calcium levels from injured animals (closed circles) did not improve above 0.54 mM during this time. Note the reversal in the calcium recovery curve from 2 hr 15 min to 2 hr 45 min.

7.3.4. CALCIUM RECOVERY: A HYPOTHESIS

The consequences of calcium entry into cells during the ischemic injury after spinal injury have been well described.[127] It is now clear also that up to four times the original calcium moves into the impact site from surrounding tissues, the CSF, or the vascular system during the first few hours after injury. By as early as 3 hr after injury, up to 70% of the calcium at the impact site has actually come from surrounding tissues. Much of this calcium is continuing to enter marginally injured and dying cells during this period. The entry of calcium into the interstitial space of the spinal cord is no doubt facilitated by the low extracellular calcium in the injured areas.

The paradox therefore presents itself that recovery of extracellular calcium to normal levels is associated with functional recovery whether occurring spontaneously or by drug manipulation. Such recovery might be expected to exacerbate calcium entry into cells by creating a favorable diffusion gradient from the extracellular space to the cell interior. It does not follow, however, that restoration of extracellular calcium necessarily causes an influx of calcium, particularly into marginally injured cells. The ability of the plasmalemmal calcium ATPase and the sodium–calcium exchanger to handle intracellular free calcium overloads is not well understood,[92] but it appears to be dependent on energetic considerations (i.e., ATP depletion). In those cells that may survive the initial insult, such circumstances could prevent massive calcium entry under these conditions.[65] In addition, the rate at which extracellular calcium is restored may be critical in the temporal sequence of marginally surviving cells; i.e., early restoration of the extracellular space could precipitate calcium or oxygen paradox phenomena such as that which occurs in the myocardium.[26] Finally, the early restoration of ionic stability of the extracellular space, particularly the normalization of ECF calcium, could prevent further diffusional entry of calcium from surrounding tissues. If such entry is important to the continuing pathology,[130] its prevention may be a major factor in the accumulation of calcium salts and their pathological consequences.

8. FUTURE STRATEGIES FOR PHARMACOLOGICAL INTERVENTION

Advances in the use of drug treatments to ameliorate experimental and subsequently clinical spinal cord trauma will depend on continuing study of the basic biological mechanisms of tissue degradation and regeneration. We do not yet know enough about the way in which the normal or perturbed nervous system functions to predict with any accuracy which simple, or complex, treatment strategies might be used to restore function after various types of injuries to the brain and spinal cord. However, a number of avenues available for advancing our knowledge in the near term seem open. In keeping with the convenient distinction in spinal cord injury between acute and chronic phases, these are discussed below.

8.1. IN THE ACUTE PHASE

Continuing progress in understanding the early events leading to membrane phospholipid degradation, its relationship to membrane permeability, and the possible role of arachidonic acid metabolites (e.g., the prostaglandins and leukotrienes) in the putative progression of tissue destruction after trauma should serve both to clarify the progressive injury hypothesis and to suggest new protective agents that might be used to arrest or reverse membrane breakdown[4,62] (also see P. Demediuk and A. I. Faden, Chapter 2). Many of the agents that have shown some promise in this regard are antioxidants or inhibitors of lipid hydrolysis. An exception is TRH, which has been reported to be one of the most effective agents (e.g., T. K. McIntosh and A. I. Faden, Chapter 5). One strategy that may be used with increasing frequency, then, is to target multiple events in the progression of injury in the acute phase. Hall and Wolfe[62] suggest, for example, that in CNS ischemia, at least three factors play a role: injury-induced increases in intracellular Ca^{2+}, increased synthesis of vasoactive prostanoids, and progressive microvascular lipid peroxidation. Each of these could be treated with different drugs, e.g., calcium channel blockers, cyclooxygenase inhibitors (e.g., ibuprofen), and antioxidants such as vitamin E.

Although such approaches may eventually be useful, we would caution that until more is known about the mechanisms of action of agents in isolation and their interactions, interpretation of results will be most difficult. We would stress again that physiological, anatomic, and behavioral measures of the immediate and long-term consequences of drug administration are necessary to assess future relevance to the treatment of CNS trauma. Nevertheless, screening the vast numbers of potential agents may well be aided by simple-systems approaches such as tissue culture. Multiple drug approaches might be best evaluated, at this stage, using such techniques, and then particularly promising combinations can be subjected to the more rigorous, long-term *in vivo* studies we advocate. Recently, gangliosides have been reported to exert some of their effects on CNS damage by a protective effect rather than by the previously invoked effects of enhancing sprouting and axonal regeneration[55] (S. E. Karpiak *et al.*, Chapter 11). These studies suggest that gangliosides may be a good candidate for enhancing the sparing of neural tissue and thus function in spinal cord impact experiments. Indeed, the ability of our injury and testing protocols to distinguish between early sparing and chronic recovery might be particularly suited to such studies.

8.2. IN THE CHRONIC PHASE

Attempts to ameliorate the chronic effects of spinal cord injury have centered on the issue of CNS regeneration. Numerous studies have examined the fate of spinal axons after transection or impact trauma; the conclusions of most recent studies have suggested the notion that without treatment of some kind, these axons will not regenerate in the adult mammal. The search for the appropriate treatment has included detailed studies of successful regeneration in lower vertebrate forms, studies of the partially successful growth of axons after injury in the developing mammal, and surgical attempts to graft appropriate substrates or replacement tissue into the cord. It now seems likely that some spinal cord regeneration or reconnection might be possible, perhaps using fetal tissue grafts or some artificial extracellular matrix substrate for growth. The pharmacological aspects of such future treatments will perhaps include agents that alter the glial response to injury,[93] enhance the growth of implanted neural tissue (e.g., NGF), and promote host–graft integration. It should be noted that these treatments, given at the time of surgical repair, constitute attempts to retard the acute response to the new injury produced by surgery as well as an attempt to promote recovery after chronic injury.

If the formation of new connections does become possible through combined grafting and pharmacological therapies, the question still arises as to the utility of the newly formed connections. Such new growth will encounter an altered distal spinal cord, and there is no assurance that usable connections will be made. Certainly, such new connections will not simply reconstitute the original nervous system of the organism, and it is likely that the number of axons that can be encouraged to cross the lesion will be relatively small. In that regard, such new pathways might be functionally equivalent to the small rim of fibers left after most contusion injuries; indeed, new growth might complement the functions of remaining fibers. It is thus likely that the issue of promoting regeneration cannot be considered in isolation from the other features of chronic spinal cord injury, i.e., the distributed nature of the lesion, and the role of pharmacological treatments in maximizing the utility of spared and altered residual systems.

We have already considered recent studies that show alterations in chronic, isolated spinal cord segments with a number of agents. Future treatments are likely to build on increasing knowledge of the properties of the denervated caudal spinal cord. For example, the work of Robinson and Goldberger[97] suggests that the positive effects of bicuculline on spinal stepping in chronic spinal-cord-transected cats may be caused in part by a reversal of increased inhibition provided by GABAergic neurons in the isolated cord. This increase could be caused by reactive synaptogensis. Thor et al.[116] have suggested that several peptidergic systems in the sacral cord may sprout in response to spinal lesions and have in fact provided an example of the potential for successful pharmacological intervention in chronic spinal cats: naloxone can initiate micturition in animals with spastic bladders. This effect might occur by the blockade of opiate systems that have hypertrophied in response to the lesion. Clearly, a more complete understanding of the role of sprouting, altered reflex circuits, and neurotransmitter receptor changes in the reorganization of the spinal cord after trauma will suggest additional pharmacological interventions that may promote the usefulness of the remaining nervous system.

We have proposed that amphetamine, which has been shown to promote recovery after some forebrain injuries (Section 6.2; D. M. Feeney and R. L. Sutton, Chapter 7), might have a similar effect after partial spinal cord lesions produced by experimental impact. This proposal is based on the hypothesis that the amphetamine effect represents a generalized enhancement of behavioral recovery, which should extend to the ability of the animal to use remaining systems throughout the neuraxis. There is, however, the possibility that amphetamine effects can be related to the alterations in noradrenergic systems consequent to a lesion. Feeney and Sutton (Chapter 7) present data suggestive of the role of noradrenergic mediation of amphetamine's effects on recovery. A cortical lesion "prunes" the ascending collaterals of noradrenergic fibers located in the locus coeruleus (LC) and other brainstem regions. Such pruning of LC fibers has been shown by Reis's group[94] to decrease tyrosine hydroxylase activity in LC neurons and collateral terminal fields. We note that the LC projects to the spinal cord as well and that these fibers will be pruned by impact or transection lesions. If amphetamine does contribute to recovery in chronic spinal-lesioned animals, this general effect on recovery of function may have a common underlying explanation on anatomic and biochemical grounds. Hypotheses on the mechanisms underlying the practice effects in amphetamine-induced recovery may be more difficult to generate. The amphetamine data available to date point to future strategies that exploit pharmacological agents that have effects not only on the repair of neural tissue or on altered reflexes but also to enhance behavioral compensation and learning to maximize residual capacities. Surely, more specific agents with fewer undesirable side effects will also be explored. Finally, conduction via the spared fibers in impact injury or new fiber growth in small quantities may prove to be a useful target for drugs.

9. SUMMARY AND CONCLUSIONS

It is now clear that the stage has been set for detailed trials to investigate the acute and chronic effects of pharmacological agents in spinal cord injury. This is because of both established animal model systems and the better understanding of mechanisms of drug action on both acute and chronic phases of injury. The need for accurate and reliable modeling and its relationship to human trauma is paralleled by the requirement for controlled, well-planned clinical trials (e.g., see ref. 15). Help from the pharmacologists and pharmacokineticists is an absolute prerequisite for designing the experimental and clinical aspects of such studies. The strategies for intervention, however, can still be expected to come from basic understanding of the inherent capacities of the CNS to repair itself.

REFERENCES

1. Afelt, Z., 1974, Functional significance of ventral descending tracts of the spinal cord in the cat, *Acta Neurobiol. Exp.* **34**:393–407.
2. Allen, A. R., 1911, Surgery of experimental lesion of spinal cord equivalent to crush injury or fracture dislocation of spinal column. A preliminary report, *J.A.M.A.* **57**:870–880.
3. Amassian, V. E., Ross, R., Wertenbaker, C., and Weiner, H., 1972, Cerebellothalamocortical interrelations in contact placing and other movements in rats, in: *Corticothalamalic Projections and Sensorimotor Activities* (T. L. Frigyesi, E. Rinvik, and M. D. Yahr, eds.), Raven Press, New York, pp. 395–444.
4. Anderson, D. K., Demediuk, P., Saunders, R. D., Dugan, L. L., Means, E. D., and Horrocks, L. A., 1985, Spinal cord injury and protection, *Ann. Emerg. Med.* **14**:816–821
5. Anderson, D. K., Saunders, R. D., Demediuk, P., Dugan, L. L., Braughler, J. M., Hall, E. D., Means, E. D., and Horrocks, L. A., 1985, Lipid hydrolysis and peroxidation in injured spinal cord: Partial protection with methylprednisolone or vitamin E and selenium, *CNS Trauma* **2**:257–267.
6. Balentine, J. D., 1978, Pathology of experimental spinal cord trauma. I. The necrotic lesion as a function of vascular injury, *Lab. Invest.* **39**:236–253.
7. Balentine, J. D., 1978, Pathology of experimental spinal cord trauma. II. Ultrastructure of axons and myelin, *Lab. Invest.* **39**:254–66.
8. Balentine, J. D., 1985, Hypotheses in spinal cord trauma research, in: *Central Nervous System Trauma Status Report 1985* (D. P. Becker and J. T. Povlishock, eds.), NIH-NINCDS, Washington, pp. 455–461.
9. Balentine, J. D., and Hilton, C. W., 1980, Ultrastructural pathology of axons and myelin in calcium induced myelopathy, *J. Neuropathol. Exp. Neurol.* **39**:339.
10. Beattie, M. S., Gray, T. S., Rosenfield, J., Meyer, P. M., and Meyer, D. R., 1978, Residual capacity for avoidance learning in decorticate rats: Enhancement of performance and demonstration of latent learning with *d*-amphetamine, *Physiol. Psychol.* **6**:279–287.

11. Bernstein, J. J., Gelderd, J., and Bernstein, M. E., 1974, Alteration of neuronal synaptic complement during regeneration and axonal sprouting in mammalian spinal cord, *Exp. Neurol.* **44:**470–482.

12. Blight, A., and Decrescito, V., 1986, Morphometric analysis of experimental spinal cord injury in the cat: The relation of injury intensity to survival of myelinated axons, *Neuroscience* **19:**321–341.

13. Blight, A. R., 1983, Cellular morphology of chronic spinal cord injury in the cat: Analysis of myelinated axons by line-sampling, *Neuroscience* **10:**521–543.

14. Bracken, M. B., Collins, W. F., Eisenberg, H. M., Flamm, E. S., Perot, P. L., Shepard, M. J., and Wagner, F. C., 1986, Response letter to: "High-dose" methylprednisolone and CNS injury, *J. Neurosurg.* **64:**986.

15. Bracken, M. B., Collins, W. F., Freeman, D. F., Shepard, M. J., Wagner, F. W., Silten, R. M., Hellenbrand, K. G., Ransohoff, J., Hunt, W. E., Perot, P. L., Grossman, R. G., Green, B. A., Eisenberg, H. M., Rifkinson, N., Goodman, J. H., Meagher, J. N., Fischer, B., Clifton, G. L., Flamm, E. S., and Rawe, S. E., 1984, Efficacy of methylprednisolone in acute spinal cord injury, *J.A.M.A.* **25:**45–52.

16. Braughler, J. M., Duncan, L. A., and Chase, R. L., 1985, Interaction of lipid peroxidation and calcium in the pathogenesis of neuronal injury, *CNS Trauma* **2:**269–284.

17. Braughler, J. M., and Hall, E. D., 1982, Correlation of methylprednisolone levels in cat spinal cord with its effect on (Na$^+$ + K$^+$)-ATPase, lipid peroxidation, and alpha motor neuron function, *J. Neurosurg.* **56:**838–844.

18. Braughler, J. M., and Hall, E. D., 1984, Effects of multi-dose methylprednisolone sodium succinate administration on injured cat spinal cord neurofilament degradation and energy metabolism, *J. Neurosurg.* **61:**290–295.

19. Braughler, J. M., and Hall, E. D., 1985, Current application of "high-dose" steroid therapy for CNS injury, *J. Neurosurg.* **62:**806–810.

20. Braughler, J. M., and Hall, E. D., 1986, "High-dose" methylprednisolone and CNS injury. Letter, *J. Neurosurg.* **64:**985–986.

21. Braun, J. J., 1966, The neocortex and visual placing in rats, *Brain Res.* **1:**381–394.

22. Braun, J. J., Meyer, P. M., and Meyer, D. R., 1966, Sparing of brightness habits in rats following visual decortication, *J. Comp. Physiol. Psychol.* **61:**79–82.

23. Bresnahan, J. C., 1978, An electron microscopic analysis of axonal alterations following blunt contusion of the spinal cord of the rhesus monkey (*Macaca mulatta*), *J. Neurol. Sci.* **37:**59–82.

24. Bresnahan, J. C., Beattie, M. S., Todd, F., and Noyes, D. H , 1987, A behavioral and anatomical analysis of spinal cord injury produced by a feedback-controlled impaction device, *Exp. Neurol.* **95:**548–570.

25. Bresnahan, J. C., King, J. S., Martin, G. F., and Yashon, D., 1976, A neuroanatomical analysis of spinal cord injury in the rhesus monkey (*Macaca mulatta*), *J. Neurol. Sci.* **28:**521–542.

26. Brierley, G. P., Wenger, W. C., and Altschuld, R. A., 1986, Heart cells as models of the cellular response to ischemia, *Adv. Exp. Med.* **194:**303–314.

27. Cajal, S. R. Y., 1959, *Degeneration and Regeneration of the Nervous System*, Volume 1, Hafner Publishing, New York, p. 396.

28. Clendenon, N. R., Allen, N., Gordon, W. A., and Bingham, W. G., 1978, Inhibition of Na$^+$K$^+$-activated ATPase activity following experimental spinal cord trauma, *J. Neurosurg.* **49:**563–568.

29. Cotman, C. W., 1985, *Synaptic Plasticity*, The Guilford Press, New York, p. 579.

30. De La Torre, J. C., 1981, Spinal cord injury. Review of basic and applied research, *Spine* **6:**315–335.

31. De La Torre, J. C., Johnson, C. M., Goode, D. J., and Mullan, S., 1975, Pharmacologic treatment and evaluation of permanent experimental spinal cord trauma, *Neurology (Minneap.)* **25:**508–514.

32. Demopoulos, H. B., Flamm, E., Pietronigro, D. D., and Seligman, M. L., 1980, The free radical pathology and the microcirculation in the major central nervous system disorders, *Acta Physiol. Scand.* **492:**91–119.
33. Dimitrijevic, M., 1983, Neurophysiological evaluation and epidural stimulation in chronic spinal cord injury patients, in: *Spinal Cord Reconstruction* (C. Kao, R. Bunge, and P. Reier, eds.), Raven Press, New York, pp. 465–474.
34. Eidelberg, E., Staten, E., Watkins, C. J., and Smith, J. S., 1976, Treatment of experimental spinal cord injury in ferrets, *Surg. Neurol.* **6:**243–246.
35. Eidelberg, E., Staten, E., Watkins, J., McGraw, D., and McFadden, C., 1976, A model of spinal cord injury, *Surg. Neurol.* **6:**35–38.
36. Eidelberg, E., Story, J. L., Walden, J. G., and Meyer, B. L., 1981, Anatomical correlates of return of locomotor function after partial spinal cord lesions in cats, *Exp. Brain Res.* **42:**81–88.
37. Eidelberg, E., Straehley, E., Erspamer, R., and Watkins, C., 1977, Relationship between residual hindlimb-assisted locomotion and surviving axons after incomplete spinal cord injuries, *Exp. Neurol.* **56:**312–322.
38. Faden, A. I., 1985, Pharmacologic therapy in acute spinal cord injury: Experimental strategies and future directions, in: *Central Nervous System Trauma Status Report 1985* (D. P. Becker and J. T. Povlishock, eds.), NIH-NINCDS, Washington, pp. 481–487.
39. Faden, A. I., and Jacobs, T. P., 1983, High dose corticosteroid therapy in experimental spinal injury: Increased mortality and failure to improve neurologic recovery, *Neurology (N.Y.)* **33:**192.
40. Faden, A. I., and Jacobs, T. P., 1985, Effect of TRH analogs on neurologic recovery after experimental spinal trauma, *Neurology* (N.Y.) 35: 1331–1334.
41. Faden, A. I., Jacobs, T. P., Patrick, D. H., and Smith, M. T., 1984, Megadose corticosteroid therapy following experimental traumatic spinal injury, *J. Neurosurg.* **60:**712–717.
42. Faden, A. I., Jacobs, T. P., and Smith, M. T., 1984, Evaluation of the calcium channel antagonist nimodipine in experimental spinal cord ischemia, *J. Neurosurg.* **60:**796–799.
43. Feeney, D. M., and Hovda, D. A., 1983, Amphetamine and apomorphine restore tactile placing after motor cortex injury in the cat, *Psychopharmacology* **79:**67–71.
44. Finger, S., and Almli, C. R., 1985, Brain damage and neuroplasticity: Mechanisms of recovery or development? *Brain Res. Rev.* **10:**177–186.
45. Flamm, E., Young, W., Demoupolos, H., DeCresito, V., and Tomasula, J., 1982, Experimental spinal cord injury: Treatment with naloxone, *Neurosurgery* **10:**227–31.
46. Ford, R. W., 1983, A reproducible spinal cord injury model in the cat, *J. Neurosurg.* **59:**268–275.
47. Ford, R. W. J., and Malm, D. N., 1984, Failure of tetracaine to reverse spinal cord injury in the cat, *J. Neurosurg.* **60:**1269–1274.
48. Ford, R. W. J., and Malm, D. N., 1985, Failure of nimodipine to reverse acute experimental spinal cord injury, *CNS Trauma* 2:9–16.
49. Forssberg, H., and Grillner, S., 1973, The locomotion of the acute spinal cat injected with clonidine i.v., *Brain Res.* **50:**184–186.
50. Gale, K., Kerasidis, H., and Wrathall, J., 1985, Spinal cord contusion in the rat: Behavioral analysis of functional neurologic impairment, *Exp. Neurol.* **88:**123–134.
51. Gamache, F. W., Myers, R. A. M., Ducker, T. B., and Cowley, R. A., 1981, The clinical application of hyperbaric oxygen therapy in spinal cord injury: A preliminary report, *Surg. Neurol.* **15:**85–87.
52. Gelfan, S., Kao, C., and Ling, H., 1972, The dendritic tree of spinal neurons in dogs with experimental hindlimb rigidity, *J. Comp. Neurol.* **146:**143.
53. Glick, S. D., 1974, Changes in drug sensitivity and mechanisms of functional recovery following brain damage, in: *Plasticity and Recovery of Function in the Central Nervous System* (D. G. Stein, J. J. Rosen, and N. Butters, eds.), Academic Press, New York, pp. 339–372.

EXPERIMENTAL SPINAL CORD INJURY

54. Goldberger, M. E., and Murray, M., 1985, Recovery of function and anatomical plasticity after damage to the adult and neonatal spinal cord, in: *Synaptic Plasticity* (C. W. Cotman, ed.), The Guilford Press, New York, pp. 77–110.
55. Gorio, A., Di Giulio, A. M., Young, W., Gruner, J., Blight, A., De Crescito, V., Dona, M., Lazzaro, A., Figliomeni, B., Fusco, M., Hallman, H., Johnson, G., Panozzo, C., Zanoni, R., and Vantini, G., 1986, G_{M1} effects on chemical, traumatic and peripheral nerve including lesions to the spinal cord, in: *Development and Plasticity of the Mammalian Spinal Cord*, Volume 3 (M. E. Goldberger, A. Gorio, and M. Murray, eds.), Springer-Verlag, New York, pp. 227–242.
56. Green, S. B., Byar, D. P., Walker, M. D., Pistenmaa, D. A., Alexander, E., Batzdorf, U., Brooks, W. H., Hunt, W. E., Mealey, J., Odom, G. L., Paolett, R., Ransohoff, J., Robertson, J. T., Selker, R. G., Shapiro, W. R., Smith, K. R., Wilson, C. B., and Strike, T. A., 1983, Comparisons of carmustine, procarbazine, and high-dose methylprednisolone as additions to surgery and radiotherapy for the treatment of malignant glioma, *Cancer Treat. Rep.* **67:**121–132.
57. Grillner, S., 1986, Locomotion in spinal vertebrates physiology and pharmacology, in: *Development and Plasticity of the Mammalian Spinal Cord*, Volume 3 (M. E. Goldberger, A. Gorio, and M. Murray, eds.), Springer-Verlag, New York, pp. 311–321.
58. Grillner, S., and Zangger, P., 1979, On the central generation of locomotion in the low spinal cat, *Exp. Brain Res.* **34:**241–261.
59. Gruner, J. A., Young, W., and DeCrescito, V., 1984, The vestibulospinal free fall response: A test of descending function in spinal-injured cats, *CNS Trauma* **1:**139–159.
60. Guth, L., Albuquerque, E. X., Deshpande, S. S., Barrett, C. P., Donati, E. J., and Warnick, J. E., 1980, Ineffectiveness of enzyme therapy on regeneration in the transected spinal cord of the rat, *J. Neurosurg.* **52:**73–86.
61. Guth, L., Brewer, C. R., Collins, W. F., Goldberger, M. E., and Perl, E. R., 1980, Criteria for evaluating spinal cord regeneration experiments. Editorial commentary, *Exp. Neurol.* **69:**1–3.
62. Hall, E. D., and Wolf, M. S., 1986, A pharmacological analysis of the pathophysiological mechanisms of post traumatic spinal cord ischemia, *J. Neurosurg.* **64:**951–961.
63. Hansebout, R. R., Tanner, J. A., and Romero-Sierra, C., 1984, Current status of spinal cord cooling in the treatment of acute spinal cord injury, *Spine* **9:**508–511.
64. Happel, R. D., Smith, K. P., Banik, M. L., Powers, J. M., Hogan, E. L., and Balentine, J. D., 1981, Ca^{++} accumulation in experimental spinal cord trauma, *Brain Res.* **211:**476–479.
65. Haworth, R. A., Goknur, A. B., Hunter, D. R., Hegge, J. O., and Berkoff, H. A., 1986, Inhibition of CA influx in isolated adult rat heart cells by ATP depletion, *J. Mol. Cell. Cardiol.* **18**(Suppl):33.
66. Hedeman, L. S., and Sil, R., 1974, Studies in experimental spinal cord trauma. Part 2. Comparison of treatment with steroids, low-molecular weight dextran and catecholamine blockade, *J. Neurosurg.* **40:**44–51.
67. Higgins, A. C., Pearlstein, R. D., Mullen, J. B., and Nashold, B. S., 1981, Effects of hyperbaric oxygen therapy on long-tract neuronal conduction in the acute phase of spinal cord injury, *J. Neurosurg.* **55:**501–510.
68. Hogan, E. L., Hsu, C. Y., and Banik, N. L., 1986, Calcium-activated mediators of secondary injury in the spinal cord, *CNS Trauma* **3:**175–179.
69. Hollinden, G., and Stokes, B. T., 1988, Blood flow alterations after spinal injury: Effects of naloxone (submitted).
70. Kao, C. C., Wrathall, J. R., and Kyoshima, K., 1983, Axonal reaction to transection, in: *Spinal Cord Reconstruction* (C. C. Kao, R. P. Bunge, and P. J. Reier, eds.), Raven Press, New York, pp. 41–58.
71. Kazda, S., Garthoff, B., Krause, H. P., and Schlobmann, K., 1982, Cerebrovascular effects of

the calcium antagonistic dihydropyridine derivative nimodipine in animal experiments, *Arzneim Forsch.* **32**:331–338.

72. Koreh, K., Seligman, M. L., Flamm, K. E. S., and Demoupoulos, H. B., 1981, Lipid antioxidant properties of naloxone *in vitro, Biochem. Biophys. Res. Commun.* **102**:1317–1322.

73. Kuchner, E. F., and Hansebout, R. R., 1976, Combined steroid and hypothermia treatment of experimental spinal cord injury, *Surg. Neurol.* **6**:371–376.

74. LaMotte, C., 1980, Early spinal cord trauma assessed by diffuse axonal uptake of HRP, *Soc. Neurosci.* **6**:734.

75. Lasek, R. J., McQuarrie, I. G., and Wujek, J. R., 1981, The central nervous system regeneration problem: Neuron and environment, in: *Posttraumatic Peripheral Nerve Regeneration: Experimental Basis and Clinical Implications* (A. Gorio, ed.), Raven Press, New York, pp. 59–70.

76. Levy, W., McCaffrey, M., and York, D., 1986, Motor evoked potential in cats with acute spinal cord injury, *Neurosurgery* **19**:9–19.

77. Lux, W. E., Feuerstein, G., and Faden, A. I., 1983, Alteration of leukotriene D_4 hypotension by thyrotropin-releasing hormone, *Nature* **302**:822–824.

78. Means, E. D., Anderson, D. K., Waters, T. R., and Kalaf, L., 1981, Effects of methylpred nisolone in compression trauma to the feline spinal cord, *J. Neurosurg.* **55**:200–208.

79. Melzack, R., and Loeser, J. D., 1978, Phantom body pain in paraplegics: Evidence for a central "pattern generating mechanism" for pain, *Pain* **4**:195–211.

80. Meyer, D. R., and Beattie, M. S., 1977, Some properties of substrates of memory, in: *Neuropeptide Influences of the Brain and Behavior* (L. H. Miller, C. A. Sandman, and A. J Kastin, eds.), Raven Press, New York, pp. 145–162.

81. Meyer, P., and Meyer, D., 1982, Memory, remembering and amnesia, in: *Expressions of Knowledge* (R. Isaacson and N. Spear, eds.), Plenum Press, New York, pp. 145–162.

82. Meyer, P. M., Horel, J. A., and Meyer, D. R., 1963, Effects of *dl*-amphetamine upon placing responses in neodecorticate cats, *J. Comp. Physiol. Psychol.* **56**:402.

83. Monakow, C. V., 1914, *Die Lokalisation im Grosshirm und der Abbau der Funktion Durch Kortikale Herde.* J. F. Bergmann, Wiesbaden, p. 333.

84. Moore, R. Y., 1974, Central regeneration and recovery of function: The problem of collateral reinnervation, in: *Plasticity and Recovery of Function in the Central Nervous System* (D. G. Stein, J. J. Rosen, and N. Butters, eds.), Academic Press, New York, pp. 111–128.

85. Naftchi, N. F., 1982, Functional restoration of the traumatically injured spinal cord in cats by clonidine, *Science* **217**:1042–1047.

86. Noyes, D., 1987, An electromechanical impactor for producing experimental spinal cord injury in animals, *Med. Biol. Eng. Comp.* **25**:335–340.

87. Noyes, D., 1987, Correlation between parameters of spinal cord impact and resultant injury, *Exp. Neurol.* **95**:535–547.

88. Osterholm, J. L., and Mathews, G. J., 1972, Altered norepinephrine metabolism following experimental spinal cord injury. Part 2. Protection against traumatic spinal cord hemorrhagic necrosis by norepinephrine synthesis blockade with alpha-methyltyrosine, *J. Neurosurg.* **36**:395–401.

89. Pant, N. C., and Gainer, H., 1980, Properties of calcium-activated protease in squid axoplasm which selectively degrades neurofilament proteins, *J. Neurobiol.* **11**:1–12.

90. Peckham, P. H., Mortimer, J. T., and Marsolais, E. B., 1980, Controlled prehension and release in the C5 quadriplegic elicited by functional electrical stimulation of the paralyzed forearm musculature, *Ann. Biomed. Eng.* **8**:369–388.

91. Rawe, S. E., Roth, R. H., Boadle-Biber, M., and Collins, W. F., 1977, Norepinephrine levels in experimental spinal cord trauma. Part 1. Biochemical study of hemorrhagic necrosis, *J. Neurosurg.* **46**:342–349.

92. Reeves, J. P., 1985, The sarcolemmal sodium–calcium exchange system, *Curr. Top. Membr. Transp.* **25**:77–127.

93. Reier, P. J., Stensaas, L. J., and Guth, L., 1983, The astrocytic scar as an impediment to regeneration in the central nervous system, in: *Spinal Cord Reconstruction* (C. C. Kao, R. P. Bunge, and P. J. Reier, eds.), Raven Press, New York, pp. 163–196.

94. Reis, D. J., Ross, R. A., Gilad, G., and Joh, T. H., 1978, Reaction of central catecholaminergic neurons to injury: Model systems for studying the neurobiology of central regeneration and sprouting, in: *Neuronal Plasticity* (C. W. Cotman, ed.), Raven Press, New York, pp. 197–226.

95. Rivlin, A., and Tator, C., 1977, Objective clinical assessment of motor function after experimental spinal cord injury in the rat, *J. Neurosurg.* **47**:577–581.

96. Rivlin, A. S., and Tator, C. H., 1978, Effect of duration of acute spinal cord compression in a new acute cord injury model in the rat, *Surg. Neurol.* **10**:39–43.

97. Robinson, G. A., and Goldberger, M. E., 1986, The development and recovery of motor function in spinal cats. II. Pharmacological enhancement of recovery, *Exp. Brain Res.* **62**:387–400.

98. Rossignol, S., Barbeau, H., and Julien, C., 1986, Locomotion of the adult chronic spinal cat and its modification by monoaminergic agonists and antagonists, in: *Development and Plasticity of the Mammalian Spinal Cord*, Volume 3 (M. E. Goldberger, A. Gorio, and M. Murray, eds.), Springer-Verlag, New York, pp. 323–345.

99. Sandler, A. N., and Tator, C. H., 1976, Review of the effect of spinal cord trauma on the vessels and blood flow in the spinal cord, *J. Neurosurg.* **45**:638–646.

100. Schlaepfer, W. W., 1979, Nature of mammalian neurofilaments and their breakdown by calcium, in: *Progress in Neuropathology*, Volume 4 (H. Zimmerman, ed.), Raven Press, New York, pp. 101–123.

101. Schramm, J., Hashizume, K., Fukushima, T., and Takahashi, H., 1979, Experimental spinal cord injury produced by slow, graded compression: Alterations of cortical and spinal evoked potentials, *J. Neurosurg.* **50**:48–57.

102. Sherrington, C., 1947, *The Integrative Action of the Nervous System*, 2nd ed., Murray Printing, Forge Village, MA.

103. Smith, J. L., Bradley, N. S., Carter, M. C., Giuliani, C. A., Hoy, M. G., Koshland, G. F., and Zernicke, R. F., 1986, Rhythmical movements of the hindlimbs in spinal cat: Considerations for a controlling network, in: *Development and Plasticity of the Mammalian Spinal Cord*, Volume 3 (M. E. Goldberger, A. Gorio, and M. Murray, eds.), Springer-Verlag, New York, pp. 347–361.

104. Somerson, S., and Stokes, B. T., 1987, Functional analysis of an electromechanical spinal cord injury device, *Exp. Neurol.* **90**:82–96.

105. Somerson, S., and Stokes, B. T., 1986, Behavioral and morphometric studies using a computerized spinal injury device, *Soc. Neurosci.* **12**:1422.

106. Stavraki, G. W., 1961, *Supersensitivity following Lesion of the Nervous System*, University of Toronto Press, Toronto, p. 205.

107. Steen, P. A., Newberg, L. A., Milde, J. H., and Michenfelder, J. D., 1983, Nimodipine improves cerebral blood flow and neurologic recovery after complete cerebral ischemia in the dog, *J. Cereb. Blood Flow Metab.* **3**:38–43.

108. Stein, D. G., Rosen, J. J., and Butters, N., 1974, *Plasticity and Recovery of Function in the Central Nervous System*, Academic Press, New York, p. 516.

109. Stewart, W., Kaczmar, T., Collins, W., and LaMotte, C. C., 1983, The relationship between the distribution of damaged axons and neurologic deficit in a rat model of spinal cord injury, *Soc. Neurosci.* **9**:1037.

110. Stokes, B. T., Fox, P., and Hollinden, G., 1983, Extracellular calcium activity in the injured spinal cord, *Exp. Neurol.* **80**:561–572.

111. Stokes, B. T., Fox, P., and Hollinden, G., 1985, Extracellular metabolites: Their measurement and role in the acute phase of spinal cord injury, in *Trauma of the Central Nervous System* (R. G. Dacey, ed.), Raven Press, New York, pp. 309–323.

112. Stokes, B. T., Hollinden, G., and Fox, P., 1984, Improvement in injury induced hypocalcia by high-dose naloxone intervention, *Brain Res.* **290**:187–90.
113. Stokes, B. T., and Somerson, S., 1988, The spinal cord microenvironment: Can the changes due to trauma be graded? *Neurochem. Pathol.* (in press).
114. Sugigama, S., Kitazawa, M., Ozawa, T., Suzuki, K., and Izawa, Y., 1980, Anti-oxidative effect of coenzyme Q_{10}, *Experientia* **36**:1002–1003.
115. Tarlov, I., 1957, *Spinal Cord Compression: Mechanisms of Paralysis and Treatment*, Charles C. Thomas, Springfield, IL.
116. Thor, K., Kawatani, M., and de Groat, W. C., 1986, Plasticity in the reflex pathways to the lower urinary tract of the cat during postnatal development and following spinal cord injury, in: *Development and Plasticity of the Mammalian Spinal Cord*, Volume 3 (M. E. Goldberger, A. Gorio, and M. Murray, eds.), Springer-Verlag, New York, pp. 65–80.
117. Tsubokawa, T., Nakamura, S., and Hayashi, N., 1975, The circulatory disturbance of spinal cord injury and its response to local cooling therapy, *Neurol. Med. Chir.* **15**:87–93.
118. Vierck, C. J., and Cooper, B. Y., 1984, Guidelines for assessing pain reactions and pain modulation in laboratory animal subjects, in: *Advances in Pain Research and Therapy: Neural Mechanisms of Pain*, Volume 6 (L. Kruger and J. C. Liebeskind, eds.), Raven Press, New York, pp. 305–322.
119. Wall, P. D., 1986, Changes in adult spinal cord induced by changes in the periphery, in: *Development and Plasticity of the Mammalian Spinal Cord*, Volume 3 (M. E. Goldberger, A. Gorio, and M. Murray, eds.), Springer-Verlag, New York, pp. 101–110.
120. Wallace, M. C., and Tator, C. H., 1986, Failure of naloxone to improve spinal cord blood flow and cardiac output after spinal cord injury, *Neurosurgery* **18**:428–432.
121. Windle, W., Smart, J., and Beers, J., 1958, Residual function after subtotal spinal cord transection in adult cats, *Neurology (Minneap.)* **8**:518–521.
122. Windle, W. F., 1980, *The Spinal Cord and Its Reaction to Traumatic Injury*, Volume 18, Marcel Dekker, New York, p. 384.
123. Wrathall, J., Pettegrew, R., and Harvey, F., 1985, Spinal cord contusion in the rat: Production of graded, reproducible, injury groups, *Exp. Neurol.* **88**:108–122.
124. Yeo, J. D., 1984, The use of hyperbaric oxygen to modify the effects of recent contusion injury in the spinal cord, *CNS Trauma* **1**:161–165.
125. Young, W., 1984, A critical overview of spinal injury research presented at the First International Symposium on CNS Trauma, *CNS Trauma* **1**:75–79.
126. Young, W., 1985, Blood flow, metabolic and neurophysiological mechanisms in spinal cord injury, in: *Central Nervous System Trauma Status Report 1985* (D. P. Becker and J. T. Povlishock, eds.), NIH–NINCDS, Washington, pp. 463–473.
127. Young, W., 1985, The role of calcium in spinal cord injury, *CNS Trauma* **2**:109–114.
128. Young, W., Flamm, E., Demoupolos, H., Tomasula, J., and DeCresito, V., 1981, Effect of naloxone on post-traumatic ischemia in experimental spinal contusion, *J. Neurosurg.* **55**:209–219.
129. Young, W., and Flamm, E. S., 1982, Effect of high-dose corticosteroid therapy on blood flow, evoked potentials and extracellular calcium in experimental spinal injury, *J. Neurosurg.* **57**:667–673.
130. Young, W., and Koreh, I., 1986, Potassium and calcium changes in injured spinal cords, *Brain Res.* **365**:42–53.
131. Young, W., Yen, V., and Blight, A. R., 1982, Extracellular calcium activity in experimental spinal contusion, *Brain Res.* **253**:115–125.

4

Serotonin Antagonists Reduce Central Nervous System Ischemic Damage

Justin A. Zivin

ABSTRACT. We have demonstrated that serotonin antagonists preserve neurological function in two different animal models. In one model, reversible occlusion was studied; in the other, irreversible ischemia was produced. In both instances, the protective effects were unequivocal. Alterations of the tissue concentrations of serotonin and its primary metabolite were not demonstrated during the stages of ischemia when irreversible damage was occurring. Thus, a new approach to the understanding of the mechanisms of action of serotonin is required. Although the mechanisms of injury reduction are not yet known, these findings make a compelling case for the utility of serotonin antagonists in the emergency therapy of such problems as cardiac arrest to prevent cerebral damage while the cardiac status is stabilized, and possibly for stroke-in-evolution to prevent continued progressive extension of damage. It may also be possible to give such therapy prophylactically in high-risk situations such as increasingly frequent transient ischemic attacks or before high-risk surgical procedures.

1. Introduction

Although there are a number of strategies that may be useful for pharmacological treatment of stroke, there is not yet a proven therapy that specifically reduces the damage caused by stroke in patients. It is possible to attempt to prevent CNS ischemia, but there is no method of minimizing destruction after focal ischemia has occurred. During ischemia, it is probable that destruction of the CNS proceeds in a series of stages. There is reason to suspect that this process can be interrupted or at least partially limited. It may not be possible to reverse all of the damage caused by acute CNS injuries, but salvaging marginally viable tissue can be crucial because, in the nervous system, important functions are frequently

JUSTIN A. ZIVIN • Department of Neurology, San Diego Veterans Administration Medical Center, and Department of Neurosciences, University of California, San Diego, La Jolla, California 92093.

controlled by small regions. Saving such regions can make an enormous difference in the ultimate degree of functional recovery.

To understand how potential treatments might work and to design more effective therapies, a detailed understanding of the pathophysiological mechanisms of stroke is necessary. Such studies are, for the most part, ethically impossible in patients, and consequently the use of animal models is required. For a variety of reasons, we decided that the cerebral vascular occlusion models that have usually been used for such studies were not optimal for pharmacological studies. Most previously available models were developed to simulate the clinical and pathological features of stroke. In essence, regardless of species, the infarcts produced vary unpredictably in size and distribution.[18,27] The large degree of variability makes therapeutic trials rather expensive because large numbers of animals are required, and biochemical studies are markedly complicated by the difficulty of predicting precisely where lesions will occur. Therefore, we have developed several methods that are more reproducible. Although these models do not simulate the most frequent types of strokes, similar central nervous system ischemic events do occur naturally, and these models allow us to correlate clinical histopathological, biochemical, and physiological phenomena in great detail. Of greatest value is our ability to use these models as bioassay systems for evaluation of therapeutic regimens. Using these complementary systems, we are able to define irreversible damage in a very practical clinical sense.

2. REVIEW OF THE EFFECTS OF SEROTONIN IN STROKE

Serotonin is a putative neurotransmitter that has potent vasoconstrictive properties. For many years, there has been speculation about its influences on the development of CNS injury.[21] Since it is present in neuronal tissue throughout the CNS and in high concentration in platelets, it has been postulated that serotonin might cause increased tissue damage when released at the site of an infarction and produce vasospasm in surrounding areas, or it might have adverse direct actions at a cellular level by mechanisms that have not yet been characterized. Since several classes of drugs are available that can specifically modify serotonin actions, we can study alterations of this monoamine with relatively selective pharmacological tools. Based on these types of conjectures, a number of investigators have studied the effects of ischemia on serotonin, and several groups have reported changes of serotonin tissue concentrations during stroke.

Welch et al.[26] measured serotonin concentrations of gerbils 3 to 4 hr after unilateral carotid ligation. They reported decreased concentrations on the infarcted side, but the time periods studied were long after irreversible damage had occurred. In another article,[5] they reported that unilateral common carotid artery occlusion in gerbils resulted in decreased serotonin within 5 min in both hemispheres, which persisted essentially unchanged for up to 1 hr. Subsequently, they also reported that 1 hr after occlusion of the blood supply to the hemisphere with multiple large emboli, serotonin remained unchanged, and 5-hydroxyindoleacetic acid (5-HIAA, the principal metabolic breakdown product of serotonin) increased.[12]

Brown et al.[1] reported decreased serotonin concentrations during global ischemia produced by raised intracranial pressure. These decreases were observed after 7.5 min of ischemia, and the decline continued after 30 min of subsequent restoration of flow. The "bloodless" global ischemia produced by raising the intracranial pressure is quite unlike either focal or global ischemia, which are the most common medical problems.

Calderini et al.[2] exposed rats to bilateral carotid occlusion plus hypovolemia for 15 min. They found no changes in serotonin and 5-HIAA, but serotonin concentration declined in some groups during 30 min of subsequent recirculation.

Mrsulja and associates[15,20] measured neurotransmitters in cerebral tissue of gerbils during infarction produced by unilateral carotid occlusion. Serotonin concentrations were shown to decrease relative to those of the opposite hemisphere. These results are difficult to interpret because the concentrations of monoamines in the perfused hemisphere may change after infarction of the opposite side.[6,14] In another paper,[4] this group found that after 15 min of cerebral ischemia produced by bilateral carotid occlusion in gerbils, serotonin declined to 78% of control in frontal cortex but was unchanged in basal ganglia.

Harrison and associates[8,9] studied serotonin and 5-HIAA in gerbils 3.5 hr after carotid ligation and found decreased concentrations in both the infarcted and control hemispheres. These studies were conducted after damage was irreversible.

Matsumoto et al.[17] made regional measurements of serotonin concentration after 1 hr of bilateral carotid occlusion in gerbils. They found that serotonin decreased in all regions in which blood flow decreased. These measurements were made substantially after irreversible damage would be expected in this animal model.

Harik et al.[7] studied serotonin changes in a model of incomplete cerebral ischemia in the rat. Ischemia was produced by a combination of halothane-induced hypotension, bilateral carotid occlusion, and increased intracranial pressure produced by infusion of mock CSF into the cisterna magna. At 45 min of ischemia, no significant changes in serotonin were found in any of the regions studied. Some inconsistent serotonin decreases were found after 30 min of recirculation. No systematic 5-HIAA changes were reported either during ischemia or after subsequent reperfusion.

To summarize, although a number of groups studied various aspects of the effects of serotonin on CNS ischemia, most of these models of focal ischemia were not particularly reproducible, and several models did not simulate human strokes. A number of these reports indicated that serotonin concentrations declined rapidly after the onset of ischemia, but most of the studies were not designed to evaluate the early time periods, when changes were becoming irreversible and therapeutic intervention might be expected to be most effective.

3. NEW METHODS FOR THE STUDY OF CNS ISCHEMIA

As noted in Section 1, previously available animal models of stroke were not well designed for biochemical and pharmacological studies. To remedy this deficiency, we developed two new methods for such studies: (1) a rabbit spinal cord ischemia model[30] and (2) a microsphere embolic stroke model. I describe these models in some detail because their use has made it possible to establish some important aspects of the effects of serotonin in CNS ischemia.

3.1. RABBIT SPINAL CORD ISCHEMIA MODEL

In the rabbit spinal cord ischemia model (RSCIM), spinal cord is produced by occlusion of the aorta just below the renal arteries. The relatively long spinal cord of rabbits and its highly segmental vascular supply in the caudal regions allows production of spinal cord ischemia without interference with the vascular supply of the viscera. Blood flow is obstructed in the hind limbs, but occlusion of the aorta for as long as several hours does not result in any permanent damage in the hind quarters. We are thus able to produce focal spinal cord destruction without causing permanent injury to any other structures.

We were able to adapt a snare ligature[3] for use in this model. A snare ligature consists of a loop of thin material that can be implanted around an artery and tightened or loosened externally after the animal has recovered from the implantation procedure. It is then possible to produce reversible obstruction of that vessel in an unanesthetized animal. In the RSCIM, the ligature is implanted around the abdominal aorta just below the renal arteries. We then allow the animals to recover from anesthesia for several hours. Spinal cord ischemia can then be induced in fully awake animals. With the arrangement that we use, the snare ligature can be cut and removed without further anesthesia.[30] All rabbits become paraplegic while the aorta is occluded, and we can conduct our experiments without the complications of anesthesia, artificial ventilation, manipulation of blood gases and pH, temperature maintenance, etc. There is relatively little surgical intervention at a site distant from nervous tissue. Because the animals are awake (occlusion of the aorta causes no apparent pain), we can make repeated neurological assessments during the ischemic period and thus ensure disruption of neurological function. We can also accurately assess the animals during all phases of the postischemic period. When required, it is possible for us to perform invasive surgical procedures and artificially control relevant physiological functions. However, such interventions may potentially alter the responses of intact animals to CNS ischemia and the effects of proposed therapies. Thus, we intentionally reduce our manipulations of the animals to the minimum. Pharmacological interventions can be administered at any time prior to, during, or after the ischemic period.

We developed a simplified three-point grading scale for evaluation of neurological impairment: grade N, normal; grade P, any partial neurological deficit; grade T, total paraplegia. The scale is so simple that there is essentially no intraobserver variation in grading. Functional activity of the rabbits is assessed 24 hr after the ischemic insult. We analyze the results by use of a quantal dose–response analysis technique[25] that allows us to generate a curve of the effect of the duration of ischemia on the fraction of animals that sustain neurological damage (see Fig. 1) and permits estimation of the location parameter, which is the duration of ischemia required to produce neurological deficits in 50% of the rabbits (ET_{50}). If the treatment curve is shifted to the right relative to the control curve (ET_{50} increases), the treatment has produced a protective effect; if the treatment curve is shifted to the left, the treatment has produced an adverse effect. The ET_{50} for control animals used in the RSCIM has been approximately 25 ± 2 min. (mean $\pm$ standard error). We have repeated this control curve in detail numerous times in the past several years, and the results have not significantly changed. Along with the highly reproducible ET_{50}s, the relatively low variance makes this a highly sensitive technique because even relatively small changes from control can be readily detected.

This model can be used for a wide variety of biochemical studies as well. We can inject radiolabeled iodoantipyrine as a marker of regional blood flow. At any time after the onset of ischemia, we can anticipate the clinical status of a group of animals, and using the blood flow tracer, we can identify the location of

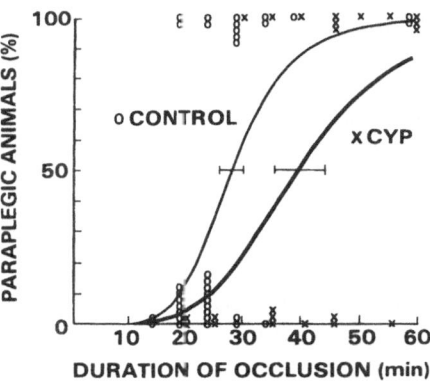

FIGURE 1. Paraplegia as a function of the duration of aortic occlusion. The curve on the left shows the time course of development of paraplegia in control animals. Paraplegia was present 24 hr after the insult in 50% of the rabbits occluded for 28.26 ± 2.28 min ($n = 35$). The curve on the right shows that 2.0 mg/kg of cyproheptadine given 5 min after the onset of occlusion resulted in an increase in the ET_{50} to 40.03 ± 4.55 min ($n = 22$). The Os at the bottom of the graph indicate the number of control animals that had some neurological function at the times indicated. The numbers of paraplegic animals are indicated at the top of the graph. The Xs indicate the numbers of functional and paraplegic animals treated with cyproheptadine. These data were used to generate the related curves. The horizontal bar on each curve at the ET_{50} indicates the standard error.

lesions that will ultimately develop. We can occlude the aorta and wait for any length of time after the onset of ischemia or after restoration of blood flow. At the end of the predetermined period, we inject the iodoantipyrine tracer over a 1-min interval and then collect appropriate blood samples to allow us to determine regional blood flow.[33] In the process the animal is sacrificed, and the spinal cord is rapidly removed and frozen. We can then section the cord and use the regional blood flow measurement to identify locations within the ischemic, marginally perfused, or normal areas of the cord. Biochemical measurements in these regions of interest allow us to correlate, in considerable detail, the clinical condition, regional blood flow, and biochemical profile of lesion development during or after CNS ischemia.

3.2. MICROSPHERE EMBOLIC STROKE MODEL

To corroborate some of the findings that were obtained using the RSCIM, we developed an embolic stroke model that is specifically designed for pharmacological studies. Previous studies of putative CNS ischemia therapies have usually involved use of reversible ischemia models. In most of these models (including the RSCIM), the blood supply to a portion of the CNS is obstructed for a period of time, and then blood flow is restored. Therapeutic efficacy is demonstrated if the tolerable duration of ischemia can be increased or the extent of damage produced by a fixed period of ischemia is reduced. Such reversible ischemia is a less frequent clinical problem than irreversible arterial occlusion.

Injection of microspheres allows us to study irreversible ischemia. Furthermore, for pharmacological trials, a method of producing incremental grades of damage is desirable. Most previously reported cerebral stroke models were intended to mimic the clinical and pathological features of human strokes and are not readily adaptable for production of graded degrees of damage. Although it is extremely difficult to predict where any given embolus will lodge, it is possible to predict, with a very high degree of precision, what will happen when numerous small emboli enter the cerebral circulation. Rapid intraarterial injection of small embolic particles will result in relatively random distribution of the particles within the territory supplied by that artery. It is important that the embolic particles be small because it is necessary for them to penetrate to terminal vessels. If large embolic particles are injected, they will obstruct just a few large vessels, and a random distribution of small lesions will not occur. It is essential that numerous small lesions be produced so that there is a correlation between the number of particles that are trapped in the brain and the amount of tissue destruction that results. When only large vessels are occluded, such a close correspondence does not exist. If only a few small particles are injected, it is unlikely that any detectable behavioral changes will be produced. Injection of many particles will almost certainly cause severe damage. Consequently, it can be predicted that a dose–response curve for the effect of the number of emboli on the neurological status of a group of animals can be generated (the form of the curve is analogous to that shown in Fig. 1 except that the fraction of abnormal animals is plotted as a function of the number of microspheres that are trapped in the brain). Effective therapy will reduce the amount of tissue destruction associated with each microsphere that is lodged in the brain. Thus, although treated animals will have the same number of lesions as control animals, the individual lesions will be smaller, and the aggregate tissue destruction will be reduced. In animals, the most reliably detectable behavioral endpoints are severe neurological damage and death. Such curves can be generated for any type of animal, but use of a species that has a relatively distinct separation between the external and internal carotid circulations is most efficient. The most readily available laboratory animals that have this property are rabbits and rats.

This technique can be used to detect whether therapy has neurologically meaningful effects. A curve of neurological response as a function of the amount of radiolabeled microspheres in the brain is determined. The test treatment is given to another set of animals, and a similar curve is produced. If the treatment causes a significant shift of the treatment curve, then a neurologically detectable effect is demonstrated. The ES_{50} is the quantity of microspheres required to produce severe neurological damage or death in 50% of the animals, and its interpretation is analogous to that used for the ET_{50} in the RSCIM. We then test for significant differences between the ES_{50}s of the treatment and control curves.

Over the years, a wide variety of materials have been used for cerebral embolism studies, but recently the most commonly utilized materials have been carbonized microspheres, which are available in a variety of sizes and can be labeled with radioactive tracers. In most instances, 15-μm spheres have been used for studies of regional blood flow rates, although a few experiments have concentrated on the pathological and physiological consequences of infarction.[10,13,16,22,23] The advantage of the microspheres is that they can be readily quantified and do not change in size or position after they have lodged in the cerebral arterial circulation.

Under surgical anesthesia, the external carotid circulation is ligated on one side, and a cannula is placed in the common carotid artery. The cannula is arranged so it is accessible externally, and the animals are allowed to recover. At the time of embolization, the awake animal is restrained, and the radiolabeled embolus particles are injected rapidly. Treatment of the animals with the agent under study can be started at any time before or after embolization. We have found that we can reliably classify the animals as either normal, grossly abnormal, or dead. Abnormalities consist of an encephalopathy most prominently characterized by reduced level of consciousness and highly uncoordinated movements. The rabbits or rats rarely show tonic or clonic postures and are otherwise appropriately responsive to noxious stimuli, indicating that seizure activity is quite uncommon, even in severely neurologically impaired animals. At the end of the study, the animals are sacrificed, and the brain is removed from each animal and cut into properly sized pieces for radioactivity measurements in a γ counter.

We found that 50-μm microspheres penetrate well into the small arteries of the brain, and pathological studies showed that they were well dispersed throughout the brain. Microspheres that are 80 μm or larger remain confined to the surface vessels, are not randomly distributed, and cannot be used for these types of studies. Relelatively smaller numbers of 50-μm microspheres are required, so they are much less costly to use than the 15-μm microspheres for these types of studies. Using these methods we have been able to generate highly reproducible embolus versus neurological damage curves using ^{125}I-labeled microspheres in rabbits.

4. BIOCHEMICAL STUDIES OF THE EFFECTS OF SEROTONIN IN CNS ISCHEMIA

We first began our studies by attempting to determine whether there were any measurable changes in spinal cord concentrations of serotonin and 5-HIAA during the first hour of ischemia.[31] The rationale was that if any changes were found it might indicate which pharmacological interventions would be most likely to alter the consequences of CNS ischemia. We found that serotonin changes did occur in the most severely damaged region of the gray matter but that the decline was modest and occurred somewhat after clinical damage became permanent. In the marginally perfused region, the changes were more complex. During the times when irreversible changes were occurring in more ischemic areas, there was a substantial decline in serotonin concentrations. However, when the damage finally became permanent in the most ischemic regions, serotonin in the marginal areas returned to normal. No systematic changes were observed in spinal cord 5-HIAA concentrations at any time during the early stages of ischemia. We subsequently conducted some studies of the effects of ischemia for 25 min or 1 hr and restoration of flow for periods of up to 1 hr.[29] We did not observe any large or consistent alterations of serotonin or 5-HIAA concentrations in these studies.

We concluded that biochemical aspects of spinal cord ischemia can be studied in great detail by using a combination of very precise spinal cord blood flow measurements in combination with very sensitive serotonin measurement methods. We confirmed that spinal cord blood flow responded in a fashion similar to cerebral blood flow during and after ischemic conditions. At the level of resolution we were able to achieve, there were no substantial changes in serotonin concentrations in ischemic or marginally perfused tissue at the durations of ischemia that would cause infarction during the early stages of irreversible tissue damage. These results suggested that studies of tissue serotonin concentrations during the early stages of ischemia and infarction are unlikely to shed any additional light on the understanding of the mechanism of serotonin involvement in tissue injury during CNS ischemia.

5. Pharmacological Studies of the Effects of Serotonin Antagonists and Agonists in CNS Ischemia

Although the biochemical studies we conducted did not elucidate the role of serotonin in ischemia, we conducted a series of pharmacological investigations that did yield a number of therapeutic insights.[28,32] Initially, we attempted to raise CNS serotonin concentrations by intravenous infusion of 5-hydroxytryptamine (5-HTP), the immediate precursor of serotonin (systemically administered serotonin will not cross the blood–brain barrier, but 5-HTP does). We found that we were able to elevate CNS 5-HTP and 5-HIAA concentrations, but nearly fatal doses of 5-HTP did not increase spinal cord serotonin concentrations. We then tried lysergic acid diethylamide (LSD), a potent serotonin blocker that is known to penetrate the blood–brain barrier. We used the RSCIM as a bioassay system for these studies. Giving the LSD 5 min after the onset of ischemia resulted in statistically significant improvement in neurological function. However, the improvement lasted only a few hours, and by 24 hr after the insult the neurological function of the LSD-treated animals was not significantly different from controls.

We then proceeded to try bromlysergic acid diethylamide (BOL), which, although a potent serotonin competitive inhibitor, lacks the psychedelic properties of LSD and is substantially less toxic. We were able to administer much higher doses of BOL and, as shown in Table I, found that at high doses the ET_{50} was increased by over 40%, and this improvement was permanent. We then were able to demonstrate that the protection afforded by BOL was dose dependent, and substantially lower doses could give protection when the drug was administered 15 min prior to the onset of ischemia. It should be noted that an improvement of this magnitude does not simply represent a minimal gain. To take one example, if the rabbits were subjected to approximately 30 min of ischemia, only 20% of the control animals were normal, and 70% were paraplegic. By comparison, treatment with BOL resulted in normal neurological function in 50% of the rabbits, and paraplegia was reduced to 20%. These results were achieved when the drug was administered 5 min after the onset of ischemia.

When BOL was administered in high doses 20 min after the onset of ischemia in the RSCIM, no protective effects could be demonstrated. Therefore, BOL does not "rescue" the spinal cord from damage after the ligature is released and does not restore function in tissue that has already suffered severe damage. The protection afforded by BOL both increased the number of animals that maintained at least some neurological functions and also increased the

TABLE I. Effects of Serotonin Agonists on ET_{50} for Ischemia-Induced Paraplegia[a]

Drug	Treatment time (min)	Dose (mg/kg)	ET_{50} (min)	n
Control			28.26 ± 2.28	35
LSD	5	0.15	25.12 ± 1.23	29
BOL	−15	0.06	28.80 ± 5.98	15
	−15	0.375	32.87 ± 4.48	24
	−15	1.5	36.62 ± 4.29*	19
	5	1.5	30.29 ± 4.51	17
	5	3.0	38.48 ± 3.95*	23
	20	1.5	25.71 ± 5.17	16
Cinanserin	−15	2.0	35.11 ± 1.40*	19
	5	10.0	37.68 ± 2.96*	14
Cyproheptadine	−15	1.0	39.28 ± 1.41*	17
	5	1.0	34.46 ± 4.02	21
	5	2.0	40.03 ± 4.55*	22
Methysergide	−15	4.0	25.32 ± 1.98	14
Bufotenine	−15	2.5	29.40 ± 7.29	20
Quipazine	−15	5.0	29.44 ± 3.87	10
Cyproheptadine and		1.0		
bufotenine	−15	1.25	32.44 ± 1.60	18

[a]Drugs were administered intravenously, either (−) 15 min before or 5 or 20 min after the onset of ischemia. The duration of ischemia required to produce paraplegia in 50% of a group is indicated by the ET_{50}. The number of animals in each group is indicated by n. Significance levels compared with control are *$P < 0.05$. The data are mean ± S.E.

number that returned to normal after ischemic insults. The lowest doses that showed protective effects were ten times the highest doses that have safely been given to humans,[11] and there were no apparent toxic effects in the rabbits. To our knowledge, detailed BOL toxicity studies have not yet been conducted in humans.

We subsequently conducted a series of trials using cinanserin, another serotonin competitive inhibitor, which has a chemical structure that is unrelated to that of LSD or BOL. As shown in Table I, this drug was almost identical to BOL in its protective effects both when given prior to and after the onset of ischemia. We were, therefore, able to demonstrate that several drugs that differ in chemical structure but have serotonin-blocking effects provide effective protection against spinal cord ischemia in a dose-dependent fashion and with increased potency when given prophylactically. These data provided strong evidence that serotonin competitive inhibitor effects were responsible for the beneficial effects.

We subsequently tried to use methysergide, another analogue of LSD, which is currently approved for use in humans in the United States. Because of low solubility, we were unable to give substantial doses without a large fluid load, and we were unable to demonstrate a protective effect for this drug. This may have been because of the relatively low doses we were able to administer, or it is possible that other as yet unknown factors prevented this drug from being effective.

To establish whether the effects of BOL were produced by increasing the residual blood flow in the ischemic portion of the spinal cord, we utilized the iodoantipyrine tracer technique. In untreated animals, spinal cord blood flow rostral to the level of aortic occlusion was 20.7 ± 2.66 ml/100 g per min ($n = 3$), and in the most ischemic regions, spinal cord blood flow was 0.39 ± 0.13. In animals given high doses of BOL, blood flow above the occlusion was 22.8 ± 5.0, and in the ischemic area it was 0.51 ± 0.04. Analysis of variance did not reveal any significant differences between treated and untreated animals. Thus, ischemia reduced blood flow to approximately 2% of normal in both treated and untreated animals, and the hypothesis that function was preserved by drug-induced increased residual blood flow was rejected. This study does suggest that the drugs may reach the ischemic regions of the spinal cord in the residual blood flow.

These initial studies were conducted with drugs that have relatively well-characterized serotonin inhibition properties without many side effects, and we were able to establish that such agents would be likely to preserve neurological function. However, with the exception of methysergide, these drugs have not been approved for use in patients in the United States. We therefore proceeded to test cyproheptadine.[28] This drug has many actions in addition to serotonin inhibition properties, but it is currently available for use in patients and is known to be relatively well tolerated in high doses in humans. We found (as shown in Table I) that administration of cyproheptadine 5 min after the onset of ischemia at 2 mg/kg or 15 min prior to the onset of ischemia at 1 mg/kg produced comparable degrees of reduction of CNS injury and that these results were in the same range as those we had found for BOL (see Table I). Cyproheptadine, at these doses, was well tolerated by the animals, and even higher doses have been accidentally ingested by patients without life-threatening consequences.

Since agents that are thought to be competitive antagonists of serotonin produced beneficial effects, we attempted to determine whether serotonin agonists would increase ischemic damage.[28] Intravenously administered serotonin will not reach the CNS, so we used bufotenine or quipazine.[28] These two drugs are pharmacologically similar to serotonin but readily enter the CNS. We found that neither drug alone caused any alteration in the ET_{50} from control values (see Table I). However, when bufotenine was administered simultaneously with cyproheptadine, the protective effects of the cyproheptadine were reversed.

In an attempt to determine how the serotonin antagonists produced the protective effects, we studied the effects of ischemia on serotonin and 5-HIAA concentrations after treatment with cyproheptadine and BOL.[29] We compared rabbits that were made ischemic but not treated with subjects that were given cyproheptadine therapy at a dose that had reduced clinically apparent neurological damage (1 mg/kg 10 min prior to the onset of ischemia). Cyproheptadine did not alter spinal cord blood flow significantly at any spinal cord level within or outside of the ischemic regions. Similarly, we could not detect any alterations in the serotonin or 5-HIAA concentrations at any location in treated ischemic animals versus untreated ischemic rabbits. We conducted similar studies of the microscopically observable changes that were present 1 week after ischemia in cyproheptadine- and BOL-treated animals. We found that in treated animals, the correlation between the severity of the clinical deficits and the topographical extent and histological completeness of tissue distruction was weaker than in untreated animals. Thus, although treatment did prevent loss of neurological function in some animals, the improvement was not always apparent histologically.

The results of these biochemical studies do not prove that serotonin is unrelated to production of CNS infarction, and alterations may be occurring in a fashion that cannot be detected by the methods that were employed in these studies. The histopathological findings suggest that although serotonin antagonists preserve neurological function, the cause of this beneficial effect is not always apparent on light microscopic examination of the tissue. Such a lack of unequivocal correlations has also been observed in other CNS ischemia models.[19,24] The reason for this interesting finding is still unclear.

6. Microsphere Studies of the Effects of Serotonin Antagonists on Stroke

Although the results of the RSCIM studies were reasonably unequivocal in indicating the beneficial pharmacological actions of serotonin antagonist on reducing CNS ischemic damage, the biochemical mechanisms were not resolved by the studies we conducted. It could be argued that these pharmacological effects were an artifact of the particular ischemia model (the RSCIM) we employed for our initial studies. To increase the probability that our findings were valid, we conducted similar studies in an entirely different CNS injury system using the microsphere embolus model in rabbits. In control rabbits the ES_{50} for 50-μm microspheres was 306.6 ± 37.2 μg ($n = 32$). When cyproheptadine was administered intravenously at a dose of 2 mg/kg 2 min after the emboli were injected, the ES_{50} for the treated group increased to 633.1 ± 137.0 μg ($n = 22$). This is a significant difference by group t-test ($P < 0.05$). Therefore, similar protective effects of serotonin antagonists can be demonstrated in unrelated models of CNS injury. In the embolic ischemia model, irreversible occlusion of blood vessels is induced. It is probable that the reduction of neurological damage was caused by salvaging the marginally perfused tissue surrounding the areas of damage produced by the emboli.

REFERENCES

1. Brown, R. M., Carlson, A., Ljunggren, B., Siesjo, B. K., and Snider, S. R., 1974, Effect of ischemia on monoamine metabolism in the brain, *Acta Physiol. Scand.* **90**:789–791.
2. Calderini, G., Carlsson, A., and Norstrom, C. H., 1978, Influence of transient ischemia in monoamine metaoblism in the rat brain during nitrous oxide and phenobarbitone anesthesia, *Brain Res.* **157**:303–310.
3. Crowell, R. M., Marcoux, F. W., and DeGirolami, U., 1981, Variability in reversibility of focal cerebral ischemia in unanesthetized monkeys, *Neurology (N.Y.)* **31**:1295–1302.
4. Cvejie, V., Micic, D. V., Djuricic, B. M., Mrsulja, B. J., and, Mrsulja, B. B., 1980, Monoamines and related enzymes in cerebral cortex and basal ganglia following transient ischemia in gerbils, *Acta Neuropathol.* **51**:71–77.
5. Gaudet, R., Welch, K. M. A., Chabi, E., and Wang, T.-P., 1978, Effect of transient ischemia on monoamine levels in the cerebral cortex of gerbils, *Neurochemistry* **30**:751–757.
6. Ginsberg, M. D., Reivich, M., Giandomenico, A., and Greenberg, J. H., 1977, Local glucose utilization in acute focal cerebral ischemia: Local dysmetabolism and diaschisis, *Neurology (Minneap.)* **27**:1042–1048.
7. Harik, S. I., Yoshida, S., Busto, R., and Ginsberg, M. D., 1986, Monoamine neurotransmitters in diffuse reversible forebrain ischemia and early recirculation: Increased dopaminergic activity, *Neurology (N.Y.)* **36**:971–977.
8. Harrison, M. J. G., and Ellam, L. D., 1981, Role of 5HT in the morbidity of cerebral infarction—a study in the gerbil stroke model, *J. Neurol. Neurosurg. Psychiatry* **44**:140–143.
9. Harrison, M. J. G., Marsden, C. D., and Jenner, P., 1979, Effect of experimental ischemia on neurotransmitter amines in the gerbil brain, *Stroke* **10**:165–168.
10. Hossmann, K. A., Hossmann, V., and Takagi, S., 1978, Microsphere analysis of local cerebral and extracerebral blood flow after complete ischemia of cat brain for one hour, *J. Neurol.* **218**:275–285.
11. Isbell, H., Miner, E. J., and Logan, C. R., 1959, Cross tolerance between D-2-brom-lysergic acid diethylamide (BOL 148) and the D-diethylamide of lysergic acid (LSD-25), *Psychopharmacologia* **1**:109–116.
12. Ishihara, N., Welch, K. M. A., Meyer, J. S., Chabi, E., Nartomi, H., Wang, T.-P., Nell, J. H., Hsu, M.-C., and Miyakawa, Y., 1979, Influence of cerebral embolism on brain monoamines, *J. Neurol. Neurosurg. Psychiatry* **42**:847–853.
13. Kogure, K., Busto, R., Scheinberg, P., and Reinmuth, O. M., 1974, Energy metabolites and water content in rat brain during the early stage of development of cerebral infarction, *Brain* **97**:103–114.
14. Kogure, K., Scheinberg, P., Matsumoto, A., Busto, R., and Reinmuth, O. M., 1975, Catecholamines in experimental brain ischemia, *Arch. Neurol.* **32**:21–24.
15. Lust, D. W., Mrsulja, B. B., Mrsulja, B. J., Passonneau, J. V., and Klatzo, I., 1975, Putative neurotransmitters and cyclic nucleotides in prolonged ischemia of the cerebral cortex, *Brain Res.* **98**:394–399.
16. Marcus, M. L., Heistad, D. D., Ehrhardt, J. C., and Abboud, F. M., 1976, Total and regional cerebral blood flow measurement with 7-, 10-, 15-, 25-, and 50-μm microspheres, *J. Appl. Physiol.* **40**:501–507.
17. Matsumoto, M., Kimura, K., Fujisawa, A., and Matsuyama, T., 1984, Differential effect of cerebral ischemia on monoamine content of discrete brain regions of the Mongolian gerbil (*Meriones unguiculatus*), *J. Neurochem.* **42**(3):647–651.
18. Molinari, G. F., and Laurent, J. P., 1976, A classification of experimental models of brain ischemia, *Stroke* **7**:14–17.
19. Moossy, J., 1979, Morphological validation of ischemic stroke models, in: *Cerebrovascular*

Diseases (R. T. Price and E. Nelson, eds.), 11th Princeton Conference, Raven Press, New York, pp. 3–10.

20. Mrsulja, B. B., Mrsulja, B. J., Spatz, M., and Klatzo, I., 1976, Brain serotonin after experimental vascular occlusion, *Neurology (Minneap.)* **26**:785–787.

21. Schmidt, C. F., 1960, Central nervous system circulation fluids and barriers, in: *Handbook of Physiology*, Volume 3 (J. Field, H. W. Magoun, and V. E. Hall, eds.), American Physiological Society, Washington, pp. 1745–1750.

22. Siegel, B., A., Meidinger, R., Elliott, A. J., Studer, R., Curtis, C., Morgan, J., and Potchen, E. J., 1972, Experimental cerebral microembolism—multiple tracer assessment of brain edema, *Arch. Neurol.* **26**:73–77.

23. Vise, W. M., Schuier, F., Hossmann, K.-A., Takagi, S., and Zulch, K. J., 1977, Cerebral microembolization. I. Pathophysiological studies, *Arch. Neurol.* **34**:660.

24. Waltz, A. G., 1979, Comparative pathophysiology of ischemic stroke models: An evaluation, in: *Cerebrovascular Diseases* (R. T. Price and E. Nelson, eds.), 11th Princeton Conference, Raven Press, New York, pp. 11–17.

25. Waud, D. R., 1972, On biological assays involving quantal responses, *J. Pharmacol. Exp. Ther.* **183**:577–607.

26. Welch, K. M. A., Wang, T. P. F., and Chabi, E., 1978, Ischemia-induced seizures and cortical monoamine levels, *Ann. Neurol.* **3**:152–155.

27. Yatsu, F. M., 1976, Biochemical mechanisms of ischemic brain infarction, in: *Handbook of Clinical Neurology*, Volume 27 (P. J. Vinken and G. W. Bruyn, eds.), American Elsevier, New York, pp. 27–37.

28. Zivin, J. A., 1985, Cyproheptadine reduces or prevents ischemic central nervous system damage, *Neurology (N.Y.)* **35**:584–587.

29. Zivin, J. A., and DeGirolami, U., 1986, Studies of the influence of biogenic amines on central nervous system ischemia, *Stroke* **17**:509–514.

30. Zivin, J. A., DeGirolami, U., and Hurwitz, E. L., 1982, Spectrum of neurological deficits in experimental CNS ischemia, *Arch. Neurol.* **39**:408–412.

31. Zivin, J. A., and Stashak, J., 1983, The effect of ischemia on biogenic amine concentrations in the central nervous system, *Stroke* **14**:556–562.

32. Zivin, J. A., and Venditto, J. A., 1984, Experimental CNS ischemia: Serotonin antagonists reduce or prevent damage, *Neurology (N.Y.)* **34**:469–474.

33. Zivin, J. A., and Waud, D. R., 1983, A precise and sensitive method for measurement of spinal cord blood flow, *Brain Res.* **258**:197–200.

5

Opiate Antagonists in CNS Injury

Tracy K. McIntosh and Alan I. Faden

ABSTRACT. Traumatic insults to the central nervous system (CNS) may produce tissue injury through both direct and indirect (secondary) mechanisms. This secondary injury process appears to result from the release or activation of endogenous "autodestructive" factors in response to the original insult. Delayed injury may be associated with reduction in blood flow and/or an alteration of the local metabolic environment. Recently, endogenous opioids have been implicated as secondary injury factors following CNS trauma. The rationale for this hypothesis has been based primarily on the therapeutic effects of opiate-receptor antagonists in a variety of experimental CNS trauma models. This review summarizes the use of opiate-receptor antagonists in the treatment of CNS injury.

1. INTRODUCTION

During the past decade a number of endogenous opioid peptides have been discovered within the central nervous system (CNS).[1,49] Three distinct opioid prohormone systems have now been identified: (1) preproenkephalin A, from which enkephalins are derived; (2) preproenkephalin B, from which leucine-enkephalin and the dynorphin family of peptides are derived; and (3) preproopiomelanocortin, from which β-endorphin is derived. These peptide systems have differential anatomic distributions within the CNS[51] and may subserve different physiological roles.[11]

Present evidence also supports the existence of at least three opiate receptor types: μ, δ, and κ.[68] The μ receptor has been best characterized; morphine is the prototypic ligand for this receptor, and β-endorphin is an endogenous opioid with potent μ effects. Leucine-enkephalin is the endogenous ligand with greatest specificity for the δ-receptor, whereas dynorphin has been proposed as the endogenous ligand for the κ-receptor.[3] The possible existence of additional types of

TRACY K. MCINTOSH AND ALAN I. FADEN • Department of Neurology, University of California, San Francisco, and Center for Neural Injury, Veterans Administration Medical Center, San Francisco, California 94121. *Present address of T. K. M.*: Laboratory for Neuroscience Research, Department of Surgery, University of Connecticut Health Center, Farmington, Connecticut 06032.

opioid binding sites (e.g., σ, ε, and λ) as well as isoreceptors for several of these receptor classes further complicates interpretation of studies examining the potential physiological or pathophysiological roles of endogenous opioids.[11]

Traumatic insults to the CNS may produce tissue injury through both direct and indirect (secondary) mechanisms.[2,6,10,13] Direct effects are caused by immediate disruption of neural connections or injury to nerve cells, whereas secondary effects develop over a period of minutes to hours following injury. This delayed injury process appears to result from the release or activation of endogenous autodestructive factors in response to the original insult, associated with a reduction in blood flow and alteration of the local metabolic environment.[5,58,61,62] Recently, endogenous opioids have been proposed as secondary injury factors following CNS trauma,[13,14,29,57] largely on the basis of the therapeutic effects of opiate-receptor antagonists. In the present review we summarize the use of these opiate-receptor antagonists in the treatment of CNS injury.

2. Opiate Antagonists

A variety of opiate-receptor antagonists have been developed, the majority through modification of the structure of potent opiate alkaloids. Among the best-known and most widely utilized of these antagonists is naloxone. Although naloxone has been considered a pure and specific opiate-receptor antagonist and, as such, has been used to infer the actions of endorphins, naloxone is neither a pure antagonist under all conditions nor completely selective. Thus, at low doses naloxone has selectivity for the μ receptor, but at higher doses it also acts on δ and κ sites.[9,63]

Actions of naloxone, particularly at high doses, may, in fact, not be opiate receptor mediated. Instead, naloxone may exert effects on calcium flux, lipid peroxidation, and γ-aminobutyric acid systems.[11] For these reasons, it is inappropriate to conclude, from observation of a naloxone effect alone, that a specific action is mediated through opiate receptors or occurs through the action of endogenous opioids. Such a conclusion requires other evidence: that multiple, structurally different antagonists produce similar effects; that effects are stereospecific; and that opiate agonists produce opposite actions.[63]

During the past few years a number of receptor-selective opiate antagonists have been developed. These include the μ-receptor antagonists β-funaltrexamine (β-FNA) and naloxonazine, the δ-selective antagonists ICI-154,129 and ICI-174,864, and antagonists with increased activity at κ sites such as WIN44,441-3, MR2266, and nalmefene (Table I). Stereoisomers have been developed for several of these antagonists. Since dextroisomers of opiate antagonists such as d-naloxone or WIN44,441-2 [WIN(+)] have no activity at the opiate receptor, they may be used in combination with the receptor-active levoisomer to determine whether activity is mediated by opiate receptors and to provide information regarding the potential role of specific opiate receptors in pathological states.

TABLE I. Selective Opiate Agonists
and Antagonists[a]

Receptor	Agonist	Antagonist
μ	Morphine	β-FNA
	DAGO	Naloxonazine
δ	DADLE	ICI-154,129
	DSTLE	ICI-174,864
κ	EKC	WIN44,441-3
	Dynorphin A	MR2266
	U50,488H	Nalmefene
		BNI

[a]DADLE, [D-Ala^2-D-Leu^5]enkephalin; DSTLE, [D-Ser^2-Leu^5-Thr^6]enkephalin; DAGO, [D-Ala^2-MePhe^4-Gly-ol] enkephalin; EKC, ethylketocyclazocine; β-FNA, β-funaltrexamine; BNI, binaltorphamine.

3. RATIONALE FOR USE OF OPIATE ANTAGONISTS IN CNS INJURY

There is considerable evidence that central opioid systems are involved in the regulation of cardiovascular function under both physiological and pathophysiological conditions.[15,18,45] Endogenous opioids and opiate receptors have been found in a large number of central cardioregulatory sites including limbic cortex, hypothalamus, brainstem, and spinal cord.[4,7,8,37,44,49,50,59,64] Intracerebroventricular (i.c.v.) or intraparenchymal injections of endogenous opioids in brain cardioregulatory sites cause cardiorespiratory changes at very low concentrations.[18] κ agonists, including dynorphin, have been found to produce hypotension when injected into both forebrain and hindbrain cardioregulatory nuclei.[35,36,41] In contrast, μ and δ agonists generally produce hypertension, particularly at low doses and in unanesthetized animals.[35]

Faden and Holaday first demonstrated that administration of the opiate antagonist naloxone hydrochloride significantly improved physiological variables and survival of animals subjected to experimental hemorrhagic[16] and endotoxic shock[17,46] and proposed that endogenous opioids contribute to the pathophysiology of shock.[12] Because of the effectiveness of naloxone in the treatment of hemorrhagic and endotoxic shock, Faden and colleagues[22,23,47] examined the effectiveness of naloxone in "spinal shock" produced by spinal cord transection; intravenous (i.v.) or i.c.v. administration of naloxone reversed hypotension following spinal transection in rats and cats. On the basis of these studies, these authors postulated that endogenous opioids are released following acute spinal trauma and contribute to secondary injury through actions on microcirculatory blood flow.[23] These hypotheses provided the rationale for the initial examination of opiate antagonists in the treatment of traumatic spinal cord injury.

3.1. Opiate Antagonists in the Treatment of Spinal Cord Injury

Early experiments utilized a model in which the cervical spinal cord was damaged by dropping a specific weight from a fixed distance onto the exposed spinal cord of anesthetized cats.[24,25] The impact energy was chosen to yield a severe but incomplete degree of injury that might be amenable to pharmacological manipulation. The injury was associated with a tenfold increase in β-endorphin-like immunoreactivity in plasma within the first hour after trauma; during this period there was a significant reduction in both gray (20%) and white (24%) matter matter blood flow, particularly at the injury level during the first 45 min after trauma.[24] Treatment with naloxone at high doses (2 mg/kg bolus followed by 2 mg/kg per hr for 4 hr) at 1 hr after injury resulted in significant recovery of spinal cord blood flow (SCBF).[24] The improvement in blood flow after naloxone treatment was greatest over the injured segment (C-7) but extended over the entire length of spinal cord (C-1 to T-5) (Fig. 1). Additionally, such treatment significantly improved neurological outcome at 6 weeks following injury as compared with saline-treated controls that demonstrated marked spastic quadriparesis (Fig. 2). These beneficial effects of naloxone treatment in experimental spinal injury were confirmed by another laboratory using a related feline injury model in which damage was produced at the level of the thoracic spinal cord.[38,66] Naloxone treatment in these studies was also associated with significant recovery of the somatosensory evoked response across the injury segment, recovery of SCBF, and enhanced neurological recovery.[38,66] In later studies it was found that naloxone treatment significantly improved neurological outcome even when treatment was delayed for 4 hr following trauma.[28] These observations are consistent with the view that the neurological deficit following spinal injury results, in part, from progressive ischemia of descending white matter tracts and supports the findings of Albin et al.[2] that the pathophysiological changes following spinal cord trauma are reversible as long as 4 hr after injury. These data also confirm that even delayed administration of opiate antagonists may have therapeutic efficacy in treatment of spinal trauma.

Other studies have examined the effects of naloxone treatment on spinal cord injury resulting from occlusion of the descending thoracic aorta in experimental animals (spinal ischemia). Such injury produces infarction of the lumbar spinal cord and leads to irreversible paralysis.[67] Naloxone, administered after reversal of the occlusion, significantly enhanced motor recovery and reduced histopathological changes in rabbits.[27,31] The beneficial effects of naloxone were dose related, with significant improvement found at doses above 0.2 mg/kg per hr (total dose 1.0 mg/kg), and optimal effects at the highest dose tested (2

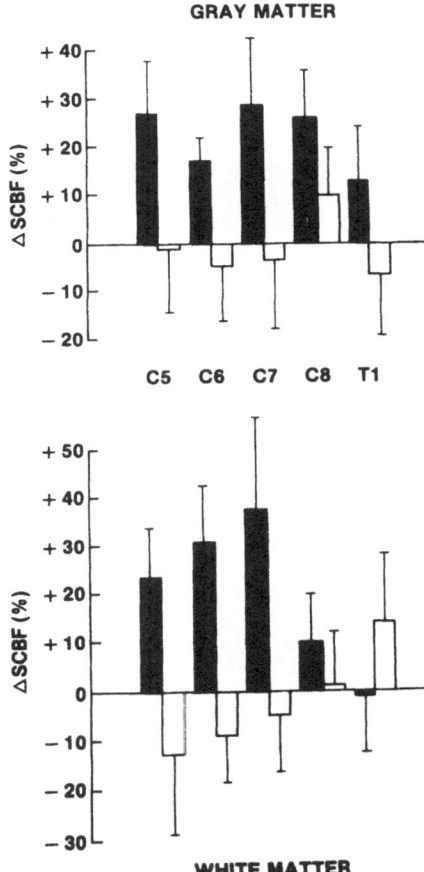

FIGURE 1. Changes in spinal cord blood flow (SCBF) at 15 min after treatment, expressed as a percentage change ($\pm$ S.E.M.) from postinjury, pretreatment values. Hatched bars represent naloxone-treated animals, and open bars saline-treated animals. C7 is the injury segment. The SCBF was measured using radioactive microspheres.

mg/kg for four hourly injections; total dose 10 mg/kg).[31] Interestingly, very-high-dose naloxone therapy (10 mg/kg for four hourly injections) appears to be less effective than the 2 mg/kg for four hourly injections (unpublished observation); another opiate-receptor antagonist {WIN44,441-3[WIN(−)], *vide infra*} also showed an inverted-U dose−response curve, with diminishing effects at very high and very low doses.[21]

The high doses of naloxone required to produce a beneficial effect in spinal cord injury and ischemia suggested that the effects might be through actions at non-μ or naloxone-insensitive receptors. To investigate this possibility, the effects of receptor-selective opiate antagonists were compared using a model of spinal cord ischemia in unanesthetized rabbits. Antagonists included ICI-154,129 (ICI), which has increased activity at δ-receptor sites, and WIN(−), which has somewhat increased activity at κ-receptor sites. In contrast to ICI, which proved

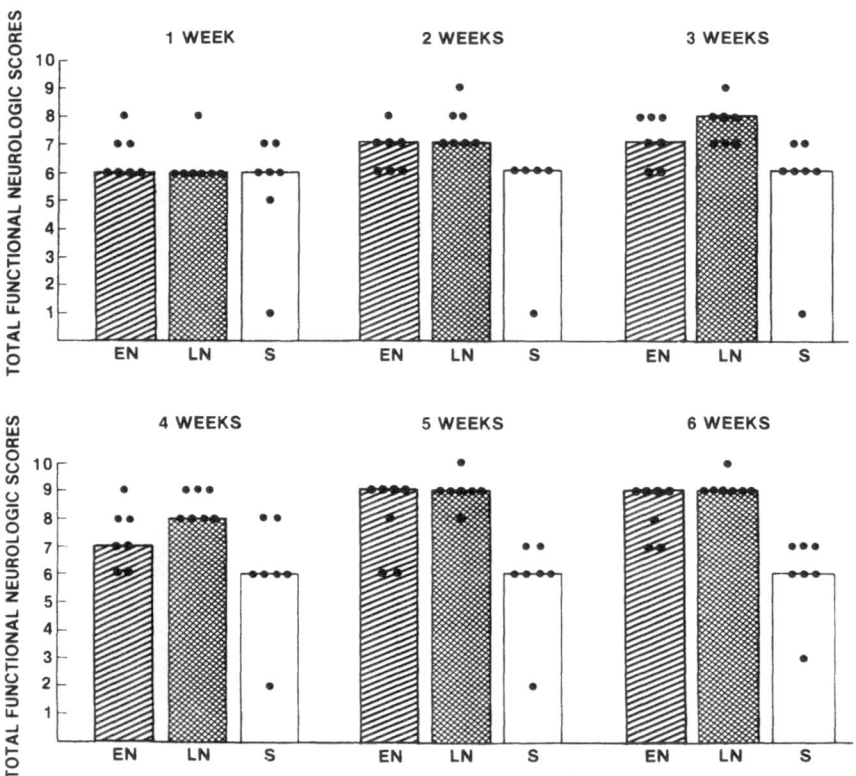

FIGURE 2. Effect of early naloxone (EN), late naloxone (LN), and saline (S) treatment on neurological recovery after cervical spinal injury. Both naloxone groups showed significantly higher
neurological scores than saline controls over the 6-week follow-up period. No significant differences
in neurological recovery were observed between the EN and LN animals. Points represent the sum of
forelimb and hindlimb neurological scores for individual animals; histograms represent median
scores. Differences between naloxone- and saline-treated animals are particularly striking when these
median scores are translated into functional equivalents: at 6 weeks, the median naloxone-treated
animals showed nearly normal motor function, whereas the median saline animal exhibited marked
spasticity or ataxia or both in both forelimbs and hindlimbs. (Reprinted with permission from Faden
et al.[28])

entirely ineffective in this model,[30] WIN(−) was highly effective and far more
potent than naloxone in improving outcome; WIN(−) improved motor recovery
and reduced histopathological changes at doses as low as 40 μg/kg given systemically, a dose approximately 50 times less than that required by naloxone for
equivalent efficacy.[21] WIN(−), but not the dextrostereoisomer WIN(+), also
proved effective following traumatic spinal cord injury in cats.[21] These observations that structurally distinct opiate antagonists produced the same physiological

action, combined with the stereospecificity of the effect, strongly support the conclusion that the beneficial effects of opiate antagonists in experimental spinal injury are through actions at opiate receptors, and suggest that the effects may be at the κ receptor.

Most recently, Faden and colleagues (A. Faden, I. Sacksen, and L. Noble, unpublished results) have examined another opiate-receptor antagonist, nalmefene, which also has increased activity at κ-receptor sites, in experimental spinal cord injury. In a newly developed model of traumatic thoracic spinal injury in anesthetized cats, nalmefene treatment significantly improved somatosensory evoked responses and long-term motor recovery compared to saline-treated control animals (A. I. Faden, unpublished observation).

3.2. OPIATE ANTAGONISTS AND TRAUMATIC BRAIN INJURY

Utilizing a fluid percussion head injury model in cats, Hayes et al.[42] were the first to observe that naloxone at high doses (10 mg/kg) significantly improved cardiovascular function, respiratory function, brain perfusion pressure, and electroencephalographic (EEG) activity. More recently, McIntosh et al.[56] observed that the opiate antagonist WIN(−) stereospecifically improves mean arterial pressure (MAP), CBF, and EEG activity following fluid percussion head injury in cats. In this study, administration of the levoisomer WIN(−), but not the dextroisomer WIN(+), caused a significant and prolonged improvement in EEG compressed spectral edge and EEG amplitude (as measured by power band analysis) within 5 min of drug treatment. Regional CBF measured at 2 hr following injury was also significantly increased by WIN(−) in those areas demonstrating greatest histopathological changes on gross examination. WIN(+) was without effect on the posttraumatic decline in CBF. These effects on regional CBF and EEG activity were subsequently observed to be independent of the systemic pressor action of the WIN(−) compound.[57] Again, the observation that multiple opiate antagonists produce the same effect and that the action is stereospecific strongly points to an opiate-receptor mechanism of action. These studies are also consistent with the hypothesis that the κ receptor mediates pathophysiological consequences of traumatic brain injury.

4. ROLE OF SPECIFIC OPIOIDS AND OPIATE RECEPTORS IN CNS INJURY

The high doses of naloxone required to show beneficial effect in CNS injury have suggested that the beneficial actions may be at non-μ opiate receptors. Findings utilizing WIN(−) and nalmefene have provided circumstantial evidence to support this hypothesis. Further experimental evidence for this conclusion has been obtained from studies in experimental spinal injury: dynorphin, the proposed endogenous ligand for the κ-opiate receptor, has been found to be unique among opioids or opiates in producing paralysis following intrathecal administration in rats.[19,20,43,60] The paralytic effects of dynorphin are dose related with transitory paralysis at low doses and permanent paralysis at high doses. Moreover, the appearance of the paralysis is similar to that after trauma; thus, dynorphin causes flaccid paralysis in the first days after administration, followed by development of spastic paraparesis. The paralytic effects of dynorphin are more pronounced with the longer dynorphin fragments, which have increased affinity at κ receptors, and less pronounced for smaller dynorphin fragments, which are more active at μ receptors.[43] In addition, traumatic injury to the spinal cord caused up-regulation of κ receptors but not μ or δ receptors[52] (Fig. 3). Finally, tissue concentrations of dynorphin increase, in a dose-related manner, at the

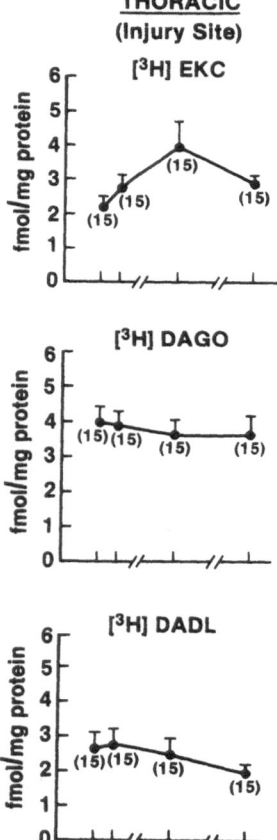

FIGURE 3. Time course of opiate binding in the rat spinal cord after traumatic injury of the thoracic region. The values are the mean ± S.E.M. of total number of rats studied, indicated at each time point. Specific binding of [³H]ethylketocyclazocine ([³H]EKC) was significantly increased at the injury site ($P < 0.02$), with the greatest changes observed at 24 hr after injury. [³H]DAGO, [³H][D-Ala²,MePhe⁴,Gly-(ol)⁵]enkephalin; [³H]DADL, [³H][D-Ala²,D-Leu⁵]enkephalin. (Reprinted with permission from Krumins and Faden.[52])

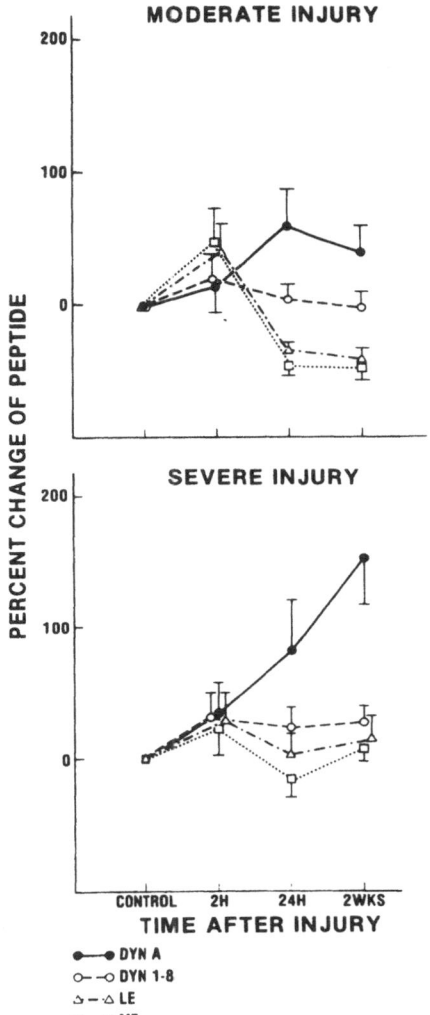

FIGURE 4. Percentage of change in peptide immunoreactivity in the rat thoracic spinal cord (injury level) at various times after traumatic injury. Moderate injury produced a significant time-dependent decrease in both leucine- and methionine-enkephalin immunoreactivity (regression analysis of variance: $F = 6.46$, $P < 0.05$ and $F = 12.24$, $P < 0.01$, respectively). Severe injury produced a significant time-dependent increase in dynorphin A (Dyn A) immunoreactivity (regression analysis of variance: $F = 16.19$, $P < 0.01$). Neither degree of injury produced significant alterations in the immunoreactivity of Dyn A-(1–8). (Reprinted with permission from Faden et al.[34])

injury site with increasing degrees of traumatic injury[34] (Fig. 4). The pattern of changes observed with dynorphin after spinal trauma is not observed for a variety of other endogenous opioids and other peptides; thus, substance P and somatostatin decrease at and below the injury site, whereas methionine- and leucine-enkephalin show little change.[33,34]

Similar patterns of opioid changes have also been confirmed in experimental head injury. A selective increase in regional concentration of dynorphin but not leucine-enkephalin was found following traumatic brain injury specifically in those areas that showed a significant decrease in regional CBF.[57] Taken together, the above data support the conclusion that pathophysiological effects of endogenous opioids in spinal cord and brain injury are mediated by dynorphin and/or the κ receptor. Further evaluation of this hypothesis will come from studies currently in progress. These include examinations of the effects of upregulation of selective opiate receptors and of the production of dynorphin tolerance.

5. OPIATE ANTAGONISTS IN CNS INJURY: CLINICAL STUDIES

A Phase I study of naloxone in human spinal cord injury has recently been published.[39] Naloxone was administered in doses ranging from 0.14 to 5.4 mg/kg for up to 48 hr after acute spinal cord injury in 29 patients. Neurological examinations were performed, and somatosensory evoked potentials (SEPs) were obtained as soon as possible after admission and again at 1 day, 2 days, 3 days, 7 days, 3 weeks, and 6 weeks to 6 months after admission. In these escalating dose studies, it was observed that patients treated with naloxone at doses above 1 mg/kg ($n = 8$), but not those treated at doses below this level, showed a dose-dependent improvement of somatosensory evoked responses. With the exception of increased awareness of pain in four patients, no difficulties were encountered in the patient's ability to tolerate large doses of naloxone. Although the numbers are small, this observation is consistent with experimental data and justified the implementation of a multiinstitutional Phase III randomized controlled study currently in progress. The use of naloxone or other opiate antagonists in human head injury has not as yet been reported.

6. FUTURE DIRECTIONS

Thyrotropin-releasing hormone (TRH) has been reported to have the ability to act *in vivo* as a partial physiological antagonist of endorphin systems. Recent studies have reported that TRH improves cardiovascular function in various shock states[55] as well as improving neurological recovery following spinal trauma in cats,[26] even when treatment was delayed up to 24 hr after injury.[32] Since administration of TRH, unlike opiate-receptor antagonists, does not block the analgesic effects of endogenous opioids or exogenous opiates, it has potential advantages over drugs like naloxone for treatment of acute spinal cord and head injury. Future studies should examine the efficacy of TRH in traumatic brain injury.

In addition to its effects as a physiological antagonist of opioid systems, TRH has been found to antagonize certain pathophysiological effects of such vasoactive lipids as leukotrienes[53] and platelet-activating factor.[54] Since these substances may play a role in the secondary injury process, the action of TRH on these systems should be elucidated. Furthermore, TRH analogues that are far more potent than TRH and less susceptible to metabolic degradation may prove particularly useful in treating spinal cord and brain injury. Preliminary studies show that these analogues are effective in experimental spinal cord injury.[14] Similarly, newer opiate-receptor antagonists possessing higher potency, longer biological half-life, and greater selectivity than naloxone may be more effective than naloxone in experimental studies and may ultimately replace naloxone in clinical testing.

REFERENCES

1. Akil, H., Watson, S. J., Young, E., Lewis, M. E., Khachaturian, H., and Walker, M. J., 1984, Endogenous opioids: Biology and function, *Annu. Rev. Neurosci.* **7**:223–225.
2. Albin, M. S., While, R. J., Yashon, D., and Harris, L. S., 1969, Effects of localized cooling on spinal cord trauma, *J. Trauma* **9**:1000–1008.
3. Cox, B., 1982, Endogenous opioid peptides: A guide to structures and terminology, *Life Sci.* **31**:1655–1658.
4. Della-Bella, D., Casacci, F., and Sassi, A., 1978, Opiate receptors: Different ligand affinity in various brain regions, *Adv. Biochem. Psychopharmacol.* **18**:271–277.
5. Demopoulos, H. B., Flamm, E. S., and Pietronigro, D. D., 1980, The free radical pathology and the microcirculation in the major central nervous system disorders, *Acta Physiol. Scand. [Suppl.]* **492**:91–119.
6. Ducker, T. B., Kindt, G. W., and Kempe, L. G., 1971, Pathological findings in acute experimental spinal cord trauma, *J. Neurosurg.* **35**:700–708.
7. Dupont, A., Lepine, J., Langelier, P., Merand, Y., Rouleau, D., Vaudry, H., Gros, C., and Barden, N., 1980, Differential distribution of β-endorphin and enkephalins in rat and bovine brain, *Regul. Peptides* **1**:43–52.
8. Elde, R., Hokfelt, T., Johansson, O., and Terenius, L., 1976, Immunohistochemical studies using antibodies to leucine–enkephalin: Initial observations on the nervous system of the rat, *Neuroscience* **1**:349–351.
9. Faden, A. I., 1983, Neuropeptides in shock and neural injury, in *The Pharmacologic Approach to the Critically Ill Patient* (B. Chernow and C. R. Lake, eds.), Williams & Wilkins, Baltimore, pp. 636–649.
10. Faden, A. I., 1983, Recent pharmacological advances in experimental spinal injury, *Trends Neurosci.* **6**:375–377.
11. Faden, A. I., 1984, Endogenous opioids: Physiologic and pathophysiologic actions, *J.A.M.A.* **84**:129–134.
12. Faden, A. I., 1984, Opiate antagonists and thyrotropin-releasing hormone. I. Potential role in the treatment of shock, *J.A.M.A.* **9**:1177–1180.
13. Faden, A., 1984, Opiate antagonists and thyrotropin-releasing hormone. II. Potential role in the treatment of central nervous system injury, *J.A.M.A.* **252**:1452–1454.
14. Faden, A. I., 1986, Neuropeptides and central nervous system injury: Clinical implications, *Arch. Neurol.* **43**:501–504.
15. Faden, A. I., and Feuerstein, G., 1983, Hypothalamic regulation of the cardiovascular and respiratory systems. Role of specific opiate receptors, *Br. J. Pharmacol.* **79**:997–1002.

16. Faden, A. I., and Holaday, J. W., 1979, Opiate antagonists: A role in the treatment of hypovolemic shock, *Science* **205**:317–318.
17. Faden, A. I., and Holaday, J. W., 1980, Naloxone treatment of endotoxic shock: Stereospecificity of physiologic and pharmacologic effects in the rat, *J. Pharmacol. Exp. Ther.* **212**:441–447.
18. Faden, A. I., and McIntosh, T. K., 1986, Endogenous opioids and central cardiovascular control, in: *Central Nervous System Control of the Heart* (T. Stober, K. Schimrigk, D. Ganten, and D. Sherman, eds.), Martin Nijhoff, Boston, pp. 123–136.
19. Faden, A. I., and Jacobs, T. P., 1983, Dynorphin induced partially reversible paraplegia in the rat, *Eur. J. Pharmacol.* **91**(2/3):321–324.
20. Faden, A. I., and Jacobs, T. P., 1984, Dynorphin-related peptides cause motor dysfunction in the rat through a non-opiate action, *Br. J. Pharmacol.* **81**:271–276.
21. Faden, A. I., and Jacobs, T. P., 1985, Opiate antagonist WIN44,441-3 stereospecifically improves neurologic recovery after ischemic spinal injury, *Neurology (N.Y.)* **35**:1311–1315.
22. Faden, A. I., Jacobs, T. P., and Holaday, J. W., 1980, Endorphin–parasympathetic interaction in spinal shock, *J. Auton. Nerv. Syst.* **2**:295–304.
23. Faden, A. I., Jacobs, T. P., and Holaday, J. W., 1980, A possible pathophysiologic role for endorphins in spinal injury, *Fed. Proc.* **39**:762.
24. Faden, A. I., Jacobs, T. P., and Holaday, J. W., 1981, Endorphins in experimental spinal injury: Therapeutic effect of naloxone, *Ann. Neurol.* **10**:326–332.
25. Faden, A. I., Jacobs, T. P., and Holaday, J. W., 1981, Opiate antagonist improves neurologic recovery after spinal injury, *Science* **211**:493–494.
26. Faden, A. I., Jacobs, T. P., and Holaday, J. W., 1981, Thyrotropin-releasing hormone improves neurologic recovery after spinal trauma in cats, *N. Engl. J. Med.* **305**:1063–1067.
27. Faden, A. I., Hallenbeck, J. M., and Brown, C. Q., 1982, Treatment of experimental stroke: Comparison of naloxone and thyrotropin-releasing hormone, *Neurology (N.Y.)* **32**:1083–1087.
28. Faden, A. I., Jacobs, T. P., and Holaday, J. W., 1982, Comparison of early and late naloxone treatment in experimental spinal injury, *Neurology (N.Y.)* **32**:677–681.
29. Faden, A., Jacobs, T. P., Smith, G. P., Green, B., and Zivin, J. A., 1983, Neuropeptides in spinal cord injury: Comparative experimental models, **4**:631–634.
30. Faden, A. I., Jacobs, T. P., and Zivin, J. A., 1983, Comparison of naloxone and a delta-selective antagonist in experimental spinal "stroke," *Life Sci.* **33**(Suppl. I):707–710.
31. Faden, A. I., Jacobs, T. P., Smith, M. T., and Zivin, J. A., 1984, Naloxone in experimental spinal cord ischemia: Dose–response studies, *Eur. J. Pharmacol.* **103**:115–120.
32. Faden, A. I., Jacobs, T. P., and Smith, M. T., 1984, Thyrotropin releasing hormone in experimental spinal injury: Dose response and late treatment, *Neurology (N.Y.)* **34**:1280–1284.
33. Faden, A. I., Jacobs, T. P., and Helke, C. J., 1985, Changes in substance P and somatostatin in the spinal cord after traumatic spinal injury in the rat, *Neuropeptides* **6**:215–225.
34. Faden, A. I., Molineaux, C. J., Rosenberger, J. G., Jacobs, T. P., and Cox, B. M., 1985, Endogenous opioid immunoreactivity in rat spinal cord following traumatic injury, *Ann. Neurol.* **17**:386–390.
35. Feuerstein, G., and Faden, A. I., 1982, Differential cardiovascular effects of μ, δ and κ opiate agonists at discrete hypothalamic sites in the anesthetized rat, *Life Sci.* **31**:2197–2200.
36. Feuerstein, G., and Faden, A., 1984, Cardiovascular effects of dynorphin A-(1–8), dynorphin A-(1–13) and dynorphin A-(1–17) microinjected into the preoptic medialis of the rat, *Neuropeptides* **5**:295–298.
37. Feuerstein, G., Molineaux, C. J., Rosenberger, J. G., Faden, A. I., and Cox, B. M., 1983, Dynorphin and Leu-enkephalin in brain nuclei and pituitary of WKY and SHR rats, *Peptides* **4**:225–229.
38. Flamm, E. S., Young, W., Demopoulos, H. B., DeCrescito, V., and Tomasula, J. J., 1982, Experimental spinal cord injury: Treatment with naloxone, *Neurosurgery* **10**:227–231.

39. Flamm, E. S., Young, W., Collins, W. F., Piepmeier, J., Clifton, G. L., and Fischer, B., 1985, A Phase I trial of naloxone treatment in acute spinal cord injury, *J. Neurosurg.* **63**:390–397.
40. Fukuda, N., Yoshiaki, S., and Nagawa, Y., 1979, Behavioral and EEG alterations with brain stem compression and effect of thyrotropin-releasing hormone (TRH) in chronic cats, *Folia Pharmacol. Jpn.* **75**:321–331.
41. Hassen, A. H., Feuerstein, G. Z., and Faden, A. I., 1984, Kappa opioid receptors modulate cardiorespiratory function in hindbrain nuclei of the rat, *J. Neurosci.* **4**:2213–2221.
42. Hayes, R. L., Galinet, B. J., Kulkarne, P., and Becker, D., 1983, Effects of naloxone on systemic and cerebral responses to experimental concussive brain injury in cats, *J. Neurosurg.* **58**:720–728.
43. Herman, B. H., and Goldstein, A., 1985, Antinociception and paralysis induced by intrathecal dynorphin A, *J. Pharmacol. Exp. Ther.* **232**:27–32.
44. Hokfelt, T., Elde, R., Johansson, O., Terenius, L., and Stein, L., 1977, The distribution of enkephalin immunoreactie cell bodies in the rat central nervous system, *Neurosci. Lett.* **5**:25–31.
45. Holaday, J., 1983, Cardiovascular effects of endogenous opiate systems, *Annu. Rev. Pharmacol. Toxicol.* **23**:541–594.
46. Holaday, J. W., and Faden, A. I., 1978, Naloxone reversal of endotoxin hypotension suggests role of endorphins in shock, *Nature* **275**:450–451.
47. Holaday, J. W., and Faden, A. I., 1980, Naloxone acts at central opiate receptors to reverse hypotension, hypothermia, and hypoventilation in spinal shock, *Brain Res.* **189**:295–299.
48. Hsu, C. Y., Halushka, P. V., Hogan, E. L., Banik, N. L., Lee, W. A., and Perot, P. L., 1985, Alteration of thromboxane and prostacyclin levels in experimental spinal cord injury, *Neurology (N.Y.)* **35**:1003–1009.
49. Hughes, J., Kosterlitz, H. W., Marley, J. S., and Smith, T. W., 1983, Opioid peptides, *Br. Med. Bull.* **39**:1–103.
50. Khachaturian, H., Watson, S. J., Lewis, M. E., Coy, D., Goldstein, A., and Akil, H., 1982, Dynorphin immunocytochemistry in the rat central nervous system, *Peptides* **3**:941–945.
51. Khachaturian, H., Lewis, M. E., Schafer, M. K.-H., and Watson, S. J., 1985, Anatomy of the CNS opioid systems, *Trends Neurosci.* **1**:111–119.
52. Krumins, S. A., and Faden, A. I., 1986, Traumatic injury alters opiate receptor binding in spinal cord, *Ann. Neurol.* **19**:498–501.
53. Lux, W. E., Feuerstein, F., and Faden, A., 1983, Alteration of leukotriene D_4 hypotension by thyrotropin releasing hormone, *Nature* **302**:822–824.
54. Lux, W. E., Feuerstein, G., Snyder, F., and Faden, A., 1983, Effect of TRH on hypotension produced by platelet activating factor, *Circ. Shock* **10**:262–266.
55. McIntosh, T., and Faden, A., 1986, Thyrotropin-releasing hormone (TRH) and circulatory shock: A review, *Circ. Shock* **18**:241–258.
56. McIntosh, T. K., Agura, V. M., Hellgeth, M., Rittner, H., Faden, A. I., and Hayes, R. L., 1985, Stereospecific efficacy of the opiate antagonist WIN44,441-3 in the treatment of head injury in the cat, *Neurosci. Abstr.* **11**(2):1200.
57. McIntosh, T. K., Hayes, R. L., Dewitt, D. S., Agura, V., and Faden, A. I., 1987, Endogenous opioids may mediate secondary damage after experimental brain injury, *Am. J. Physiol.* **253**:E565–E574.
58. Osterholm, J. L., 1974, The pathophysiological response to spinal cord injury, *J. Neurosurg.* **40**:5–33.
59. Pfeiffer, A., and Herz, A., 1982, Discrimination of three opiate-receptor binding sites with the use of computerized curve fitting techniques, *Mol. Pharmacol.* **21**:266–271.
60. Przewlocki, R., Shearman, G. T., and Herz, A., 1983, Mixed opioid/nonopioid effects of dynorphin and dynorphin-related peptides after their intrathecal injection in rats, *Neuropeptides* **3**:233–240.

61. Rawe, S. E., Lee, W. A., and Perot, P. L., 1981, Spinal cord glucose utilization after experimental spinal cord injury, *Neurosurgery* **9**:40–47.
62. Sandler, A. N., and Tator, C. H., 1967, Review of the effect of spinal cord trauma on the vessels and blood flow in the spinal cord, *J. Neurosurg.* **5**:638–646.
63. Sawynok, J., Pinsky, C., and LaBella, F. A., 1979, Mini review on the specificity of naloxone as an opiate antagonist, *Life Sci.* **25**:1631–1642.
64. Simantov, R., Kuhar, M. J., Uhl, G. R., and Snyder, S. H., 1977, Opioid peptide enkephalin: Immunohistochemical mapping in rat central nervous system, *Proc. Natl. Acad. Sci. U.S.A.* **74**:2167–2172.
65. Stokes, B. T., Fox, P., and Hollinden, G., 1983, Extracellular calcium activity in injured spinal cord, *Exp. Neurol.* **80**:561–572.
66. Young, W., Flamm, E. S., Demopoulos, H. B., Tomasula, J. J., and DeCrescito, V., 1981, Naloxone ameliorates posttraumatic ischemia in experimental spinal contusion, *J. Neurosurg.* **55**:209–219.
67. Zivin, J. A., Doppman, J. L., Reid, J. L., Toppaz, M. L., Saavedra, J. M., Kopin, I. J., and Jacobowitz, D. M., 1982, Biochemical and histochemical studies of biogenic amines in spinal cord trauma, *Neurology (N.Y.)* **26**:99–107.
68. Zukin, R. S., and Zukin, S. R., 1981, Multiple opiate receptors: Emerging concepts, *Life Sci.* **29**:2681–2690.

6

Adaptive Changes in Central Dopaminergic Neurons after Injury
Effects of Drugs

Franz Hefti and William J. Weiner

ABSTRACT. Central dopaminergic neurons play an important role in motor, emotional, and cognitive behavior. These dopaminergic systems are affected both by normal aging and by various diseases. The most prominent of these diseases is Parkinson's disease, which is associated with a gradual and progressive loss of dopaminergic neurons in the human brain. Studies on human brain have revealed a remarkable ability of these neurons to compensate for partial destruction of their systems, and these findings have prompted numerous investigations of the adaptive changes of dopaminergic neurons to experimental injury. The findings reveal that dopaminergic neurons react to a partial lesion of their pathways with several adaptive changes. Dopaminergic neurons surviving a partial lesion respond by increasing transmitter synthesis and release. Furthermore, after near-total lesions, a supersensitivity of postsynaptic transmitter receptors develops. Because of these biochemical adaptive changes, few surviving neurons are able to compensate for the loss of a majority of other dopaminergic neurons. Recent findings indicate that biochemical adaptive processes can be further stimulated by pharmacological manipulation. The possible mechanisms of actions of these pharmacological agents are discussed.

1. Introduction

Several neurological diseases are characterized by the loss of specific populations of neurons in the brain. In Parkinson's disease there is a selective degeneration of dopaminergic cells (for review see refs. 14, 57, 60). Alzheimer's disease has been associated with the loss of cholinergic neurons of the basal forebrain, ascending noradrenergic and serotoninergic neurons, somatostatin-containing

FRANZ HEFTI AND WILLIAM J. WEINER • Department of Neurology, University of Miami School of Medicine, Miami, Florida 33101.

103

cortical neurons, hippocampal neurons, and other peptide-containing neurons.[58,69] In Huntington's disease cortical and striatal neurons degenerate,[72] and
amyotrophic lateral sclerosis is characterized by the loss of large motor neurons.[21,22] The standard pharmacological treatment of these diseases attempts to
replace the "missing" neurotransmitter. This approach has been very successful
in the case of Parkinson's disease, where dopaminergic agonists effectively
alleviate the symptoms[14,60]; however, it has not been as successful for the other
degenerative diseases. Even in Parkinson's disease, substitution therapy is not
able to compensate for complete loss of the dopaminergic neuronal system at
later stages of the disease.

A different and potentially more useful pharmacological approach to these
neurodegenerative diseases is to exploit their gradual progressive nature. The
slow degenerative processes may induce adaptive changes that compensate to a
certain extent for the primary deficit produced by the lesion. Such compensatory
changes might involve the remaining population of the affected neuronal system
as well as neurons postsynaptic to them. Very little attention has been given so
far to the possibility of promoting such compensatory changes pharmacologically. This chapter discusses the events occurring during the gradual and progressive degeneration of the ascending dopaminergic system of the mesencephalon and the pharmacological possibilities of influencing these processes.

Mesencephalic dopaminergic neurons are involved in many aspects of brain
function. These systems are primarily related to motor control but are also
involved with cognitive and emotional behavior. These dopaminergic systems
degenerate selectively in Parkinson's disease, giving rise to specific movement
and behavioral deficits. Degenerative changes characteristic of Parkinson's disease can be reproduced in experimental animals. In humans and animals progressive degeneration results first in increased transmitter release by surviving
dopaminergic neurons and second, in more advanced stages of degeneration, in
changes in the postsynaptic receptors mediating the actions of dopamine (DA).
In animals, regeneration of severed dopaminergic neurons represents a third
possible compensatory change. The following sections describe compensatory
changes in transmitter release and postsynaptic receptors and discusses the possibility of promoting these processes pharmacologically. Special emphasis is
given to the stimulation of transmitter release by dopaminergic neurons surviving
a degenerative process. The chapter is preceded by a brief description of the
anatomy and function of mesencephalic dopaminergic neurons.

2. ANATOMY AND FUNCTION OF MESENCEPHALIC DOPAMINERGIC NEURONS

Cell bodies of the ascending dopaminergic neurons of the mammalian mesencephalon are located in the zona compacta of the substantia nigra and in the

ventral tegmental area medioventral to the substantia nigra. These cell bodies innervate the caudate nucleus and putamen (corpus striatum), nucleus accumbens, olfactory tubercle, septum, hippocampus, amygdala, and various cortical areas. Traditionally, the ascending dopaminergic systems are divided into two pathways. Dopaminergic cell bodies located in the zona compacta innervate mainly the corpus striatum, forming the nigrostriatal dopaminergic projection. The axons of this pathway constitute part of the medial forebrain bundle, from which they enter the internal capsule and radiate into the corpus striatum. Cell bodies located in the ventral tegmental area innervate the nucleus accumbens, olfactory tubercle, amygdala, and cortex. The axons of these neurons course through the medial forebrain bundle and the internal capsule. These pathways are referred to as the mesolimbic dopaminergic systems. However, it is more appropriate to look at the nigrostriatal and mesolimbic pathways as parts of a topographically organized ascending dopaminergic projection originating in the mesencephalon. Cell bodies located in the caudolateral part of the substantia nigra project to the lateral corpus striatum, and the cell bodies located anteromedially in the tegmentum project to anteromedial forebrain areas (e.g., frontal cortex). The vast majority of the dopaminergic nigrostriatal fibers innervate target areas on the ipsilateral side of the brain. The anatomy of dopaminergic projections has been the subject of several excellent reviews.[23,55,56,63]

The nigrostriatal and mesolimbic dopaminergic projections of the mesencephalon represent the main and most extensive dopaminergic projections in the central nervous system. Besides these pathways there are minor dopaminergic pathways. There are a dopaminergic nigrothalamic pathway and several groups of short dopaminergic neurons in the diencephalon. These neurons are mainly located in the periaqueductal areas of the diencephalon. The principal group of these cells originates in the arcuate nucleus and innervates the median eminence and the infundibular stalk of the pituitary. In addition, there are descending dopaminergic projections innervating the spinal cord and dopaminergic interneurons in the olfactory bulb and the retina.[56]

Transmitter biochemistry of the dopaminergic neurons has been well characterized and described in many reviews.[12,36,63,71] Dopamine is synthesized by two enzymes that transform the precursor amino acid tyrosine first into 3,4-dihydroxyphenylalanine (dopa, catalyzed by tyrosine hydroxylase, TH) and then to DA (catalyzed by aromatic amino acid decarboxylase, AAAD). In the terminals of the dopaminergic neurons, DA is stored in vesicles and is released on stimulation. The action of DA is terminated by an uptake system and by enzymatic metabolism of the transmitter. The enzymatic breakdown is catalyzed by monoamine oxidase (MAO) and catechol-O-methyltransferase (COMT). These two enzymes form DA's principal metabolites, 3,4-dihydroxyphenylacetic acid (DOPAC) and homovanillic acid (HVA). Dopamine receptors are divided into two classes, D_1 and D_2 receptors (for review see refs. 16, 18, 41). D_1 receptors are coupled to adenylate cyclase, whereas D_2 receptors are not or are negatively coupled to this enzyme. Apparently, most behavioral effects of DA are mediated by D_2 receptors. The function of the D_1 receptors remains to be elucidated. Progress in this field can be expected in the next few years, since selective agonists for the two types of receptors have recently become available. Several lines of evidence suggest the possibility that dopaminergic neurons contain auto-receptors for dopamine. These receptors might be located both on cell bodies in the mesencephalon and on the terminals in the corpus striatum.[15,66] However these autoreceptors were never directly demonstrated, and their pharmacological characteristics remain unclear.[34,47,48,52]

The role of dopaminergic neurons in behavior has been studied with various experimental tools that either interfere with or stimulate dopaminergic functions (for review see refs. 12, 36, 63, 71). The most frequently used experimental tool is 6-hydroxydopamine, a neurotoxic agent that selectively destroys cate-cholaminergic neurons. This toxin, when injected locally in the areas of the cell bodies of dopaminergic neurons, results in a selective destruction of these cells.[74,75] In recent years, another compound, 1-methyl-4-phenyl-1,2,3,6-tetrahydropyridine (MPTP), which was discovered as a by-product of synthetic heroin, was found to destroy nigrostriatal dopaminergic neurons selectively in primates and man.[14,49,50] Although MPTP reduces DA levels in mice, it is still not clear whether MPTP results in destruction of dopaminergic neurons in rodents and other nonprimate animals. The function of dopaminergic neurons can also be inhibited with metabolic inhibitors such as α-methyltyrosine, an inhibitor of TH, which produces a blockade of DA synthesis. Several antagonists are available that selectively block DA receptors on postsynaptic neurons.[16,18,41] A potentiation of dopaminergic functions can be achieved by inhibiting the catabolic enzyme MAO, resulting in higher concentrations of DA at synaptic sites. Furthermore, dopaminergic functions can also be potentiated by the administration of direct-acting DA receptor agonists or by the administration of dopa. Dopa elevates DA synthesis by bypassing the blood–brain barrier and the rate-limiting enzyme TH.

Because mesencephalic dopaminergic neurons are involved in motor, cognitive, and emotional behavior in rats (for review see ref. 9), their destruction results in hypokinesia, aphagia, adipsia, and sensory neglect. Motor functions are thought to be mediated mainly by the nigrostriatal neurons, given the integration of the corpus striatum in the extrapyramidal system. The projection of mesolimbic neurons to the nucleus accumbens also participates in motor control, whereas the other projections of this pathway to septum, amygdala, and cortex are believed to be responsible for the emotional and cognitive behavioral effects of dopamine. Dopaminergic afferents to the cortex have been shown to be involved in positive reinforcement. The crucial role of ascending mesencephalic dopaminergic neurons is best illustrated by human Parkinson's disease.[14,57,60] This disease is characterized by the primary motor symptoms hypokinesia, rigidity, and tremor, which very often are accompanied by behavioral depression. Dopaminergic neurons undergo a selective degeneration in this disease, and it is generally accepted that most, if not all, of the behavioral deficits are caused by the loss of dopaminergic neurons. The behavioral symptoms may be modified by pharmacological manipulations increasing dopaminergic function. Excessive stimulation of DA receptors in parkinsonian patients very often results in in involuntary movements and visual hallucinations.

3. COMPENSATORY CHANGES IN TRANSMITTER RELEASE

Transmitter synthesis and release by mesencephalic dopaminergic neurons is controlled by several factors that are dependent on the activity of the neurons.[46] This activity is a function of neuronal input to both the mesencephalon and other neurons that influence dopaminergic neurons by acting on presynaptic receptors.[48] Furthermore, synthesis and release are dependent on the status of the dopaminergic system itself. Loss of part of the nigrostriatal system results in compensatory adjustments in the remaining neurons. These interactions have been studied in animals with partial lesions of the nigrostriatal system produced by applying various amounts of 6-hydroxydopamine directly into the substantia nigra. This experimental approach results in a dose-dependent reduction of the number of dopaminergic cells within the nigrostriatal system.

Rats were then taken for the measurement of DA synthesis by measuring the conversion of [³H]tyrosine to [³H]DA[3] or the accumulation of DOPA after inhibition of AAAD.[30,33] Dopamine release was assessed by measuring the levels of the principal DA metabolites, DOPAC and HVA.[1,30,33,78] The ratios of DOPA, DOPAC, and HVA levels to that of DA itself served as an index of DA synthesis or release per surviving dopaminergic neurons. The use of these ratios is justified because DA levels are not affected by most induced changes in activity of dopaminergic neurons[46] and therefore serve as an index of the number of surviving dopaminergic neurons.

Agid et al.[3] first reported that partial dopaminergic lesions resulted in elevated ratios of newly formed [³H]DA to DA and concluded that the partial lesions resulted in an elevated rate of DA synthesis by remaining dopaminergic neurons. This was later confirmed by studies showing that partial lesions also elevated the ratio of DOPA accumulating after AAAD inhibition to DA.[30,33] Elevated DA release in striata of animals with partial nigrostriatal lesions was indicated by increased DOPAC/DA and HVA/DA ratios.[1,30,33,78]

There is still some controversy on whether the rate-limiting enzyme of DA synthesis, TH, exhibits greater activity in neurons surviving partial lesions. Zigmond et al.[78] found increased TH/DA ratios 2 days after 6-hydroxydopamine administration. However, this was only the case when TH activity was measured under "suboptimal" conditions, i.e., in the presence of subsaturating concentrations of the cofactor. This increase disappeared after more than 2 days. In contrast, TH activity measured under optimal conditions (i.e., in the presence of saturating concentrations of cofactor) was normal 2 days after 6-hydroxydopamine lesions but increased later and remained elevated for more than 2 months. In contrast to these results, Hefti et al.[30] found no elevation in TH/DA 2 weeks after lesion formation and using optimal conditions in the enzyme assay. Tyrosine hydroxylase is normally believed to be the rate-limiting enzyme in dopamine synthesis. It can therefore be anticipated that an increase in release and synthesis has to be accompanied by an elevation in TH activity. However, TH activity in vivo is influenced by the concentrations of oxygen, cofactor (tetrahydropteridine), tyrosine, DA, and the state of phosphorylation.[11,51] Any of these factors can influence the hydroxylation of tyrosine in vivo in a way not reflected by in vitro measurements of TH activity.

The increases in DA synthesis and release are dependent on the size of lesion of the nigrostriatal system. Increases become apparent when lesions destroy more than approximately two-thirds of the dopaminergic neurons. Larger lesions are accompanied by a gradual increase of these ratios. With lesions destroying more than 90% of nigrostriatal neurons, DOPA/DA, DOPAC/DA, and HVA/DA ratios are elevated up to fourfold.[1,30,33,78] Increases in transmitter synthesis and release induced by partial nigrostriatal lesions seem to be permanent, since elevated ratios have been observed 1 to 2 months after lesioning.[78]

Various mechanisms might cause the increase in striatal DA synthesis and release after partial nigrostriatal lesions. First, the inhibitory action of the GABAergic striatonigral feedback system[60] might be decreased because less DA is impinging on postsynaptic receptors in the damaged striatum. Second, striatal cholinergic interneurons, which are inhibited by DA release from nigrostriatal neurons, probably had increased their activity after the partial removal of the dopaminergic input. Release of acetylcholine from the striatal interneurons could increase striatal DA release by stimulating presynaptic receptors located on dopaminergic terminals.[25–27] Third, if DA autoreceptors on striatal dopaminergic terminals are accessible to DA released from neighboring neurons, partial nigrostriatal lesions might diminish the inhibition of DA synthesis mediated by these receptors. Fourth, the self-inhibition of nigrostriatal neurons, mediated by autoreceptors localized on dendrites or cell bodies,[2] could be diminished by the loss of dendrites on neighboring dopaminergic cells, leading to an increased firing rate and transmitter release from the terminals.

The increase in DA released from surviving neurons seems to compensate physiologically for the loss of the other neurons, since lesions producing up to 90% loss of the nigrostriatal neurons induced no behavioral manifestations.[30,31,33] Changes in postsynaptic receptors (discussed in Section 5) only occur with lesions affecting more than 90% of dopaminergic neurons. In an autopsy study of patients with Parkinson's disease, even those with mild symptoms were shown to have lost at least 70% of the DA normally found in the corpus striatum.[10,35] These authors proposed that during the preclinical phase of Parkinson's disease, residual dopaminergic neurons compensate for the degenerated neurons.

Is it possible to accelerate further the dopamine release from the remaining dopaminergic neurons by pharmacological manipulation? Effective drugs might postpone the appearance of behavioral deficits in Parkinson's disease. To address this problem, studies were initiated with experimental animals in which the effects of various drug treatments on DA release of neurons surviving a partial nigrostriatal lesions were tested. These studies are described in the following section.

4. PHARMACOLOGICAL STIMULATION OF DA SYNTHESIS AND RELEASE IN DOPAMINERGIC NEURONS SURVIVING PARTIAL NIGROSTRIATAL LESIONS

As outlined in Section 3, 6-hydroxydopamine injected into the substantia nigra of rats produces a dose-dependent destruction of the nigrostriatal pathway. The findings obtained from experiments with rats having experimentally induced partial lesions correspond closely to those from postmortem studies of brains from parkinsonian patients. In such brains, the HVA/DA ratio is elevated in the caudate nucleus.[10,39] The increase in release of transmitter per surviving dopaminergic neuron probably represents an adaptive mechanism that helps to compensate for the loss of dopaminergic neurons projecting to the caudate nucleus. It was not known whether the rates of synthesis and release of transmitter reached by surviving neurons represent maximal values or whether they could be further enhanced by pharmacological manipulation. This question was studied in recent years in our laboratories. Rats were produced with lesions of the dopaminergic nigrostriatal system that resulted in elevated turnover and release of surviving dopaminergic neurons, and the effects of drugs that were known to accelerate DA turnover and release in such animals were studied.

Methods used for these studies were described in detail elsewhere.[28–34] Briefly, rats were injected with 2–10 μg of 6-hydroxydopamine into the right anteromedial substantia nigra (level A2400, 2.6 mm ventral, 1.6 mm lateral[45]). These injections produced partial lesions of the dopaminergic nigrostriatal pathway of variable severity. Dopamine metabolism was measured in the corpus striatum after treatment of the animals with various drugs. To assess synthesis of DA *in vivo,* the accumulation of DOPA was measured after administration of *m*-hydroxybenzylhydrazine dihydrochloride (NSD 1015; an inhibitor of AAAD, 100mg/kg, administered 30 min before death). The concentrations of DOPAC and HVA in the striatum were determined to assess release of DA *in vivo.* Dopamine and its metabolites were determined using high-performance liquid chromatography with electrochemical detection.

The unilateral injection of 6-hydroxydopamine into the substantia nigra reduced the concentration of DA in ipsilateral striata of individual animals to various degrees. The DOPA/DA ratio as well as DOPAC/DA and HVA/DA ratios remained unaffected in ipsilateral striata in those animals with DA levels reduced by less than two-thirds of the concentrations measured on the contralateral sides. In animals in which the lesions had reduced DA concentrations in the striatum more than two-thirds of contralateral values, DOPA/DA, DOPAC/DA, and HVA/DA ratios were increased up to fourfold higher than the corresponding ratios measured in control striata, indicating elevated rates of DA synthesis and release in dopaminergic neurons surviving a partial nigrostriatal lesion (Fig. 1).

To test whether the elevated rates of DA synthesis and release on lesioned sides could be further increased by pharmacological manipulation, various drugs were applied that are known to increase DA synthesis and release in an intact nigrostriatal dopaminergic system. The first compound to be tested was γ-butyrolactone (GBL), which blocks the firing of nigrostriatal neurons and results in a brief increase in DA synthesis in the corpus striatum.[76,77] The effects on DA metabolism are thought to be mediated by presynaptic DA receptors, which exert an inhibitory control on DA synthesis. In animals treated with GBL, these receptors are not stimulated because of the absence of impulse-mediated release of DA, resulting in an acceleration of DA synthesis. (In animals treated with GBL alone, newly synthesized DA accumulates in the terminals, resulting in an elevation of DA levels in the striatum. This effect would normally preclude the use of DA levels as an index for the number of dopaminergic neurons. Animals taken for the measurement of DA synthesis were pretreated with an inhibitor of AAAD, which prevented the transformation of additionally synthesized DOPA into DA and the increase in DA levels.)

In rats with nigrostriatal lesions reducing the dopaminergic innervation by less than 75%, DOPA/DA ratios were similar in striata ipsi- and contralateral to the lesion. Administration of GBL elevated these ratios approximately threefold on both ipsi- and contralateral sides. In control rats with nigrostriatal lesions reducing the dopaminergic innervation by more than 75%, the DOPA/DA ratio was increased fourfold on the lesioned side compared to control values. Administration of GBL further elevated this ratio to a level 22-fold higher than that in control striata of untreated animals, i.e., to a level significantly higher than that produced by the lesion itself (Fig. 1). These findings indicate that the rate of DA synthesis reached by dopaminergic neurons surviving in a damaged nigrostriatal system does not represent a maximal level but can be further elevated by pharmacological manipulation.

To test whether DA release from dopaminergic neurons surviving a partial nigrostriatal lesion can be elevated further, lesioned animals were treated with morphine, haloperidol, or nicotine. These compounds were chosen because they had previously been shown to increase striatal concentrations of DOPAC and HVA. Morphine increases the firing rate of nigrostriatal neurons, most probably by acting on opiate receptors in the substantia nigra.[38,61] The increase in activity

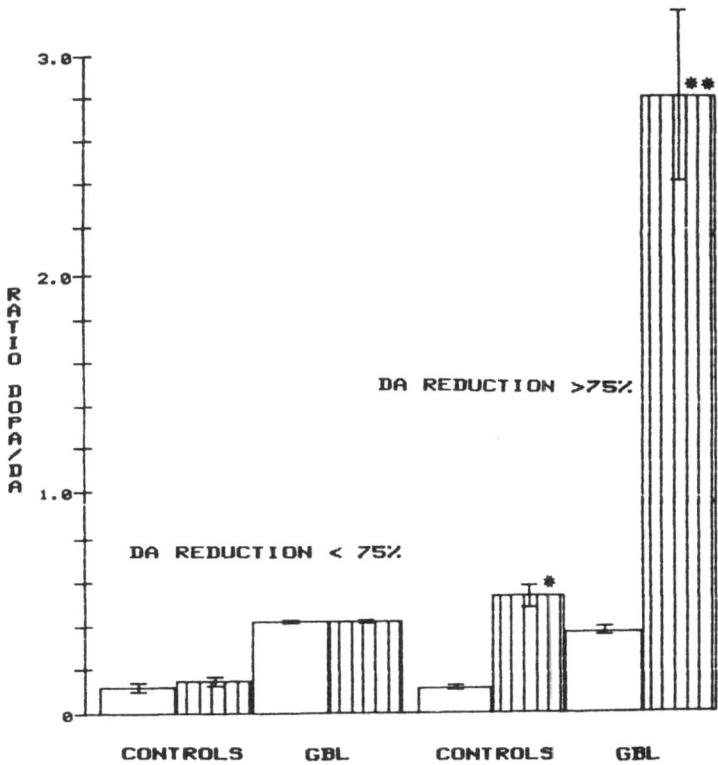

FIGURE 1. Synthesis of DA by nigrostriatal neurons surviving a unilateral partial nigrostriatal lesion induced by 6-hydroxydopamine, and the effect of γ-butyrolactone (GBL). Synthesis of DA was assessed by measuring the accumulation of dopa after inhibition of aromatic amino acid decarboxylase by NSD 1015 (100 mg/kg, 30 min). Striatal DA concentrations served as an index of the severity of the lesion. Animals were assigned to one of the following groups: (1) rats in which the striatal DA levels on the lesioned side were reduced less than 75% as compared to the control side (DA reduction <75%; columns on the left), and (2) rats with reductions in striatal DA levels larger than 75% of control values (DA reduction >75%; columns on the right). The ratio of DOPA/DA served as an index for synthesis of DA per neuron; GBL (750 mg/kg) was given 35 min before death. Open bars represent DOPA/DA ratios measured in striata contralateral to the lesion. Striped bars represent values measured in striata of the lesioned side. Lesions reducing DA concentrations by more than 75% elevated the DOPA/DA ratio in lesioned striata above levels measured on control sides and on both sides of control animals with the smaller lesions (*$P < 0.01$, t-test). The DOPA/DA ratio was further increased by GBL administration (**different from values measured on corresponding control sides and from values of lesioned sides of control animals, $P < 0.01$). Bars represent means ± S.E.M. of 8–15 animals per group. Dopamine and dopa levels in control striata of animals receiving NSD 1015 only (controls) were 59.5 ± 2.3 and 7.7 ± 0.3, respectively (pmol/g wet weight, means ± S.E.M.).

is accompanied by an acceleration of synthesis and release of DA in the corpus striatum.[4,5] Animals whose striatal DA levels ipsilateral to the lesion were reduced by more than 75% of control values were used for these experiments. The lesions elevated the DOPAC/DA and HVA/DA ratios in ipsilateral striata 1.3- and 1.9-fold, respectively, relative to those in contralateral striata. A single injection of morphine further increased these ratios to levels 1.8 and 3.1 times control values, respectively (Table I). These findings indicate that DA release, like DA synthesis, by dopaminergic neurons surviving a partial nigrostriatal lesion can be further elevated by pharmacological manipulation.

Like morphine, haloperidol increases the firing rate, synthesis, and release of DA in nigrostriatal neurons.[13,20,67] The effect of haloperidol, however, appears to be a consequence of its ability to block DA receptors in the brain. The blockade of pre- and postsynaptic DA receptors in the striatum is thought to result in a compensatory increase in electrical and metabolic activity of these neurons.[6] In striata ipsilateral to the partial nigrostriatal lesion, haloperidol increased the DOPAC/DA ratio 4.5-fold and the HVA/DA ratio 4.3-fold above values measured in untreated and unlesioned control striata (Table I). Values reached were significantly higher than those produced by the nigrostriatal lesion alone (1.3-fold and 1.9-fold, respectively).

Nicotine is known to increase the firing rate of nigrostriatal neurons by directly stimulating cholinergic receptors in the substantia nigra.[53,54] This electrophysiological activation is accompanied by increases in striatal HVA but not DOPAC concentrations.[53,54] A single injection of nicotine increased the

TABLE I. Effect of Morphine, Haloperidol, and Nicotine on DA Release by Dopaminergic Neurons Surviving a Partial Nigrostriatal Lesion[a]

	DA	DOPAC	HVA	DOPAC/DA	HVA/DA
Controls					
Con. side	64.2 ± 5.7	3.5 ± 0.5	3.6 ± 0.4	0.06 ± 0.01	0.07 ± 0.02
Les. side	8.9 ± 2.5	0.7 ± 0.3	1.0 ± 0.2	0.08 ± 0.01†	0.13 ± 0.01†
Morphine					
Con. Side	72.6 ± 8.8	5.3 ± 0.7	5.2 ± 0.8	0.08 ± 0.01	0.08 ± 0.01
Les. side	9.3 ± 1.4	1.0 ± 0.2	1.7 ± 0.3	0.11 ± 0.01*	0.22 ± 0.03*†
Haloperidol					
Con. side	60.6 ± 8.0	16.0 ± 1.4	17.5 ± 1.3	0.29 ± 0.02	0.36 ± 0.04
Les. side	9.8 ± 1.6	2.4 ± 0.3	2.5 ± 0.5	0.27 ± 0.02*	0.30 ± 0.04*
Nicotine					
Con. side	67.0 ± 2.4	4.8 ± 0.3	3.0 ± 0.2	0.08 ± 0.01	0.06 ± 0.01
Les. side	4.7 ± 1.4	0.5 ± 0.2	0.6 ± 0.1	0.13 ± 0.04*	0.21 ± 0.04*†

[a]Rats had partial unilateral lesions of the dopaminergic nigrostriatal systems induced by injection of 6 μg of 6-hydroxydopamine into the substantia nigra. Two weeks after lesioning they were injected with morphine (20 mg/kg, 30 min before death), haloperidol (2.5 mg/kg, 60 min), or nicotine (1 mg/kg, 30 min). Concentrations are given in picomoles per gram wet weight (means ± S.E.M.; $n = 9$–11). *Different from corresponding side of control animals; †different from contralateral side; $P < 0.01$ (t-test).

DOPAC/DA and HVA/DA ratios to levels 2.2 and 3.0 times control values, respectively, i.e., to levels higher than those produced by the nigrostriatal lesion alone (Table I).

The findings indicate that dopaminergic neurons surviving a partial lesion of the nigrostriatal tract synthesize and release their transmitter at an elevated but still submaximal rate. Thus, pharmacological manipulation can further increase synthesis and release of DA by surviving neurons. Such increases were induced by drugs stimulating dopaminergic neurons by various mechanisms of action.

These findings prompt the speculation that synthesis and release of DA by nigrostriatal dopaminergic neurons remaining in a brain affected by neurodegenerative processes could be considerably increased by pharmacological manipulation above the elevated rates produced by the degeneration alone. Such increases in release of DA might postpone the appearance of behavioral deficits. These findings have special relevance to Parkinson's disease, which is characterized by a selective and progressive degeneration of the dopaminergic nigrostriatal neurons. Apparently, 80% of dopaminergic neurons have to be lost before parkinsonian symptoms become evident.[10,39] The adaptive increase in DA release by surviving dopaminergic neurons is believed to compensate for the lost DA up to this percentage of cell loss. With lesions affecting more than 80% of dopaminergic neurons, this adaptive process is insufficient, and behavioral deficits become manifest. Compounds further accelerating DA release from the surviving dopaminergic neurons might be able to extend the capacity of dopaminergic neurons for compensation and further postpone the appearance of clinical symptoms.

There is good evidence indicating that DA release by nigrostriatal neurons surviving in a parkinsonian brain can be further accelerated in a similar way as shown in rats with experimental lesions. In the human brain, rates of release of DA per neuron (as indicated by HVA/DA ratios) vary considerably among brain regions.[39] The rates are greatest in hippocampus and cortex, i.e., in areas with a small density of dopaminergic fibers. In the caudate nucleus, which receives a very dense dopaminergic innervation, the HVA/DA ratio is 10–30 times smaller than in cortical areas.[39] In brains from parkinsonian patients in whom a large proportion of dopaminergic neurons have degenerated, the HVA/DA ratio is elevated in the caudate nucleus[10,39] but not in cortex and hippocampus.[39] It therefore appears that nigrostriatal neurons of the human brain synthesize and release DA at rates far below the maximal rate for human dopaminergic neurons. The maximal rates might be reached by dopaminergic neurons innervating the cortex and hippocampus. Pharmacological manipulation might elevate synthesis rates in nigrostriatal neurons to the high levels at which dopaminergic cells projecting to the cortex operate.

Drugs used in the animal studies discussed were experimental tools that are, for various reasons, not useful in the treatment of Parkinson's disease. Therapeutically useful drugs would selectively stimulate synthesis and release of DA without acting on postsynaptic DA receptors and without interfering with other functions of the brain. As a first possibility, this might be achieved with selective antagonists of DA autoreceptors, which are thought to have an inhibitory influence on the synthesis and release of DA. However, the existence and selectivity of presynaptic DA receptors are still disputed.[34,47,48,52] Svensson *et al.*[73] have recently reported the development of selective antagonists for DA autoreceptors, which stimulated DA synthesis of neurons surviving a partial nigrostriatal lesion.[29]

Dopamine release by surviving nigrostriatal neurons could also be accelerated indirectly by drugs acting on other systems that exert an excitatory influence on dopaminergic neurons. Nicotine represents an example of such a compound, since it activates nigrostriatal neurons by a direct action in the substantia nigra.[53,54] A clinical trial with nicotine carried out in 1926 revealed significant improvement after nicotine in some patients.[62] However, the beneficial effects of nicotine were limited to a reduction in muscle rigidity, whereas other typical parkinsonian symptoms were not affected. Nicotine is consumed regularly by smokers, and several studies published during the last 20 years have shown that there are fewer smokers among parkinsonian patients than among healthy controls.[7,40,43,44,59,64] Smokers seem to have a smaller risk of being affected by Parkinson's disease. The cause for the protective effect of smoking is not known, but it can be speculated that nicotine is able to stimulate DA release from the remaining dopaminergic neurons so that persons with sufficiently large reductions in the number of dopaminergic neurons to become parkinsonian under normal conditions might not exhibit these symptoms when smoking. This would then result in a reduction of the percentage of smokers in the population of parkinsonian patients. However, the protective effect of smoking might be caused by other mechanisms.

The two possibilities discussed represent just the beginning approach to attempt to stimulate transmitter synthesis in the population of dopaminergic neurons that remain after an extensive lesion of the ascending mesencephalic DA system. Compounds selectively accelerating DA release of these neurons might help to alleviate Parkinson's disease.

5. Compensatory Changes in Postsynaptic Receptor Sensitivity

The actions of DA are mediated by specific receptors located on neurons postsynaptic to the dopaminergic cells. The corpus striatum contains D_1 receptors located on striatal interneurons and D_2 receptors located on interneurons and probably also on cortical afferents.[16] These subtypes are identified by specific ligands.[16,18,41] In addition, D_1 but not D_2 receptors are characterized by their ability to stimulate adenylate cyclase.[41,42] As is the case for several other examples of ligand–receptor interactions, it was shown that expression of DA receptors is influenced by the ligand concentration. In the absence of exposure to DA after lesions of nigrostriatal fibers, DA receptors in the striatum develop "supersensitivity." Initial evidence for this concept was derived from behavioral studies on animals with unilateral nigrostriatal lesions. Anden et al.[6] described rotational behavior in rats with unilateral electrolytic lesions that destroyed the nigrostriatal pathway. In subsequent studies, Ungerstedt and Arbuthnott[75] showed that the unilateral injection of 6-hydroxydopamine into the substantia nigra produced rotational behavior when animals were treated with DA agonists. They proposed a widely accepted model in which denervation of the striatum resulted in supersensitivity of dopaminergic receptors on the lesioned side, and DA agonists induced a behavioral asymmetry because of differential stimulation of DA receptors in the two striata. Despite many studies, the exact mechanism leading to the expression of rotational behavior is still not understood.[19,24,70]

The concept of DA receptor supersensitivity, which was derived from behavioral studies, was later confirmed using biochemical methods. Creese and Snyder[17] found that nigrostriatal lesions that support rotational behavior result in an elevation of the number of striatal D_2 receptor sites. In these studies receptors were analyzed in membrane fractions under equilibrium conditions. Denervation-induced supersensitivity of DA receptors in damaged striata in vivo was found by Neve et al.[65] but not by Bennett and Wooten,[8] who found no difference in accumulation of a DA ligand, injected intravenously, between lesioned and control striata. The difference between these results might reflect methodological aspects discussed by Perlmutter and Raichle.[68]

Behavioral and biochemical supersensitivity of DA receptors develops when more than 90% of the nigrostriatal neurons are destroyed. Apomorphine and other DA agonists, which induce circling by directly stimulating the supersensitive receptors in the striatum, were effective only in animals with reductions in DA levels larger than 90% of control values.[30,33] Similar findings were obtained in animals given L-dopa, which stimulates DA receptors by elevating striatal DA levels.[30,33] In addition, binding to postsynaptic DA receptors was reported to increase after nigrostriatal lesions of the same severity.[17]

Supersensitivity of postsynaptic DA receptors may represent an adaptive mechanism that contributes to the amelioration of deficits caused by a nigrostriatal lesion. However, the extent of this compensation is not clear. Rats with massive destruction in the nigrostriatal system associated with receptor supersensitivity show little behavioral deficit or asymmetry unless challenged pharmacologically or by behavioral stimulation.[30,33] These observations point to the possibility that postsynaptic receptor supersensitivity might contribute to the behavioral compensation. In contrast, in parkinsonian patients, behavioral deficits become apparent when approximately 70% of the dopaminergic neurons are destroyed, which is considerably earlier than the postsynaptic supersensitivity seen in the experimental model.[10,39]

The mechanism is not known by which reduced stimulation by DA leads to increased expression of DA receptors. Elucidation of this mechanism might

116   FRANZ HEFTI AND WILLIAM J. WEINER

reveal possibilities to enhance receptor expression pharmacologically. If available, such treatments might be used to enhance the expression of DA receptors in brains with smaller nigrostriatal lesions. In Parkinson's disease, drugs inducing the expression of DA receptors might postpone the manifestations of symptoms.

ACKNOWLEDGMENT. The authors gratefully acknowledge the support of the National Parkinson Foundation, Miami Florida.

REFERENCES

1. Acheson, A. L., Zigmond, M. J., and Stricker, E. M., 1979, Tyrosine hydroxylase and DOPAC in striatum after 6-hydroxydopamine, *Trans. Am. Soc. Neurochem.* **10**:142.
2. Aghajanian, G. K., and Bunney, B. S., 1977, Dopamine 'autoreceptors': Phrmacological characterization by microiontophoretic single cell recording studies, *Naunyn Schmiedebergs Arch. Exp. Pathol. Pharmacol.* **297**:1–7.
3. Agid, Y., Javoy, F., and Glowinski, J., 1973, Hyperactivity of remaining dopaminergic neurons after partial destruction of the nigrostriatal dopaminergic system in the rat, *Nature (New Biol.)* **245**:150–151.
4. Ahtee, L., and Kaarianen, J., 1973, The effect of narcotic analgesics on the homovanillic acid content of rat nucleus caudatus, *Eur. J. Pharmacol.* **22**:206–208.
5. Alper, R. H., Demarest, K. T., and Moore, K. E., 1980, Morphine differentially alters synthesis and turnover of dopamine in central neuronal systems, *J. Neural Transm.* **48**:157–165.
6. Anden, N. E., Corrodi, H., Fuxe, K., and Ungerstedt, U., 1971, Importance of nervous impulse flow for the neuroleptic induced increase in amine turnover in central dopamine neurons, *Eur. J. Pharmacol.* **15**:193–199.
7. Baumann, R. J., Jameson, H. D., McKean, H. E., Haack, D. G., and Weisberg, L. M., 1980, Cigarette smoking and parkinson disease: 1. A comparison of cases with matched neighbors, *Neurology (N.Y.)* **30**:839–843.
8. Bennet, J. P., and Wooten, G. F., 1986, Dopamine denervation does not alter in vivo 3H-spiperone binding in rat striatum: Implications for external imaging of dopamine receptors in Parkinson's disease, *Ann. Neurol.* **19**:378–383.
9. Benninger, R. J., 1983, The role of dopamine in locomotor activity and learning, *Brain Res. Rev.* **6**:173–196.
10. Bernheimer, H., Birkmayer, W., and Hornykiewicz, O., 1973, Brain dopamine syndromes of Parkinson and Huntington, *J. Neurol. Sci.* **20**:415–455.
11. Bullard, W. P., and Capson, T. L., 1983, Steady-state kinetics of bovine striatal tyrosine hydroxylase, *Mol. Pharmacol.* **23**:104–111.
12. Bunney, B. S., and Aghajanian, G. K., 1978, Mesolimbic and mesocortical dopaminergic systems; physiology and pharmacology, in: *Psychopharmacology—A Generation of Progress* (M. E. Lipton, K. C. Killam, and A. DiMascio, eds.), Raven Press, New York, pp. 159–186.
13. Bunney, B. S., Walters, J. R., Roth, R. H., and Aghajanian, G. K., 1973, Dopaminergic neurons: Effect of antipsychotic drugs and amphetamine on single cell activity, *J. Pharmacol. Exp. Ther.* **185**:560–568.
14. Calne, D. B., and Langston, J. W., 1983, Aetiology of Parkinson's disease, *Lancet* **2**:1457–1458.
15. Clark, D., Hjorth, S., and Carlsson, A., 1985, Dopamine-receptor agonists: Mechanism underlying autoreceptor selectivity. I. Review of the evidence, *J. Neural Transm.* **62**:1–52.

16. Creese, I., 1982, Dopamine receptors explained, *Trends Neurosci.* **5**:40–43.
17. Creese, I., and Snyder, S. H., 1979, Nigrostriatal lesions enhance striatal [³H]apomorphine and [³H]spiroperidol binding, *Eur. J. Pharmacol.* **56**:277–281.
18. Creese, I., Sibley, D. R., Hamblin, M. W., and Leff, S. E., 1983, The classification of DA receptors: Relationship to radioligand binding, *Annu. Rev. Neurosci.* **6**:43–71.
19. Crossman, A. R., Sambrook, M. A., Gorgies, S. W., and Salter, P., 1977, The neurological basis of motor asymmetry following unilateral 6-hydroxydopamine brain lesions in the rat: The effect of motor decortication, *J. Neurol. Sci.* **34**:407–414.
20. DiChiara, G., Porceddu, M. L., Spano, P. F., and Gessa, G. L., 1977, Haloperidol increases and apomorphine decreases striatal dopamine metabolism after destruction of striatal dopamine-sensitive adenylate cyclase by kainic acid, *Brain Res.* **130**:374–382.
21. Dyck, P. J., Stevens, J. C., and Mulder, D. W., 1975, Frequency of nerve fiber degeneration of peripheral motor and sensory neurons in amyotrophic lateral sclerosis: Morphometry of deep and superficial peroneal nerve, *Neurology (Minneap.)* **25**:781–785.
22. Engel, W. K., 1977, Motor neuron disorders, in: *Scientific Approaches to Clinical Neurology* (E. S. Goldensohn and S. H. Appel, eds.), Lea & Febiger, Philadelphia, pp. 1322–1346.
23. Fuxe, K., Hokfelt, T., and Ungerstedt, U., 1970, Morphological and functional aspects of central monoamine neurons, *Int. Rev. Neurobiol.* **13**: 93–115. Press, New York, p. 93.
24. Garcia-Munoz, M., Patino, P., Wright, A. J., and Arbuthnott, G. W., 1983, The anatomical substrate of the turning behavior seen after lesions in the nigrostriatal dopamine system, *Neuroscience* **8**:87–95.
25. Giorguieff, M. F. R., LeFloch, M. L., Westfall, T. C., Glowinski, J., and Besson, M. D., 1976, Nicotine effect of acetylcholine on the release of newly synthesized [³H]dopamine in rat striatal slices and cat caudate nucleus, *Brain Res.* **106**:117–131.
26. Giorguieff, M. F. R., LeFloch, M. I., Glowinski, J., and Besson, M. J., 1977, Involvement of cholinergic presynaptic receptors of nicotinic and muscarinic types in the control of the spontaneous release of dopamine form striatal dopaminergic terminals in the rat, *J. Pharmacol. Exp. Ther.* **200**:535–544.
27. Giorguieff-Chesselet, M. F., Kemel, M. L., Wandscheer, D., and Glowinski, J., 1979, Regulation of dopamine release by presynaptic nicotinic receptors in rat striatal slices: Effect of nicotine in a low concentration. *Life Sci.* **25**:1257–1262.
28. Hefti, F., 1980, A simple, sensitive method for measuring 3,4-dihydroxyphenylacetic acid and homovanillic acid in rat brain tissue using high-performance liquid chromatography with electrochemical detection, *Life Sci.* **25**:775–781.
29. Hefti, F., 1987, (1S, 1R)-5-Methoxy-1-methyl-2-(n-propylamino)tetralin ([+]-AJ-76) elevates transmitter synthesis in dopaminergic neurons surviving a partial nigrostriatal lesion, *Neuropharmacology,* 26:1239–1241.
30. Hefti, F., Melamed, E., and Wurtman, R. J., 1980, Partial lesions of the dopaminergic nigrostriatal system in rat brain: Biochemical characterization, *Brain Res.* **195**:123–137.
31. Hefti, F., Melamed, E., and Wurtman, R. J., 1980, Circling behavior in rats with partial, unilateral nigro-striatal lesions: Effect of amphetamine, apomorphine, and DOPA, *Pharmacol. Biochem. Behav.* **12**:185–188.
32. Hefti, F., Melamed, E., and Wurtman, R. J., 1981, The site of dopamine formation in rat striatum after L-DOPA administration, *J. Pharmacol. Exp. Ther.* **217**:189–197.
33. Hefti, F., Enz, A., and Melamed, E., 1985, Partial lesions of the nigrostriatal pathway in the rat. Acceleration of transmitter synthesis and release of surviving dopaminergic neurons by drugs, *Neuropharmacology* **24**:19–23.
34. Helmreich, I., Reimann, W., Hertting, G., and Starke, K., 1982, Are presynaptic dopamine autoreceptors and postsynaptic receptors in the rabbit caudate nucleus pharmacologically different? *Neuroscience* **7**:1559–1566.

35. Hornykiewicz, O., 1982, Brain neurotransmitter changes in Parkinson's disease, in: *Movement Disorders* (C. D. Marsden and S. Fahn, eds.), Butterworths, London, pp. 41–58.
36. Iversen, L. L., 1975, Biochemistry of biogenic amines, in: *Handbook of Psychopharmacology*, Volume 3, (L. L. Iverson, S. D. Iverson, and S. H. Snyder), Plenum Press, New York, pp. 381–411.
37. Iversen, S. D., 1977, Brain dopamine systems and behavior, in: *Handbook of Psychopharmacology*, Volume 8 (L. L. Iversen, S. D. Iversen, and S. H. Snyder, eds.), Plenum Press, New York, pp. 333–384.
38. Iwatsubo, K., and Clouet, D. H., 1977, Effects of morphine and haloperidol on the electric activity of rat nigrostriatal neurons, *J. Pharmacol. Exp. Ther.* **202**:429–436.
39. Javoy-Agid, F., Ruberg, M., Taquet, H. Y., Bobobza, B., Agid, Y., Gaspar, P., Berger, F., N'Guyen-Legros, J., Alvarez, C., Gray, F., Escourolle, R., Scatton, B., and Rouquier, L., 1984, Biochemical neuropathology of Parkinson's disease, *Adv. Neurol.* **40**:189–190.
40. Kahn, H. A., 1966, The Dorn study of smoking and mortality among U.S. veterans: A report on eight and one-half years of observation, in: *Epidemiological Approaches to the Study of Cancer and Other Chronic Diseases (National Cancer Institute Monograph No. 19)*, (W. Haenszel, ed.), Government Printing Office, Washington, D. C., pp. 127–204.
41. Kebabian, J. W., and Calne, D. B., 1979, Multiple receptors for DA, *Nature* **277**:93–96.
42. Kebabian, J. W., Agui, T., VanOene, J. C., Shigematsu, K., and Saavedra, J. M., 1986, The D_1 receptor: New perspectives, *Trends Pharmacol. Sci.* **3**:14–18.
43. Kessler, I. I., and Diamond, K. L., 1971, Epidemiologic studies of Parkinson's disease. I. Smoking and Parkinson's disease, *Am. J. Epidemiol.* **94**:16–25.
44. Kessler, I. I., 1972, Epidemiologic studies of Parkinson's disease. III. A communitiy based survey, *Am. J. Epidemiol.* **96**:242–254.
45. Koenig, J. F. R., and Klippel, R. A., 1963, *The Rat Brain. A Stereotaxic Atlas of the Forebrain and Lower Parts of the Brain Stem.* Williams & Wilkins, Baltimore.
46. Korf, J., Graddijk, L., and Westerink, B. H. C., 1976, Effects of electrical stimulation of the nigrostriatal pathway of the rat on dopamine metabolism, *J. Neurochem.* **26**:579–584.
47. Laduron, P. M., 1984, Lack of evidence for adrenergic and dopaminergic autoreceptors, *Trends Pharmacol. Sci.* **11**:459–461.
48. Laduron, P. M., 1985, Presynaptic heteroreceptors in regulation of neuronal transmission, *Biochem. Pharmacol.* **34**:467–470.
49. Langston, J. W., 1985, MPTP and Parkinson's disease, *Trends Neurosci.* **2**:79–83.
50. Langston, J. W., 1985, MPTP neurotoxicity: An overview and characterization of phases of toxicity, *Life Sci.* **36**:201–206.
51. Lazar, M. A., Lockfeld, A. J., Truscott, R. J. W., and Barchas, J. D., 1982, Tyrosine hydroxylase from bovine striatum: Catalytic properties of the phosphorylated and nonphosphorylated forms of the purified enzyme, *J. Neurochem.* **39**:409–422.
52. Leff, S. E., and Creese, I., 1983, Dopaminergic D-3 binding sites are not presynaptic autoreceptors, *Nature* **306**:586–589.
53. Lichtensteiger, W., Felix, D., Lienhart, R., and Hefti, F., 1976, A quantitative correlation between single unit activity and fluorescence intensity of dopamine neurons in zona compacta of substantia nigra, as demonstrated under the influence of nicotine and physostigmine, *Brain Res.* **117**:85–103.
54. Lichtensteiger, W., Hefti, F., Felix, D., Huwyler, T., Melamed, E., and Schlumpf, M., 1982, Stimulation of nigrostriatal dopamine neurons by nicotine, *Neuropharmacology* **21**:963–968.
55. Lindvall, O., and Bjorklund, A., 1978, Organization of catecholamine neurons in the rat central nervous system, in: *Handbook of Psychopharmacology*, Volume 9 (L. L. Iversen, S. D. Iversen, and S. H. Snyder, eds.), Plenum Press, New York, p. 139.
56. Lindvall, O., and Bjorklund, A., 1983, Dopamine- and norepinephrine-containing neuron systems: Their anatomy in the rat brain, in: *Chemical Neuroanatomy* (P. C. Emson, ed.), Raven Press, New York, pp. 229–255.

57. Lloyd, K. G., Davidson, L., and Hornykiewcz, O., 1975, The neurochemistry of Parkinson's disease: Effects of L-dopa therapy, *J. Pharmacol. Exp. Ther.* **195**:453–464.
58. Marchbanks, R. M., 1982, Biochemistry of Alzheimer's disease, *J. Neurochem.* **39**:9–15.
59. Martila, R. J., and Rinne, U. K., 1980, Smoking and Parkinson's disease, *Acta Neurol. Scand.* **62**:322–325.
60. Marsden, C. D., 1982, Basal ganglia disease, *Lancet* 1141–1146.
61. Matthews, R. T., and German, D. C., 1984, Electrophysiological evidence for excitation of rat ventral tegmental area dopamine neurons by morphine, *Neuroscience* **11**:617–625.
62. Moll, H., 1926, The treatment of post-encephalitic parkinsonism by nicotine, *Br. J. Med.* **26**:1079–1081.
63. Moore, R. Y., and Bloom, F. E., 1978, Central catecholamine neuron systems: Anatomy and physiology of dopamine systems, *Annu. Rev. Neurosci.* **1**:129–169.
64. Nefzger, M. D., Quadfasel, F. A., and Karl, V. C., 1967, A retrospective study of smoking and Parkinson's disease, *Am. J. Epidemiol.* **88**:149–158.
65. Neve, K. A., Kozlowski, M. R., and Marshall, J. F., 1982, Plasticity of neostriatal dopamine receptors after nigrostriatal injury: Relationship to recovery of sensorimotor functions and behavioral supersensitivity, *Brain Res.* **244**:33–44.
66. Nowycky, M. C., and Roth, R. H., 1978, Dopaminergic neurons: Role of presynaptic receptors in the regulation of transmitter biosynthesis, *Prog. Neuropsychopharmacol.* **2**:139–158.
67. Nowycky, M. C., Walters, J. R., and Roth, R. H., 1978, Dopaminergic neurons: Effect of acute and chronic morphine administration on single cell activity and transmitter metabolism, *J. Neural Transm.* **42**:99–116.
68. Perlmutter, J. S., and Raichle, M. E., 1986, *In vitro* and *in vivo* receptor binding: Where does the truth lie? *Ann. Neurol.* **19**:384–385.
69. Price, D. L., Struble, R. G., Whitehouse, P. J., Kitt, C. A., and Cork, L. C., 1985, Neuropathological processes in Alzheimer's disease, *Drug Dev. Res.* **5**:59–67.
70. Pycock, C. J., 1980, Turning behavior in animals, *Neuroscience* **5**:461–514.
71. Roberts, P. J., Woodruff, G. N., and Iversen, L. L. (eds.), 1978, *Dopamine. Advances in Biochemical Psychopharmacology,* Volume 19, Raven Press, New York.
72. Shoulson, I., and Chase, T. N., 1976, Huntington's disease, *Annu. Rev. Med.* **26**:419–426.
73. Svensson, K., Carlsson, A., Johansson, A. M., Arvidsson, L. K., and Nilsson, J. L. G., 1986, A homologous series of N-alkylated cis-(+)-(1S,2R)-5-methoxy-1-methyl-2-aminotetralins: Central dopamine receptor antagonists showing profiles ranging from classical antagonism to selectivity for autoreceptors, *J. Neural Transm.* **65**: 29–38.
74. Tranzer, J. P., and Thoenen, H., 1968, An electron microscopic study of selective, acute degeneration of sympathetic nerve terminals after administration of 6-hydroxydopamine, *Experientia* **24**:155–156.
75. Ungerstedt, U., and Arbuthnott, G. W., 1970, Quantitative recording of rotational behavior in rats after 6-hydroxydopamine lesions of the nigrostriatal system, *Brain Res.* **24**:485–493.
76. Walters, J. R., and Roth, R. H., 1974, Dopaminergic neurons: Drug induced antagonism of the increase in tyrosine hydroxylase activity produced by cessation of impulse flow, *J. Pharmacol. Exp. Ther.* **191**:82–91.
77. Walters, J. R., and Roth, R. H., 1976, Dopaminergic neurons: *In vivo* system for measuring drug interactions with presynaptic receptors, *Naunyn Schmiedebergs Arch. Pharmacol.* **296**:5–14.
78. Zigmond, M. J., Acheson, A. L., Stachowiak, M. K., and Stricker, E. M., 1984, Neurochemical compensation after nigrostriatal bundle injury in an animal model of preclinical parkinsonism, *Arch. Neurol.* **41**:856–861.

7

CATECHOLAMINES AND RECOVERY OF FUNCTION AFTER BRAIN DAMAGE

DENNIS M. FEENEY AND RICHARD L. SUTTON

ABSTRACT. Amphetamine (AMP) induces a temporary restoration of tactile placing responses in cats with unilateral sensorimotor cortex injury and an enduring acceleration of recovery in the hemiplegic rat and cat. Improved locomotor ability occurs within hours after a single dose of the drug, but only if experience is provided during the period of drug action. Following bilateral visual cortex ablation in cats, binocular depth perception is restored by four doses of AMP only if visual experience is given during the period of drug intoxication. These beneficial effects of AMP are blocked by haloperidol, which also retards recovery when given alone, implicating the catecholamines in recovery. The AMP effect on recovery has also been extended to rat models of stroke and cortical contusion. Although AMP analogues are beneficial in rat and cat hemiplegia models, drugs affecting primarily the dopamine system were not effective. Additional studies have implicated norepinephrine (NE) in the AMP effect. The maintenance of recovery may also depend on NE, since some α-noradrenergic antagonists reinstate hemiplegic symptoms in recovered animals. The cortical injuries produce a widespread metabolic depression, which is improved by AMP and worsened by haloperidol. The effects of AMP plus relevant experience treatment are most compatible with the theory of diaschisis or the concept of a "remote functional depression" after brain injury that is reversible by drug intervention. Preliminary data indicate that similar drug effects are produced in humans with brain injury, since some catecholamine antagonists retard recovery from aphasia, and AMP combined with physical therapy improves motor performance in hemiplegic stroke patients.

1. HISTORICAL BACKGROUND

1.1. TACTILE PLACING

Occasionally serendipity can play as important a role in furthering scientific progress as does a well-planned series of experiments. But, as has been said, "serendipity favors the prepared mind," and as a beginning assistant professor

DENNIS M. FEENEY AND RICHARD L. SUTTON • Departments of Psychology and Physiology, The University of New Mexico, Albuquerque, New Mexico 87131.

one of us (D.M.F.) was not prepared to recognize the importance of a research observation. I had been fascinated by the very short report on the transient restoration of visual and tactile placing in decorticate cats induced by amphetamine (AMP) as described by Meyer et al.[37] These data contradicted what I had been taught about brain function and was not incorporated into any modern conceptions of recovery of function to help explain the phenomenon (but see ref. 38). Meyer et al.[37] had used racemic AMP, and in the early 1970s it was widely accepted that the two isomers of AMP had markedly different actions on norepinephrine (NE) and dopamine (DA).

1.2. VISUAL CLIFF

In an unpublished study, I attempted to analyze the apparent restoration of the visual–motor reflex by administering the d or l isomers of AMP to cats with bilateral visual cortex ablations. To determine if the effect was on the visual or motor component of the reflex, I tested the cats on a visual cliff and gave the d or l isomers of AMP once a week (using a within-subjects design) to study the relative importance of the catecholamines (CA) in this effect. This seemed economical and appropriate, since the effect of AMP on the placing reflexes reportedly lasted only 12 hr, which we have verified quite recently for tactile placing.[17] Disappointingly, all of the cats completely recovered visual cliff performance after the second dose of AMP, an effect we attributed to incomplete lesions. Others[9] later reported no effect of AMP on this task. Failing to recognize a potentially important observation, we dropped the experiment and did not return to it for many years.

1.3. HEMIPLEGIC RAT MODEL

In the late 1970s our laboratory was investigating the behavioral, electrophysiological, and anatomic changes that correlate with spontaneous recovery of motor function after unilateral motor cortex contusion in the rat.[10,14] An undergraduate assistant, Abel Gonzalez, suggested that we put neurotransmitters into the wound to see if we could promote recovery of function (which R.L.S. recently did using transplants in the cat with striking results; see Section 3.5). Since we were conducting other experiments with AMP in the laboratory at that time, and this drug affects so many neurotransmitters, we decided to give AMP systemically. Much to our amazement, a single dose of AMP produced an immediate and enduring acceleration of recovery from hemiplegia as measured on a beam-walking task. This task reveals hemiplegic symptoms in animals with unilateral sensorimotor cortex injury quite clearly compared to observations of motor performance on a flat surface. In the beam-walk task, an animal is placed at one end of a narrow elevated beam close to a bright light and loud noise, and its ability to traverse the beam to a dark goal box is rated on a seven-point scale (see refs. 16 and 19 for details). In most of our subsequent experiments on recovery from hemiplegia in the rat, we have used a single dose of drug given 24 hr following suction ablation of the sensorimotor cortex.[15,16,19] Testing for any effects of drugs on recovery of this motor function is conducted over the following 2 to 3 weeks. In this paradigm AMP was so effective in alleviating symptoms that we stopped almost all other projects to investigate this phenomenon.

1.4. NOREPINEPHRINE AND THE IMPORTANCE OF EXPERIENCE

It is most important to note that a single dose of AMP alone was not effective in promoting recovery from hemiplegia.[16] To obtain the acceleration of recovery, the animals had to be tested on the beam-walking task during intoxication. If rats were confined in a small box to prevent major ballistic movements during the period of AMP action, no promotion of recovery was obtained. Furthermore, an enduring retardation of recovery was observed if a single dose of haloperidol (HAL) was given in place of AMP. This effect was also blocked by restricting motor experience during intoxication (see Fig. 1).

A dose–response study[15,19] using rats with unilateral motor cortex ablations indicated that 2 mg/kg of AMP was quite effective in promoting recovery from hemiplegia, but at 4 mg/kg, stereotypies appeared, and this dose was no more effective than the 2 mg/kg dose. A 1 mg/kg dose produced some promotion of recovery, but treated animals were not significantly different from saline controls. Because of the well-established link between the motor system and DA, the marked effect of AMP on DA, and the observation that the AMP promotion of recovery from hemiplegia was blocked by the CA antagonist HAL (see Fig. 1), we decided to test systematically the involvement of DA in this AMP effect. We examined the effect of the specific DA agonist apomorphine at a wide range of doses (0.02–20 mg/kg) in the rat beam-walking model and did not obtain any effect on recovery of function. A preliminary study with methylphenidate indicated no effect, but more recent work suggests beneficial effects on the hemiplegic rat.[48] Although methylphenidate affects both NE and DA,[42] results discussed in the following paragraph and the lack of any effect with apomorphine suggest that DA may not be mediating the AMP-induced recovery from hemiplegia.

Subsequent to some of this work we began to test for the role of NE in recovery of function and began to think that this drug modulation of recovery might be a general manifestation of neuroplasticity as proposed by Kasamatsu and Pettigrew[29,30] (but see refs. 3 and 50 for recent developments in this area). In his doctoral dissertation, Michael Boyeson noted that after a single intraventricular dose (100 μg/10 μl) of NE, but not DA, significant recovery of beam-walking ability was obtained in rats with unilateral sensorimotor cortex ablation. More recent dose–response studies (our laboratory and M. G. Boyeson, personal communication) indicate that higher doses of DA promote recovery from hemiplegia. However, the observation that the beneficial effects of 150 μg/μl of DA is blocked by pretreatment with FLA-57 (30 mg/kg i.p.; a

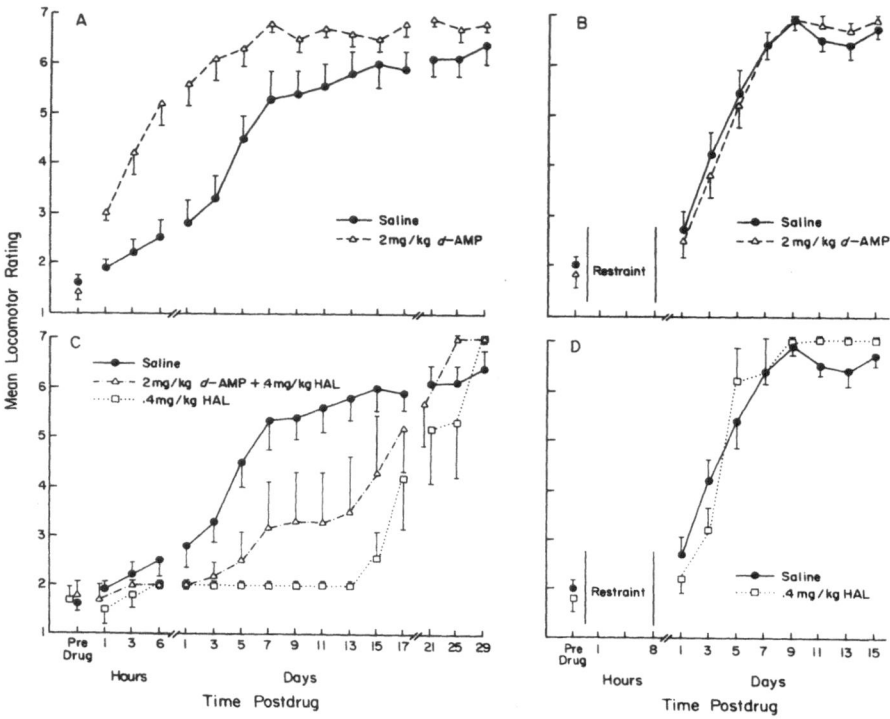

FIGURE 1. Mean ratings of beam walking after unilateral ablation of the rat sensorimotor cortex. Prior to surgery all animals received scores of 7. Note the enduring acceleration of recovery in animals given a single dose of *d*-amphetamine (AMP) 24 hr after surgery (A). This effect was blocked by preventing locomotion during drug intoxication (B) or by administering haloperidol (HAL) (C). The retardation of spontaneous recovery by HAL was also blocked by preventing locomotion (D). Vertical bars represent standard errors of the mean (S.E.M.). (Reproduced from Feeney *et al.*[16] Copyright 1982 by AAAS.)

dopamine–β-hydroxylase inhibitor) suggests that this effect is mediated by NE (M. G. Boyeson, personal communication). The time course of recovery induced by NE was almost identical to the AMP effect depicted in Fig. 1.[4,5] Compared to saline controls, animals given a single dose of AMP 24 hr after a right cortical lesion had reduced levels of NE but markedly higher levels of the NE metabolite 4-hydroxy-3-methoxyphenolglycol (MOPEG) in the left cerebellum at 18 days post-surgery. Based on proportional measures of NE/MOPEG, Boyeson suggested that the cerebellar NE system was turning over several times faster in AMP-treated animals, and this may have enabled the left cerebellum to compensate for the injured right sensorimotor cortex.

Boyeson[4] also replicated in the rat some interesting observations first made in cats after administration of the α-adrenergic antagonist phenoxybenzamine.[26] In animals recovered on the beam-walking task, a single dose of phenoxybenzamine reinstated the symptoms of hemiplegia. This reinstatement of deficits did not occur after administration of propranolol, a β-adrenergic antagonist. These data suggested that NE was involved in both recovery of function and the maintenance of that recovery after sensorimotor cortex injury.

1.5. HEMIPLEGIC CAT MODEL

David Hovda replicated and extended to cats the basic effect of a single dose of AMP plus experience on promoting recovery from hemiplegia.[24] After unilateral sensorimotor cortex ablation, the cat is much more severely impaired than the rat, and the hemiplegic symptoms on a beam-walking task (similar to that used in the rat) endure for months. Multiple injections of AMP, beginning on day 10 post-surgery (four treatments of 5 mg/kg spaced at 4-day intervals), were more effective in accelerating recovery than was a single dose. After each injection of AMP, some cats did not receive beam-walking experience during intoxication but were returned to a very large group cage rather than being restrained during intoxication. The lack of beam-walking experience after AMP administration prevented the beneficial effect of a single dose compared to animals tested under AMP influence. However, the multiple-injection regimen overrode this necessity for specific beam-walking experience. After the third dose of AMP, cats that were not tested on the beam during intoxication showed a significant improvement in their ability to walk the beam (during drug-free test sessions) and further improved after the fourth dose.

This finding suggested that the locomotor experience during AMP intoxication in the large home cage had eventually generalized to the beam-walking task, thus allowing for the recovery from hemiplegia.[24] The saline controls never recovered during the 60-day test period, whereas all of the treated groups recovered within the first 30 days. This study has several important clinical implications: (1) treatment can be effective even if delayed for days after injury; (2) multiple doses are much more effective than a single dose; (3) drug treatment may induce recovery to a level that could not be attained spontaneously; (4) physical therapy during AMP intoxication need not be tailored to all of the deficits exhibited by patients if multiple doses of AMP are administered.

1.6. BINOCULAR VISION

After extending our findings to the cat and developing the hypothesis that the AMP-plus-experience effect may be mediated by NE, we began to consider that the AMP effect on recovery of function was perhaps a subset of plasticity rather than an effect specific to the motor system. With this in mind, we reinvestigated the effect of AMP on visual cliff performance after bilateral visual cortex lesions in the cat.[18] This time we used a between-subjects design and housed some of the cats in the dark during intoxication to examine the role of experience in recovery of function after visual system injury. Only those cats that were housed in the light and tested on the visual cliff shortly after AMP injections (four doses given at 4-day intervals beginning 10 days after injury) showed any recovery of depth perception. This recovery depended on utilization of binocular cues, since these treated and recovered cats, as do normal cats, performed at chance levels during tests under monocular viewing conditions. Like the AMP effect after sensorimotor cortex ablations, this AMP-induced recovery of depth perception was also blocked by HAL.[25] Additionally, the effect in reinstating depth perception was dependent on visual experience during intoxication, since even after seven injections of AMP the animals kept in the dark after AMP administration showed no recovery[18]; unlike motor behavior, visual experience can be completely controlled.

This effect of AMP on recovery of depth perception after cortical lesions in cat was later replicated and extended using a visual cliff apparatus designed to determine visual thresholds and more extensive cortical ablations including the lateral suprasylvian gyrus.[22,27] These observations of restoration of depth perception by drug treatments may be clinically relevant, since these experiments are the first we know of that show an enduring restoration of a "permanently" lost behavior by short-term drug treatment combined with experience. Thus, patients may not only recover more quickly but also may attain a higher level of ultimate function if they are given appropriate treatment after brain trauma.

2. THEORETICAL BASES

As described above, this treatment approach was initially a serendipitous observation and not tied to any theoretical position of recovery of function (see ref. 21 for discussion of theories of recovery of function). However, with continuing research we have considered (and discarded) some theoretical explanations and developed some working hypotheses.

2.1. MORPHOLOGICAL CHANGES

Since the promotion of recovery is so rapid, appearing on the first testing session 1 hr after a single AMP treatment (see Fig. 1), this would exclude morphological changes such as sprouting to explain these effects. This leaves several other hypotheses: (1) the taking over of function by some homologous brain region and this process of vicariation being accelerated by drug-plus-experience treatment; (2) the AMP-plus-experience regimen possibly unmasking "silent synapses"; (3) the acquisition of new behavioral strategies or "behavioral substitution"; (4) drug-induced alterations in cerebral blood flow (CBF); or (5) a treatment-induced alleviation of a "remote functional depression" (RFD) of cerebral metabolism,[20] a revision of some aspects of von Monakow's[13,52] theory of diaschisis. We have focused on the latter hypothesis since our data appear to reduce the importance of, if not exclude, the other theories (although other mechanisms may play some role in these effects).

2.2. VICARIATION

If intact cortical tissue is somehow stimulated by drug treatment to assume "vicariously" the functions of ablated tissue, the contralateral homologous cortex would be the most likely candidate to mediate recovery of function. Since the AMP-induced recovery is obtained after bilateral visual cortex ablation,[18,27] this would argue against that interpretation. Additionally, this hypothesis of cortical vicariation has been tested for the locomotor system using cats with bilateral frontal cortex ablations.[47] Saline-treated cats showed no significant recovery of beam-walking ability in 30 days after these lesions, whereas cats given three injections of AMP showed marked and significant recovery. This effect was obtained in cats with lesions restricted to the sensorimotor cortex as well as in cats with massive frontal ablations, indicating that neither the contralateral cortex nor tissue immediately adjacent to sensorimotor regions is needed for the AMP-induced recovery of locomotor ability.

The unmasking of silent synapses has not been directly investigated in our models of recovery but seems an unlikely explanation since after some CNS lesions the effect takes some time to appear, although rapid cortical reorganization has been reported following peripheral nerve section (see ref. 53 for a partial review). Interestingly, drugs (including the CA precursor L-dopa) can transiently modify the dermatomes in the monkey using the classical isolated dorsal root model,[12] and similar drug-induced alterations may be occurring in cortically damaged animals.

2.3. BEHAVIORAL SUBSTITUTION

Similarly, the acquisition of new behavioral strategies by brain-damaged animals would take at least two, if not multiple, trials. In our rat and cat hemiplegia models, the treated animals given task-relevant experience are significantly better than the saline controls on the very first trial after AMP injection. Experience during the period of drug action may serve to make recovery enduring rather than transient. However, this explanation cannot account for the AMP effect on placing reflexes after cortical ablation,[17,37] where only transient reinstatement of behavioral function is obtained.

2.4. CEREBRAL BLOOD FLOW AND CHOLINERGIC SYSTEM

The dosage of AMP used in our rat hemiplegia model studies does increase CBF,[43] which may cause changes that interact with experience to produce immediate and enduring changes in brain function. To test this hypothesis, Michael Boyeson (personal communication) has examined the AMP effect in the rat hemiplegia model after pretreatment with atropine, which blocks the AMP increase in CBF.[43] As illustrated in Fig. 2, AMP (2 mg/kg) significantly acceler-

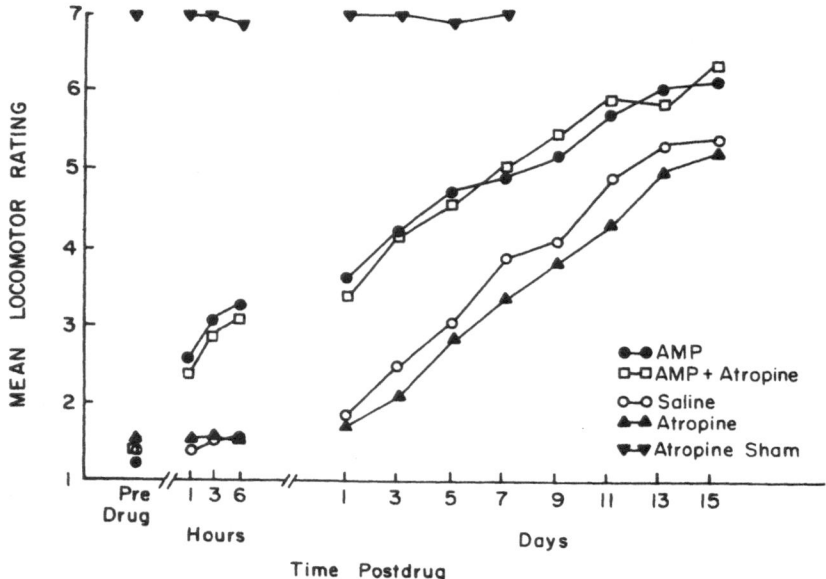

FIGURE 2. Mean ratings of beam walking after unilateral ablation of the rat sensorimotor cortex. Prior to surgery all animals received scores of 7. Note the enduring acceleration of recovery in animals given a single dose of *d*-amphetamine (AMP; 2 mg/kg) or a dose of AMP plus atropine (4 mg/kg), which would block the effect of AMP on CBF. This dose of atropine alone did not affect recovery rate as compared to spontaneous recovery exhibited by saline controls. The possibility that this effect is caused by sedation seems unlikely, since atropine (4 mg/kg) given to sham operates did not affect beam-walking ability. (These data are reproduced with permission from Dr. Michael G. Boyeson.)

ated recovery compared to saline controls ($F_{1,14} = 5.69$, $P < 0.039$), and the combined atropine (4 mg/kg)-plus-AMP (2 mg/kg) group also showed significantly better recovery on the beam-walking task compared to saline controls ($F_{1,14} = 4.93$, $P < 0.043$). Atropine (4 mg/kg) alone did not alter the rate of recovery from that observed in saline controls with unilateral sensorimotor cortex ablation. These data indicate that the AMP effect is not caused by alterations in CBF or by effects of AMP on cholinergic muscarinic receptors, reinforcing our interpretation that the basis for the AMP effect in promoting recovery from hemiplegia is the drug's effect on the CAs. Furthermore, muscarinic receptor blockade does not appear to influence, positively or negatively, spontaneous recovery from hemiplegia (Fig. 2).

2.5. DIASCHISIS, RFD, AND METABOLIC STUDIES

Based on preliminary data, we[19,20] have proposed that recovery after cortical injury may depend on the alleviation of RFD, which is a modern revision of von Monakows'[13,52] theory of diaschisis. Unilateral sensorimotor cortex injury evokes a widespread depression of cortical metabolism in the ipsilateral hemisphere as revealed by staining for the oxidative enzyme α-glycerophosphate dehydrogenase[10] (α-GPDH; see Fig. 3). This injury-induced depression of metabolism is blocked by AMP, and this effect is prevented if HAL is administered concomitant with AMP.[20] Lesions of the locus coeruleus (LC) prior to cortical injury shortened the time to onset of α-GPDH cortical paling, indicating that NE and projections from this noradrenergic nucleus mediate the metabolic depression.[20] Apomorphine, which does not enhance behavioral recovery,[48] also did not alter cortical paling of the enzyme stain in the hemiplegic rat model.[20]

Additionally, preliminary evidence from the ablation model of hemiplegia revealed a global reduction of cerebral [^{14}C]2-deoxyglucose utilization 48 hr

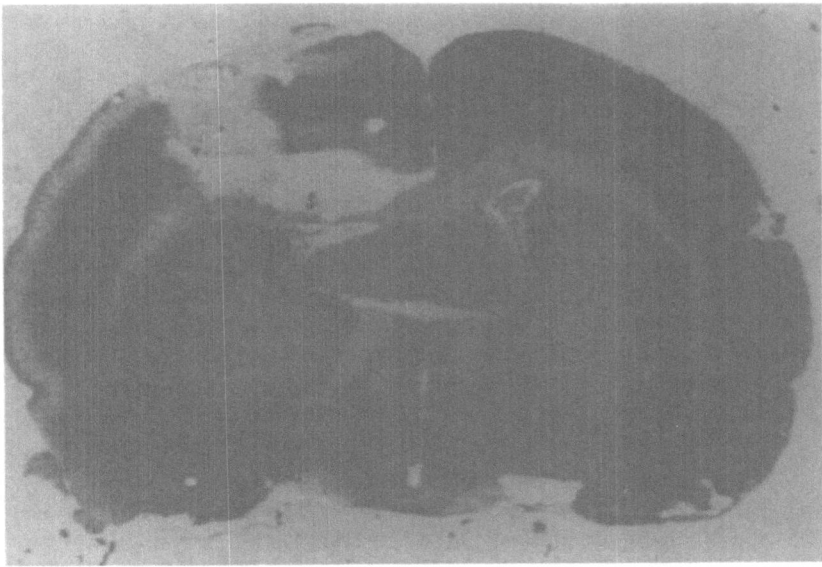

FIGURE 3. Histochemical stain for α-glycerophosphate dehydrogenase (α-GPDH) of a section through the area of a contusion injury to rat cortex. The cortical contusion produced an area of necrotic cavitation at the top of the cortex of the left hemisphere that expanded into the underlying white matter. Note the reduced staining for the oxidative enzyme α-GPDH through the entire cortex ipsilateral to the injury (compared to the contralateral cortex) but remote from the locus of primary damage. This reduced α-GPDH cortical staining was observed throughout the cortex of the entire hemisphere even at sites quite remote from areas of morphological damage. This widespread reduction of metabolism ipsilateral to cortical injury could be blocked by amphetamine (but not apomorphine), and this amphetamine effect is prevented by concomitant haloperidol administration. Thus, the α-GPDH response to cortical injury reacts to drug manipulation in parallel with recovery from the behavioral symptoms of hemiplegia after cortical damage. Lesions of the locus coeruleus alone had no effect on α-GPDH but, when made prior to the cortical injury, shortened the time to onset of the α-GPDH paling. This suggests a role for this noradrenergic nucleus in the behavioral and α-GPDH responses to focal cortical injury. (See refs. 10 and 20 and the text for details.)

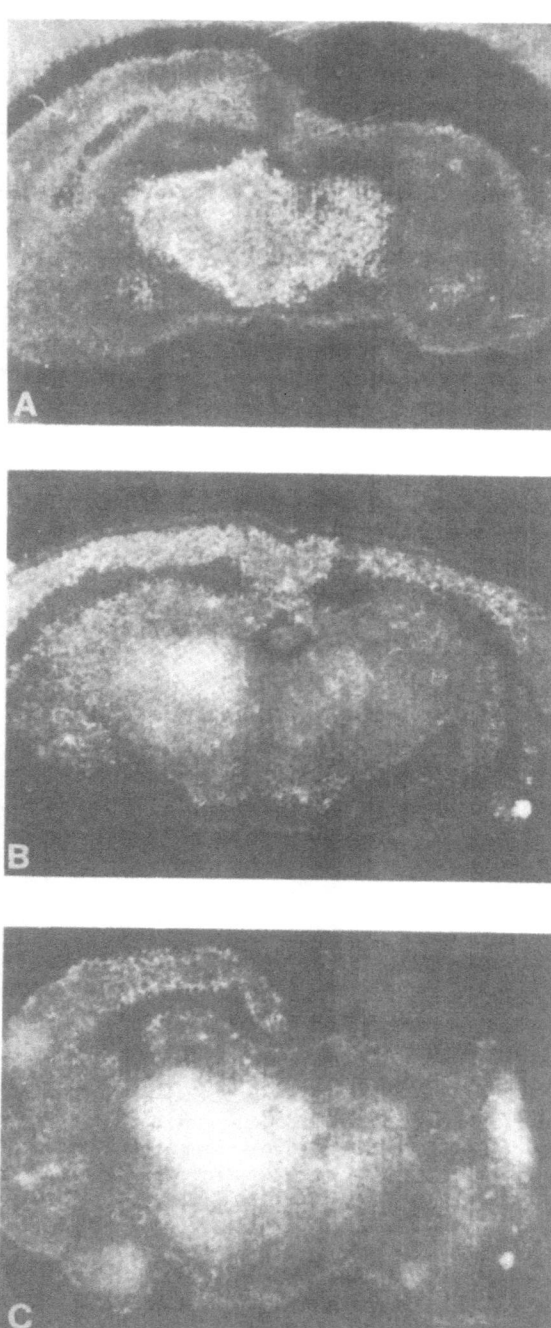

after cortical injury.[20] The effects of HAL and AMP on this measure of glycolytic metabolism parallel their effects on recovery of function. That is, HAL worsens the metabolic depression, and AMP greatly improves glucose utilization after this injury in the rat (see Fig. 4). The effect of AMP on the postinjury cerebral metabolic depression is most prominent in the cerebellum, red nucleus, and vicinity of the LC, thus alleviating a metabolic depression that may be related to the "crossed cerebellar diaschisis" or RFD seen in humans with hemiplegia secondary to supratentorial infarcts.[1,2] However, it should be noted that hypometabolism in the cerebellum contralateral to supratentorial infarct or tumor does not consistently correlate with behavioral symptoms such as hemiplegia.[13,31,39]

Based on this set of data, one general working hypothesis is that after cortical injuries there is a metabolic depression in systems remote from the site of injury, involving circuitry implicated in the performance of some of the functions lost after injury. Behavioral function may spontaneously recover with time as this RFD dissipates, much like von Monakow's hypothetical diaschisis, or this process may be accelerated and/or retarded by pharmacological manipulations. Diaschisis[13,19,52] was circularly defined—i.e., its presence and dissipation were based solely on the clinical observation of the spontaneous remission of some symptoms after brain injury—and as originally proposed was nothing more than a descriptive term for this phenomenon.[52] However, modern techniques may be useful for determining potential underlying physiological mechanisms for this concept.[13] The construct of RFD is a more limited and modern construct and may be preferable to the more global and often misused concept of diaschisis.[13,19] Additionally, RFD has been anchored to depressed cerebral metabolism that is alleviated by drugs that facilitate behavioral recovery and worsened by drugs slowing recovery in the rat hemiplegia model.[20] However, RFD only applies to depressed function after brain injury, although pathological excitation may also produce behavioral symptoms and should be included in a modern revision of the theory of diaschisis.[13]

The CAs are also known to be depressed after cortical injuries (see refs. 19

FIGURE 4. Black-and-white photographs of computer-enhanced color images of autoradiographs. Darker regions indicate low glucose utilization, whereas lighter regions indicate higher metabolic activity. (A) [^{14}C]2-Deoxyglucose (2-DG) utilization 48 hr after unilateral sensorimotor cortex ablation in a saline-treated animal. Note darkened cortex ipsilateral (right) and contralateral (left) to injury, indicating widespread reduction of 2-DG uptake and metabolism. This section was taken approximately 0.5 mm posterior to ablation. (B) 2-Deoxyglucose utilization in an uninjured rat. This section was taken approximately 1.5 mm posterior to bregma. (C) 2-Deoxyglucose utilization 48 hr after unilateral sensorimotor cortex ablation in an amphetamine (2 mg/kg)-treated animal. Note the increased 2-DG uptake throughout cortical and subcortical areas compared with the saline-treated animal, indicating that amphetamine is alleviating a widespread metabolic depression. This section was taken approximately 0.5 mm posterior to injury. (Reproduced from Feeney et al.[20] Copyright 1986 by Psychonomic Society Inc.).

and 20 for a partial review and references), and alleviation of a CA RFD by AMP may "enable" intact "performance" structures to respond to the environment. This interaction seems to produce an enduring change in these performance structures and accelerate spontaneous recovery. The reinstatement of "permanently" lost behaviors may reflect a similar process, or the drug may be correcting a system imbalance analogous to that demonstrated by Sprague[45] after unilateral cortical ablation. We stress that this formulation can only be considered a working hypothesis at present, and such a process may only account for some types of recovery of function.

3. RECENT DATA

3.1. CYTOCHROME OXIDASE

We[46] have just completed work on the effects of unilateral sensorimotor cortex ablations and/or AMP treatment in the rat using another measure of cerebral oxidative metabolism, the cytochrome oxidase (CYO) histochemical stain developed by Wong-Riley.[55] In this study, rats were given AMP (2 mg/kg) or saline 24 hr after surgery and sacrificed for CYO histochemistry 24 hr later. Spot densitometry readings in various structures indicated that unilateral brain injury produced bilateral reductions in CYO activity in many regions including the globus pallidus, subthalamic and red nuclei, LC, and the cerebellum. Amphetamine (2 mg/kg) reversed this effect of the injury, increasing CYO activity bilaterally in all of these structures. Thus, these data are consistent with the notion of RFD of metabolic function occurring in structures involved with locomotor performance that are remote from the site of injury, and this RFD is alleviated by AMP administration. We have also found a similar restitution of CYO activity long after discontinuation of AMP treatment,[22,28] which indicates that the AMP-induced alterations of oxidative metabolism do not simply reflect an immediate postintoxication effect of drug treatment.

3.2. IDAZOXAN

Other recent experiments have provided additional evidence that NE mediates the AMP effect on recovery of locomotor ability after sensorimotor cortex ablation. Tyson et al.[51] have replicated the basic effect of AMP (2 mg/kg) in the hemiplegic rat model. Administration of the selective α_2 antagonist idazoxan (1 mg/kg), which should enhance NE release by disinhibiting presynaptic NE terminals and/or autoreceptors of the LC, did not enhance recovery of function compared to saline controls (see Fig. 5). However, when idazoxan (1 mg/kg) was given prior to AMP (2 mg/kg), it blocked the AMP effect in rats with unilateral sensorimotor cortex ablations (Fig. 5). These preliminary data suggest that the NE released by AMP may be affecting recovery through actions on α_2 receptors. It may be that the released NE is acting on presynaptic α_2 receptors,

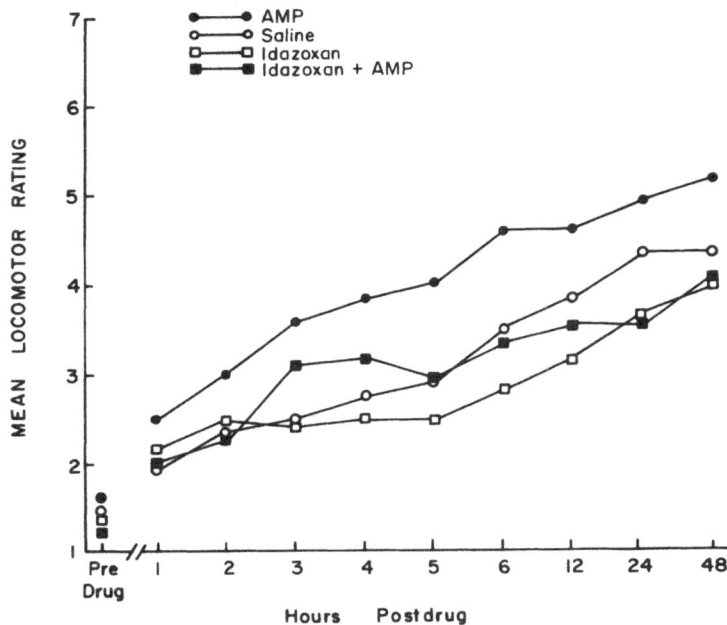

FIGURE 5. Mean beam-walking scores for rats after unilateral ablation of the sensorimotor cortex. All animals scored 7 prior to injury. Note the acceleration of recovery from hemiplegia after a single dose of *d*-amphetamine (AMP; 2 mg/kg) as compared to saline controls. Administration of a single dose of the selective α_2 antagonist idazoxan (1 mg/kg) did not affect spontaneous recovery rate. Coadministration of this dose of idazoxan with AMP blocked the AMP-induced acceleration of recovery, indicating that noradrenergic α_2 receptors may be mediating the AMP effect. (See text for more recent data and comments on interpretation of these results.)

shutting down the LC and other noradrenergic nuclei via feedback inhibition mechanisms, although effects on postsynaptic α_2 adrenoceptors cannot be ruled out at this time. To clarify the role of various noradrenergic receptors in the NE mediation of the AMP effect,[5,51] dose–response studies using a variety of noradrenergic agonists and antagonists are in progress. The importane of dose–response studies is underscored by the recent observation that a 2 mg/kg dose of idazoxan does promote recovery of the hemiplegic rat. Additionally, careful behavioral analyses are crucial even when using apparently simple behavioral tasks. For example, recent work indicates that idazoxan-induced blockade of the AMP effect on recovery is due to the induction of stereotypies (L. B. Goldstein and J. N. Davis, personal communication).

3.3. LOCUS COERULEUS AND CEREBELLUM

Boyeson *et al.*[6] have gathered preliminary data that support the notion that the LC and NE are critically involved in the recovery of beam-walking ability.

They made unilateral (or sham) lesions of the LC in rats (which did not affect beam-walking), followed by ablation of the ipsilateral sensorimotor cortex 2 weeks later. Animals were given a single infusion of NE or vehicle into the cerebellum contralateral to injury 24 hr after cortical ablation. This NE treatment permanently accelerated recovery above vehicle control levels when the LC was intact. The LC-lesioned and ablated rats that received NE infusion into the cerebellum recovered beam-walking ability within 6 hr of this treatment, but the effect was drug dependent. These data suggest that the hypothesis[20] of an NE-induced alleviation of RFD (e.g., in the cerebellum after cortical injury) is viable.

In an effort to determine if AMP would prove beneficial in cases of stroke, Ann Salo[44] developed an animal model of embolic stroke for her doctoral dissertation research. Using a morbidity index modified from McGraw et al.[36] and a peg-walking locomotor task such as developed by Watson and McElligott,[54] Salo found that continuous minipump infusion of AMP at 1 mg/kg per day for 7 days reduced both morbidity and mortality in infarcted rats. None of the animals given AMP died from the experimental strokes (homologous blood clots injected via chronic cannulae into the carotid artery without anesthesia), whereas half of the animals given saline via the minipumps died. The beneficial effects of AMP on morbidity (including locomotor ability) and mortality in this experimental model of stroke were both significantly different from saline controls. The prevention of mortality was both an unexpected and exciting finding and needs further investigation.

3.4. Phentermine and Phenylpropanolamine

Given the frequency of human cases of trauma or hemhorrhagic stroke, where any increase of blood pressure would be an undesirable risk factor, the use of CA agonists that have weaker cardiovascular side effects than AMP would seem desirable. We have tested some of these drugs using the beam-walking paradigm and found that some can also promote recovery from hemiplegia in rat and cat. For example, a single injection of phentermine (6, 12, or 24 mg/kg) given 24 hr after unilateral sensorimotor cortex ablation in rat produces effects similar to those reported for AMP, particularly at the 12 mg/kg dose. Phentermine (15 mg/kg) was also tested in cats with unilateral sensorimotor cortex lesions, and, like AMP, this drug produces an enduring acceleration of recovery from hemiplegia and transiently reinstates tactile placing responses in the forelimb contralateral to injury.[23,48]

The effect of phenylpropanolamine (PPA) has also been examined in the rat hemiplegia model.[19] This drug significantly accelerated recovery from hemiplegia above that of saline controls, although PPA was not as effective in this model as is AMP or phentermine. This may reflect the use of less than optimal doses (10 to 20 mg/kg) or the fact that PPA exerts fewer CNS effects than do the more effective drugs. However, these findings are promising, and this drug and other AMP analogues need further investigation.

3.5. Transplants

As was mentioned above, AMP only temporarily restores visual or tactile placing responses in brain-injured animals. To determine whether or not prolonged exposure to CAs would extend the recovery of such responses, we transplanted CA-secreting adrenal medulla chromaffin cells to the injury site of unilateral frontal cortex-ablated cats.[49] This treatment proved effective for inducing recovery from hemiplegia, as cats receiving transplants at 21 days after cortical injury recovered to presurgical levels on the beam-walking task earlier than did cats given chromaffin cell grafts 12 days post-injury or an adrenalectomy control animal. Furthermore, these "late" transplant cats also showed variable but enduring restoration of tactile placing responses (up to 10 months after grafting was performed). We proposed that the surviving grafted cells acted as endogenous minipumps, actively secreting CAs, and thus produced an enduring behavioral recovery.

3.6. Cortical Contusion

Since traumatic brain injury may respond to treatments differently than ablation or stroke models, we have begun to investigate the basic AMP effect in a model of cortical contusion, using a weight-drop method.[14] We have studied recovery of beam-walking ability in rats with unilateral contusion injury to the sensorimotor cortex using various impact forces. As can be seen in Fig. 6, a single dose of AMP given 24 hr after a 400 g-cm contusion injury was effective in accelerating recovery from hemiplegia compared to the spontaneous recovery rates for saline controls with this type of injury ($F_{1,8} = 16.99$, $P < 0.01$). However, AMP was not effective in accelerating recovery after a contusion injury of 800 g-cm, even when a second injection was administered to rats on day 3 post-injury. Although histological and biochemical analyses are not yet completed on these animals, we suspect that the additional subcortical damage (e.g., to the caudate, hippocampus, or brainstem) induced by the 800 g-cm impact force is preventing any beneficial effects of drug treatment.

We have also tested for drug effects on recovery of forepaw dexterity after contusion injury of the right sensorimotor cortex. For these studies, rats on a 22:2 hr food deprivation schedule were trained to reach for food pellets with their left forepaw to a criterion of nine out of ten successes (i.e., reaching for, grasping, and retrieving the pellets) on 3 successive days prior to surgery. After injury, errors on this task consisted primarily of inability to grasp the food pellets or successful reach and grasping of pellets but subsequent dropping of the pellets when the rats attempted to retrieve and consume the pellet. A trauma dose–response effect on deficits in forepaw dexterity was observed (see Fig. 7), with more severe deficits and slower spontaneous recovery evident after an 800 g-cm

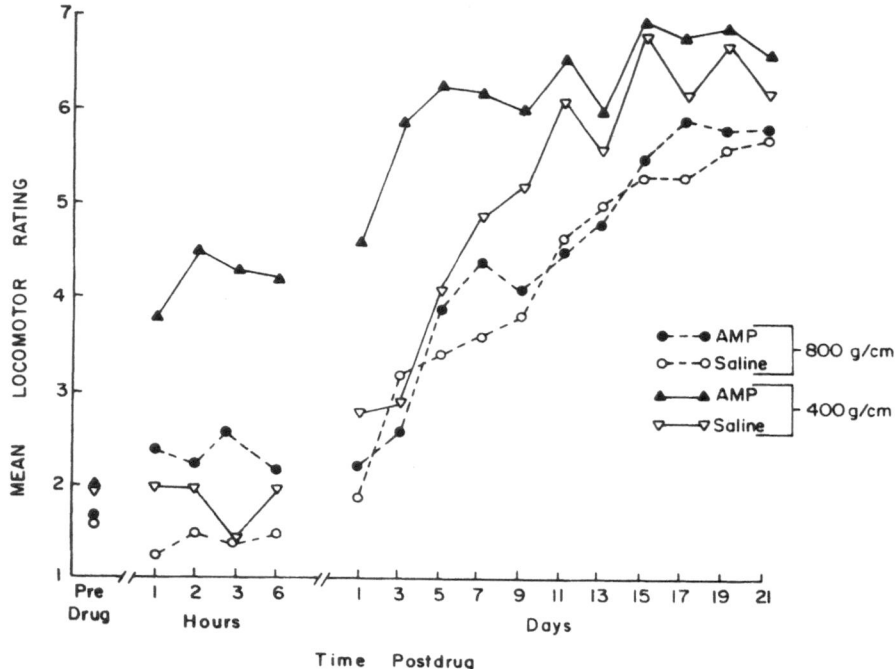

FIGURE 6. Mean ratings of beam walking after unilateral contusion injury to the sensorimotor cortex of rat. Note that a single dose of d-amphetamine (AMP; 2 mg/kg) given 24 hr after a 400 g-cm injury force was effective in accelerating recovery as compared to spontaneous recovery shown by saline-treated animals with this degree of injury. However, this dose of AMP did not affect recovery after an 800 g-cm contusion injury even though a second injection was given to these animals on day 3 postinjury (hourly testing data after the second injection are not shown).

as compared to a 400 g-cm contusion impact. As can be seen in Fig. 7, a single dose of AMP (2 mg/kg) given to animals with a 400 g-cm contusion 24 hr post-injury did not significantly alter recovery of forepaw dexterity as compared to saline controls ($P > 0.05$). Similarly, as compared to saline controls, no beneficial effects of AMP on performance of this task was observed in rats with an 800 g-cm contusion injury even though AMP was administered at both 24 and 72 hr after injury ($P > 0.10$). Furthermore, no additional improvement in animals' ability to reach, grasp, and retrieve food pellets was seen beyond the period illustrated in Fig. 7, although testing was continued through day 85 after injury.

3.7. CLINICAL DATA

There have been a few reports that pharmacological agents employed in our animal models have similar effects in patients with brain injury. Two case reports

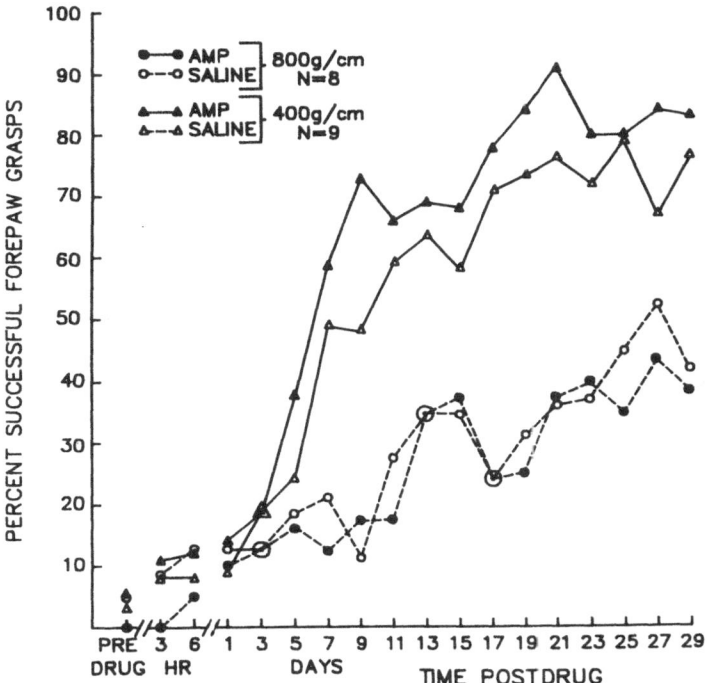

FIGURE 7. Mean percentage successful retrieval of food pellets with the left forepaw by rats with contusion injury of the right sensorimotor cortex. Note the greater initial deficits and slower rates of recovery by animals in the 800 g-cm impact groups as compared to those in the 400 g-cm groups. Administration of AMP (2 mg/kg) 24 hr after a 400 g-cm contusion and at 24 and 72 hr after an 800 g-cm contusion did not significantly affect recovery of forepaw dexterity.

have noted that AMP reduces some symptoms in brain-injured humans.[7,32] One study reported beneficial effects of AMP on a very mixed sample of patients including some with stroke but did not use placebo controls or objective measures of recovery.[8] Only recently has a double-blind, placebo-controlled study examined the effect of AMP on recovery in stroke patients with objective tests of recovery.[11] Eight highly selected patients with hemiparesis were followed for 24 hr post-drug in this pilot study. Within 10 days of a first ischemic stroke, patients were randomly assigned to receive either a single oral dose of 10 mg of AMP or placebo. To provide the necessary experience during intoxication, drug and placebo patients were given approximately 1 hr of intensive physical therapy. Compared to placebo controls, the patients receiving AMP showed significant improvement on objective measures of motor performance when retested the day after treatment. Importantly, AMP had no effect on blood pressure or heart rate in these patients. Like the effect in the rat, this motor improvement is not likely a result of an AMP-induced increase in CBF, since even higher doses of AMP in normal volunteers do not significantly increase regional CBF.[35]

3.8. DRUG CONTRAINDICATIONS

Other retrospective studies on recovery from aphasia after stroke have suggested that thiazides, some antihypertensives, and HAL may retard recovery and are contraindicated in stroke cases.[40,41] These patients were receiving speech therapy and monthly testing for aphasia, and those receiving some drugs scored significantly lower than patients not receiving medication and also scored below their expected levels of spontaneous recovery. In one patient, administration of HAL worsened aphasic symptoms, and his recovery of language ability was slowed (compared to predicted ability) for months after discontinuation of drug treatment (see Fig. 6 in ref. 19). This finding is reminiscent of the HAL-induced reinstatement of tactile placing deficits in cats that had spontaneously recovered this reflex after small unilateral sensorimotor cortex ablation.[17]

4. FUTURE DIRECTIONS

4.1. MECHANISMS

There are two complementary lines of research that should be undertaken to further our understanding of the role of the CAs in recovery of function. First, more basic research investigating the underlying mechanisms of the AMP effect in animal models of recovery of function is needed. This would include behavioral, biochemical, histochemical, pharmacological, and neurophysiological investigations. Second, long-term clinical trials must be undertaken using patients with various types of cerebral injuries and deficits to determine fully the potential clinical utility of this treatment (such trials with stroke patients are currently under way at several centers). Animal studies indicate that this treatment is not a panacea. The AMP-plus-experience treatment has no beneficial effect on recovery of locomotor function after cerebellar injury[5] or on recovery of forepaw dexterity (see Fig. 7) or on locomotor recovery after more severe (i.e., 800 g-cm) cortical contusion (see Fig. 6). The spectrum of symptoms of brain injury that may benefit from this treatment regimen as well as the limiting factors remain to be fully delineated.

Although our pharmacological data indicate an important, and perhaps central, role for NE in recovery after cortical injury, there are substantial gaps in our understanding of the mechanisms of the AMP effect in recovery of function. Others have shown beneficial effects of CAergic agents on recovery from septal nucleus lesions[34] or after amygdaloid lesions,[33] and these drug effects are apparently mediated by DA. Our pharmacological data indicate a primary role of NE in the recovery of some symptoms after sensorimotor cortex injuries. However, firm conclusions can only be reached after additional biochemical studies are conducted and by observing similar behavioral effects of several purported agonists and opposite actions of antagonists, and such studies are ongoing.

To accelerate recovery, AMP plus experience has been given early (within 10 days post-injury in cat and post-stroke in man) after injury, and some data suggests that this may be essential.[18] Whether or not this treatment regimen must be initiated early after injury to benefit recovery of function needs to be systematically studied. Furthermore, we have only limited data directly measuring drug effects on the proposed RFD, although these data do suggest that only those pharmacological manipulations affecting behavioral recovery after brain injury also affect RFD. To test the CA–RFD hypothesis, drugs that affect recovery of behavior after cortical trauma must be further studied together with direct and quantifiable indices of neuronal function (metabolic, biochemical, and electrophysiological).

4.2. OPTIMIZING THERAPY

Finally, it is most likely that pharmacotherapy will have to be tailored to the particular conditions of each patient. Relevant factors will include the severity and pattern of behavioral deficits, the locus and extent of CNS injury, the mode of brain damage (e.g., hemhorrhagic or ischemic stroke, trauma, tumor), the time after injury, and the age of the person. Perhaps a sequence of different (or combinations of) pharmacological treatment regimens (such as those discussed in other chapters of this book) will be necessary, dependent on these considerations. Such clinical problems must be addressed by experimental studies in order to establish a scientific basis for obtaining optimal recovery of function in the brain-injured patient. Finding the answer to these clinical questions will take considerable effort and extensive interdisciplinary investigation.

ACKNOWLEDGMENTS. We would like to thank Dr. David A. Hovda for his careful reading and comments on an early draft of this manuscript. We also would like to acknowledge the contributions of our colleagues, Drs. D. A. Hovda, M. G. Boyeson, and A. A. Salo, who spent many long hours in the laboratory collecting much of the data presented in this chapter. This work and preparation of this manuscript were supported by the U.S. Army Medical Research Acquisition Activity, Contract No. DAMD17-86-C-6144, DHHS Grant 3-S06-RR08139, and DHHS grant #1 R01 NS20220-01A2.

REFERENCES

1. Baron, J. C., Bousser, M. G., Comar, D., and Castaigne, P., 1980, "Crossed cerebellar diaschisis" in human supratentorial brain infarction, *Trans. Am. Neurol. Assoc.* **105**:459–461.

2. Baron, J. C., Bousser, M. G., Comar, D., Duquesnoy, N., Sastre, J., and Castaigne, P., 1981, "Crossed cerebellar diaschisis:" A remote functional depression secondary to supratentorial infarction of man, *J. Cereb. Blood Flow Metab. [Suppl.]* **1**:S500–S501.

3. Bear, M. F., and Daniels, J. D., 1983, The plastic response to monocular deprivation persists in kitten visual cortex after chronic depletion of norepinephrine, *J. Neurosci.* **3**:407–416.

4. Boyeson, M. G., 1983, *The Role of Norepinephrine in Recovery of Function following Unilateral Sensorimotor or Neocortical Cerebellar Lesions in the Rat,* Ph.D. Dissertation, University of New Mexico, Albuquerque.

5. Boyeson, M. G., and Feeney, D. M., 1984, The role of norepinephrine in recovery from brain injury, *Soc. Neurosci. Abstr.* **10**:68.

6. Boyeson, M. G., Krobert, K. A., and Hughes, J. M., 1986, Norepinephrine infusions into cerebellum facilitate recovery from sensorimotor cortex injury in the rat, *Soc. Neurosci. Abstr.* **12**:1120.

7. Bugiani, O., and Gatti, R., 1980, L-Dopa in children with progressive neurological disorders, *Ann. Neurol.* **7**:93.

8. Clark, A. N. G., and Manikar, G. D., 1979, D-Amphetamine in elderly patients refractory to rehabilitation procedures, *J. Am. Geriatr. Soc.* **27**:174–177.

9. Cornwell, P., Overman, W., Levitsky, C., and Shipley, J., 1976, Performance on the visual cliff by cats with marginal gyrus lesions, *J. Comp. Physiol. Psychol.* **90**:996–1010.

10. Dail, W. G., Feeney, D. M., Murray, H. M., Linn, R. T., and Boyeson, M. G., 1981, Responses to cortical injury: II. Widespread depression of the activity of an enzyme in cortex remote from focal injury, *Brain Res.* **211**:79–89.

11. Davis, J. N., Crisostomo, E. A., Duncan, P., Propst, M., and Feeney, D. M., 1987, Amphetamine and physical therapy facilitate recovery from stroke: Correlative animal and human studies, in: *Cerebrovascular Diseases* (M. E. Raichle and W. J. Powers, eds.), Raven Press, New York, pp. 297–306.

12. Denny-Brown, D., Kirk, E. J., and Yanagasawa, N., 1973, The tract of Lissauer in relation to sensory transmission in the dorsal horn of spinal cord in the macaque monkey, *J. Comp. Neurol.* **151**:175–200.

13. Feeney, D. M., and Baron, J.-C., 1986, Diaschisis, *Stroke* **17**:817–830.

14. Feeney, D. M., Boyeson, M. G., Linn, R. T., Murray, H. M., and Dail, W. G., 1981, Responses to cortical injury: I. Methodology and local effects of contusions in the rat, *Brain Res.* **211**:67–77.

15. Feeney, D. M., Gonzales, A., and Law, W. A., 1981, Amphetamine restores locomotor function after motor cortex injury in the rat, *Proc. West. Pharmacol. Soc.* **24**:15–17.

16. Feeney, D. M., Gonzalez, A., and Law, W. A., 1982, Amphetamine, haloperidol and experience interact to affect rate of recovery after motor cortex injury, *Science* **217**:855–857.

17. Feeney, D. M., and Hovda, D. A., 1983, Amphetamine and apomorphine restore tactile placing after motor cortex injury in the cat, *Psychopharmacology* **79**:67–71.

18. Feeney, D. M., and Hovda, D. A., 1985, Reinstatement of binocular depth perception by amphetamine and visual experience after visual cortex ablation, *Brain Res.* **342**:352–356.

19. Feeney, D. M., and Sutton, R. L., 1987, Pharmacotherapy for recovery of function after brain injury, *CRC Crit. Rev. Neurobiol.* **3**:135–197.

20. Feeney, D. M., Sutton, R. L., Boyeson, M. G., Hovda, D. A., and Dail, W. G., 1985, The locus coeruleus and cerebral metabolism: Recovery of function after cortical injury, *Physiol. Psychol.* **13**:197–205.

21. Finger, S., and Stein, D. G., 1982, *Brain Damage and Recovery: Research and Clinical Perspectives,* Academic Press, New York.

22. Hovda, D. A., 1985, *Effects of Amphetamine on Recovery of Binocular Depth Perception and Tactile Placing after Visual Cortex Ablation in the Cat,* Ph.D. Dissertation, University of New Mexico, Albuquerque.

23. Hovda, D. A., Bailey, B., Montoya, S., Salo, A. A., and Feeney, D. M., 1983, Phentermine accelerates recovery of function after motor cortex injury in rats and cats, *Fed. Proc.* **42**:1157.

24. Hovda, D. A., and Feeney, D. M., 1984, Amphetamine with experience promotes recovery of locomotor function after unilateral frontal cortex injury in the cat, *Brain Res.* **298**:358–361.

25. Hovda, D. A., and Feeney, D. M., 1985, Haloperidol blocks amphetamine induced recovery of binocular depth perception after bilateral visual cortex ablation in cat, *Proc. West. Pharmacol. Soc.* **28**:209–211.

26. Hovda, D. A., Feeney, D. M., Salo, A. A., and Boyeson, M. G., 1983, Phenoxybenzamine but not haloperidol reinstates all motor and sensory deficits in cats fully recovered from sensorimotor cortex ablations, *Soc. Neurosci. Abstr.* **9**:1002.

27. Hovda, D. A., Sutton, R. L., and Feeney, D. M., 1985, Asymmetry of bilateral visual cortex lesions affect amphetamine's ability to produce recovery of depth perception, *Soc. Neurosci. Abstr.* **11**:1016.

28. Hovda, D. A., Sutton, R. L., and Feeney, D. M., 1987, Recovery of tactile placing after visual cortex ablation in cats: A behavioral and metabolic study of diaschisis, *Exp. Neurology* **97**: 391–402.

29. Kasamatsu, T., and Pettigrew, J. D., 1976, Depletion of brain catecholamines: Failure of ocular dominance shift after monocular occlusion in kittens, *Science* **194**:206–208.

30. Kasamatsu, T., and Pettigrew, J. D., 1979, Preservation of binocularity after monocular deprivation in the striate cortex of kittens treated with 6-hydroxydopamine, *J. Comp. Neurol.* **185**:139–162.

31. Kurshner, M., Alavi, A., Reivich, M., Dann, R., Burke, A., and Robinson, G., 1984, Contralateral cerebellar hypometabolism following cerebral insult: A positron emission tomographic study, *Ann. Neurol.* **15**:425–434.

32. Lipper, S., and Tuchman, M. M., 1976, Treatment of chronic post-traumatic organic brain syndrome with dextroamphetamine: First reported case, *J. Nerv. Ment. Dis.* **162**:366–371.

33. Maeda, H., and Maki, S., 1986, Dopaminergic facilitation of recovery from amygdaloid lesions which affect hypothalamic defensive attack in cats, *Brain Res.* **363**:135–140.

34. Marotta, R. F., Logan, N., Potegal, M., Glusman, M., and Gardner, E. L., 1977, Dopamine agonists induce recovery from surgically-induced septal rage, *Nature* **269**:513–515.

35. Mathew, R. J., and Wilson, W. H., 1985, Dextroamphetamine-induced changes in regional cerebral blood flow, *Psychopharmacology* **87**:298–302.

36. McGraw, C. P., Pashyan, A. G., and Wendell, O. T., 1976, Cerebral infarction in the Mongolian gerbil exacerbated by phenoxybenzamine treatment, *Stroke* **7**:485–488.

37. Meyer, P. M., Horel, J. A., and Meyer, D. R., 1963, Effects of d,l-amphetamine upon placing responses in neodecorticate cats, *J. Comp. Physiol. Psychol.* **56**:402–404.

38. Meyer, P. M., and Meyer, D. R., 1982, Memory, remembering and amnesia, in: *The Expression of Knowledge* (R. L. Isaacson and N. E. Spear, eds.), Plenum Press, New York, pp. 179–212.

39. Patronas, N. J., Chiro, G. D., Smith, B. H., De La Paz, R., Brooks, R. A., Milam, H. L., Kornblith, P. L., Bairamian, D., and Mansi, L., 1984, Depressed cerebellar glucose metabolism in supratentorial tumors, *Brain Res.* **291**:93–101.

40. Porch, B. E., and Feeney, D. M., 1986, Effects of antihypertensive drugs on recovery from aphasia, in: *Clinical Aphasiology*, BRK Publishers, Minneapolis Vol. 16, pp. 309–314.

41. Porch, B., Wyckes, J., and Feeney, D. M., 1985, Haloperidol, thiazides and some antihypertensives slow recovery from aphasia, *Soc. Neurosci. Abstr.* **11**:52.

42. Ross, S. B., 1979, The central stimulatory action of inhibitors of the dopamine uptake, *Life Sci.* **24**:159–168.

43. Rovere, A. A., Raynald, A. C., and Scremin, O. U., 1977, On the mechanism of the amphetamine induced vasodilatation at the rat's cerebral cortex, *Experientia* **33**:1461–1462.

44. Salo, A. A., 1986, *Development of a Model of Cerebral Infarction in Rats and Evaluation of*

Treatment with Continuous Infusion of Amphetamine or Naloxone, Ph.D. Dissertation, University of New Mexico, Albuquerque.

45. Sprague, J. M., 1966, Interaction of cortex and superior colliculus in mediation of visually guided behavior in the cat, *Science* **153:**1544–1547.

46. Sutton, R. L., Chen, M. J., Hovda, D. A., and Feeney, D. M., 1986, Effects of amphetamine on cerebral metabolism following brain damage as revealed by quantitative cytochrome oxidase histochemistry, *Soc. Neurosci. Abstr.* **12:**1404.

47. Sutton, R. L., Hovda, D. A., and Feeney, D. M., 1984, Multiple doses of *d*-amphetamine accelerate recovery of locomotion following bilateral frontal cortex injury in cat, *Soc. Neurosci. Abstr.* **10:**67.

48. Sutton, R. L., Hovda, D. A., and Feeney, D. M., 1988, Effect of catecholamine agonists on recovery of motor ability after unilateral frontal cortex ablation in rat and cat (submitted for publication).

49. Sutton, R. L., Hovda, D. A., Feeney, D. M., and Dail, W. G., 1985, Intracerebral autografts of adrenal medulla chromaffin cells in adult cats with unilateral frontal cortex ablations (UFCA): Beneficial effects on recovery of locomotor and tactile placing (TP) abilities, *Soc. Neurosci. Abstr.* **11:**614.

50. Trombley, P., Allen, E. S., Soyke, J., Blaha, C. D., Lane, R. F., and Gordon, B., 1986, Doses of 6-hydroxydopamine sufficient to deplete norepinephrine are not sufficient to decrease plasticity in the visual cortex, *J. Neurosci.* **6:**266–273.

51. Tyson, A., Miller, G., Feeney, D., and Davis, J., 1986, Amphetamine and recovery of function: Use of an alpha-2 antagonist provides further evidence that norepinephrine mediates the amphetamine-induced acceleration of recovery of motor function after motor cortex lesions, *Soc. Neurosci. Abstr.* **12:**1120.

52. von Monakow, C., 1914, "Diaschisis," Localization in the cerebrum and functional impairment by cortical loci, in: *Brain and Behavior:* Volume 1. *Mood States and Mind* (K. H. Pribram, ed.), Penguin, Baltimore, pp. 27–36, (partial translation of original work by G. Harris, published in 1969).

53. Wall, J. T., and Kaas, J. H., 1985, Cortical reorganization and sensory recovery following nerve damage and regeneration, in: *Synaptic Plasticity* (C. W. Cotman, ed.), Guilford Press, New York, pp. 231–260.

54. Watson, M., and McElligott, J. G., 1984, Cerebellar norepinephrine depletion and impaired acquisition of specific locomotor tasks in rats, *Brain Res.* **296:**129–138.

55. Wong-Riley, M., 1979, Changes in the visual system of monocularly sutured or enucleated cats demonstrable with cytochrome oxidase histochemistry, *Brain Res.* **171:**11–28.

8

Ganglioside Involvement in Membrane-Mediated Transfer of Trophic Information
Relationship to G_{M1} Effects following CNS Injury

R. Dal Toso, S. D. Skaper, G. Ferrari, G. Vantini, G. Toffano, and A. Leon

Abstract. The systemic administration of G_{M1} monosialoganglioside has been shown to ameliorate outcome following injury to the adult mammalian central nervous system. In addition, cultured neurons, both primary and clonal, are known to respond to the ganglioside with pronounced morphological changes characteristic of cell differentiation. In cells with an absolute requirement for a neuronotrophic factor for survival and/or neurite outgrowth, the G_{M1} effects are associated with amplification of the effects of the trophic factor on its target neuronal cells.

In an attempt to elucidate the underlying mechanisms *in vitro* and their relationship to G_{M1} effects *in vivo*, the present chapter analyzes the information now available concerning (1) the role of neuronotrophic factors following brain injury, (2) the function of gangliosides in the process of membrane-mediated transfer of information, in particular, trophic information, and (3) the relationship between neuronotrophic factors and neuritogenic properties of the G_{M1} ganglioside in clonal and primary neuronal cells *in vitro*. In addition, the possible relevance of neuronotrophic factors in G_{M1} effects *in vivo* is discussed.

R. Dal Toso, G. Ferrari, G. Vantini, G. Toffano, and A. Leon • Fidia Research Laboratories, 35031 Abano Terme, Italy. S. D. Skaper • Fidia Research Laboratories, 35031 Abano Terme, Italy, and Department of Biology and School of Medicine, University of California at San Diego, La Jolla, California 92023.

1. INTRODUCTION

In the central nervous system (CNS), neurons are known to communicate with one another as well as with nonneuronal elements (e.g., astroglial cells). One form of communication results from the ability of neurons to modulate the physiological activity of other neurons by means of electrically linked neurotransmitter release. Another form of communication occurs through trophic signals (i.e., neuronotrophic factors) derived from the target neurons and/or nonneuronal cells in close physical association with the former.[62,65,83] These signals have long been known to regulate neuronal numbers and synaptic connections in early life. More recent evidence now indicates that trophic signals, although less apparent, persist in maturity. During this stage it has been suggested that trophic factors control the neuronal survival and synaptic readjustments that occur in response to neuropathological situations.[115]

1.1. NEURONOTROPHIC ACTIVITY AFTER INJURY

In the adult, trophic signals are most readily detectable following CNS injury. Many laboratories have shown that injury elicits an increase of neuronotrophic activity in the denervated tissue.[7,14,34,35,64,75,76,119] A good example is the sprouting of sympathetic fibers into the denervated hippocampus following damage to the cholinergic septal–hippocampal pathway.[14] This sympathetic ingrowth is induced by sufficiently increased levels of nerve growth factor (NGF)-like activity in the denervated hippocampus, suggesting that the hippocampus produces an endogenous NGF-like protein that acts as a neuronotrophic factor for the septal cholinergic neurons. Its content in the hippocampus appears to reflect the degree of cholinergic innervation. Moreover, these trophic effects are more readily revealed in the adult following CNS injury, e.g., the axonal sprouting that may occur following partial target denervation.[16,64,76,77] These and other evidence have led to the hypothesis that neuronotrophic signals, in sufficient amounts, play a key role in determining the outcome following injury to the adult brain.[115] A corollary of this hypothesis is that a trophic deficit (perhaps as a result of an increase in the trophic needs of the neurons at early postlesion stages) may well be one of the underlying causes of the progressive axonal degeneration and neuronal cell death that occur after the insult. If so, an increased trophic availability should enhance neuronal cell survival and facilitate repair processes.

1.2. TROPHIC EFFECTS AND EXOGENOUS FACTORS

One experimental mode for increasing trophic availability is the exogenous supplementation of an appropriate trophic factor to the injured brain area. In this context, intracerebral injections of NGF, beginning before the lesion or at early postlesion times, to adult rats with lesions of the septal–hippocampal cholinergic pathway have been shown to increase choline acetyltransferase (ChAT) activity in the septum and hippocampus[44] and to partially prevent the injury-induced death of the septal cholinergic neurons.[43,54,121] It is noteworthy that NGF has been shown to behave as a neuronotrophic factor in adult rodents for only the cholinergic neurons of the basal forebrain.[52] Other neuronotrophic factors effective on diverse neuronal cell types *in vitro* have been detected in the CNS.[4,19,20,47,69,72,117] It is likely that the further purification of some of these factors as well as the characterization of their effects *in vitro* and *in vivo* will add considerably to our understanding of their role in CNS repair in the adult.

1.3. TROPHIC EFFECTS AND MEMBRANE CONSTITUENTS

Another means for increasing trophic effects is to enhance neuronal cell responsiveness to endogenous trophic signals.[115] The efficacy of trophic factors depends not only on their quantity but also on the capability of the neurons to respond to the signal(s). The operations that translate an external signal into an intracellular biochemical event take place at the level of the cell plasma membrane and involve a sequential multistep process, namely: (1) binding to specific receptors on the external surface of the cell (signal recognition); (2) generation of active intracellular messengers (signal transduction); and (3) generation of a cascade of biochemical reactions eliciting the appropriate cellular response (signal translation). In addition, many components of the membrane (e.g., proteins, lipids) appear to be involved in this process whereby each component is part of a dynamic ensemble that is responsible, as a whole, for the physiological response. Understanding the role of neuronal membrane components in the processes of transmembrane signaling of neuronotrophic factors may well lead to novel ways of enhancing trophic efficacy in the lesioned brain.

Among the neuronal components that may be involved in trophic factor-mediated transmembrane signaling, increasing attention is being paid to gangliosides, in particular monosialoganglioside G_{M1} (nomenclature according to Svennerholm[108]). There is now considerable evidence indicating that this ganglioside is effective in modulating neuronal cell responsiveness to neuronotrophic factors *in vitro* and, most important, in ameliorating the outcome following CNS injury to adult rodents. Since the latter aspect is described and discussed in the accompanying chapters by Dunbar and Stein (Chapter 10) and by Sabel (Chapter 9), the aim here is to outline briefly and discuss the general considerations and evidence concerning the involvement of gangliosides in cell-surface-mediated events and, in particular, the involvement of G_{M1} in neuronal transmembrane signaling of neuronotrophic cues. For this purpose, we have subdivided this chapter into three major sections. In the first section, we provide some background information (chemical features, cellular distribution, membrane organization, etc.) supporting the concept that the gangliosides are involved in the process of neuronal membrane-mediated transfer of information. In the second section, we review the studies utilizing cell cultures that suggest or are compatible with a ganglioside role in modulation of neuronal cell responsiveness to neuronotrophic factors. In the third section, we discuss the possibility that neuronotrophic factors may also be involved in the G_{M1} effects observed following CNS injury *in vivo*.

2. Evidence for Ganglioside Involvement in the Biotransduction of Membrane-Mediated Information

Gangliosides, sialic-acid-containing glycosphingolipids, are normal components of the plasma membrane of vertebrate cells.[55] Although their functions remain largely obscure, the possibility that gangliosides are involved in the process of transmembrane signaling essentially derives from knowledge of their chemical characteristics, cellular localization, and membrane organization.[109] In addition, the fact that gangliosides are particularly abundant in CNS gray matter suggests that these molecules contribute significantly to the structural–functional features of neuronal membranes.

Although it is beyond the scope of this chapter to describe the above aspects, some general comments concerning peculiar features of gangliosides that make them potential candidates for modulation of neuronotrophic signals at the level of the neuronal membrane are briefly discussed below. Particular reference is given to the ganglioside G_{M1}.

2.1. Chemical Diversity of the Gangliosides

Gangliosides are a heterogeneous group of glycosphingolipids characterized by the presence of sialic acid.[109] Each ganglioside molecule consists of a hydrophobic ceramide moiety and a hydrophilic sialosyloligosaccharide moiety (Fig. 1). The ceramide consists of a long-chain fatty acid (primarily C18:0) linked by an amide bond to a long-chain base (C_{18} or C_{20}), unsaturated (sphingenine) or

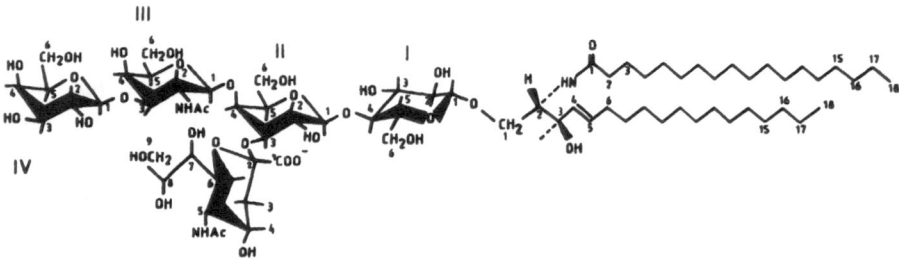

FIGURE 1. Chemical structure of G_{M1} ganglioside.

saturated (sphinganine). The sialosyloligosaccharide is β-glycosidically linked to the ceramide. It consists of a neutral oligosaccharide core to which one or more sialic acids are attached.[109]

The type of neutral oligosaccharide core and sialic acid residue (primarily N-acetylneuraminic acid), as well as the number and position of the sialic acids per molecule, varies among the different gangliosides.[109] For example, the following neutral oligosaccharide cores have been found to occur in gangliosides: (1) galactose (Gal), (2) lactose (Galβ1 → 4Glc), (3) gangliotriose (GalNAcβ1 → 4Galβ1 → 4Glc), (4) gangliotetraose (Galβ1 → 3GalNAcβ1 → 4Galβ1 → 4Glc), (5) globotetraose (GalNAcβ1 → 3Galαl → 4Galβ1 → 4Glc), and (6) neolactotetra (hexa-, octa-)ose [(Galβ1 → 4GlcNAcβ1 → 3) Galβ1 → 4Glc]. This has led to classification of the gangliosides into gangliosides of the ganglio, globo, or lacto series. In addition, the number of sialic acid residues may vary from one to seven. In the ganglio series, the single or multiple sialic acids are α-glycosidically attached to the galactose moiety(ies) or one to another by a 2α → 8 ketoside linkage. This variability of the ganglio series has led to classification according to Svennerholm[108] of the gangliosides into monosialoganglioside (G_{M1}), disialoganglioside G_{D1a}, etc. (see Table I and note that this classification also takes into consideration the position of the sialic acid, e.g., G_{D1a} versus G_{D1b}, as well as the length of the oligosaccharide core e.g., G_{M1} versus G_{M2}). For further information concerning ganglioside structure and nomenclature, see the recent reviews by Wiegandt,[120] Ledeen,[55] and Ando[2] and the report of the IUPAC–IUB Commission on Biochemical Nomenclature.[46]

TABLE 1. Chemical Structure and Nomenclature (According to Svennerholm[108]) of the Major Gangliosides of the Ganglio Series

Svennerholm nomenclature	Schematic structure
G_{M4}	NeuAcα2 → 3Galβ1 → 1'Cer
G_{M3}	NeuAcα2 → 3Galβ1 → 4Glcβ1 → 1'Cer
G_{D3}	NeuAcα2 → 8NeuAc2 → 3Galβ1 → 4Glcβ1 → 1'Cer
G_{M2}	GalNAcβ1 → 4Gal (3 ← 2αNeuAc)β1 → 4Glcβ1 → 1'Cer
G_{D2}	GalNAcβ1 → 4Gal (3 ← 2αNeuAc8 ← 2αNeuAc)β1 → 4Glcβ1 → 1'Cer
G_{M1}	Galβ → 3GalNAcβ1 → 4Gal (3 ← 2αNeuAc)β1 → 4Glcβ1 → 1'Cer
G_{D1a}	NeuAcα2 → 3Galβ1 → 3GalNAcβ1 → 4Gal (3 ← 2αNeuAc)β1 → 4Glcβ1 → 1'Cer
G_{D1b}	Galβ1 → 3GalNAcβ1 → 4Gal (3 ← 2αNeuAc8 ← 2αNeuAc)β1 → 4Glcβ1 → 1'Cer
G_{T1a}	NeuAcα2 → 8NeuAcα2 → 3Galβ1 → 3GalNAcβ1 → 4Gal (3 ← 2αNeuAc)β1 → 4Glcβ1 → 1'Cer
G_{T1b}	NeuAcα2 → 3Galβ1 → 3GalNacβ1 → 4Gal (3 ← 2αNeuAc8 ← 2αNeuAc)β1 → 4Glcβ1 → 1'Cer
G_{Q1b}	NeuAcα2 → 8NeuAcα2 → 3Galβ1 → 3GalNAcβ1 → 4Gal (3 ← 2αNeuAc8 ← 2αNeuAc)β1 → 4Glcβ1 → 1'Cer

The gangliosides, thus, are a crowded family of compounds differing in both their sialosyloligosaccharide and ceramide compositions.[120] Different molecular species are known to occur in different tissues and organs. In addition, the proportion among the different ganglioside species varies among different organs and tissues. A study of the functional roles of gangliosides implies comprehension of the specific role played by the individual gangliosides in a particular cell type.

2.2. Tissue Distribution and Cellular Localization

Unlike other glycosphingolipids in mammals, the highest concentrations of gangliosides are found in the gray matter of the nervous system.[2,55,56,109,120] The gangliosides found in this region differ qualitatively from those found in other tissues as well as within the same tissue. For example, whereas the gangliosides present in the CNS belong mostly to the ganglio series, those of the PNS and extraneuronal tissues contain high amounts of gangliosides of the lacto and globo series. Furthermore, the predominant gangliosides detected in the mature brain gray matter are G_{M1}, G_{D1a}, G_{D1b}, G_{T1b}, and G_{Q1b}, whereas the major gangliosides of brain white matter are G_{M1} and G_{D1a}.

Gangliosides have been shown to be almost exclusively localized on the outer leaflet of the lipid bilayer of the plasma membrane. The ceramide portion is inserted into the lipid bilayer, whereas the sialosyloligosaccharide head group protrudes towards the external environment. Because of their abundance in mammalian brain gray matter, the ganglioside content in the outer membrane layer of neuronal cells has been calculated to be about one-fifth that of phospholipids. Gangliosides comprise a major part of the glycoconjugate network extending from the neuronal membrane surface, with high concentrations having been found to occur in synaptic plasma membranes. However, it is not yet clear whether or not they are evenly distributed over the plasma membrane (see also section 2.3).

Their asymmetric distribution, together with the chemical diversity of the protruding oligosaccharide portion, makes gangliosides particularly subject to interactions with a variety of different extracellular substances. It has been suggested that gangliosides may function as binding sites for various bioactive factors.[9,45] Although a number of agents have been shown to interact with the sialosyloligosaccharide portion of gangliosides,[40,41,109] the most specific interaction is that of cholera toxin with G_{M1}.[32] With the exception of the latter ganglioside, in most cases the receptor has been characterized as a protein (binding to gangliosides is generally of much lower affinity and specificity).[41] Because of this, gangliosides have been suggested as being able either to affect receptor—ligand interactions indirectly by forming secondary auxiliary cell surface binding sites or to act as modulators of protein-receptor function.[41] The first view is based on the assumption that gangliosides may behave as ligand sites that affect in a positive cooperative manner their binding to the protein receptor. This has recently been demonstrated in the case of fibronectin binding to its cell surface protein receptor.[110] In addition, a similar situation appears to occur in the case of tetanus toxin binding to the cell surface.[70] The second view, i.e., the role of gangliosides as modulators of receptor proteins, is based on the assumption that receptors are allosteric proteins and have a site that interacts with gangliosides directly or indirectly, with consequent modification of receptor function[41] (and not necessarily ligand interaction). An example of the latter is the recent demonstration that gangliosides affect the tyrosine kinase activity associated with growth factor receptors.[10,11]

2.3. MEMBRANE ORGANIZATION

Studies utilizing both artificial and biological membranes have shown that the concentration of gangliosides in a given region of the membrane is not static but depends on dynamic interactions among ganglioside polar head groups, divalent cations such as calcium, and other cell surface glycoproteins.[109] For example, when ganglioside micelles are incubated at 37°C with phosphatidylcholine bilayers or vesicles (artificial membranes), the gangliosides spontaneously incorporate in the phospholipid structure without disrupting the bilayer organization.[111] All the incorporated gangliosides are present on the outer surface. Once incorporated, the gangliosides appear to have a lateral mobility comparable to that measured for phospholipids and can interact with phospholipids and other gangliosides either through hydrophobic interactions of the hydrocarbon chains or head group interactions.[97] Furthermore, the presence of Ca^{2+}, Mg^{2+}, or other cations and molecules that depress the repulsive electrostatic forces between the negatively charged sialic acids enhances processes of cross linking and condensing of ganglioside head groups.[74,97] The gangliosides tend to concentrate into clusters, thereby affecting the curvature, local composition, and stability of the membranes.[63]

2.3.1. DYNAMIC PROPERTIES OF GANGLIOSIDES IN BIOLOGICAL MEMBRANES

The examination of ganglioside organization in biological membranes is technically more difficult than in artificial membranes. Such studies imply the use of very specific probes, and, unfortunately, antibodies or lectins may also recognize glycoproteins on the cell surface. In addition, endogenously occurring gangliosides are known to be cryptic on the cell surface of most normal cells[80] and thus not readily accessible to foreign molecules such as antibodies.

To date the B subunit of cholera toxin is one of the most specific probes for endogenously occurring gangliosides, in particular G_{M1}.[32] Together with fluorescently labeled cholera toxin antibodies, the B subunit has been used to visualize the distribution of endogenous G_{M1} molecules on the surface of living cells.[104] Human and murine lymphocytes, when labeled at 4°C with cholera toxin, show a fluorescence either evenly distributed or in small aggregates.[86] At 37°C there is a redistribution of the label into a cap at one pole of the cell. The mechanism underlying the capping phenomenon is not known but is energy dependent, associated with cocapping of the cytoskeletal actin protein, and inhibited by cytochalasin B.[51] These observations have led to the suggestion that G_{M1} may be associated with membrane proteins, which in turn are linked to the cytoskeletal system.[51,86]

Another approach to the study of the dynamic interactions of gangliosides on the cell surface utilizes radiolabeled, fluorescent, or chemically modified exogenous gangliosides. It is assumed that, once incorporated into the plasma membrane, their behavior will mimic that of endogenous gangliosides. Most of these studies have been done utilizing G_{M1}. The radiolabeled ganglioside is known to associate readily with both membrane preparations[112] and cells[13,29,84] in a temperature-, time-, and concentration-dependent manner. Other than a labile type of association with the cell surface, there occurs a stable, trypsin-insensitive type of association. Indirect evidence indicates that this form of associated ganglioside is intercalated into the outer layer of the membrane.[96] Furthermore, headgroup interactions have been reported to occur between the exogenously inserted gangliosides themselves and Ca^{2+} as well as with cell surface glycoproteins.[30] The formation of caps on the cell surface has also been observed after addition of exogenous, fluorescently labeled G_{M1} molecules to lymphocytes treated with the B subunit of cholera toxin.[104] This suggests that (1) the inserted G_{M1} ganglioside may self-associate to form microdomains in the lipid bilayer and (2) exogenous gangliosides, once inserted into the plasma membrane, display a dynamic behavior similar to that of endogenous gangliosides. In addition, the stably associated ganglioside is both functionally and metabolically active.[33,73,101]

2.3.2. GANGLIOSIDES AND CELLULAR RESPONSE

The formation of compositional domains and phases with high or low ganglioside content may be of functional significance. Membrane function is dependent on many factors, including cell surface charge density, membrane fluidity, and local interactions between cell surface proteins and other components present in the plasma membrane. Gangliosides contribute significantly to the cell surface charge density, and the sialic acid on the cell surface is known to affect cell behavior.[94] In opportune conditions, gangliosides tend to concentrate into clusters on the cell surface. This causes local changes in membrane fluidity, thereby indirectly influencing several processes taking place at the cell surface as well as at the intramembrane level. In addition, gangliosides can interact both with cell surface glycoproteins (by mutual carbohydrate–carbohydrate interactions) and membrane-embedded proteins (hydrophobically).

It is thus apparent that gangliosides can influence the processes of transmembrane signaling in several different ways. They may affect signal recognition by directly or indirectly modulating ligand–receptor binding (see Section 2.3.1). In addition, they may affect the process of signal transduction[5,6,10,11] by directly or indirectly modulating receptor coupling to second messenger systems, membrane-bound enzyme systems,[21,37,60,79] and/or ion permeability.[116] Evidence is available supporting all these possibilities. Furthermore, the possibility that ganglioside clusters may be associated with intramembrane proteins connected with the cytoskeletal system suggests that gangliosides may be involved in the regulation of the metabolic response of the cell to external stimuli. In this context it is noteworthy that gangliosides have also been implicated in cell adhesion.[8,110]

3. Evidence for Ganglioside Involvement in Neuronal Cell Responsiveness to Neuronotrophic Factors

The quantitative and qualitative features of gangliosides in neuronal cells have raised a fundamental question: how do these high ganglioside concentrations and structural complexities serve the special needs of the neuron? The answer to this question remains largely unknown. This is mainly due to the fact that specific inhibitors of ganglioside synthesis or metabolism as well as specific tools (apart from choleragenoid and certain monoclonal antibodies) for perturbating gangliosides on the cell surface are still lacking. Because of this, ganglioside studies at present fall into two categories. The first is the study of ganglioside patterns, both quantitative and qualitative, of neuronal cells in various conditions (e.g., immature versus mature neurons) that seek to establish relationships among the gangliosides and particular cellular functions. The second is the study of the effects following the addition of exogenous gangliosides to neuronal membranes or cells, with the assumption that once incorporated into the plasma membrane, they will mimic the endogenously occurring gangliosides. The latter approach is used presently in studying both basic aspects of ganglioside function as well as the relationship between the effects of the gangliosides in neuronal cells *in vitro* and their pharmacological effects *in vivo*.

Recent findings utilizing both of the abovementioned approaches have led to the suggestion that gangliosides, in particular G_{M1}, may somehow function in the process of neuritogenesis in the embryo and/or neurite repair in the adult. Because extrinsic trophic influences are also known to be involved in these phenomena, the major findings supporting a neuritogenic effect of gangliosides and its relationship to trophic influences are briefly discussed in the following section.

3.1. Studies in Normal Neuronal Development and "Accidents of Nature"

Much of the current interest concerning ganglioside involvement in the process of neuritic outgrowth derives from studies of ganglioside composition and distributional pattern during brain development. During the latter process, the expression of gangliosides changes in parallel with CNS differentiation.[53,122] For example, intense expression of ganglioside G_{D3} has been shown to be a common feature of mitotically active neuroectodermal cells.[38,92] With transition to a postmitotic phase of neuronal development, G_{D3} drops to a much lower level with an accompanying accretion of the more complex gangliosides.[90,91] At discrete periods of brain development, such as exodendritic sprouting, there occurs a substantial increase in ganglioside complexity and in net amount of lipid-bound sialic acid.[90] Also noteworthy is the study of Willinger and Schachner[122] reporting expression of G_{M1} on maturing postmitotic cerebellar granule cell neurons and their growing neurites. As the granule cell matures, G_{M1} gradually becomes restricted to the cell body. These studies have led workers to postulate that gangliosides, and in particular G_{M1}, play a distinctive role in neurite growth and sprouting during development. This hypothesis is consistent with evidence indicating that anti-G_{M1} antibodies produce long-lasting morphological and behavioral abnormalities when administered to developing animals.[49]

Another indication of the neuritogenic properties of gangliosides derives from ultrastructural studies of mature neurons in humans and animals with genetically determined ganglioside storage diseases, namely, G_{M1} and G_{M2} gangliosidosis ("accidents of nature").[81,82,118] Affected neurons display aberrant sprouting of neurites from axon hillocks (meganeurites). These observations have been interpreted as evidence of an effect of the altered cell surface ganglioside patterns, with the excess ganglioside being viewed as a possible agent capable of affecting neurite outgrowth long after the genetic program for such development has ceased. The potential importance of genotypic variations in these diseases, however, has not been excluded. Nonetheless, the evidence documenting that anti-G_{M1} antibodies inhibit neurite regeneration *in vitro*[105] and axonal elongation *in vivo*[102] is consistent with the hypothesis that the normal membrane G_{M1} ganglioside may be involved in the process of axonal outgrowth.

In order to test the abovementioned hypothesis, many workers have assessed ganglioside patterns in both clonal and primary neuronal cells *in vitro*.[22,28,66] In addition, in an attempt to comprehend the underlying mechanisms, the ability of exogenous gangliosides to induce morphological and/or biochemical differentiation of these cells has also been investigated. For obvious reasons, the following section focuses on the latter aspect.

3.2. STUDIES UTILIZING NEUROBLASTOMA CELLS

Neuroblastoma cells have been extensively applied as a model system for examining the roles of plasma membrane constituents in the regulation of neurite outgrowth and cellular differentiation. In comparison to primary neurons, many of these cell types possess a relatively smaller amount and a simplified pattern of gangliosides on their cell surface.[22,66,85] In addition, although they are malignant-transformed cells, under suitable experimental conditions, e.g., in the presence of dibutyryl cAMP or in the absence of serum, neuroblastoma cells may be induced to form neuritelike processes and to express biochemical properties characteristic of mature neurons.[23] Such differentiation is usually accompanied by profound changes in membrane architecture and properties, including changes of membrane fluidity[23] and increases in ganglioside content and complexity.[18,22,85]

Furthermore, several neuroblastoma cell lines have been shown to undergo morphological differentiation on addition of mixed or single ganglioside species, including G_{M1}, to the culture medium.[12,14,24,48,59,61,68,71] This effect is (1) not mimicked by the addition of neutral glycolipids, sulfatides, or free sialic acid,[12,59] (2) not caused by the presence of contaminants in the gangliosides,[12] (3) correlated with a stable insertion of the ganglioside on the cell surface (studies limited to G_{M1}),[29] and (4) associated with changes in biochemical parameters (e.g., decreased proliferation) characteristic of cellular differentiation.[59] There is evidence that the individual gangliosides differ in their ability to affect different neuroblastoma cell lines[12,48,87,114] (perhaps because of species differences, differences in dedifferentiation stage, and/or the endogenous ganglioside pattern of the cells) as well as the various phases of neurite formation, e.g., neurite elongation, neurite branching, and synapse formation.[61,68,89] For example, the ganglioside-induced neurite outgrowth in mouse neuroblastoma N_2A cells has been reported, under selected conditions, to be associated with the appearance of maturelike synapses.[106,107] Interestingly, this effect occurs only when the G_{M1} ganglioside is present. G_{M1} has also been reported to facilitate the development of neuromuscular junctions in spinal cord–muscle preparations *in vitro*.[78]

In these cells it appears as if the accretion, via synthesis or exogenous supplementation, of gangliosides on the cell surface may by itself be a stimulus for neurite outgrowth and development. A difficulty with this interpretation, however, is that several distinct mechanisms, including inhibition of cell division, can promote the morphological and biochemical differentiation of neuroblastoma cells. The above interpretation is also in contrast to results obtained in other cell types, e.g., pheochromocytoma PC_{12} and primary sensory neurons (see Section 3.3). The latter cells are known to require NGF for survival and/or neurite outgrowth, gangliosides being unable to substitute for NGF. On the other hand, loss of specific growth factor control on cell behavior is a common finding in many types of cancer cells. It is thus possible that in the neuroblastoma cells, gangliosides may mediate neuritic outgrowth by activating a postreceptor pathway that bypasses the requirement for the trophic factor–receptor interaction. In mouse neuroblastoma N_2A cells, there is evidence that the neuritogenic response to the exogenously supplemented G_{M1} ganglioside is characterized by a series of temporally related biochemical events, e.g., increases in cAMP content and protein phosphorylation.[89] Furthermore, in the SB21B1 neural hybrid clonal cell line, ganglioside-induced neurite outgrowth is associated with a severalfold increase in the expression of mRNA for tubulin but not for actin, suggesting a possible ganglioside involvement in the regulation of tubulin gene expression.[93] Alternative possibilities to the above phenomena include ganglioside effects on modulation of cellular responsiveness to yet unidentified trophic or neurite-promoting factor(s) present in the culture medium.

3.3. Studies Utilizing Primary PNS Neurons and PC_{12} Cells

Following the studies utilizing neuroblastoma cells, gangliosides came to be viewed as potential neuronotrophic or neuritogenic agents. A critical question, thus, is whether gangliosides, in particular exogenous G_{M1}, behave as a signal in their own right or operate through modification of a ligand-induced membrane behavior. A related question concerns the role played by the individual gangliosides in the process of neurite outgrowth.

3.3.1. G_{M1} and NGF

In an attempt to answer the first question, many laboratories have evaluated the effects of exogenous gangliosides, in particular G_{M1}, in cultured PC_{12} cells and primary neurons from the peripheral nervous system (PNS), i.e., fetal chicken E8 dorsal root ganglia and E11 sympathetic ganglia. The latter neurons are known to require NGF for survival, neurite outgrowth, and development *in vitro* as *in vivo*.[62] Likewise, PC_{12} cells, a clonal line from rat pheochromocytoma, respond to NGF with expression of properties characteristic of mature sympathetic neurons, which include arrested proliferation and extension of neurites.[39]

The addition of G_{M1} to the culture medium of chicken DRG (E8) or sympathetic ganglia (E11) explants has been reported, under the appropriate conditions, to facilitate NGF-induced neurite outgrowth.[57,99] No appreciable G_{M1} effects were observed in the absence of NGF. This indicates that the G_{M1} effect in these cells (1) is dependent on NGF and (2) involves G_{M1} potentiation of the acquisition and/or maintenance of the NGF-triggered effects. Similar results were also observed in the corresponding dissociated primary neuronal cell cultures[25,57,98] (see Fig. 2) as well as in PC_{12} cells.[31,50,68,89]

As with neuroblastoma cells, asialo-G_{M1}, sulfatide, and free sialic were totally ineffective.[31,89] This suggests that the G_{M1} effects are directly linked to the integrity of the G_{M1} molecule and presumably are not the result of aspecific ionic interactions. G_{M1} was also shown to facilitate NGF effects in adult mouse

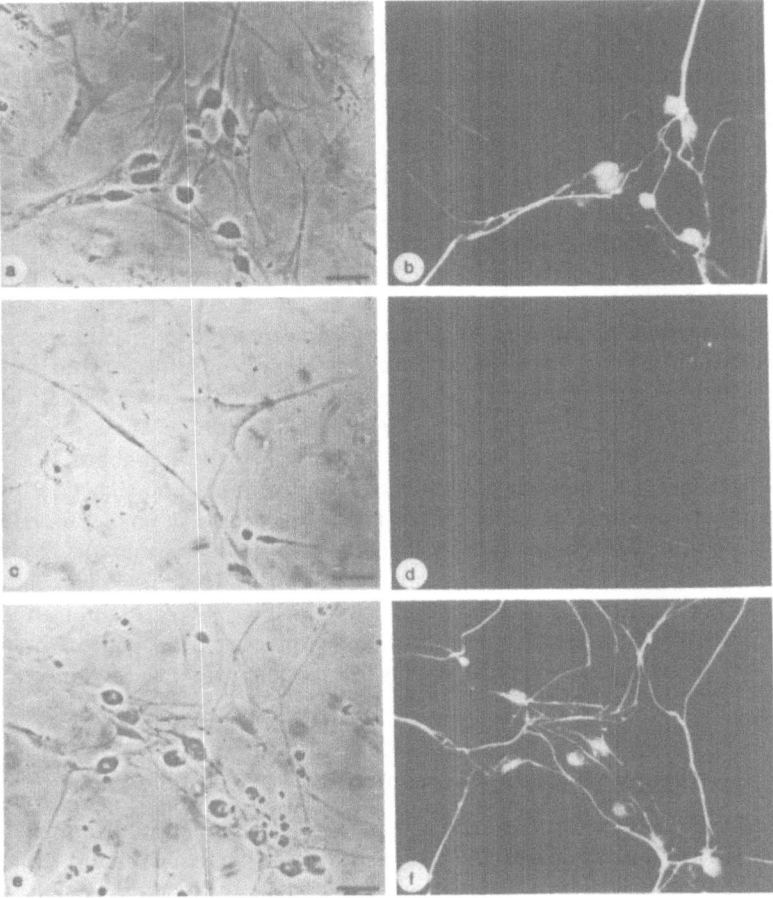

FIGURE 2. Example of G_{M1}-induced potentiation of NGF effects in fetal chicken dissociated DRG (E8) neurons *in vitro*. NGF $\pm$ G_{M1} was added to the cells at plating time. After 5 days, the cells were fixed, stained with monoclonal antibody to neurofilament protein (RT 97), as reported by Doherty *et al.*,[25] and observed under phase contrast (left panel) and fluorescence microscopy (right pannel). a,b, NGF (5 ng/ml); c,d, G_{M1} (100 μg/ml); e,f, NGF (5 ng/ml) + G_{M1} (100 μg/ml). Photograph kindly provided by P. Doherty and F. Walsh, Institute of Neurology, the National Hospital, Queen Square, London WC1N 3BG, England.

superior cervical ganglia explants, indicating that the action of G_{M1} is not limited to fetal tissue.[107]

Thus, in cells with an absolute NGF requirement for survival and/or neurite outgrowth, the exogenously supplied G_{M1}, although not in itself possessing intrinsic trophic activity, is able to facilitate the neuronal cell responsiveness to NGF. This is consistent with the observation that the addition of G_{M1} together with NGF is associated with a ganglioside-induced increase in the expression of neurofilament protein.

3.3.2. UNDERLYING MECHANISMS

Most likely the G_{M1}-induced potentiation of NGF effects on its target cells involves a modification of cell surface properties consequent to the stable insertion of the ganglioside. However, the biochemical mechanisms by which G_{M1} exerts its effects have yet to be identified. Binding studies have not revealed increased NGF binding by G_{M1}-treated cells.[31] Possible explanations could involve modulation of cell surface transduction mechanisms or enhancement of specific NGF-induced posttranslational events. In this context, the stable insertion of very small amounts of G_{M1} is known to modify enzymatic activities of neuronal membranes.[60] Analogously, very small amounts of exogenously inserted G_{M1} have been reported to affect platelet-derived growth factor (PDGF)-induced receptor phosphorylation in fibroblast 3T3 cells.[10] This may indicate that the exogenous G_{M1} molecules are inserted into the membrane (or subsequently packed via interaction with membrane proteins and phospholipids) at well-defined and preferential sites, the result of which is a change in the functional properties of defined microdomains in the plasma membrane.[103,109] Another possibility is that stable membrane-associated G_{M1} may then be internalized and recycled into more complex gangliosides.[36,101] This in turn may be responsible for the resulting modification in membrane properties. Which of these two alternative mechanisms plays a predominant role is currently unknown.

3.3.3. G_{M1} VERSUS OTHER GANGLIOSIDES

The second question, i.e., the role played by the individual gangliosides in the process of neurite outgrowth, has also been addressed utilizing the above-mentioned culture systems. Two different approaches have been applied. One is the comparison of the effects of different exogenously supplemented single ganglioside species. The other is the study of the effects of antiganglioside antibodies.

In both PC_{12} cells and primary fetal (E8) chicken neurons, none of the other major ganglioside species (e.g., G_{D1a}, G_{D1b}, and G_T), as with G_{M1}, were effective in the absence of NGF, although all were able to potentiate the NGF-mediated effects.[31,68,89] There is, however, no clear consensus about the potencies of the different gangliosides. Some authors report that G_{M1} is the most effective in potentiating the action of NGF,[68,89] but others show that the polysialogangliosides (G_{T1b} and G_Q) are more effective in facilitating neurite outgrowth (studies mainly conducted in older ganglia).[26,42] This discrepancy may be caused by differences in species and age of the cells or by culture conditions and parameters used in assessing the ganglioside effects. Since neuronal cell association studies have not been conducted with ganglioside species other than G_{M1}, one cannot exclude the possibility that different exogenous gangliosides may interact differently with the surface of neuronal cells. Their metabolic fate may differ as well.

The second approach, although limited by the availability of ganglioside antibodies, has provided some insight into the role played by the individual gangliosides in the process of neurite outgrowth. Affinity-purified antibodies to G_{M1} were shown to be able to block the NGF-induced neurite sprouting of chicken embryo DRG explants, whereas antibodies to G_{M2} and the monoclonal antibody A2B5 (presumably directed to more complex gangliosides) were less effective.[88,89,95] This suggests that, in comparison to other gangliosides, both the endogenously occurring and exogenously inserted G_{M1} molecules on the surface play a role in mediating the NGF effects. An important step will be the identification of molecular steps affected by the exogenously inserted G_{M1} molecules and determination of whether such events are affected by anti-G_{M1} antibodies.

3.4. Studies Utilizing Primary CNS Neurons

Another important question is whether the exogenously supplied G_{M1} is also effective in promoting survival and/or neurite outgrowth in CNS neurons *in vitro*. For this purpose the effects of exogenous gangliosides, including G_{M1}, were evaluated in primary dissociated neuronal cell cultures obtained from different areas (e.g., mesencephalon, cortex) of fetal rat, mouse, or chicken brain. Although nonneuronal cells can be minimized in these cultures by proper selection of embryonic age and culture conditions, these cultures contain many neuronal cell types, some of which may serve as potential innervation targets.[3] In addition, both the survival and development of these cells are known to be highly dependent on the cell density. In particular, when seeded at relatively high cell densities, the CNS neurons survive, extend neurites, and express properties of mature nerve cells even without any additional exogenous trophic support.[3,19] This has been taken as an indication of the presence of yet unidentified self-supportive trophic influences produced *in vitro* by the cultured cells themselves.

The addition of gangliosides, including G_{M1}, has been reported to facilitate neurite outgrowth in a variety of primary dissociated CNS neurons *in vitro*.[27,67,98] In addition, in fetal mouse dissociated mesencephalic neurons maintained in serum-free conditions, exogenously supplied G_{M1} but not asialo-G_{M1}, has been shown to enhance the biochemical development and survival of at least the dopaminergic and GABAergic neurons present.[58] This effect (1) is correlated with stable insertion of the ganglioside molecules on the cell surface and (2) requires the presence of adequate titers of cell-density-derived trophic influences. Thus, as occurs with NGF in primary sensory (E8) and sympathetic (E11) neurons, G_{M1} seems unable to substitute for the trophic influences but can potentiate their action and/or exert independent influences to which CNS neurons can only respond if appropriately supported. However, NGF is totally without effect on the dopaminergic and GABAergic neurons in the mesencephalic culture system. This suggests that G_{M1} potentiation of the neuronotrophic efficacy on neuronal cells is not limited to NGF. Such a conclusion is consistent with the observations that the exogenously supplied G_{M1} also amplifies the ciliary neuronotrophic factor (CNTF)-dependent effects in fetal chick (E8) ciliary ganglia neurons *in vitro*.[98]

4. G_{M1} Effects *in Vivo:* Possible Relationship with Neuronotrophic Factors

As discussed earlier, the systemic administration of G_{M1} has been reported to ameliorate outcome following injury to the CNS. In several studies, these effects have been associated with promotion of neuronal cell survival. Furthermore, G_{M1} ganglioside affects neuronal behaviors *in vitro*. In cells with an absolute requirement for a neuronotrophic factor for survival and/or neurite outgrowth, G_{M1} cannot substitute for the trophic factor but can enhance the effects of the trophic factor. The question then arises of the relationship between the ganglioside effects *in vitro* and *in vivo*.

As exemplified by NGF, neuronotrophic factors are present in the adult brain and may be essential components in the regulation of neuronal cell survival and repair after an insult. However, even though trophic activity has been reported to increase after brain injury, it appears that this increase is either insufficient or reaches efficacious levels only at a time subsequent to most neuronal cell death (see Fig. 3). We thus suggest that the G_{M1}-induced potentiation of CNS recovery *in vivo* may be related to the G_{M1} enhancement of the neuronotrophic factor effects, as found *in vitro*. This implies that the potentiating effect of G_{M1} *in vivo* is presumably related to an enhancement of neuronotrophic activity already present in the damaged tissue and undergoing a process of slow increase. Thus, such trophic activity is inadequate *per se* after injury, at least at early postlesion times, but is rendered adequate by the treatment with G_{M1}.

Although much work is still necessary to establish the validity of the above-mentioned hypothesis, some *in vivo* results indirectly support such a possibility. The concentrations of G_{M1} effective on CNS neurons *in vitro* are compatible with those obtainable in the brain after systemic administration *in vivo*.[58] Early postlesion treatment with G_{M1} has been reported to facilitate neuronal cell survival not only of dopaminergic[1,113] and noradrenergic neurons[15] but also of

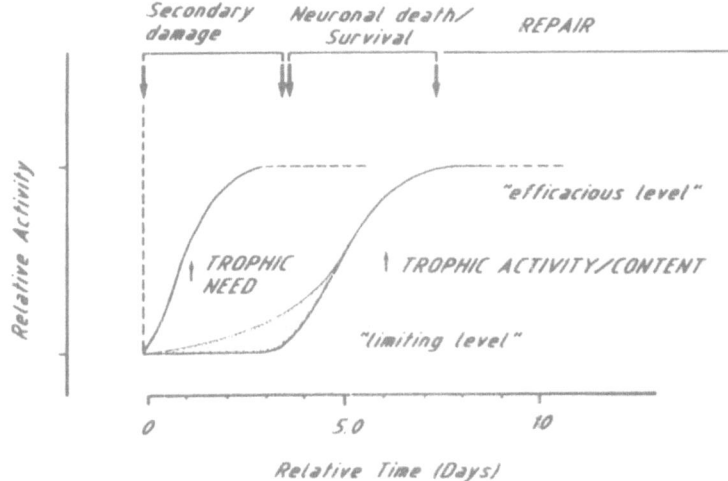

FIGURE 3. Theoretical graphic representation of neuronotrophic titers and activity following adult mammalian CNS injury: the working hypothesis of G_{M1} effects *in vivo* (see text for further elucidation and also Varon[115])

cholinergic neurons[17,100] known to be NGF responsive. Furthermore, initial *in vivo* experiments conducted utilizing NGF ± G_{M1} treatment in neonatal rats following vinblastine-induced sympathectomy indicate that G_{M1} enhances the NGF effects on the maintenance of noradrenergic innervation in the target organs.[114A] Analogous experiments are currently being conducted in adult rats following injury to cholinergic neurons of the basal forebrain.

ACKNOWLEDGMENTS. We thank Dr. G. Kirschner (Fidia Research Laboratories, Abano Terme, Italy) for expertise and helpful discussions concerning the chemistry of gangliosides.

REFERENCES

1. Agnati, L. F., Fuxe, K., Calzà, L., Benfenati, F., Cavicchioli, L., Toffano, G., and Goldstein, M., 1983, Gangliosides increase the survival of lesioned nigral dopamine neurons and favour the recovery of dopaminergic synaptic function in the striatum of rats by collateral sprouting, *Acta Physiol. Scand.* **119**:347–363.
2. Ando, S., 1983, Gangliosides in the nervous system, *Neurochem. Int.* **5**:507–537.
3. Barbin, G., Selak, I., Manthorpe, M., and Varon, S., 1984, Use of central neuronal cultures for the detection of neuronotrophic agents, *Neuroscience* **12**:33–43.
4. Barde, Y.-A., Edgar, D., and Thoenen, H., 1982, Purification of a new neurotrophic factor from mammalian brain, *EMBO J.* **1**:549–553.
5. Bar-Sinai, A., Aldouby, Y., Chorev, M., and Levitzki, A., 1986, Association of turkey erythrocyte β-adrenoceptors with a specific lipid component, *EMBO J.* **5**:1175–1180.
6. Berry-Kravis, E., and Dawson, G., 1985, Possible role of gangliosides in regulating an adenylate cyclase-linked 5-hydroxytryptamine (5-HT) receptor, *J. Neurochem.* **45**:1739–1747.

7. Björklund, A., and Stenevi, U., 1981, *In vivo* evidence for a hippocampal adrenergic neuronotrophic factor specifically released on septal deafferentation, *Brain Res.* **229:**403–428.
8. Blackburn, C. C., Swank-Hill, P., and Schnaar, R. L., 1986, Gangliosides support neural retina cell adhesion, *J. Biol. Chem.* **261:**2873–2881.
9. Brady, O., and Fishman, P. H., 1979, Biotransducers of membrane-mediated information, *Adv. Enzymol.* **50:**303–323.
10. Bremer, E. G., Hakomori, S., Bowen-Pope, D. F., Raines, E., and Ross, R., 1984, Ganglioside-mediated modulation of cell growth, growth factor binding, and receptor phosphorylation, *J. Biol. Chem.* **259:**6818–6825.
11. Bremer, E. G., Schlessinger, J., and Hakomori, S., 1986, Ganglioside-mediated modulation of cell growth. Specific effects of G_{M3} on tyrosine phosphorylation of the epidermal growth factor receptor, *J. Biol. Chem.* **261:**2434–2440.
12. Byrne, M. C., Ledeen, R. W., Roisen, F. J., Yorke, G., and Scalafani, J. R., 1983, Ganglioside-induced neuritogenesis: Verification that gangliosides are the active agents, and comparison of molecular species, *J. Neurochem.* **41:**1214–1222.
13. Callies, R., Schwarzmann, G., Radsak, K., Seigert, R., and Wiegandt, H., 1977, Characterization of the cellular binding of exogenous gangliosides, *Eur. J. Biochem.* **80:**425–432.
14. Collins, F., and Crutcher, K. A., 1985, Neuronotrophic activity in the adult rat hippocampal formation: Regional distribution and increase after septal lesion, *J. Neurosci.* **5:**2809–2814.
15. Commissiong, J. W., and Toffano, G., 1986, The effect of G_{M1} ganglioside on coerulospinal noradrenergic, adult neurons and on fetal monoaminergic neurons transplanted into the transected spinal cord of the adult rat, *Brain Res.* **380:**205–215.
16. Cotman, C. W., and Nieto-Sampedro, M., 1984, Cell biology of synaptic plasticity, *Science* **225:**1287–1294.
17. Cuello, A. C., Stephens, P. H., Tagari, P. C., Sofroniew, M. V., and Parson, R. C. A., 1986, Retrograde changes in the nucleus basalis of the rat, caused by cortical damage, are prevented by exogenous ganglioside G_{M1}, *Brain Res.* **376:**373–377.
18. Dahms, N. M., and Schnaar, R. L., 1983, Ganglioside composition is regulated during differentiation in the neuroblastoma × glioma hybrid cell line NG108-15, *J. Neuroci.* **3:**806–817.
19. Dal Toso, R., Giorgi, O., Soranzo, C., Kirschner, G., Ferrari, G., Favaron, M., Benvegnù, D., Vicini, S., Toffano, G., Azzone, G. F., and Leon, A., Development and survival of neurons in dissociated fetal mesencephalic serum-free cultures: I. Effects of cell density and of an adult mammalian striatal derived neuronotrophic factor (SDNF), *J. Neurosci.* (in press).
20. Davies, A. M., Thoenen, H., and Barde, Y.-A., 1986, Different factors from the central nervous system and periphery regulate the survival of sensory neurons, *Nature* **319:**497–499.
21. Davis, C. W., and Daly, J. W., 1980, Activation of rat cerebral cortical 3′,5′-cyclic nucleotide phosphodiesterase activity by gangliosides, *Mol. Pharmacol.* **17:**206–211.
22. Dawson, G., 1979, Complex carbohydrates of cultured neuronal and glial cell lines, in: *Complex Carbohydrates of Nervous Tissue* (R. U. Margolis and R. K. Margolis, eds.), Plenum Press, New York, p. 29.
23. de Laat, S. W., and van der Saag, P. T., 1982, The plasma membrane as a regulatory site in growth and differentiation of neuroblastoma cells, *Int. Rev. Cytol.* **74:**1–54.
24. Dimpfel, W., Moller, W., and Mengs, U., 1981, Ganglioside-induced neurite formation in cultured neuroblastoma cells, in: *Gangliosides in Neurological and Neuromuscular Function, Development and Repair* (M. M. Rapport and A. Gorio, eds.), Raven Press, New York, pp. 119–134.
25. Doherty, P., Dickson, J. G., Flanigan, T. P., and Walsh, F. S., 1985, Ganglioside G_{M1} does not initiate, but enhances neurite regeneration of nerve growth factor-dependent sensory neurones, *J. Neurochem.* **44:**1259–1265.
26. Doherty, P., Dickson, J. G., Flanigan, T. P., and Walsh, F. S., 1986, Molecular specificity of ganglioside action on neurite regeneration in cell cultures of sensory neurons, in: *Gangliosides*

and Neuronal Plasticity, Fidia Research Series, Volume 6 (G. Tettamanti, R. W. Ledeen, K. Sandhoff, Y. Nagai, and G. Toffano, eds.), Liviana Press, Padua, pp. 335–345.

27. Dreyfus, H., Ferret, B., Harth, S., Gorio, A., Freysz, L., and Massarelli, R., 1984, Effect of exogenous gangliosides on the morphology and biochemistry of cultured neurons, in: *Gangliosides Structure, Function and Biochemical Potential* (R. W. Ledeen, R. K. Yu, M. M. Rapport, and K. Suzuki, eds.), Plenum Press, New York, pp. 513–524.

28. Dreyfus, H., Louis, J. C., Harth, S., and Mandel, P., 1980, Gangliosides in cultured neurons, *Neuroscience* **5:**1647–1655.

29. Facci, L., Leon, A., Toffano, G., Sonnino, S., Ghidoni, R., and Tettamanti, G., 1984, Promotion of neuritogenesis in mouse neuroblastoma cells by exogenous gangliosides. Relationship between the effect and the cell association of ganglioside G_{M1}, *J. Neurochem.* **42:**299–305.

30. Felgner, P. L., Thompson, T. E., Barenhozz, Y., and Lichtenberg, D., 1983, Kinetics of transfer of gangliosides from their micelles to dipalmitoylphosphatidylcholine vesicles, *Biochemistry* **22:**1670–1674.

31. Ferrari, G., Fabris, M., and Gorio, A., 1983, Gangliosides enhance neurite outgrowth in PC12 cells, *Dev. Brain Res.* **8:**215–222.

32. Fishman, P. H., 1982, Role of membrane gangliosides in the binding and action of bacterial toxin, *J. Membr. Biol.* **69:**85–97.

33. Fishman, P. H., Bradley. R. M., Hom, B. H., and Moss, J., 1983, Uptake and metabolism of exogenous gangliosides by cultured cells: Effect of choleragen on the turnover of G_{M1}, *J. Lipid Res.* **24:**1002–1011.

34. Gage, F. H., Björklund, A., and Stenevi, U., 1984, Denervation releases a neuronal survival factor in adult rat hippocampus, *Nature* **308:**637–639.

35. Gasser, U. E., Weskamp, G., Otten, U., and Dravid, A. R., 1986, Time course of the elevation of nerve growth factor (NGF) content in the hippocampus and septum following lesions of the septohippocampal pathway in rats, *Brain Res.* **376:**351–356.

36. Ghidoni, R., Sonnino, S., Chigorno, V., Venerando, B., and Tettamanti, G., 1983, Occurrence of glycosylation and deglycosylation of exogenously administered ganglioside G_{M1} in mouse liver, *Biochem. J.* **213:**321–329.

37. Goldenring, J. R., Otis, L. C., Yu, R. K., and De Lorenzo, R. J., 1985, Calcium/ganglioside-dependent protein kinase activity in rat brain membrane, *J. Neurochem.* **44:**1229–1234.

38. Goldman, J. E., Hirano, M., Yu, R. K., and Seyfried, T. N., 1984, G_{D3} ganglioside is a glycolipid characteristic of immature neuroectodermal cells, *J. Neurochem.* **7:**179–192.

39. Greene, L. A., and Shooter, E. M., 1980, The nerve growth factor: Biochemistry, synthesis and mechanism of action, *Annu. Rev. Neurosci.* **3:**353–402.

40. Hakomori, S., 1981, Glycosphingolipids in cellular interaction, differentiation and oncogenesis, *Annu. Rev. Biochem.* **50:**733–764.

41. Hakomori, S., 1983, Ganglioside receptors: A brief overview and introductory remarks, *Adv. Exp. Med. Biol.* **174:**333–339.

42. Hauw, J. J., Fenelon, S., Boutry, J.-M., Nagai, Y., and Escourolle, R., 1981, Effects of brain gangliosides on neurite growth in guinea pig spinal ganglia tissue cultures and on fibroblast cell cultures, in: *Gangliosides in Neurological and Neuromuscular Function, Development and Repair* (M. M. Rapport and A. Gorio, eds.), Raven Press, New York, pp. 171–175.

43. Hefti, F., 1986, Nerve growth factor promotes survival of septal cholinergic neurons after fimbrial transections, *J. Neurosci.* **6:**2155–2162.

44. Hefti, F., Dravid, A., and Hartikka, J., 1984, Chronic intraventricular injections of nerve growth factor elevate hippocampal choline acetyltransferase activity in adult rats with partial septo-hippocampal lesions, *Brain Res.* **293:**305–311.

45. Holmgren, J. H., Elwing, H., Fredman, P., Strannegard, O., and Svennerholm, L., 1980, Ganglioside as receptors for bacterial toxins and Sendai virus, *Adv. Exp. Med. Biol.* **125:**453–470.

46. IUPAC-IUB Commission on Biochemical Nomenclature, 1977, The nomenclature of lipids, *Lipids* **12**:455–468.
47. Johnson, J. E., Barde, Y. A., Schwab, M., and Thoenen, H., 1986, Brain-derived neurotrophic factor supports the survival of cultured rat retinal ganglion cells, *J. Neurosci.* **6**:3031–3038.
48. Jorgensen, O. S., and Dimpfel, W., 1982, Nervous system-specific protein D2 associated with neurite outgrowth in nerve cell cultures, *J. Neuroimmunol.* **2**:107–117.
49. Kasarskis, E. J., Karpiak, S. E., Rapport, M. M., Yu, R. K., and Bass, N. H., 1981, Abnormal maturation of cerebral cortex and behavioral deficit in adult rats after neonatal administration of antibodies to gangliosides, *Dev. Brain Res.* **1**:25–35.
50. Katoh-Semba, R., Skaper, S. D., and Varon, S., 1984, Interaction of G_{M1} ganglioside with PC12 pheochromocytoma cells: Serum and NGF-dependent effects on neuritic growth (and proliferation), *J. Neurosci. Res.* **12**:299–310.
51. Kellie, S., Patel, B., Pierce, E. J., and D. R. Critchley, 1983, Capping of cholera toxin-ganglioside G_{M1} complexes on mouse lymphocytes is accompanied by co-capping of α-actinin, *J. Cell Biol.* **97**:447–454.
52. Korsching, S., 1986, The role of nerve growth factor in the CNS, *Trends Neurosci.* **9**:570–573.
53. Koulakoff, A., Bizzini, B., and Berwald-Netter, Y., 1983, Neuronal acquisition of tetanus toxin binding sites: Relationship with the last mitotic cycle, *Dev. Biol.* **100**:350–357.
54. Kromer, L. F., 1987, Nerve growth factor treatment after brain injury prevents neuronal death, *Science* **235**:214–216.
55. Ledeen, R. W., 1983, Gangliosides, in: *Handbook of Neurochemistry*, Volume 3 (A. Lajtha, ed.), Plenum Press, New York, pp. 41–90.
56. Ledeen, R. W., 1985, Gangliosides of the neuron, *Trends Neurosci.* **8**:169–174.
57. Leon, A., Benvegnù, D., Dal Toso, R., Presti, D., Facci, L., Giorgi, O., and Toffano, G., 1984, Dorsal root ganglia and nerve growth factor: A model for understanding the mechanism of G_{M1} effects on neuronal repair, *J. Neurosci. Res.* **12**:277–287.
58. Leon, A., Dal Toso, R., Presti, D., Benvegnù, D., Facci, L., Kirschner, G., Tettamanti, G., and Toffano, G., Development and survival of neurons in dissociated fetal mesencephalic serum-free cell cultures: II. Modulatory effects of gangliosides, *J. Neurosci.* (in press).
59. Leon, A., Facci, L., Benvegnù, D., and Toffano, G., 1982, Morphological and biochemical effects of gangliosides in neuroblastoma cells, *Dev. Neurosci.* **5**:108–114.
60. Leon, A., Facci, L., Toffano, G., Sonnino, S., and Tettamanti, G., 1981, Activation of (Na^+, K^+) ATPase by nanomolar concentrations of G_{M1} ganglioside, *J. Neurochem.* **37**:350–357.
61. Leskawa, K. C., and Hogan, E. L., 1985, Quantitation of the in vitro neuroblastoma response to exogeneous, purified gangliosides, *J. Neurosci. Res.* **13**:539–550.
62. Levi-Montalcini, R., and Callissano, P., 1986, Nerve growth factor as a paradigm for other polypeptide growth factors, *Trends Neurosci.* **9**:473–477.
63. Maggio, B., 1985, Geometric and thermodynamic restrictions for the self-assembly of glycosphingolipid–phospholipid systems, *Biochim. Biophys. Acta* **815**:245–258.
64. Manthorpe, M., Nieto-Sampedro, M., Skaper, S. D., Lewis, E. R., Barbin, G., Longo, F. M., Cotman, C. W., and Varon, S., 1983, Neuronotrophic activity in brain wounds of the developing rat. Correlation with implant survival in the wound cavity, *Brain Res.* **267**:47–56.
65. Manthorpe, M., Rudge, J. S., and Varon, S., 1986, Astroglial cell contributions to neuronal survival and neuritic growth, in *Astrocytes*, Volume 2 (S. Fedoroff and A. Vernadakis, eds.), Academic Press, New York, pp. 315–376.
66. Margolis, R. K., Salton, S. R. J., and Margolis, R. V., 1983, Complex carbohydrates of cultured PC12 pheochromocytoma cells. Effects of nerve growth factor and comparison with neonatal and mature rat brain, *J. Biol. Chem.* **258**:4110–4117.
67. Massarelli, R., Ferret, B., Gorio, A., Durand, M., and Dreyfus, H., 1985, The effect of

exogenous gangliosides on neurons in culture: A morphometric analysis, *Int. J. Dev. Neurosci.* **3**:341–348.

68. Matta, S. G., Yorke, G., and Roisen, F. J., 1986, Neuritogenic and metabolic effects of individual gangliosides and their interaction with nerve growth factor in cultures of neuroblastoma and pheochromocytoma, *Dev. Brain Res.* **27**:243–252.
69. Mizrachi, Y., Rubinstein, M., Kimbi, Y., and Schwartz, M., 1986, A neuronotrophic factor from goldfish brain: Characterization and purification, *J. Neurochem.* **46**:1675–1682.
70. Montecucco, C., 1986, How do tetanus and botulinum toxins bind to neuronal membranes? *Trends Biochem. Sci.* **11**:314–317.
71. Morgan, J. I., and Seifert, W., 1979, Growth factors and gangliosides: A possible new perspective in neuronal growth control, *J. Supramol. Struct.* **10**:111–124.
72. Morrison, R. S., Sharma, A., DeVellis, J., and Bradshaw, R. A., 1986, Basic fibroblast growth factor supports the survival of cerebral cortical neurons in primary culture, *Proc. Natl. Acad. Sci. U.S.A.* **83**:7537–7541.
73. Moss, J., Fishman, P. ., Manganiello, V. C., Vaughan, M., and Brady, R. O., 1976, Functional incorporation of gangliosides into intact cells: Induction of choleragen responsiveness, *Proc. Natl. Acad. Sci. U.S.A.* **73**:1034–1037.
74. Myers, M., Wortman, C., and Freire, E., 1984, Modulation of neuraminidase activity by the physical state of phospholipid bilayers containing gangliosides Gd_{1a} and GT_{1b}, *Biochemistry* **23**:1442–1448.
75. Needels, D. L., Nieto-Sampedro, M., Whittemore, S. R., and Cotman, C. W., 1985, Neuronotrophic activity for ciliary ganglion neurons. Induction following injury to the brain of neonatal, adult and aged rats, *Dev. Brain Res.* **18**:275–284.
76. Nieto-Sampedro, M., Manthorpe, M., Barbin, G., Varon, S., and Cotman, C. W., 1983, Injury-induced neuronotrophic activity in adult rat brain. Correlation with survival of delayed implants in a wound cavity, *J. Neurosci.* **3**:2219–2229.
77. Nieto-Sampedro, M., Whittemore, S. R., Needels, D. L., Larson, J., and Cotman, C. W., 1984, The survival of brain transplants is enhanced by extracts from injured brain, *Proc. Natl. Acad. Sci. U.S.A.* **81**:6250–6254.
78. Obata, K., Oide, M., and Handa, S., 1977, Effects of glycolipids on *in vitro* development of neuromuscular junction, *Nature* **266**:369–371.
79. Partington, C. R., and Daly, J. W., 1979, Effect of gangliosides on adenylate cyclase activity in rat cerebral cortical membranes, *Mol. Pharmacol.* **15**:484–491.
80. Peters, M. W., Singleton, C., Barber, K. R., and Grant, C. W. M., 1983, Glycolipid crypticity in membranes—not a simple shielding effect of macromolecules, *Biochim. Biophys. Acta* **731**:475–482.
81. Purpura, D., 1978, Ectopic dendritic growth in mature pyramidal neurons in human ganglioside storage disease, *Nature* **276**:520–521.
82. Purpura, D. P., and Baker, H. J., 1977, Neurite induction in mature cortical neurones in feline G_{M1}-ganglioside storage disease, *Nature* **266**:553–554.
83. Purves, D., 1986, The trophic theory of neural connections, *Trends Neurosci.* **9**:486–489.
84. Radsak, K., Schwarzmann, G., and Weigandt, H., 1982, Studies on the cell association of exogenously added sialoglycolipids, *Hoppe Seylers Z. Physiol. Chem.* **263**:243–272.
85. Rebel, G., Robert, J., and Mandel, P., 1980, Glycolipids and cell differentiation, in: *Structure and Function of Gangliosides* (L. Svennerholm, P. Mandel, H. Dreyfus, and J. Urban, eds.), Plenum Press, New York, p. 159.
86. Revesz, T., and Greaves, M., 1975, Ligand-induced distribution of lymphocyte membrane ganglioside G_{M1}, *Nature* **257**:103–106.
87. Roisen, F. J., Bartfeld, H., Nagele, R., and Yorke, G., 1981, Ganglioside stimulation of axonal sprouting *in vitro*, *Science* **214**:577–578.
88. Roisen, F. J., Bartfeld, H., Rapport, M., Huang, Y., and Yorke, G., 1984, Ganglioside

164 R. Dal Toso *et al.*

modulation of nerve growth factor stimulated neuronal development, *Anat. Rec.* **208**:150A–151B.

89. Roisen, F. J., Matta, S. G., Yorke, G., and Rapport, M. M., 1986, The role of gangliosides in neurotrophic interaction *in vitro*, in: *Gangliosides and Neuronal Plasticity, Fidia Research Series*, Volume 6 (G. Tettamanti, R. W. Ledeen, K. Sandhoff, Y. Nagai, and G. Toffano, eds.), Liviana Press, Padua, pp. 245–255.

90. Rösner, H., 1980, Ganglioside changes in the chicken optic lobes and cerebrum during embryonic development. Transient occurrence of "novel" multisialogangliosides, *Roux Arch. Dev. Biol.* **188**:205–213.

91. Rösner, H., 1982, Ganglioside changes in the chicken optic lobes as biochemical indicators of brain development and maturation, *Brain Res.* **236**:49–61.

92. Rösner, H., Al-Aqtum, M., and Henke-Fahle, S., 1985, Development expression of G_{D3} and polysialogangliosides in embryonic chicken nervous tissue reacting with monoclonal antiganglioside antibodies, *Dev. Brain Res.* **18**:89–95.

93. Rybak, S., Ginzburg, I., and Yavin, E., 1983, Gangliosides stimulate neurite outgrowth and induce tubulin mRNA accumulation in neural cells, *Biochem. Biophys. Res. Commun.* **116**:974–980.

94. Schauer, R., 1985, Sialic acids and their role as biological masks, *Trends Biochem. Sci.* **10**:357–360.

95. Schwartz, M., and Spirman, N., 1982, Sprouting from chicken embryo dorsal root ganglia induced by nerve growth factor is specifically inhibited by affinity-purified antiganglioside antibodies, *Proc. Natl. Acad. Sci. U.S.A.* **79**:6080–6083.

96. Schwarzmann, G., Hoffmann-Bleihauer, P., Shubert, J., Sandhoff, K., and Marsh, D., 1983, Incorporation of ganglioside analogues into fibroblast cell membranes. A spin label study, *Biochemistry* **22**:5041–5048.

97. Sharon, F. J., and Grant, C. W. M., 1978, A model for ganglioside behaviour in cell membranes, *Biochim. Biophys. Acta* **507**:280–293.

98. Skaper, S. D., Katoh-Semba, R., and Varon, S., 1985, G_{M1} ganglioside accelerates neurite outgrowth from primary peripheral and central neurons under selective culture conditions, *Dev. Brain Res.* **23**:19–26.

99. Skaper, S. D., and Varon, S., 1985, Ganglioside G_{M1} overcomes serum inhibition of neuritic outgrowth, *Int. J. Dev. Neurosci.* **3**:187–198.

100. Sofroniew, M. V., Pearson, R. C. A., Cuello, A. C., Tagari, P. C., and Stephens, P. H., 1986, Parenterally administered G_{M1} ganglioside prevents retrograde degeneration of cholinergic cells of the rat basal forebrain, *Brain Res.* **398**:393–396.

101. Sonderfeld, S., Conzelmann, E., Schwarzmann, G., Burg, J., Hinrichs, U., and Sandoff, K., 1985, Incorporation and metabolism of ganglioside G_{M2} in skin fibroblasts from normal and G_{M2} gangliosidosis subjects, *Eur. J. Biochem.* **149**:247–255.

102. Sparrow, J. R., McGuinness, C., Schwartz, M., and Grafstein, B., 1984, Antibodies to gangliosides inhibit gold-fish optic nerve regeneration *in vivo*, *J. Neurosci. Res.* **12**:233–243.

103. Spiegel, S., Fishman, P. H., and Weber, R. J., 1985, Direct evidence that endogenous G_{M1} ganglioside can mediate thymocyte proliferation, *Science* **230**:1285–1287.

104. Spiegel, S., Kassis, S., Wilchek, M., and Fishman, P. H., 1984, Direct visualization of redistribution and capping of fluorescent gangliosides on lymphocytes, *J. Cell Biol.* **99**:1575–1581.

105. Spirman, N., Sela, B. A., and Schwartz, M., 1982, Antiganglioside antibodies inhibit neuritic outgrowth from regenerating goldfish retinal explants, *J. Neurochem.* **39**:874–877.

106. Spoerri, P. E., 1983, Effects of gangliosides on the in vitro development of neuroblastoma cells: An ultrastructural study, *Int. J. Dev. Neurosci.* **6**:383–391.

107. Spoerri, E. P., 1986, Facilitated-establishment of contacts and synapses in neuronal cultures: Ganglioside-mediated neurite sprouting and outgrowth, in: *Gangliosides and Neuronal Plas-*

ticity, Fidia Research Series, Volume 6 (G. Tettamanti, R. W. Ledeen, K. Sandhoff, Y. Nagai, and G. Toffano, eds.), Liviana Press, Padua, pp. 309–325.

108. Svennerholm, L., 1963, Chromatographic separation of human brain gangliosides, *J. Neurochem.* **10:**613–623.

109. Tettamanti, G., Sonnino, S., Ghidoni, R., Masserini, M., and Venerando, B., 1985, Chemical and functional properties of gangliosides. Their possible implication in the membrane-mediated transfer of information, in: *Physics of Amphiphiles: Micelles, Vesicles and Miroemulsions* (V. de Giorgio and M. Corti, eds.), XC Corso Societa Italiana di Fisica, Bologna, pp. 607–636.

110. Thompson, L. K., Horowitz, P. M., Bentley, K. L., Thomas, D. D., Alderete, J. F., and Klebe, R. J., 1986, Localization of the ganglioside-binding site of fibronectin, *J. Biol. Chem.* **261:**5209–5214.

111. Thompson, T. E., and Tillack, T. W., 1985, Organization of glycosphingolipids in bilayers and plasma membranes of mammalian cells, *Annu. Rev. Biophys. Biophys. Chem.* **14:**361–386.

112. Toffano, G., Benvegnù, D., Bonetti, A. C., Facci, L., Leon, A., Orlando, P., Ghidoni, R., and Tettamanti, G., 1980, Interactions of G_{M1} ganglioside with crude rat brain neuronal membranes, *J. Neurochem.* **35:**861–866.

113. Toffano, G., Savoini, G., Moroni, F., Lombardi, G., Calzà, L., and Agnati, L. F., 1984, Chronic G_{M1} ganglioside treatment reduces dopamine cell body degeneration in the substantia nigra after unilateral hemitransection in rat, *Brain Res.* **296:**233–239.

114. Tsuji, S., Arita, M., and Nagai, Y., 1983, G_{Q1b}, a bioactive ganglioside that exhibits novel nerve growth factor (NGF)-like activities in the two neuroblastoma cell lines, *J. Biochem.* **94:** 303–306.

114A. Vantini, G., Fusco, M., Bigon, E., and Leon, A., G_{M1} ganglioside potentiates the effect of nerve growth factor in preventing vinblastine-induced sympathectomy in newborn rats, *Brain Res.* (in press).

115. Varon, S., Manthorpe, M., and Williams, L. R., 1984, Neuronotrophic and neurite-promoting factors and their clinical potentials, *Dev. Neurosci.* **6:**73–100.

116. Vyskocil, F., Di Gregorio, F., and Gorio, A., 1985, The facilitating effect of gangliosides on the electrogenic (Na^+/K^+) pump and on the resistance of the membrane potential to hypoxia in neuromuscular preparations, *Pflügers Arch.* **403:**1–6.

117. Walicke, P., Cowan, W. M., Ueno, N., Baird, A., and Guillemin, R., 1986, Fibroblast growth factor promotes survival of dissociated hippocampal neurons and enhances neurite extension, *Proc. Natl. Acad. Sci. U.S.A.* **83:**3012–3016.

118. Walkley, S. U., Wurzelmann, S., and Purpura, D. P., 1981, Ultrastructure of neurites and meganeurites of cortical pyramidal neurons in feline gangliosidosis as revealed by the combined Golgi–EM technique, *Brain Res.* **211:**293–398.

119. Whittemore, S. R., Nieto-Sampedro, M., Needels, D. L., and Cotman, C. W., 1985, Neuronotrophic factors for mammalian brain neurons: Injury induction in neonatal, adult and aged brains, *Dev. Brain Res.* **20:**169–178.

120. Wiegandt, H., 1985, Gangliosides, in: *New Comprehensive Biochemistry,* Volume 10 *Glycolipids* (H. Wiegandt, ed.), Elsevier Biomedical, Amsterdam, pp. 199–260.

121. Williams, L. R., Varon, S., Peterson, G. M., Wictorin, K., Fischer, W., Björklund, A., and Gage, F. H., 1986, Continuous infusion of nerve growth factor prevents basal forebrain neuronal death after fimbria fornix transection, *Proc. Natl. Acad. Sci. U.S.A.* **83:**9231–9235.

122. Willinger, M., and Schachner, M., 1980, G_{M1} ganglioside as a marker for neuronal differentiation in mouse cerebellum, *Dev. Biol.* **74:**101–117.

9

ANATOMIC MECHANISMS WHEREBY GANGLIOSIDE TREATMENT INDUCES BRAIN REPAIR

WHAT DO WE REALLY KNOW?

BERNHARD A. SABEL

ABSTRACT. Because exogenous gangliosides have repeatedly been demonstrated to reduce behavioral deficits following various types of brain injury, the anatomic alterations underlying this phenomenon are of particular interest.

Biochemical and anatomic evidence has been taken to suggest that gangliosides stimulate axon sprouting after lesions in adult rodents. Although a time-dependent increase of transmitter levels and retrograde axonal transport are certainly consistent with such a possibility, the final proof is still outstanding. In developing animals, however, direct evidence for ganglioside-induced axon sprouting has very recently been obtained in the retinotectal system of the hamster.

Because of a dissociation in the time course of axonal sprouting (about 14 days) and that of behavioral improvement (as little as 2 days post-lesion), mechanisms other than axonal sprouting may have to explain the behavioral findings. The possibility that gangliosides prevent secondary degenerative events is therefore proposed. Evidence for this hypothesis was obtained using biochemical assays of transmitter levels, uptake of transmitters or their precursors, evaluation of anterograde terminal degeneration, and retrograde morphological alterations. Similar to studies on sprouting, evidence for reduced secondary degeneration in adulthood is, in most studies, indirect. Again, more clear-cut alterations were observed in developing animals.

In order to obtain direct evidence for ganglioside-induced sprouting or prevention of secondary degeneration in adulthood, it is recommended to abandon the exclusive use of transmitter assays. Structural neuroanatomic techniques should be helpful to obtain more definite answers in future studies.

BERNHARD A. SABEL • Institute of Medical Psychology, University of Munich, School of Medicine, 8000 Munich 2, Federal Republic of Germany.

167

168 BERNHARD A. SABEL

1. INTRODUCTION

Since the early days of neurology it was believed that the brain has no capacity for structural and functional repair after damage. Perhaps Ramon y Cajal contributed to this early pessimistic view by stating, in 1928, "In adult centers, the nerve paths are something fixed and immutable; everything may die, nothing may regenerate."[37,p.750] In the last decade a new movement has emerged in the neurological sciences, and regeneration and recovery of function are now firmly established concepts.[14]

Research efforts are currently under way to understand the mechanisms involved in structural and functional brain repair and, more excitingly, to find means to manipulate these processes directly.

It is probably fair to say that, among current experimental drug therapies, the administration of gangliosides is one of the easiest approaches to treating brain injury and has, so far, produced the most consistent behavioral benefits (see G. L. Dunbar and D. G. Stein, Chapter 10). Since the earlier behavioral studies on the effects of intraperitoneal injections of gangliosides,[39,41,44] my own research interest recently focused on the anatomic alterations that accompany ganglioside treatment after brain damage.[39,42] The aim of this chapter is to summarize these findings and those of others in order to elucidate the anatomic mechanism(s) whereby ganglioside administration improves behavioral performance following brain injury.

The question of which mechanism(s) underlie any drug effect on brain repair may involve three levels of analysis.

The first level of analysis addresses molecular mechanisms. Here, it is of interest to determine (1) the metabolic fate of the drug, (2) the cellular and subcellular localization of the drug or its metabolites, (3) molecular changes and interactions in the cellular membrane or plasma, and (4) the molecular cascade (i.e., second messengers) involved in the cellular phenotypic expression.

The second level of analysis involves subcellular mechanisms, including compensatory changes in (1) receptor sensitivity, (2) axonal transport, (3) transmitter biosynthesis and release, and (4) changes in organelles, cytoskeletal organization, etc.

Finally, the third level of analysis includes cellular and supracellular mechanisms. Collectively, I refer to these as "anatomic" mechanisms, and they could include (1) morphological alterations of cells through atrophy, regeneration, sprouting, etc.; (2) the interaction of various cell types with one another (neurons versus glia); and (3) alterations of neuronal networks. The status of neuronal networks, i.e., the extent of functional connectivity, is of particular importance for understanding behavioral recovery.

Figure 1 displays several of the anatomic (cellular/supracellular) mechanisms whereby brain repair can be achieved. In this simplistic model of brain damage let us assume that a brain system, consisting of nucleus A, nucleus B,

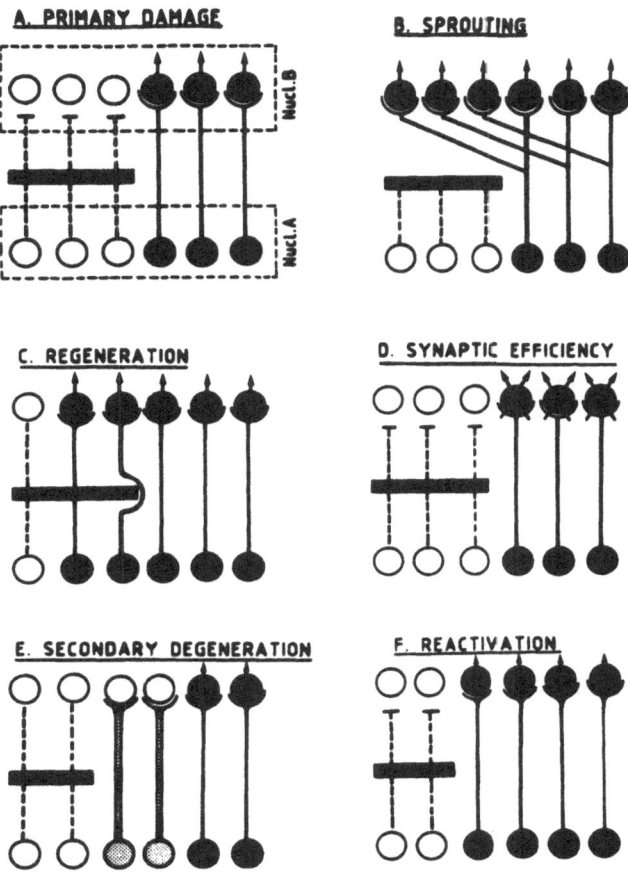

FIGURE 1. Simplified models of brain repair mechanisms. In part A the primary damage, indicated by a horizontal bar, transects a portion of the axons that connect neurons of nucleus A with those of nucleus B. The axotomy leads to anterograde as well as retrograde degeneration, with subsequent neuron death in nucleus A and partial deafferentation of nucleus B. Neurons that lost their function are indicated by open circles, whereas solid circles represent those neurons that still function properly. Let us assume that a behavioral deficit occurs only if 50% or more neurons are defective in nucleus B. Parts B to D: In principle, restoration of function can be achieved by several means. Part B: Collateral sprouts (axon branches) may form and reinnervate the denervated postsynaptic cells. Part C: True regeneration is only rarely observed, but in this case the axotomized neuron would regrow a new axon, either directly through the lesion site or by growing around the lesion site. Part D: The efficiency of the spared system could be increased by denervation supersensitivity on the postsynaptic membrane. This would lead to a more potent response of the innervated cells (indicated by the arrows). Parts E and F: Another injury model could be proposed in which the primary damage is followed by secondary axonal and neuronal distruction. This secondary event could involve either real damage or temporary functional depression in areas near the primary lesion site. In this model, brain repair could be achieved by "reactivation" of the depressed neurons via increased axoplasmic flow, transmitter synthesis, etc. Some of the molecular events in F could be similar to those in D.

and the axonal connections from A to B, only functions properly when more than half of the postsynaptic cells respond to electrophysiological inputs. If a lesion disrupts half of the connections, leaving cells in nucleus B disconnected because of the primary damage (deafferentation), only half of the cells in nucleus B function properly; a behavioral deficit is apparent.

Functional repair can be achieved by reactivating denervated postsynaptic cells. This can be accomplished through (1) sprouting of axon branches (Fig. 1B) and (2) by increasing the response of postsynaptic cells via up-regulation of postsynaptic receptors (Fig. 1D) or presynaptic transmitter synthesis/release and synaptic efficiency (see legend to Fig. 1 for details).

An alternative injury model could also be postulated in which, in addition to the primary loss of connections, there is a temporary depression of neuronal and axonal integrity in the vicinity of the lesion (Fig. 1E). This "depression" may be characterized by reduced metabolic activity, reduced axon transport, and reduced synthesis of macromolecules, transmitters, etc. In this case, functional restoration could be achieved by reactivation of cellular metabolism, axonal transport, transmitter release, etc. (Fig. 1F). Compensation in Fig. 1D and Fig. 1F may be similar.

It is the totality of events on the molecular, subcellular, and anatomic levels that determines whether a system is functionally (behaviorally) intact or deficient after injury.

Ganglioside administration has repeatedly been shown to improve behavioral performance after brain damage. It is the goal of the present chapter to discuss which anatomic mechanisms may be altered by ganglioside treatment and which of them may underlie the behavioral improvements seen after ganglioside administration.

2. REGENERATION AND SPROUTING AFTER BRAIN INJURY

Several investigators have proposed that exogenous gangliosides enhance central sprouting as the basis for behavioral recovery.[39,50,54] I examine the current evidence pertaining to the question of whether (1) gangliosides affect axonal growth, regeneration, or sprouting in the CNS and, (2) if so, whether the sprouting can mediate behavioral changes.

2.1. GANGLIOSIDES IN DEVELOPMENT AND PERIPHERAL NERVE REGENERATION

The discovery that exogenous gangliosides promote sprouting was first made in the peripheral nervous system and can be attributed to Ceccarelli and co-workers.[8] Although the gangliosides were used originally as a control substance in another study, the results triggered a vigorous research effort in the early 1980s on gangliosides and regeneration in the peripheral and central nervous system.

In their study, Ceccarelli et al.[8] performed a pre- and postganglionic anastomosis of the superior cervical ganglion axons in cats. Following such surgery, regenerating axons reinnervate the ganglion or nictitating membrane smooth muscle. This regeneration leads to a partial recovery from paralysis by postoperative day 45. When treated with daily intraperitoneal (i.p.) injections of 50 mg/kg of a ganglioside, the cats showed complete recovery, with normal functioning of the pupil and nictitating membrane. It was concluded that gangliosides enhance peripheral regeneration, which was substantiated by the demonstration of increased catecholaminergic fluorescence in the smooth muscle after postganglionic anastomosis.

In the years following this historically important finding, evidence from other studies also pointed to a possible role of gangliosides in neuronal growth phenomena. In development, G_{M1} gangliosides are expressed on the cell surface of differentiating cells as well as on their growing axonal membranes.[53] Although their differential localization at certain stages of development does not necessarily imply a direct role of gangliosides in axon growth, an experiment performed by nature does suggest a direct modulatory role for gangliosides in neuronal growth.

In G_{M1} gangliosidosis, the deficiency of the appropriate enzyme (β-galactosidase) leads to abnormally high levels of gangliosides in neuronal lysosomes.[33] As a consequence, neurons in a variety of brain structures form meganeurites that arise from the base of the ganglioside-laden neurons. These meganeurites form multiple neuritic growth processes, neurites, and spines, usually seen in earlier stages of development. Thus, the intracellular excess quantity of gangliosides appears to be causally linked to (abnormal) neuronal growth phenomena.

2.2. Sprouting in Adulthood

Because exogenous gangliosides had been shown to enhance sprouting of peripheral nerves, Oderfeld-Nowak and co-workers[30,54] thought it might be possible to find similar effects in the brain after hippocampal deafferentation. Since their first publication in 1981,[30] a number of investigators have also attempted to obtain evidence for ganglioside-induced sprouting in adult animals after lesions in the cortex, the nigrostriatal system, and the spinal cord. Unless specifies otherwise, the ganglioside treatments used in these experiments were given systemically (either intraperitoneal or intramuscular, usually between 10 and 50 mg/kg). As can be seen, the evidence that gangliosides enhance lesion-induced sprouting in adulthood is highly suggestive but nevertheless still indirect.

2.2.1. HIPPOCAMPUS

In their initial experiment, Oderfeld-Nowak *et al.*[30] created electrocoagulation lesions of the medioventral septum. After such lesions, an initial 4-day-long decrease in acetylcholinesterase (AChE) and choline acetyltransferase (ChAT) was evident in hippocampus, followed by a progressive recovery of enzyme levels from day 5 to day 21. It was assumed that the enzyme recovery reflects the growth of new axon branches originating from septal cholinergic fibers of the spared dorsal septum (intrasystem sprouting).

With daily treatment with a ganglioside mixture, the initial decline in enzyme levels was about the same for both lesion groups. However, at postoperative day 18 (P18) and P50, ganglioside-treated animals had recovered significantly more cholinergic enzymes in hippocampus, and it was concluded that gangliosides facilitated reinnervation of the hippocampus by some, yet unidentified, cholinergic afferents.

Similar effects were found when purified monosialoganglioside (G_{M1}) was used.[29] After entorhinal cortex lesions, which destroy glutaminergic input to the hippocampus, G_{M1} elevated the AChE and ChAT activity in hippocampus regio inferior and dentate gyrus. Although this effect was only studied 3 weeks after the lesion, it was concluded that G_{M1} enhanced heterotypic sprouting of the septohippocampal pathway (29). The authors also reported a significant increase in enzyme activity by 6 days after lesions (P6). This rapid elevation of enzyme activity is also consistent with a sprouting hypothesis, but the G_{M1} effect "may also be due to the influence on other mechanisms besides sprouting, such as enhancement of hyperactivity or enhancement of synaptic mechanisms in presynaptic nerve terminals or retardation of degeneration processes."[29,p.417]

Although most of the results indicate that gangliosides enhance sprouting, there is also one experiment indirectly demonstrating that gangliosides may suppress sprouting or not affect sprouting at all. Fass and Ramirez[13] made bilateral lesions of the entorhinal cortex and assessed AChE activity of the septodentate pathway histochemically. It was assumed that intensification of AChE staining in the denervated dentate gyrus would provide evidence for collateral sprouting. In untreated animals, an intial loss of AChE activity was followed by an intensification of AChE staining as early as P3, with a nearly linear increase until P10. The intensity of AChE in the ganglioside group, however, was significantly smaller at 3 days and 10 days post-lesion. If AChE activity is assumed to be an adequate measure of sprouting under treatment conditions, these findings would imply a ganglioside-induced early suppression of sprouting.

Regardless of whether gangliosides enhance or suppress sprouting in the hippocampus, changes in enzyme levels may not necessarily reflect an effect of exogenous gangliosides on collateral axon sprouting unless several alternative explanations can be ruled out.

It is conceivable, for example, that axons spared by the lesion up-regulate their transmitter biosynthesis and release. Such a compensatory mechanism is well known to occur after partial nigrostriatal lesions[1] (see also F. Hefti and W. J. Weiner, Chapter 6). Thus, ganglioside-induced elevated enzyme levels may reflect increases in transmitter synthesis independent of sprouting. There are two pieces of evidence related to the cholinergic system suggesting that this might be the case. For example, when relatively high concentrations of gangliosides are added to a cholinergic cell line *in vitro*, they were found to elevate levels of choline acetyltransferase without promoting fiber outgrowth.[23] Furthermore, the rate of synthesis and release of ACh is enhanced in cortical slices taken from cats with gangliosidosis.[25]

It may also be possible that gangliosides alter enzyme activity *per se*. Earlier observations that gangliosides do not affect enzyme levels in intact tissue had been used to discount this hypothesis. However, ganglioside-treated normal animals are not the appropriate control, because ganglioside concentrations are probably lower in the unlesioned area, where the blood–brain barrier is not disrupted. In normal brain, only a very small amount of the substance passes through the blood–brain barrier.[47]

Unless these two alternatives can be ruled out, the evidence is only "consistent" with the sprouting hypothesis but does not provide conclusive proof.

2.2.2. Nigrostriatal System

The nigrostriatal system is an attractive injury model because it lends itself to the investigation of correlations between reinnervation and behavioral performance. When the nigrostriatal pathway is severed unilaterally (either by hemitransection or intranigral injections of the neurotoxin 6-hydroxydopamine, 6-OHDA), the resulting asymmetry in dopamine neurotransmission leads to a specific behavioral deficit: rats rotate in circles. This behavioral deficit is particularly pronounced after injections of dopaminergic agonists, and behavioral sparing (i.e., reduced initial deficit) or recovery (gradual return toward normal) can conveniently be monitored.

The loss of dopaminergic innervation in the caudate nucleus after partial unilateral transections of the nigrostriatal pathway is evident by a 50% reduction in the V_{max} of tyrosine hydroxylase (TH) activity and homovanillic acid (HVA) content on P8.[50] When animals are treated with purified monosialogangliosides (G_{M1}), they show the same reduction of enzyme activity on P8.[50] Whereas on P15, saline-treated controls still show only 50% TH activity, G_{M1}-treated rats recover 80% of normal TH levels; because the increase in TH activity was further substantiated by immunofluorescence and by HVA analysis, it was concluded that G_{M1} injections increase central dopaminergic axon sprouting or regeneration.

Unfortunately, this interpretation of the data is also subject to the criticisms that increased HVA and TH activity could reflect a compensatory increase in transmitter biosynthesis and release. This is not an unreasonable alternative explanation. A possible role of some surviving neurons in mediating the ganglioside effect is supported by several findings: (1) G_{M1} reduces the loss of [^{3}H]DA uptake in striatal synaptosomes in the first few days after a lesion, indicating that more terminals are present (did not degenerate?), and (2) G_{M1} may also enhance cell survival in the substantia nigra (see Section 3). Regardless of these alternative interpretations, the current evidence is nevertheless equally consistent with the hypothesis that G_{M1} stimulates sprouting in the striatum after nigrostriatal hemitransections. However, conclusive proof for either or both hypotheses is still outstanding.

In order to address this problem with a morphological rather than a biochemical method, we injected a retrograde tracing dye (HRP) into the striatum.[39,41] We reasoned that if G_{M1} enhances collateral sprouting, an increased number of retrogradely labeled neurons should be observed in substantia nigra pars reticulata (SNr) after hemitransections. As expected, the transection led to a significant loss of labeled neurons at P3, 25% of the normal number. At P15, however, there were significantly more labeled neurons in SNr of G_{M1}-treated animals (see Fig. 2).

Although these findings strongly suggest that G_{M1} enhances reinnervation of the striatum, possibly via collateral sprouting, there is still the alternative explanation that soon after the lesion, axons may fail to transport HRP without being structurally destroyed. That gangliosides may facilitate axonal transport was indeed observed by Kalia et al.[26] However, in this study reestablishment of retrograde transport with ganglioside treatment was seen within 3 days after peroneal nerve crush.

2.2.3. OTHER SYSTEMS

The effects of gangliosides on sprouting and regeneration were also studied after lesions of the rat neocortex[24,28] and spinal cord.[4,21]

In order to create cerebral cortex lesions in adult rats, Kojima et al.[28] slowly infused 6-OHDA into cortex via an osmotic minipump. The degeneration of norepinephrine (NE)-containing terminals was clearly evident by fluorescence histochemistry and biochemical assays after 3 and 7 days. A recovery of NE levels in cortex rostral to the infusion site occurred within 5 weeks, paralleled by a reappearance of fluorescent NE nerve terminals. Although treatment with G_{M1} had no effect on the initial degeneration (defined by biochemical means), a partial but significant elevation of NE was observed to result from the treatment 7 days[24] and 2 weeks[28] after the lesion. This finding was interpreted as evidence for regrowth (regeneration or sprouting) of NE terminals. Similar to studies in the hippocampus and striatum, these results could also be interpreted as a G_{M1}-

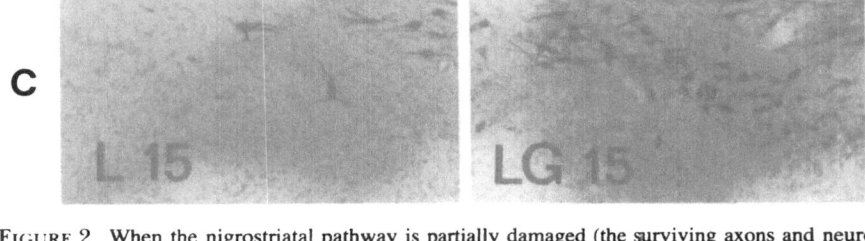

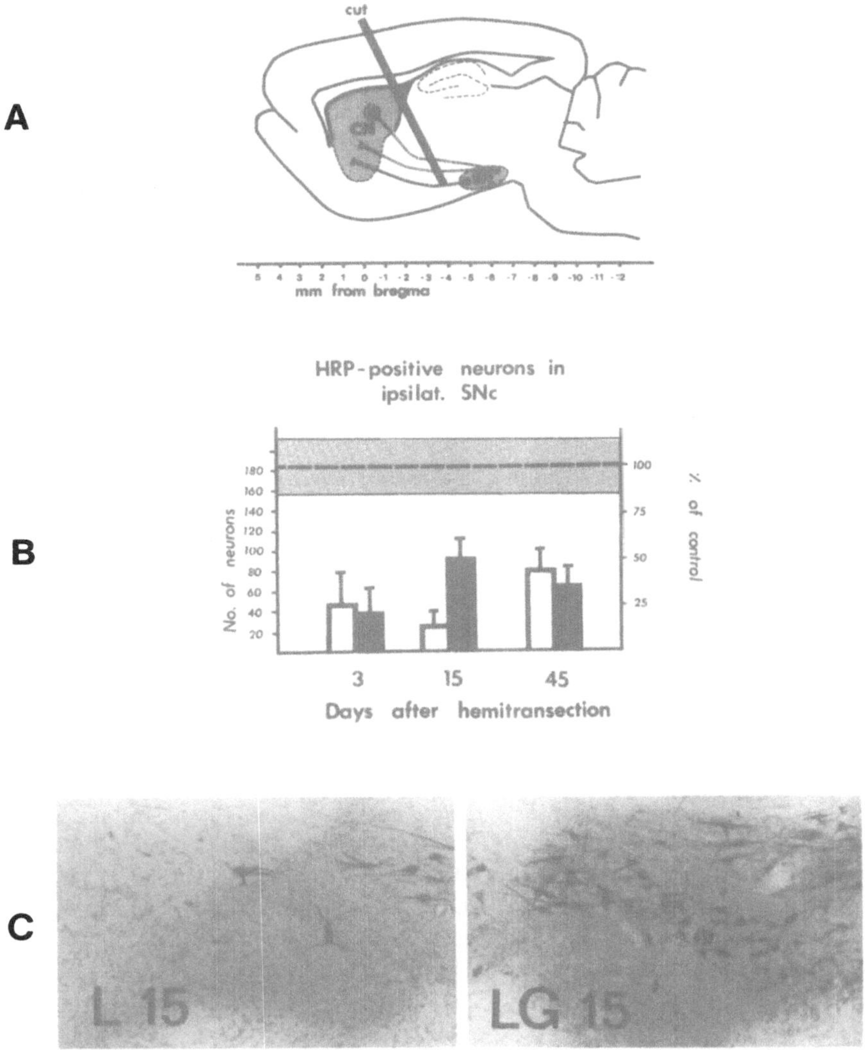

FIGURE 2. When the nigrostriatal pathway is partially damaged (the surviving axons and neurons are indicated by a solid line, part A), only the few surviving neurons in substantia nigra (SN) still maintain intact connections with the caudate nucleus (CN). Only these neurons are able to pick up and retrogradely transport HRP that had previously been injected into the caudate nucleus. Part B shows the result of counts of HRP-positive neurons in the SN. At 3 days post-lesion, only 25% of the normal number of neurons are stained in both treatment groups. At P15, however, ganglioside-treated animals (solid bar) have significantly more labeled neurons in SN than saline controls (open bar). At P45, the number of cells has also increased in saline-treated animals. Part C: Examples of labeled neurons in SN on P15 in animals treated (LG15) or not treated (L15) with G_{M1}. (From Sabel et al.[39])

induced elevation of transmitter levels because of accelerated synthesis in structurally spared fibers.

Studies in transected adult rat spinal cord revealed that when HRP was injected 10 mm below the transection, more retrogradely labeled cells were found in medulla oblongata of G_{M1}-treated rats.[9] This reestablishment of axonal transport could be interpreted in terms of either true regeneration across the cut or enhanced uptake and retrograde transport of HRP. In similar experiments,[21] the spinal cord was hemisected, resulting in a loss of 5-HT below the transection and a bilateral loss of 5-HIAA, NE, and DA. The G_{M1} treatment apparently elevated 5-HIAA and DOPAC above and below the lesion on both sides and 5-HT below the hemitransection. Again, no clear conclusions can be drawn from the experiment.

2.3. SPROUTING IN DEVELOPMENT

It is well known that sprouting and regeneration are more easily elicited in early stages of postnatal development.[46] When gangliosides are given early in life, there is indirect evidence that they enhance central regeneration or sprouting after neurotoxin lesions in neocortex[24] and spinal cord.[18] Direct evidence for enhanced sprouting has very recently been reported in the kitten red nucleus[16,17] and in the superior colliculus of golden hamsters.[42]

2.3.1. NEUROTOXIN LESIONS

Systemic injections of 5,7-HT (a serotonin neurotoxin) or 6-OHDA in neonatal rats leads to the degeneration of distal nerve terminals in various structures of the CNS. Axons and terminals degenerate in cortex, hippocampus, spinal cord, etc., evident by a loss of 5-HT.[24] Although the initial neurotoxin-induced loss of transmitter activity was not affected by G_{M1} treatment, G_{M1} partially restored serotonin levels in cortex[24] and perhaps in spinal cord.[18] This elevation of transmitter levels can be considered indirect evidence for G_{M1}-enhanced sprouting in development.

2.3.2. RED NUCLEUS

Electrophysiological evidence for ganglioside-induced sprouting at later stages of development was obtained by Tsukahara and co-workers.[16,17] Large neocortical ablations were made in kittens of various ages, and the probability of occurence of EPSPs in the red nucleus was determined following stimulation of contralateral cerebral cortex.

After large neocortical lesions, a loss of slow-rising postsynaptic potentials (EPSPs) on red nucleus neurons was observed, indicating a loss of cortical afferents on distal dendrites. When decortication was performed within the first

150 days of life, slow-rising EPSPs reappeared, indicative of sprouting of crossed corticorubral fibers onto distal dendrites. When kittens received lesions at 70–140 days of age, the probability of recording EPSPs in the red nucleus following contralateral cortex stimulation was about 20%. Ten daily injections of a crude ganglioside mixture into a gelatin sponge that was inserted into the lesion cavity increased the response probability to about 65% when kittens were tested more than 3 weeks later. Therefore, "ganglioside application appears to have a facilitatory effect on sprouting and formation of functional synapses" in the red nucleus.[16,p.45]

2.3.3. VISUAL SYSTEM

Most recently, I obtained direct anatomic evidence for ganglioside-enhanced sprouting in the developing hamster visual system.[42,43]

When early lesions of the right superior colliculus (rSC) are made on postnatal day 1 (Pn1), retinofugal fibers, which normally innervate the rSC,

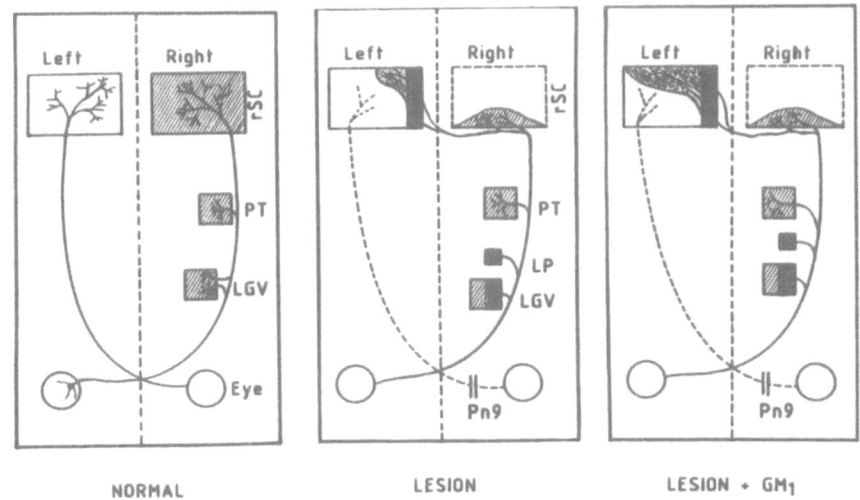

FIGURE 3. Left panel: In the subcortical visual system of the hamster, the optic tract from the left eye crosses the midline and innervates various structures on the right side, among them the ventral lateral geniculate nucleus of the thalamus (LGv), several pretectal nuclei (PT), and the superior colliculus (rSC). Middle panel: When the right superior colliculus is removed (indicated by the dashed line) on postnatal day one (Pn1), an abnormal neuronal circuit forms with dense terminal fields (indicated by the solid area) in LGv and LP (lateral posterior nucleus of the thalamus, normally not innervated by the optic tract) and with an abnormal decussation to the left tectum. Here, the optic tract innervates tissue near the midline (the hatched area). This abnormal left tectal innervation can be induced to sprout over larger areas (dotted area) when competing axons from the right eye are removed on Pn9. Right panel: When hamsters are treated with G_{M1} gangliosides, this sprouting response is significantly enhanced without reducing the abnormal innervation fields located more proximal to the retinal ganglion cells (LGv, LP).

grow abnormally to the left tectum and terminate in areas near the midline[46] (see also Fig. 3). Axons of the abnormal terminal field and those from the right eye segregate, and a sharp border between the terminal fields of both eyes is formed in the same tectum. When the right eye is removed, the abnormally formed terminal field from the left eye sprouts over a larger area of the left tectum. This sprouting response is most vigorous at birth or shortly thereafter and gradually diminishes until Pn14, when sprouting is no longer observed.[46]

In order to test for possible sprouting enhancement by G_{M1}, we induced sprouting on Pn9 (a stage of intermediate growth vigor) by right eye removal and injected G_{M1} intraperitoneally every day for 3 weeks. In order to trace and quantify the retinofugal pathway from the left eye, the left eye was removed, and, after 3 days, the brain was processed for degenerating axons and axon terminals with the Fink–Heimer procedure. If G_{M1} had a stimulatory effect on sprouting, we would expect to see a larger and/or denser termination field in the left tectum.

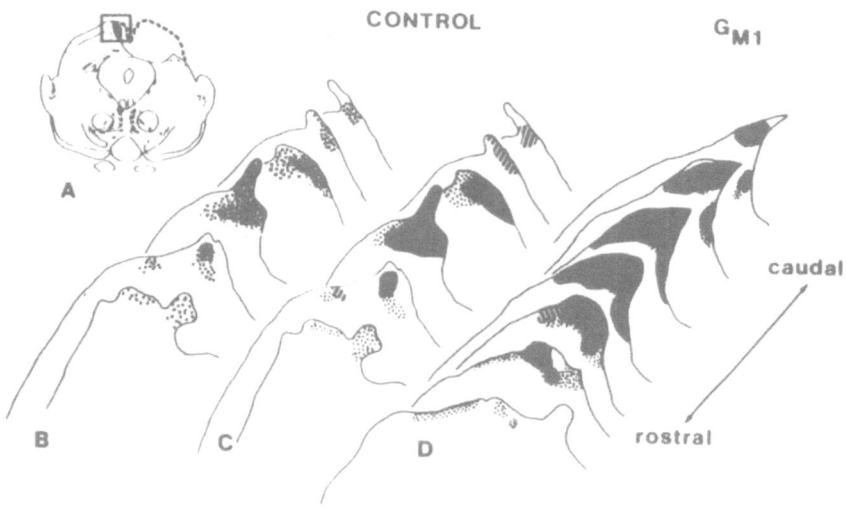

FIGURE 4. This graph shows typical examples of terminal field reconstructions. Part A is a low-magnification drawing of a coronal section through the mesencephalon, showing the position of the tectum. The dashed line indicates where the tectal surface of a normal brain, without an early lesion, would be. The area in the box represents the medial aspect of the left tectum, which, in greater magnification, is shown as a series of consecutive sections in parts B, C, and D. To visualize the retinofugal projections to these areas, the left eye was removed, and degenerating terminal fields were stained (part B). These were then quantified by tracing them on paper with the aid of a drawing tube attached to a light microscope, using a 10x objective. The size of the degenerating terminal fields of different densities (which were rated light, moderate, or heavy) were then measured with computer aid. A typical control case (i.e., closest to the group mean) is shown in C, and part D shows a typical case (defined likewise) with G_{M1} treatment. Note the larger size and greater density of the terminal field and the more extensive lateral spread in the G_{M1} case.

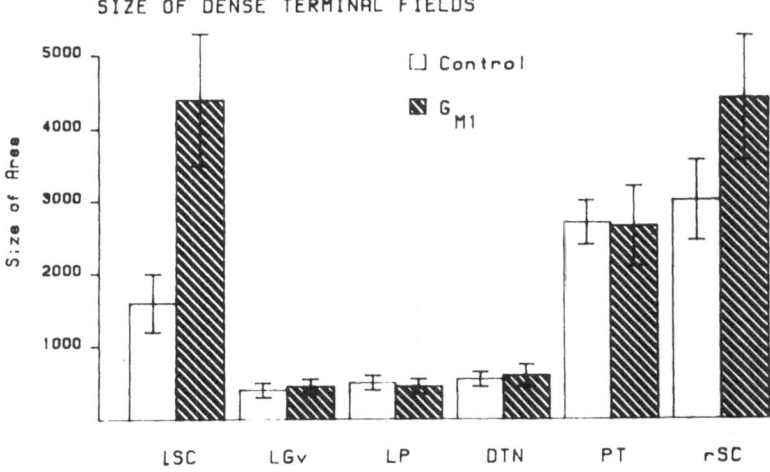

FIGURE 5. Mean and S.E.M. of the areas of heavy degeneration in the various brain structures innervated by the optic tract. Animals were either treated (shaded bars) or not treated (open bars) with G_{M1}. Significant differences were only seen in the left SC. Abbreviations are explained in legend to Fig. 3.

The quantification of the left tectal terminal field involved (1) the area measurement of the retinotectal terminal field and (2) the rating of termination density as light, moderate, or heavy with subsequent light microscopic counting of silver grains in representative areas (at 100×, oil immersion; see Fig. 4).

The total size of the terminal field in the left tectum was twice as large in G_{M1}-treated animals as in controls; this increased the number of grains from 3.2 million in controls to 7.9 million in G_{M1}-treated hamsters. Because silver grains represent axon branches and terminals, this finding directly demonstrates that the G_{M1} increases axon sprouting in developing hamsters (Fig. 5).

We also quantified the size of diencephalic terminal fields in the right hemisphere. These are structures normally innervated by the left eye, such as the dorsal and ventral lateral geniculate nuclei of the thalamus (LGd and LGv), several pretectal nuclei (PT), and spared tissue of the damaged superior colliculus (rSC). Terminal fields in these structures as well as in an abnormally innervated nucleus (the lateral posterior nucleus of the thalamus, LP) were not affected in their size by the G_{M1} treatment. Thus, G_{M1} initiates outgrowth only in areas that have recently been deafferented (as was the case in the left tectum, where deafferentation was achieved by right eye removal). Our data provide the first *in vivo* evidence for the earlier *in vitro* finding[11] that G_{M1} fails to initiate neurite sprouting. Rather, G_{M1} potentiates an ongoing sprouting response.

Two other studies are also worth mentioning in which the interaction of developing tissue with adult tissue was studied. When fetal mesencephalic tissue was grafted into the ventricles 4 weeks after caudate nucleus deafferentation in rats,[15] there was clear penetration of catecholaminergic fibers over a distance of 0.5 to 1 mm into the host brain, but G_{M1} treatment was without effect. Although it is possible that gangliosides may not be able to overcome the endogenous limitations for axon elongation, it is also conceivable that implantation was performed too late. At 4 weeks after denervation, levels of neuronotrophic substances in the host brain may not be sufficient (see M. Nieto-Sampedro, Chapter 15).

Relatively low levels of neuronotrophic factors are also encountered immediately (several hours) after the lesion. It is therefore not surprising that when fetal locus coeruleus tissue is implanted in the spinal cord at this time, tissue survival and process outgrowth are not influenced by G_{M1}.[9]

2.4. CONCLUSIONS ON SPROUTING

Currently, the two most important questions are (1) do exogenous gangliosides promote central sprouting, and (2) does the sprouting mediate behavioral changes? The information available today allows several tentative conclusions.

The data are consistent with the hypothesis that exogenous gangliosides enhance reinnervation after various types of lesion in adulthood. This conclusion is based on the observation of a time-dependent elevation of transmitter levels and their metabolites[50,54] and an increased retrograde cell labeling.[39,41] This evidence in adult animals, however, can not yet be considered conclusive proof and does not provide evidence as to whether reinnervation is through collateral sprouting or true regeneration. The possibility that gangliosides increase transmitter levels, enzyme activity, and/or axonal transport independent of sprouting has not yet been ruled out as an alternative explanation. Clearly, direct evidence is needed to obtain a firm demonstration of ganglioside-induced sprouting in adulthood. Additional studies using electron microscopy and/or anterograde axonal transport techniques may be required to accomplish this.

At least for certain brain systems, ganglioside-enhanced biochemical recovery depends on the nature of the lesion. When lesions are total, without sparing any significant number of axons, there is no G_{M1} effect[12,49] (see also G. L. Dunbar and D. G. Stein, Chapter 10). This underscores the significance of the spared fibers in the recovery process of a partially damaged system.

In development, however, direct evidence for ganglioside-enhanced sprouting has been obtained in the red nucleus and in the hamster visual system. Although gangliosides are potent stimulators of an ongoing sprouting response, they seem to be unable to initiate outgrowth by themselves. Rather, they potentiate the spontaneous outgrowth that occurs after degeneration in the target tissue. Whether this growth of distal sprouts occurs at the expense of sprouts more proximal to the soma (i.e., a "reversal" of pruning) is presently unclear.

On the surface, regeneration and sprouting are intuitively attractive mechanisms that could be responsible for brain repair. Unfortunately, behavioral correlates of sprouting (i.e., recovery of function) have been exceedingly difficult to obtain and have been subjected to various criticisms.[36]

In any case, if ganglioside-induced sprouting is the cellular mechanism whereby gangliosides stimulate behavioral improvement after injury, a gradual behavioral improvement would be expected to parallel the time course of axon outgrowth. Clearly, this has never been observed. Rather, ganglioside administrations result in behavioral sparing (reducing the initial deficit), which can not easily be explained by sprouting. Therefore, the behavioral improvement induced by gangliosides following brain lesions must be caused by the reduction of some deteriorative events that happen soon after the brain injury. It is possible that sprouting does contribute to behavioral performance at later time points, but this is still unknown.

3. PREVENTING SECONDARY DEGENERATION AFTER BRAIN INJURY

If sprouting is not the anatomic substrate for the behavioral effects of exogenous gangliosides, we need to focus our attention instead on early secondary events soon after brain injury.

For the purpose of this discussion, early ''secondary deteriorative events'' are definded as those cellular and subcellular events that occur within hours or several days after injury and are not the direct consequence of the primary insult. They include retrograde cell atrophy and degeneration, anterograde degeneration, edema (see S. E. Karpiak *et al.*, Chapter 11), and subcellular perturbation (changes in ion equilibrium, lipid peroxidation, etc.).

These secondary events are important because they are reasonable targets for pharmacological agents such as gangliosides. Indeed, in the last several years reports of gangliosides' ability to reduce secondary deteriorative events in adulthood and in developing animals following injury to different neuronal systems have appeared.

3.1. DEGENERATION IN ADULTHOOD

3.1.1. CHOLINERGIC SYSTEMS

When the magnocellular nuclei (MFN) are damaged, high-affinity choline uptake (HACU) and choline acetyltransferase (ChAT) fall to 40–50% of normal in ipsilateral frontal cortex within 4 days.[32] Because HACU is a presynaptic marker, the loss probably reflects cholinergic terminal degeneration. A subsequent increase in HACU occurs until postoperative day 20. This increase may indicate an elevation of the metabolic and firing activity of residual cholinergic neurons,[32] since increased ACh release depends on choline availability through the HACU system.

When gangliosides are given after a lesion of MFN, there is no significant loss of HACU in the ipsilateral frontal cortex at P4 as compared to a 38% loss in lesion controls.[31] In addition, G_{M1} significantly increased HACU in the contralateral cortex to above-normal levels, also not found in saline controls. Because of the spontaneous recovery of HACU in lesion controls at later time points, there were no longer any differences at P10 and P20.

This rapid time course of HACU restoration can not be explained by collateral sprouting. Instead, it may indicate either (1) prevention of terminal degeneration by G_{M1} or (2) a rapid increase in activity of residual neurons within 4 days post-lesion.

There is no spontaneous recovery of ChAT activity within 20 days after the lesion in untreated animals. When animals were treated with G_{M1} for 20 days, the fall of ChAT in ipsilateral frontoparietal cortex was not affected, but significantly more ChAT was observed in other areas of neocortex (45% increase).[7] However, because no time course was obtained for this measure, the ChAT increase could be indicative of sprouting or of increased activity of cholinergic neurons that were better able to survive the lesion because of G_{M1} treatment. Because an active avoidance response deficit after the MFN lesion was already significantly smaller on P4,[7] and because cortical ACh appears to be involved in the control of active avoidance performance, it is possible that differences in ChAT activity between G_{M1}-treated animals and lesion controls appear shortly (within hours or days) after the lesion. If this is so, the primary action of the G_{M1} would be a maintenance of the number of cholinergic connections, probably via a reduction of secondary degeneration of cholinergic neurons in MFN.

Recently, evidence has been obtained[10] that is in agreement with such a hypothesis. When unilateral cortical damage was inflicted in 30-day-old rats, G_{M1} prevented retrograde soma shrinkage and denritic loss in the basal nucleus, evident after a 30-day treatment with daily G_{M1} injections. Again, no time course was obtained, and it is therefore not possible to judge from the data whether there was an initial shrinkage soon after the lesion that was later reversed by G_{M1} or whether G_{M1} prevented the shrinkage.

Another cholinergic system, the septohippocampal pathway, has also been investigated. Partial lesions of the dorsal hippocampal afferents lead to partial loss of cholinergic (and serotoninergic) enzymes in hippocampus.[20] When the lesion encroached on dorsal aspects of the septum, the loss of AChE and ChAT was about 50 and 70%, respectively. If the lesion was restricted to areas above the septum, cholinergic deafferentation was less severe as indicated by a loss of only 15% and 25% of AChE and ChAT, respectively. In the case with the more severe lesion, G_{M1} reduced the loss of both AChE and ChAT activity compared to lesioned controls. When the lesion was less severe, however, this G_{M1} effect was not observed.

These data suggest a tight correlation between the amount of degeneration and the facilitating effects of G_{M1}. They also suggest that if the lesion placement varies slightly, the G_{M1} facilitation may be either profound or null (similar effects in the nigrostriatal system were found using behavioral assays; see ref. 12).

3.1.2. NIGROSTRIATAL SYSTEM

Following partial hemitransection of the nigrostriatal pathway, TH activity in substantia nigra (SN) drops to about 50% of control levels by P14. In animals with G_{M1} injections, there is only a 20% loss of TH activity.[51] Because a semiquanitative analysis of immunocytochemical material revealed similar findings, it was concluded that G_{M1} enhanced cell survival in SN. Unfortunately, both the measurement of TH activity and that of immunoreactivity use dopamine levels as an indicator of cell number. Therefore, an alternative interpretation of these data is possible, namely, that G_{M1} increased transmitter synthesis in surviving neurons.

Two observations are consistent with such a hypothesis. First, close inspection of recent findings[19] of increased DA utilization per neuron after G_{M1} treatment indicates that an increased synthesis may fully account for elevated TH activity in SN. Dopamine synthesis per neuron seems to be increased to above normal levels in G_{M1}-treated animals. Secondly, an increase in relative amount of TH immunoreactivity in cells located more rostrally in SN was observed after hemitransection. This DA increase was significantly more pronounced after G_{M1} treatment.[3] Because no such effect was seen more caudally, increased optical density of TH activity in caudal SNc in G_{M1}-treated animals was interpreted as enhanced cell survival. Thus, the possibility exists that cell loss is little, if at all, affected by G_{M1} but that G_{M1} elevates the compensatory up-regulation of transmitter synthesis (see discussion above). A purported increase in the "length" of nigral dendrites[51] may also be the result of the same compensatory mechanism.

Whatever the true event may be, G_{M1} enhances either cell survival or compensatory transmitter synthesis in surviving neurons. Although we cannot reach a firm conclusion yet, both mechanisms could account for the reduction of behavioral deficits after partial brain lesions and would result in the maintenance of spontaneous electrophysiological activity.[48] This interpretation would also explain why behavioral deficits after total lesions cannot be reduced by G_{M1} treatment.[12] Future studies should make use of techniques that can differentiate between cell number and levels of transmitters.

To understand the behavioral impairments after brain damage, it is also important to recognize that such deficits are not only the result of the loss of the damaged structure itself but are also caused by the deafferentation of target structures. If gangliosides do, in fact, reduce cell death, behavioral benefits can only be expected when the structural integrity of the neuronal connections is maintained.

In order to address the issue of whether gangliosides maintain the integrity of axonal connections, we directly quantified the extent of anterograde degeneration using the Fink–Heimer method.[38] Following hemitransections of the nigrostriatal pathway in the left hemisphere and a caudate nucleus lesion in the right hemisphere, we quantified the extent of anterograde degeneration in substantia nigra pars reticulata 7 days following the lesion (Fig. 6). Animals treated

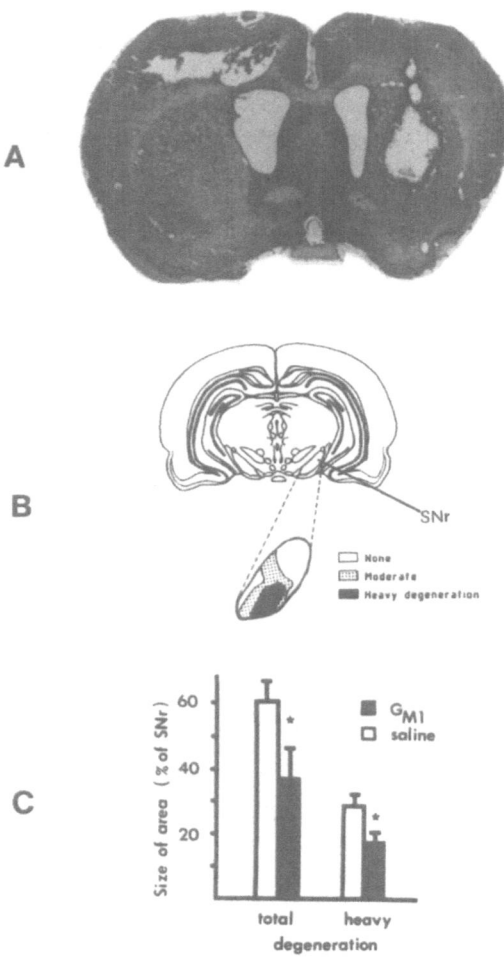

FIGURE 6. Part A: When rats receive lesions of the caudate nucleus (CN) (as shown here in a coronal brain section), anterograde degeneration can be visualized in substantia nigra pars reticulata (SNr, part B) and can be rated to be absent, light (dotted area), or heavy (solid area). Part C: Ganglioside-treated rats show significantly smaller total areas of degeneration and smaller areas of heavy terminal degeneration. (From Sabel et al.[38])

with G_{M1} had significantly smaller areas of degeneration on the side with the caudate lesion than saline-treated controls with comparable lesions. No significant differences were seen on the side with the hemitransection. Thus, G_{M1} treatment was effective in maintaining neuronal connectivity after caudate lesions. This may be the result of either prevention of secondary cell death or axon protection in areas surrounding the lesion.

In contrast to our failure to find differences in anterograde degeneration after hemitransections, Raiteri et al.[34] observed at P5 a less severe reduction of [^{3}H]dopamine uptake in striatal synaptosomes in animals that were treated with a G_{M1} derivative. Although this biochemical finding may also be interpreted in terms of increased function of spared terminals, taken together with our anatomic data it may be concluded that G_{M1} exerts some "protective" action (preventing degeneration) on neurons and their axons after lesions in the nigrostriatal system.

3.1.3. OTHER LESIONS

We have recently performed unilateral aspirations of the posterior half of neocortex in adult hamsters and have examined retrograde changes in the dorsal lateral geniculate nucleus (LGd) of the thalamus (B. A. Sabel, J. Gottlieb, and G. E. Schneider, unpublished data). Either 4 weeks or 8 weeks following the lesion, LGd had collapsed in size to about 45% of the opposite, nonlesioned hemisphere. Daily G_{M1} injections given during the entire survival time did not prevent the retrograde degenerative events in adult hamsters. Our finding is in agreement with those of Dunbar et al.,[12] who could not observe effects of G_{M1} on reducing neuron loss in LGd after the same type of lesion in adult rats.

3.2. DEGENERATION IN DEVELOPMENT

Neuronal reaction to distal injury is an age-dependent event. In early stages of development, cell death as a result of retrograde or transsynaptic degeneration is very rapid. With increasing age, however, the neuron is better able to survive the injury, although it does show signs of atrophy, i.e., shrinkage and chromatolysis. This age-dependent reaction to injury may be the consequence of growing independence of developing neurons from trophic factors in the target field. Thus, neuronal death in development is not only the direct consequence of injury but also the result of lack of trophic support from the target field. In contrast, adult neurons have the capability to store these trophic substances.

If developing neurons are particularly dependent on trophic factors, the influence of G_{M1} on degeneration in development seems to be of particular interest.

In our study of sprouting of the optic tract axons described above,[43] we removed the right superior colliculus on the day after birth (Pn1). In addition to the assessment of the optic tract sprouting, we evaluated the size of the early tectal lesion without prior knowledge of the group identity. Although the G_{M1} treatment was not started until Pn9, treated animals had significantly smaller right tectal lesions than controls and had less damage in left tectal tissue located close to the midline (Fig. 7). It thus seemed as if lesions inflicted early in life grew larger over time and that this deterioration was prevented even with delayed G_{M1} treatment.

To assess the time course and possible effects of G_{M1} in another developmental lesion paradigm, we have studied retrograde degeneration of the lateral geniculate after neocortex lesion in developing animals as described above (B. A. Sabel, J. Gottlieb, and G. E. Schneider, unpublished data). At postnatal day 14, the posterior half of the right neocortex was removed in hamsters, and the size of LGd determined 1 or 3 weeks later. If gangliosides prevent retrograde degenerative events such as atrophy and cell death, a lesion-induced shrinkage of LGd should be less severe.

One week after the lesion, control and G_{M1}-treated hamsters had compara-

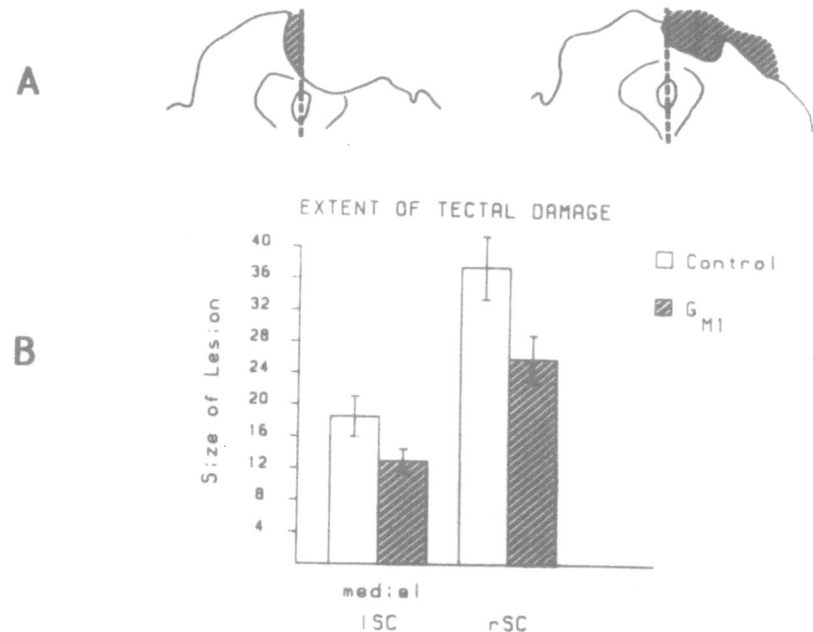

FIGURE 7. We made heat lesions of the right superior colliculus (rSC) in hamsters on postnatal day 1 (Pn1). At Pn9, a 3-week-long treatment with G_{M1} was begun. Part A shows the estimated area of the lesion in the left and right tectum (striated area). The quantitative analysis for both treatment groups is shown in part B. Treated hamsters were found to have less damage in medial tissue of the left tectum, and the right tectal damage was also significantly less severe.

ble shrinkage of about 58% (compared to the intact left hemisphere). At 3 weeks post-lesion, the difference was even larger in controls (73%) but remained the same for the G_{M1}-treated animals (59%), which now had a significantly larger volume in the right LGd than saline-injected controls ($P < .03$).

The two studies therefore provide evidence that G_{M1} treatment prevents secondary degenerative events (e.g., retrograde cell death) after lesions in developing hamsters.

Along these lines a recent finding by Carmignoto et al.[6] is noteworthy. As previously demonstrated, monocular deprivation in kittens at Pn35 results in a shift of ocular dominance in favor of the normal eye in neurons of visual cortex, evident by a loss of cells that can be excited by stimulation of the deprived eye. However, as Carmignoto et al.[6] showed, when G_{M1} is given systemically, the ocular dominance shift following monocular deprivation is partially counteracted. Here, G_{M1} may have reduced the withdrawal of deprived eye connections.

4. OTHER MECHANISMS

Although collateral sprouting and secondary degeneration have been the topic of most studies on exogenous gangliosides, there are other mechanisms of action whereby exogenous gangliosides may induce brain repair. These are (1) denervation-induced sensitivity alterations of postsynaptic receptors and (2) synaptic efficiency.

4.1. DENERVATION SUPERSENSITIVITY

When input to a structure is lost, the postsynaptic membranes compensate for the loss of transmitter by increasing the number or affinity of the receptors. There is no clear-cut a priori hypothesis whether exogenous gangliosides would increase or decrease the denervation supersensitivity. Although gangliosides have been shown to increase receptor function,[22] it is equally possible that enhanced sprouting or reduced loss of input would maintain the status of the postsynaptic membrane; i.e., gangliosides would prevent denervation supersensitivity. In a sense, prevention of supersensitivity would be an epiphenomenon of reduced denervation. The current evidence supports the latter possibility.

It has been observed, for example, that G_{M1}-treated cats in which pre- and postganglionic anastomosis has been performed do not show the expected supersensitivity of the nictitating membrane to i.v. injections of epinephrine.[8] In the CNS, a similar observation was made.[2] Here, G_{M1}-treated animals did not show as severe an increase in [³H]spiperone and [³H]NPA binding in the striatum after hemitransection as did controls.

4.2. SYNAPTIC EFFICIENCY

Gangliosides may also alter the synaptic efficiency of the neurons spared after a partial lesion. When hippocampal slices were enriched with G_{M1} by incubating them in neuraminidase or G_{M1},[52] a potentiated synaptic response was recorded from the pyramidal layer after stimulation of Schaffer collateral–commissural fibers. Obviously, it would be of interest to determine whether these or similar events are also operative in spared synapses following partial brain lesions.

5. DISCUSSION

From the behavioral studies it is clear that ganglioside treatment reduces deficits following brain damage.[40] What are the anatomic events underlying this phenomenon? Careful consideration of the current evidence, both biochemical and anatomic, allows us to reach several tentative conclusions.

Conclusion 1: Gangliosides enhance axonal sprouting in developing animals, but direct proof in mature animals has yet to be demonstrated. Among the anatomic changes, enhanced reinnervation of the target structure by regeneration or sprouting has been assumed to be the main cause for gangliosides' behavioral effects. Although direct evidence for axonal sprouting has been obtained in the developing hamster tectum and in the red nucleus of kittens, such evidence in adulthood is still outstanding. Since the enhanced recovery of transmitter levels and their enzymes as well as retrograde transport after lesions in adulthood follow the typical time course (see Fig. 8, parts A and B), the data are consistent with the sprouting hypothesis. However, studies using electron microscopy and autoradiography are needed to provide conclusive evidence for ganglioside-enhanced sprouting in mature animals.

Conclusion 2: The indirect evidence for sprouting in adulthood can be interpreted in an alternative way. If the delayed elevation of transmitter levels and axonal transport do not indicate sprouting, what do they indicate? An alternative interpretation of these findings could be as follows. It is conceivable that gangliosides elevate transmitter biosynthesis and release and enhance retrograde axonal transport without affecting sprouting at later postlesion stages. In this case, one has to consider the fact that analyses of axonal transport and transmitter levels are always performed in the structure as a whole. Thus, the compensation could be achieved in two ways: (1) either transport and transmitter rate increases per spared neuron (both treatment groups would than be assumed to have the same number of neurons and axons) or (2) gangliosides would reduce a secondary loss of neurons and their axons. These neurons would, at a later point, increase axonal transport and transmitter synthesis.

The observation of a ganglioside-induced maintenance of presynaptic ele-

1. FUNCTIONAL PARAMETERS

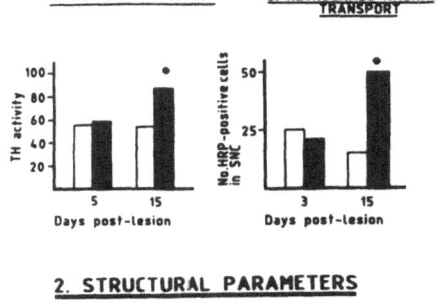

FIGURE 8. The "structural–functional paradox." The graphs are redrawn from various studies of the nigrostriatal system (A, Toffano et al.[48]; B, Sabel et al.[39]; C, Toffano et al.[48]; D, Sabel et al.[38]). Note that different scales have been used for easier comparibility between the studies. When "functional" parameters are used (levels of transmitter enzymes, part A, or retrograde axonal transport, part B), exogenous gangliosides (solid bars) do not have an effect soon after the lesion (P3 or P5) but significantly increase these parameters at a later point (P15) compared to controls (open bar). These findings have generally been interpreted in terms of enhanced sprouting/regeneration by G_{M1}. When "structural" parameters are used, which indicate the status of presynaptic elements (terminals), G_{M1}-treated animals show reduced

2. STRUCTURAL PARAMETERS

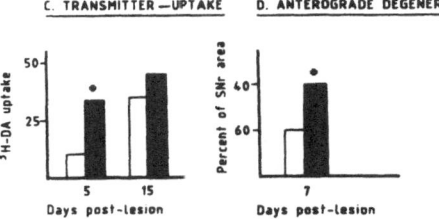

loss of transmitter uptake (part C) or reduced anterograde degeneration soon after the lesion (note that the scale in part D has been inverted; i.e., a larger bar indicates more intact terminals or less anterograde degeneration).

ments[38,49] tends to support the latter possibility, although this prevention of secondary degeneration is observed soon after the lesion (P4 to P7), well in advance of transmitter or transport recovery (P14 to P18). This discrepancy between the time course of transmitter and axonal transport elevation (functional markers) and that of reduced loss of presynaptic (structural) markers is a "structural–functional paradox" (see Fig. 8). However, this "structural–functional paradox" could be reconciled in a speculative spirit: it is conceivable that ganglioside treatment leads to a sparing of neurons and axons soon after the lesion, but a reduction of transmitter synthesis and axonal transport takes place nevertheless. Because of the enhanced survival, neurons are (at a later point) able to recover their axonal transport and transmitter production. These hypothetical "ghost neurons" would remain structurally intact after the lesion but functionally impaired, and they would die if not saved by some endogenous or exogenous trophic substance(s) (secondary degeneration; see Fig. 1).

Conclusion 3: Sprouting is not the anatomic basis of ganglioside-induced behavioral improvement. In any event, if the increased recovery of biochemical an anatomic parameters is indeed an expression of sprouting, the time course of this sprouting (within 14–18 days post-lesion) is not the same as that of behavioral improvement (as early as P2). This dissociation suggests that ganglioside-enhanced sprouting cannot account for the behavioral improvement. Instead, early events after the lesion are more likely to form the basis of behavioral sparing[35] (see also G. L. Dunbar and D. G. Stein, Chapter 10).

Conclusion 4: Gangliosides reduce secondary degenerative events. It has been suggested that gangliosides reduce retrograde cell death.[51] However, direct cell counts have not been obtained so far, and it is difficult to conceive how neurons saved from death and still disconnected from their target might contribute to behavior. Our recent finding is therefore of interest: we observed less anterograde degeneration in substantia nigra following caudate nucleus lesions when rats were treated with G_{M1}.[38] This seems to be a more useful anatomic measure of degeneration, for it expresses the extent of remaining connectivity that could be responsible for behavioral improvement.

Apparently, in developing brains, secondary degeneration following lesions can be effectively reduced with ganglioside treatment. Cortical as well as tectal lesions result in less secondary damage in hamsters treated with G_{M1}.

Although enhanced synaptic efficiency is a possible alternative mechanism. I favor the conclusion that ganglioside-induced behavioral sparing[13,27,41,48,50] results from the prevention of secondary degenerative events in a partially damaged system. This conclusion is also in agreement with the observation that G_{M1} promotes behavioral improvement only when lesions are partial and not when they are total.[12] Because these neurons are already committed to the function impaired by the lesion, their salvation by drug treatment appears to be the most fruitful approach.[45]

Gangliosides are, however, unable to counteract the primary degenerative events of neurotoxins both in development[24] and in adulthood.[49] The disruption of the blood–brain barrier, as it occurs following mechanical lesions, may be a necessary condition.

A purported reduction in denervation supersensitivity is probably an epiphenomenon of (1) enhanced cell survival, (2) reinnervation of the denervated structure, or (3) higher rates of transmitter release.

Conclusion 5: The specificity of gangliosides' action in vivo is not yet known. At the appropriate dose, purified G_{M1} gangliosides and the ganglioside mixture are equally effective in reducing behavioral deficits in brain-damaged animals. With the exception of tissue culture work,[5] the issue of treatment specificity (the question of which gangliosides are most effective, which portion of the molecule is necessary for the effects, etc.) has not yet been addressed.

6. RECOMMENDATIONS FOR FUTURE RESEARCH

There is much indirect evidence for gangliosides' ability to reduce secondary degenerative events and to enhance axon sprouting in adult animals following brain damage. Studies should now be performed to address these issues with techniques that are not prone to alternative interpretations. Perhaps the exclusive use of transmitter assays should be abandoned in favor of structural, neuroanatomic techniques.

The possible correlation of a reduction of secondary degenerative events by gangliosides with enhanced behavioral sparing also remains a great challenge for future investigations. Here, we ought to search for anatomic alterations that are behaviorally more meaningful than are reduced retrograde degeneration following axotomy. A disconnected neuron, even if saved from dying, can not be expected to contribute significantly to behavioral recovery.

We now need less experimental "phenomena" but more definite answers. This should improve our understanding of the repair-enhancing effects of exogenous gangliosides in animals with brain injury and eventually lead to the use of gangliosides in future neurology.

Having accomplished these ambitious goals, perhaps we ought to modify Ramon y Cajal's statement to say that "not everything may die, and something may regenerate."

REFERENCES

1. Acheson, A. L., Zigmond, M. J., and Stricker, E. M., 1980, Compensatory increase in tyrosine hydroxylase activity in rat brain after intraventricular injections of 6-hydroxydopamine, *Science* **207**:537–540.
2. Agnati, L. F., Fuxe, K., Calza, L., Benfenati, F., Cavicchioli, L., Toffano, G., and Goldstein, M., 1983, Gangliosides increase the survival of lesioned nigral dopamine neurons and favour the recovery of dopaminergic synaptic function in striatum of rats by collateral sprouting, *Acta Physiol. Scand.* **119**:347–363.
3. Agnati, L. F., Fuxe, K., Calza, L., Goldstein, M., Toffano, G., Giardino, L., and Zoli, M., 1984, Further studies on the effects of the G_{M1} ganglioside on the degenerative and regenerative features of mesostriatal dopamine neurons, *Acta Physiol. Scand.* **532**:37–44.
4. Bose, B., Osterholm, J. L., and Kalia, M., 1986, Ganglioside-induced regeneration and reestablishment of axonal continuity in spinal cord-transected rats, *Neurosci. Lett.* **63**:165–169.
5. Byrne, M. C., Ledeen, R. W., Roisen, F. J., Yorke, G., and Sclafani, J. R., 1983, Ganglioside-induced neuritogenesis: Verification that gangliosides are the active agent, and comparison of molecular species, *J. Neurochem.* **41**:1222.
6. Carmignoto, G., Canella, R., and Bisti, S., 1984, Can functional reorganization of area 17 following monocular deprivation be modified by G_{M1} internal ester treatment? *J. Neurosci. Res.* **12**:477–483.
7. Casamenti, F., Bracco, L., Bartolini, L., and Pepeu, G., 1985, Effects of ganglioside treatment in rats with a lesion of the cholinergic forebrain nuclei, *Brain Res.* **338**:45–52.
8. Ceccarelli, B., Aporti, F., and Finesso, M., 1975, Effects of brain gangliosides on functional recovery in experimental regeneration and reinnervation, *Adv. Exp. Med. Biol.* **71**:275–293.
9. Commissiong, J. W., and Toffano, G., 1986, The effect of G_{M1} ganglioside on coerulospinal noradrenergic, adult neurons and on fetal monoaminergic neurons transplanted into the transected spinal cord of the adult rat, *Brain Res.* **380**:205–215.
10. Cuello, A. C., Stephens, P. H., Tagari, P. C., Sofroniew, M. V., and Pearson, R. C. A., 1986,

Retrograde changes in the nucleus basalis of the rat, caused by cortical damage, are prevented by exogenous ganglioside G_{M1}, *Brain Res.* **376**:373–377.

11. Doherty, P., Dickson, J. G., Flanigan, T. P., and Walsh, F. S., 1985, Ganglioside G_{M1} does not initiate, but enhance neurite regeneration of nerve growth factor-dependent sensory neurons, *J. Neurochem.* **44**:1259–1265.

12. Dunbar, G. L., Butler, W. M., Fass, B., and Stein, D. G., 1987, Behavioral and neurochemical alterations induced by exogenous ganglioside in brain damaged animals: Problems and perspectives, in: *Gangliosides and Neuronal Plasticity* (G. Tettamanti, R. W. Ledeen, K. Sandhoff, Y. Nagai, and G. Toffano, eds.), Springer Verlag, Berlin, pp. 365–380.

13. Fass, B., and Ramirez, J. J., 1984, Effects of ganglioside treatment on lesion-induced behavioral impairments and sprouting in the CNS, *J. Neurosci. Res.* **12**:445–458.

14. Finger, S., and Stein, D. G., 1982, *Brain Damage and Recovery*, Academic Press, New York.

15. Freed, W. J., 1985, G_{M1} ganglioside does not stimulate reinnervation of the striatum by substantia nigra grafts, *Brain Res.* **14**:91–95.

16. Fujito, Y., Watanabe, S., Kobayashi, H., and Tsukahara, N., 1984, Lesion-induced sprouting in the red nucleus at the early developmental stage, in: *Early Brain Damage*, Volume 2 (S. Finger and C. R. Almli, eds.), Academic Press, New York, pp. 35–47.

17. Fujito, Y., Watanabe, S., Kobayashi, H., and Tsukahara, N., 1985, Promotion of sprouting and synaptogenesis of cerebrofugal fibers by ganglioside application in the red nucleus, *Neurosci. Res.* **2**:407–411.

18. Fusco, M., Dona, M., Tessari, F., Hallmann, H., Jonsson, G., and Gorio, A., 1986, G_{M1} ganglioside counteracts selective neurotoxin-induced lesion of developing serotonin neurons in rat spinal cord, *J. Neurosci. Res.* **15**:467–479.

19. Fuxe, K., Agnati, L. F., Benfenati, F., Zini, I., Gavioli, G., and Toffano, G., New evidence for the morphofunctional recovery of striatal function by ganglioside G_{M1} treatment following a partial hemitransection of rats. Studies on dopamine neurons and protein phosphorylation, in: *Gangliosides and Neuronal Plasticity* (G. Tettamanti, R. Ledeen, K. Sandhoff, Y. Nagai, and G. Toffano, eds.), Springer Verlag, Berlin, pp. 347–364.

20. Gradkowska, M., Skup, M., Kiedrowski, L., Calzolari, S., and Oderfeld-Nowak, B., 1986, The effect of G_{M1} ganglioside on cholinergic and serotoninergic systems in the rat hippocampus following partial denervation is dependent on the degree of fiber degeneration, *Brain Res.* **375**:417–422.

21. Hadjiconstantinou, M., and Neff, N. H., 1986, Treatment with G_{M1} ganglioside increases rat spinal cord indole content, *Brain Res.* **366**:343–345.

22. Hakomori, S., 1984, Ganglioside receptors: a brief overview and introductory remarks, in: *Ganglioside Structure, Function, and Biomedical Potential* (R. W. Ledeen, R. K. Yu, M. M. Rapport, and K. Suzuki, eds.), Plenum Press, New York, pp. 333–339.

23. Hefti, F., Hartikka, J., and Frick, W., 1985, Gangliosides alter morphology and growth of astrocytes and increase the activity of choline acetyltransferase in cultures of dissociated septal cells, *J. Neurosci.* **5**(8):2086–2094.

24. Jonsson, G., Gorio, A., Hallman, H., Janigro, D., Kojima, H., Luthman, J., and Zanoni, R., 1984, Effects of G_{M1} ganglioside on developing and mature serotonin and noradrenaline neurons lesioned by selective neurotoxins, *J. Neurosci. Res.* **12**:459–476.

25. Jope, R. S., Baker, H. J., and Conner, D. J., 1986, Increased acetylcholine synthesis and release in brains of cats with G_{M1} gangliosidosis, *J. Neurochem.* **46**:1567–1572.

26. Kalia, M., and DiPalma, J. R., 1982, Ganglioside-induced acceleration of axonal transport following nerve crush injury in the rat, *Neurosci. Lett.* **34**:1–5.

27. Karpiak, S. E., 1983, Ganglioside treatment improves recovery of alternation behaviour following unilateral entorhinal cortex lesions, *Exp. Neurol.* **81**:330–339.

28. Kojima, H., Gorio, A., Janigro, D., and Jonsson, G., 1984, G_{M1} ganglioside enhances regrowth of noradrenaline nerve terminals in rat cerebral cortex lesioned by 6-hydroxydopamine, *Neuroscience* **13**(4):1011–1022.

29. Oderfeld-Nowak, B., Skup, M., Ulas, J., Jezierska, M., Gradkowska, M., and Zaremba, M., 1984, Effect of G_{M1} ganglioside treatment on postlesion responses of cholinergic enzymes in rat hippocampus after various partial deafferentations, *J. Neurosci. Res.* **12**:409–420.

30. Oderfeld-Nowak, B., Wojcik, M., Ulas, J., and Potempska. A., 1981, Effects of chronic ganglioside treatment on recovery process in hippocampus after brain lesions in rats, in: *Gangliosides in Neurological and Neuromuscular Function, Development, and Repair* (M. M. Rapport and A. Gorio, eds.), Raven Press, New York, pp. 197–209.

31. Pedata, F., Giovannelli, L., and Pepeu, G., 1984, G_{M1} ganglioside facilitates the recovery of high-affinity choline uptake in the cerebral cortex of rats with a lesion of the nucleus basalis magnocellularis, *J. Neurosci. Res.* **12**:421–428.

32. Pedata, F., LoConte, G., Sorbi, S., Marconini-Pepeu, I., and Pepeu, G., 1982, Changes in high affinity choline uptake in rat cortex following lesions of the magnocellular forebrain nuclei, *Brain Res.* **233**:359–367.

33. Purpura, D. P., and Baker, H. J., 1977, Neurite induction in mature cortical neurons in feline G_{M1}-ganglioside storage disease, *Nature* **266**:553–554.

34. Raiteri, M., Versace, P., and Marchi, M., 1985, G_{M1} monosialoganglioside inner ester induces early recovery of striatal dopamine uptake in rats with unilateral nigrostriatal lesion, *Eur. J. Pharmacol.* **118**:347–350.

35. Ramirez, J. J., Fass, B., Kilfoil, T., Henschel, B., Grones, W., and Karpiak, S. E., 1987, Ganglioside-induced enhancement of behavioral recovery after bilateral lesions of the entorhinal cortex, *Brain Res.* **414**:85–90.

36. Ramirez, J. J. and Stein, D. G., Sparing and recovery of spatial alternation performance after entorhinal cortex lesions in rats, *Behav. Brain Res.* **13**:53–61.

37. Ramon y Cajal, S., 1928, *Degeneration and Regeneration of the Nervous System* (R. M. May, trans.), Oxford University Press, London.

38. Sabel, B. A., DelMastro, R., Dunbar, G. L., and Stein, D. G., 1987, Reduction of anterograde degeneration in brain damaged rats by G_{M1} gangliosides, *Neurosci. Lett.* **77**:360–366.

39. Sabel, B. A., Dunbar, G. L., Butler, W. M., and Stein, D. G., 1985, G_{M1} gangliosides stimulate neuronal reorganization and reduce rotational asymmetry after hemitransections of the nigro-striatal pathway, *Exp. Brain Res.* **60**:27–37.

40. Sabel, B. A., Dunbar, G. L., Fass, B., and Stein, D. G., 1985, Gangliosides, neuroplasticity, and behavioral recovery after brain damage, in: *Brain Plasticity, Learning, and Memory* (B. E. Will, P. Schmitt, and J. C. Dalrymple-Alford, eds.), Plenum Press, New York, pp. 481–493.

41. Sabel, B. A., Dunbar, G. L., and Stein, D. G., 1984, Gangliosides minimize behavioral deficits and enhance structural repair after brain injury, *J. Neurosci. Res.* **12**:429–443.

42. Sabel, B. A., and Schneider, G. E., 1986, G_{M1} ganglioside injections increase abnormal retinal projections in left tectum following early right tectal lesions, *Soc. Neurosci. Abstr.* **139**:26.

43. Sabel, B. A., and Schneider, G. E., 1988, Enhanced sprouting of retinotectal fibers after early superior colliculus lesions in hamsters treated with gangliosides. *Exp. Brain Res.* (in press).

44. Sabel, B. A., Slavin, M. D., and Stein, D. G., 1984, G_{M1} ganglioside treatment facilitates behavioral recovery from bilateral brain damage, *Science* **225**:340–342.

45. Sabel, B. A., and Stein, D. G., 1986, Pharmacological treatment of central nervous system injury, *Nature* **323**:493.

46. So, K.-F., and Schneider, G. E., 1978, Abnormal recrossing retinotectal projections after early lesions in Syrian hamsters: Age-related effects, *Brain Res.* **147**:277–295.

47. Tettamanti, G., Venerando, B., Roberti, S., Chigorno, V., Sonnino, S., Ghidoni, R., Orlando, P., and Massari, P., 1981, The fate of exogenously administered brain gangliosides, in: *Gangliosides in Neurological and Neuromuscular Function, Development and Repair* (M. M. Rapport and A. Gorio, eds.), Raven Press, New York, pp. 225–270.

48. Toffano, G., Agnati, L. F., Fuxe, K., Aldinio, C., Consolazione, A., Valenti, G., and Savoini, G., 1984, Effect of ganglioside treatment on the recovery of dopaminergic nigro-striatal neurons after different types of lesion, *Acta Physiol. Scand.* **122**:313–321.

49. Toffano, G., Savoini, G., Aporti, F., Calzolari, S., Consolazione, A., Maura, G., Marchi, M., Raiteri, M., and Agnati, L. F., 1984, The functional recovery of damaged brain: The effect of G_{M1} monosialoganglioside, *J. Neurosci. Res.* **12**:397–408.
50. Toffano, G., Savoini, G., Moroni, F., Lombardi, G., Calza, L., and Agnati, L. F., 1983, G_{M1} ganglioside stimulates the regeneration of dopaminergic neurons in the central nervous system, *Brain Res.* **261**:163–166.
51. Toffano, G., Savoini, G., Moroni, F., Lombardi, G., Calza, L., and Agnati, L. F., 1984, Chronic G_{M1} ganglioside treatment reduces dopamine cell body degeneration in the substantia nigra after unilateral hemitransection in rat, *Brain Res.* **296**:233–239.
52. Wieraszko, A., and Seifert, W., 1985, The role of monosialoganglioside G_{M1} in the synaptic plasticity: *In vitro* study on rat hippocampal slices, *Brain Res.* **345**:159–164.
53. Willinger, M., and Schachner, M., 1980, G_{M1} ganglioside as a marker for neuronal differentiation in mouse cerebellum, *Dev. Biol.* **74**:101–117.
54. Wojcik, M., Ulas, B., and Oderfeld-Nowak, B., 1982, The stimulating effect of ganglioside injections on the recovery of choline acetyltransferase and acetylcholinesterase activities in the hippocampus of the rat after septal lesions, *Neuroscience* **7**:495–499.

10

Gangliosides and Functional Recovery from Brain Injury

Gary L. Dunbar and Donald G. Stein

ABSTRACT. In the first part of this chapter, we review studies that have focused on the effectiveness of ganglioside treatments for reducing behavioral deficits following brain damage. Our review indicates that gangliosides are an effective treatment following a variety of injuries to structures and pathways of the septohippocampal system, the cerebral cortex, and the nigrostriatal system. Although the underlying mechanism of this ganglioside-induced behavioral recovery is still not understood, the observation, in most of these studies, of its early onset indicates that gangliosides are promoting functional recovery by means other than the facilitation of neuronal sprouting.

In the second part of this chapter, we present recent data comparing G_{MI} gangliosides, its inner ester, AGF2, and d-amphetamine for their efficacy in promoting functional recovery following bilateral damage to the caudate nucleus. While all of these treatments reduced the behavioral impairments caused by the injury, the intermediate dose (20 mg/kg) of AGF2 was the most effective. Since the behavioral recovery was rapid, and since there was no histological evidence of a ganglioside-enhancement of neuronal sprouting or neuronal survival, we suggest that gangliosides may promote recovery by affecting beneficial biochemical or metabolic changes, rather than inducing morphological restructuring.

We conclude this chapter by discussing possible explanations of why gangliosides are therapeutically effective in some situations but not in others. In this context, our analyses are focused primarily on the types of injury, the timing of treatment, and the behavioral parameters that are examined. We believe that a better understanding of how these variables interact can provide further insight into how gangliosides work, and ultimately will lead to the most efficacious use of gangliosides as a pharmacological treatment for brain damage.

GARY L. DUNBAR AND DONALD G. STEIN • Brain Research Laboratory, Department of Psychology, Clark University, Worcester, Massachusetts 01610. *Present address of G.L.D.:* Department of Psychology, Central Michigan University, Mt. Pleasant, Michigan 48852. *Present address of D.G.S.:* Dean of the Graduate School and Associate Provost for Research, Rutgers University at Newark, Newark, New Jersey 07102.

1. INTRODUCTION

One of the more promising approaches in the search for a phamacological treatment of behavioral deficits following brain damage involves the use of gangliosides. What makes this class of substances particularly attractive as therapeutic agents for CNS injury is that, unlike other neurotrophic substances such as nerve growth factor, gangliosides are able to penetrate the blood–brain barrier after systemic injections.[29,33,44] Furthermore, parenterally administered gangliosides appear to have no toxic side effects at therapeutically effective doses.[25] Since gangliosides offer the potential of a safe and effective pharmacological treatment for brain injury without necessitating surgical intervention, increasing attention has been focused on how they might affect behavioral recovery. Although their specific mechanism of action is not yet understood, the proposed explanations that have received the most attention are those that suggest that gangliosides stimulate regenerative and collateral sprouting[31,48] or enhance neuronal survival after injury.[2,38,49] In this chapter, we examine the question of whether ganglioside-induced sprouting or neuronal sparing affects functional recovery. We also provide an overview of the behavioral research that examines the effects of gangliosides after lesions in structures and pathways of the septohippocampal system, the cerebral cortex, and the nigrostriatal system.

2. BEHAVIORAL RECOVERY FOLLOWING DAMAGE TO THE SEPTOHIPPOCAMPAL SYSTEM

The initial studies using septohippocampal system injury as a model for evaluating the effects of ganglioside treatments focused on testing whether or not gangliosides could facilitate lesion-induced sprouting. The first attempt to relate ganglioside-enhanced hippocampal reorganization with behavioral recovery was made by Karpiak.[27] He found that ganglioside-treated rats with entorhinal cortex (EC) lesions made significantly fewer errors on a spatial alternation task by the first postoperative day. Since the behavioral recovery preceded the 5- to 7-day period considered necessary for functional reinnervation to occur,[42] Karpiak concluded that the recovery was more likely to be the result of a protective effect of gangliosides against further neuronal loss following the lesion rather than a ganglioside enhancement of sprouting.

Fass and Ramirez[18] also attempted to relate the time course of behavioral recovery to indices of neuronal sprouting. They found that ganglioside treatments reduced the hyperactivity observed in open-field behavior of rats with bilateral EC lesions. As was found in Karpiak's study, the improvement shown by the ganglioside-treated rats was apparent during the first testing session (2 days after the lesion), again suggesting that the recovery was probably independent of the sprouting response that occurs after this type of injury. Additional support for this contention was obtained in the second part of the experiment, when a reduction in hippocampal acetylcholinesterase (AChE) staining was observed in ganglioside-treated rats with unilateral EC lesions. The density of staining in the denervated dentate gyrus of these rats was significantly less than that in their untreated, brain-damaged counterparts, indicating that the gangliosides suppressed sprouting of septodentate fibers after the unilateral EC lesions.

It is tempting to suggest that the reduction in behavioral deficits observed in the treated animals may have been a result of a suppression of sprouting by the ganglioside treatments. However, a comparison of the time courses for behavioral recovery and for hippocampal AChE staining shown in this study reveals no clear correspondence. At the very least, the Fass and Ramirez experiment indicated that ganglioside treatments can facilitate a reduction in behavioral impairments, and such facilitation may well be independent of the effects they have on neuronal sprouting.

More recently, Poplawsky and Isaacson[35] have suggested that the beneficial behavioral effects of gangliosides may be dissociated from neuritogenic or neuronotrophic effects. They found that ganglioside-treated rats with septal lesions had significantly lower emotionality scores than untreated rats with the same lesions when these animals were rated on postsurgery day 2. Since gangliosides exerted their effects so early, and since the effects were greatest for the transient changes in behavior following septal lesions (e.g., emotionality) without affecting the more permanent changes, such as facilitation of avoidance behaviors and decreases in avoidance rearing, these authors argued that the effects of gangliosides observed in their study were probably biochemical in nature.

In summary, there is, at present, no evidence that directly relates ganglioside-induced neuronal sprouting with functional reinnervation of the hippocampus. Gangliosides have been shown to exert their influence on behavioral recovery very early after disruptions of hippocampal pathways. The available evidence, therefore, appears to support the notion that ganglioside-facilitated behavioral recovery is at least initially a result of neurochemical alterations that prevent further neuronal or glial degeneration and/or enhance the functioning of spared tissue.

3. BEHAVIORAL RECOVERY FOLLOWING DAMAGE OR DENERVATION OF CORTICAL STRUCTURES

3.1. RECOVERY AFTER LESIONS TO THE CHOLINERGIC FOREBRAIN NUCLEI

Casamenti and colleagues[8] have shown that gangliosides are effective in preventing reductions in cerebral choline acetyltransferase (ChAT) activity and in improving the acquisition of active avoidance but not passive avoidance responses in rats with lesions of the cholinergic forebrain nuclei. In the Casamenti *et al.* report, as was the case in most of the behavioral studies we have reviewed, the behavioral effects of gangliosides occurred early during testing, with the greatest improvement in performance taking place 4–7 days after surgery. Interestingly, gangliosides had little effect on ChAT losses in the more heavily denervated frontal–parietal area but had a significant effect in the parieto-occipital area, where a smaller number of fibers had been destroyed. This suggests that gangliosides may be more effective when more neurons are spared.

Casamenti and colleagues hypothesized that gangliosides may increase ChAT levels by promoting collateral sprouting of cholinergic neurons or that gangliosides have a stimulatory effect on residual neurons. The latter hypothesis appears to be the more likely explanation, because the greatest behavioral effects occurred during the first week of testing. This interpretation also has support from earlier work demonstrating a ganglioside-induced high-affinity choline uptake in the cortex of rats with lesions of the nucleus basalis magnocellularis.[34] Perhaps this or some other stimulatory effect on these neurons acts to prevent further damage after a traumatic insult. This could also explain the recent finding that gangliosides can prevent cell shrinkage and losses in ChAT activity in the nucleus basalis of rats with cortical damage.[9]

3.2. RECOVERY AFTER CORTICAL LESIONS

Work in our laboratory at Clark University also has indicated that gangliosides can promote behavioral recovery after cortical damage, but this effect may depend on the location and/or the size of the lesion. In one study, we made bilateral aspiration lesions of the mediofrontal cortex of rats and tested them on a spatial alternation task.[15] We found that untreated rats with these lesions were significantly impaired relative to sham-operated controls, whereas the ganglioside-treated animals were not (Fig. 1).

More recently, however, we found that gangliosides were unable to ameliorate deficits in brightness and pattern discrimination of rats with bilateral aspiration lesions of the visual cortex.[6] We hypothesized that the lack of a positive ganglioside effect in the latter study may be a result of the disruption in circadian rhythms caused by the lack of visual input or "cortical blindness" caused by these extensive lesions. A similar effect was noted by Toffano *et al.*[47] when gangliosides were found to be ineffective in restoring striatal TH levels in hemitransected rats that were deprived of light. Therefore, the differences between the results of our frontal study and our occipital experiment may be attributed to the location of the lesion; it may be the case that not all types of CNS injury are amenable to ganglioside "therapy." Alternatively, the size of the lesion may be a critical factor; our mediofrontal aspirations removed considerably less cortical tissue than did our visual cortex aspirations. If lesions are too extensive, no

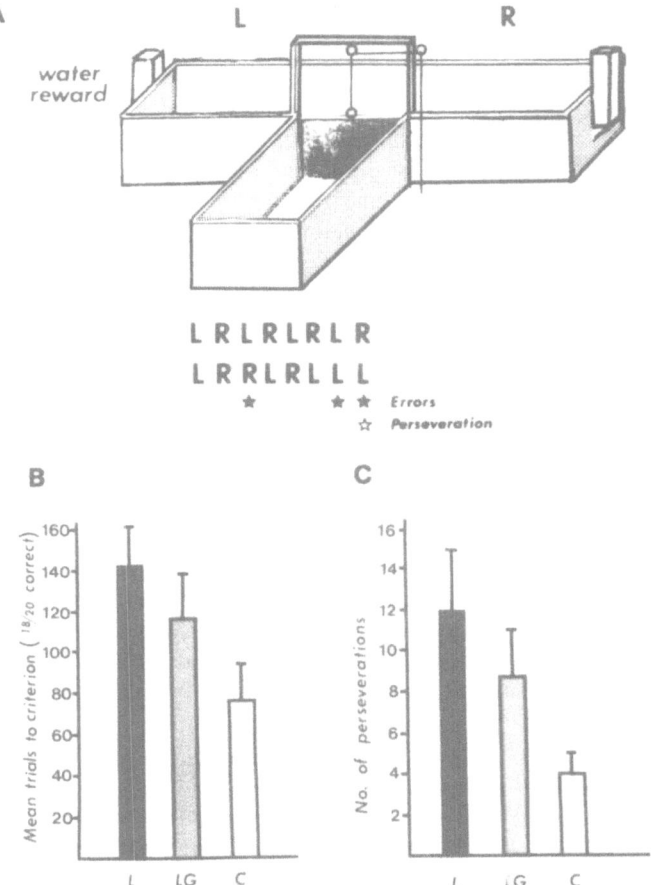

FIGURE 1. The performance of rats that received mediofrontal cortex lesions and injections of either saline (L) or 30 mg/kg G_{M1} gangliosides (LG) was compared to that of sham-operated controls (C) on a spatial alternation task (A). Ganglioside-treated rats were not as impaired as the untreated rats with lesions on trials to criterion (B) and number of perseverations (C).

treatment may be affective, and this is a factor that needs further attention in determining the limits of various treatments for CNS injuries. Finally, the dose or the number of injections given may have to be increased following extensive damage or after lesions to certain areas (i.e., the occipital cortex) in order to facilitate functional recovery.

It is important to point out that in both experiments, we found no indication of morphological changes induced by gangliosides. In our frontal study, cell counts in the lateral parts of the medial dorsal nucleus of the thalamus, a major source of afferent fibers to the mediofrontal cortex, revealed no differences between groups. In our visual cortex study, there was a significant lesion-induced loss of cells in the lateral geniculate body of the thalamus, a major source of fiber projections to the visual cortex; however, there were no differences in cell counts between the treated and untreated lesion groups. Although these findings do not preclude the possibility that gangliosides enhance sprouting after cortical damage, they do lend more support to the hypothesis that the underlying behavioral effects of gangliosides are primarily neurochemical and metabolic in nature.

3.3. RECOVERY AFTER ISCHEMIA

Much of the recent research demonstrating the facilitating effects of ganglioside treatments for behavioral recovery following cortical damage has involved the use of animal models of transient cerebral ischemia (see S. E. Karpiak *et al.*, Chapter 11) and clinical trials with human stroke patients. In one model of ischemia,[7] the two carotid arteries were occluded for 1 hr, followed by behavioral and physiological testing at 24-hr intervals. In this model, rats that were treated with gangliosides 1 hr after the occlusion performed significantly better on a passive avoidance learning task than did ischemic rats that received no treatment. This improvement was paralleled by enhanced cerebral blood flow and reductions in neurological deficits, cerebral edema, cell damage, K^+ efflux, Ca^{2+} accumulation, and electrocorticographic disturbances.

Clinical studies of the effects of gangliosides following cortical damage in human stroke patients have revealed some promising results. In one study, it was reported that the qualitative ratings of neurological functioning were higher for patients receiving gangliosides than for patients receiving placebo injections.[4] A second study reported an improvement in the EEG profiles of ganglioside-treated patients in addition to higher ratings on clinical tests of neurological functioning.[5] What is particularly interesting about these findings is that in both studies, the ganglioside treatments were still effective even though administration began during the subacute phase (at least 10 days after the stroke). This suggests that it is not necessary to administer gangliosides during the acute phase of injury in order to achieve a therapeutic effect, at least not after cerebrovascular accidents in humans. It remains to be seen whether gangliosides could exert a more powerful effect if they were administered during the acute phase. Another interesting finding in these studies was that ganglioside treatments had beneficial effects for clinical signs but had no effect on morphological changes as revealed by computerized tomography (CT). Although the absence of any morphological alterations may be the result of the limited resolution of CT or the restricted time of treatment (6 weeks), it does suggest, once again, that gangliosides may have functional effects without corresponding morphological changes.

In summary, ganglioside treatments have been shown to be effective in countering some of the behavioral deficits experienced after damage to the cerebral cortex or its afferent and efferent connections. However, this therapeutic effect may be limited by the location and/or size of the damage. Presently, there is little evidence to indicate that the beneficial effects of gangliosides on recovery from behavioral deficits can be attributed directly to enhanced neuronal sprouting in cortical pathways.

4. BEHAVIORAL RECOVERY FOLLOWING NIGROSTRIATAL DAMAGE

4.1. EARLY STUDIES ON RECOVERY FOLLOWING NIGROSTRIATAL DAMAGE

When rats with unilateral transections of the nigrostriatal pathway are challenged with injections of amphetamine or apomorphine, they show a stereotyped rotation ipsiversive to the lesion. With this rotational model developed by Ungerstedt,[50] the initial findings indicating that gangliosides facilitated behavioral recovery (i.e., reduced this rotational asymmetry) were attributed to an enhancement of the rate and extent of regenerative sprouting of dopaminergic fibers. For example, Toffano and colleagues[48] found that gangliosides reduced the number of apomorphine-induced rotations at 14 and 30 days following unilateral hemitransections of the nigrostriatal pathway. The reduction of behavioral deficits corresponded in time to the increases in tyrosine hydroxylase (TH) activity, TH-related immunofluorescence, and levels of homovanillic acid (HVA) on the transected side of the brain. The increases were evident beyond 2 weeks after the transections but not at postoperative day 8. These data correspond nicely with the expected time course for reinnervation of the striatum (e.g., about 2 weeks) by sprouting nigrostriatal axons. As a result, these authors interpreted their findings to indicate that the gangliosides enhanced functional recovery by inducing "within-system" regenerative sprouting.

Although the argument for sprouting in this model is compelling, an alternative explanation could be that gangliosides stimulate TH activity without increasing striatal dopamine levels[17] or that gangliosides may have reduced striatal dopamine supersensitivity without affecting regeneration.[22] Furthermore, since behavioral measures were not reported for postoperative day 8, it is not possible to know if a reduction in rotations could have occurred in the absence of the biochemical and histochemical indices for reinnervation.

Subsequent studies by Toffano and his co-workers[2,40,46,47] have essentially confirmed their initial findings of a ganglioside-induced behavioral recovery (i.e., reduced rotational asymmetry). Nevertheless, the data indicating that sprouting may be the underlying process of this recovery are still open to alternative interpretations. For example, the observation that gangliosides have no effect on recovery after extensive or complete mechanical hemitransections[47] was interpreted to mean that recovery is a product of collateral sprouting from remaining fibers on the side of the lesion. However, these data could also be interpreted as simply indicating that a minimal number of fibers must be spared or protected from secondary degeneration in order for behavioral recovery to occur. It has recently been shown that when striatal dopamine levels fall below 60% of their normal levels, the residual undamaged neurons increase their synthesis and release of dopamine.[32] Ganglioside treatments may act to accelerate further the metabolic activity of the fibers that remain after the partial lesions, allowing them to take over some of the functioning of the lost axons. A stimulating effect of gangliosides on the metabolism of spared neurons immediately following injury may actually facilitate the survival of these cells.[1]

There are also clues in these follow-up studies that indicate a possible temporal dissociation between the biochemical indices for sprouting and concomitant reductions in rotational activity. Specifically, behavioral findings in two of these studies[2,47] show a reduction in apomorphine-induced rotational activity at postoperative day 8, which does not correspond to the findings of no differences between treated and untreated animals in TH activity on postoperative day 8.[46,48] Not only do these new findings fail to associate TH activity with rotational behavior on the eighth day after surgery (the earliest time at which these animals were tested), the actual reductions in rotational activity during this time period are greater than at any subsequent testing session. If increased levels of TH activity accurately reflect reinnervation, these findings would cast doubt on the hypothesis that collateral sprouting accounts for the behavioral recovery observed after ganglioside treatments.

4.2. LATER STUDIES ON RECOVERY AFTER NIGROSTRIATAL DAMAGE

Work in our laboratory at Clark University has also shown a lack of correspondence between the onset of behavioral recovery and anatomic indices of neuronal reorganization. Our first study revealed that ganglioside treatments could reduce spatial alternation deficits following bilateral caudate nucleus (CN) lesions.[39] This effect appeared to be more pronounced during the initial testing sessions (postoperative days 10–40) but was still significant during retesting (postoperative days 90–104). Interestingly, cell counts of the Nissl-stained tissue revealed no differences among the brain-injured rats with no treatment, the ganglioside-treated group, and the sham controls for the number of glia and neurons medial to the lesion site or in the substantia nigra pars compacta (SNc). These data suggest that there may be a dissociation between these measurements of morphological structure and behavioral recovery that is similar to the dissociation obtained when neurochemical parameters were examined.

In another experiment, we asked whether or not ganglioside-induced behavioral recovery could be associated with a different morphological parameter for sprouting. In this context, we measured the rotational activity of animals with unilateral hemitransections of the nigrostriatal pathway at postoperative days 2, 12, or 39 and then injected horseradish peroxidase (HRP) into the denervated CN at postoperative days 3, 15, or 45.[37] Our results revealed a clear dissociation in the ganglioside-treated rats between the amphetamine-induced rotational asymmetry (at postoperative day 2) and the number of HRP-labeled neurons in the ipsilateral SNc (at postoperative day 3). Thus, as early as 2 days following the hemitransection, ganglioside-treated animals displayed significantly less rotational asymmetry than did their untreated counterparts despite the fact that there were no differences between these two groups in the reduction (from intact control levels) of HRP-labeled neurons in the ipsilateral substantia nigra pars compacta (iSNc). Although there was a correspondence between increases in HRP labeling of the iSNc and a reduction of rotational asymmetry at postoperative day 12, this recovery was temporary, and the asymmetry returned by postoperative day 39. At any rate, if HRP retrograde transport can be taken to indicate reinnervation, the early behavioral recovery observed in this study cannot be accounted for by collateral sprouting.

Recent studies by Li and his co-workers[30] have confirmed our findings that ganglioside treatments can reduce amphetamine-induced rotational asymmetry as early as 2 days after unilateral nigrostriatal transections. Furthermore, they found that only those animals receiving the ganglioside injections immediately or within the first 2 hr following surgery had significant reductions in the number of ipsiversive rotations. This behavioral effect was not significant for animals receiving injections prior to surgery or at 4, 8, or 12 hr after surgery. Li and colleagues also found that gangliosides prevented a loss of striatal Na^+, K^+-ATPase activity on the same side as the transection. Since maintenance of higher levels of Na^+, K^+-ATPase activity correlated with their previous findings of reduced levels of edema,[28] the authors suggested that functional recovery may be enhanced by the ganglioside-induced facilitation of Na^+, K^+-ATPase activity.

Although the possibility exists that gangliosides influence the reduction of behavioral impairments following nigrostriatal damage by acting on early events through one mechanism (e.g., maintaining Na^+, K^+-ATPase activity) and later events through another (e.g., promoting sprouting), the available evidence suggests that it may be the acute effects of gangliosides that are primarily responsible for reducing behavioral deficits. In those studies showing the time course of a ganglioside-induced reduction in behavioral deficits following nigrostriatal damage, either the most significant reductions have occurred during the initial testing sessions[2,47] or there have been no consistently significant improvements beyond the first day of testing.[37] If the primary behavioral benefits of gangliosides were related to their facilitation of sprouting, the expected results would be reversed (i.e., the greatest improvements should come during the later testing periods).

In summary, the available evidence to date does not unequivocally support the contention that gangliosides enhance behavioral recovery by the facilitation of sprouting following damage to the nigrostriatal pathway. Gangliosides may indeed promote sprouting of nigrostriatal fibers, but this appears to have little, if anything, to do with the reductions in behavioral deficits observed after ganglioside treatments. Instead, gangliosides may exert their effects on behavioral recovery by promoting the survival of undamaged or partially damaged fibers and/or by reducing secondary degeneration; however, evidence directly relating these events to behavioral recovery is lacking. What has been consistently shown in the studies we have reviewed is that gangliosides exert their effects very early after nigrostriatal damage. Such recovery may be accomplished by reducing lesion-induced edema, enhancing Na^+,K^+-ATPase activity, and/or increasing the dopamine uptake of spared nigrostriatal fibers. Regardless of the specific underlying mechanisms, we now think that the behavioral recovery following ganglioside treatments is primarily dependent on the early events surrounding the nigrostriatal damage.

4.3. RECENT DATA ON RECOVERY AFTER NIGROSTRIATAL DAMAGE

Recently, we examined the effects of gangliosides on rotational activity following complete nigrostriatal transections.[11,16] As we discussed previously, Toffano et al.[47] found that gangliosides were ineffective in preventing the loss of striatal TH levels after complete transections; however, no behavioral measures were taken, so it was not known whether gangliosides might reduce rotational asymmetry in spite of their inability to maintain TH levels after such extensive lesions. In addition, we were interested to see whether ganglioside treatments would affect the aphagia and adipsia commonly observed after extensive transections of the nigrostriatal pathway.

Interestingly, we found that ganglioside treatments did not reduce amphetamine-induced rotational activity (Fig. 2A) but effectively prevented the dramatic weight loss observed during the first postoperative week in the untreated brain-damaged rats (Fig. 2B). These findings support the contention of Toffano and colleagues that some residual fibers must remain after the transections in order for gangliosides to facilitate recovery (or at least reduce rotational asymmetry). Just why gangliosides were effective in preventing the loss of consummatory behavior without reducing rotational activity remains to be seen, but since gangliosides worked very early to prevent the lesion-induced suppression of eating and drinking, it is unlikely that their effects were mediated by enhancement of sprouting.

4.4. RECENT DATA ON RECOVERY AFTER BILATERAL LESIONS OF THE CAUDATE NUCLEUS

More recently, we have completed a series of experiments comparing G_{M1} ganglioside, its inner ester AGF2, and d-amphetamine for their efficacy in pro-

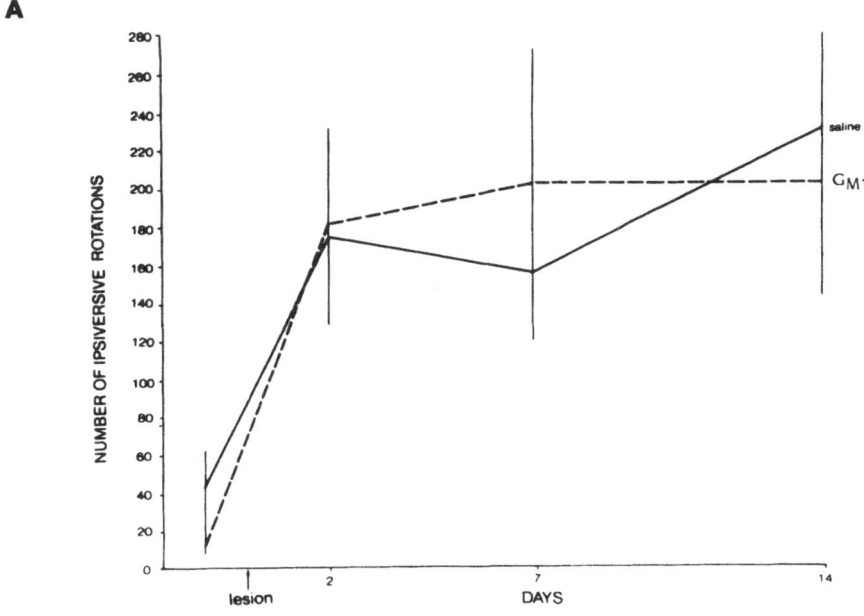

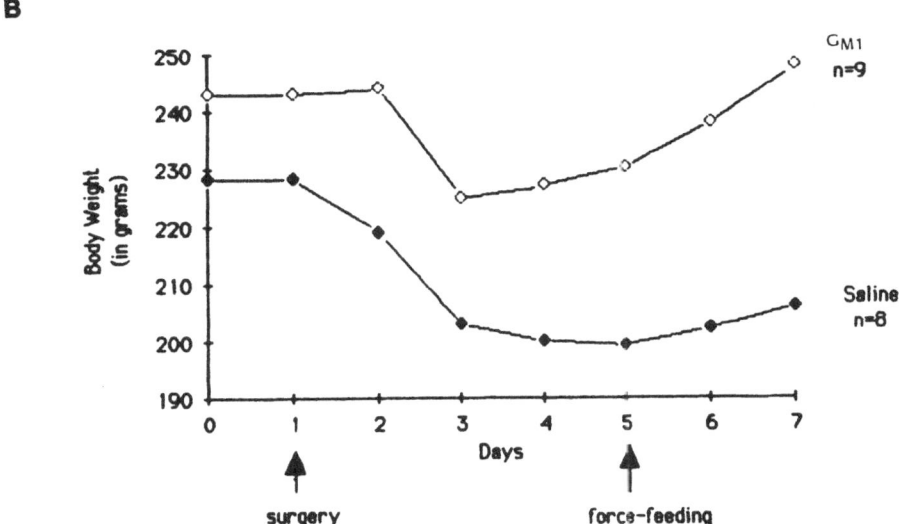

FIGURE 2. G_{M1} treatments had no effect on the rotational behavior of rats with complete transections of the nigrostriatal pathway (A) but were able to protect these rats from lesion-induced aphagia and adipsia during the first week of surgery (B).

moting recovery of spatial reversal deficits following bilateral lesions of the CN.[12–14] These experiments were designed to accomplish several goals. First, we wanted to replicate our original findings of a ganglioside-induced recovery,[39] and second, we wanted to extend our findings by monitoring the time course of the recovery to observe when the gangliosides first exerted their beneficial effects.

We also wanted to see whether or not AGF2 would be effective in attenuating symptoms caused by caudate lesions. Since AGF2, a precursor of G_{M1}, has been suggested to have a longer plasma half-life and a wider distribution volume than G_{M1} and was effective in restoring TH levels following transections of the nigrostriatal pathway,[3] we were interested in comparing its behavioral effects with G_{M1} and establishing a dose–response curve for AGF2.

In addition, we wanted to compare the effects of d-amphetamine treatments with those of gangliosides for promoting behavioral recovery. Work by Feeney and colleagues has shown that amphetamine treatments enable animals to recover from severe motor deficits following CNS damage (see D. M. Feeney and R. L. Sutton, Chapter 7). Could amphetamine treatments also facilitate brain-injured animals' ability to solve a more complex learning task? Since both gangliosides and amphetamine probably exert their effects biochemically during the acute phase of injury, we were particularly interested in comparing their behavioral effects over time. We were also interested in testing the effects of a combined ganglioside–amphetamine treatment to determine whether or not the interaction would have an additive or potentiating effect.

The procedures we used were essentially the same as those employed in our original study.[39] Prior to surgery, all the rats were trained to avoid a 0.2-mA shock by running to either of two open doors in the testing apparatus (Fig. 3A). Following training, the animals were randomly assigned to one of the following groups: controls, which received sham surgery and saline injections; group LC, which received bilateral CN lesions and saline injections; groups G_{M1}, Amph, AG10, AG20, AG30, and G_{M1}+Amph, all of which received bilateral CN lesions and treatments of, repectively, 30 mg/kg G_{M1}, 2 mg/kg d-amphetamine, 10 mg/kg AGF2, 20 mg/kg AGF2, 30 mg/kg AGF2, and combined injections of 30 mg/kg G_{M1} plus 2 mg/kg d-amphetamine. All injections were i.p. and began within 5 min after surgery and were continued daily for 15 days. In order to control for possible extraneous temporal factors, all surgery and behavioral testing were scheduled for squads of five rats on each day, three rats from a treatment group and one each from the LC and sham groups.

Spatial reversal testing began on postoperative day 5. Five seconds after a rat was placed in the start box, a guillotine door was raised, triggering a 5-sec warning tone, which was followed by a 0.2-mA footshock. In order to avoid or escape shock, the rats had to enter through the doorway into the goal area on their nonpreferred side (as determined during presurgical training). When a given rat avoided or escaped shock in ten of ten trials for two consecutive days, the goal area was reversed to the opposite side. The rats could only avoid or escape shock by learning to make this reversal. The reversals were continued throughout the 30 days of testing each time the rats attained the criterion of successfuly avoiding or escaping shock ten of ten trials for two consecutive days. On any trial that the rats failed to escape shock within 30 sec, they were forced through the correct side of the maze, and this was recorded as a failure to escape. The primary dependent measures in these experiments were the number of reversals and number of times the rats were able to avoid shock.

When the performance was assessed over the entire 30-day testing period, only the rats that received treatments of 20 mg/kg AGF2 showed significant improvement relative to untreated rats with lesions. In fact, these animals performed at a level comparable to the sham controls on measures of average reversals (Fig. 3B) and mean avoidance (Fig. 3C). Rats receiving 30 mg/kg of G_{M1} or AGF2 were statistically indistinguishable from either the sham or the LC group on average number of reversals, but they made significantly fewer avoidances compared to the sham controls. The time-course analyses comparing the G_{M1}, Amph, and G_{M1} + Amph groups with the untreated lesion and sham control groups revealed that both gangliosides and amphetamines accelerated behavioral recovery, significantly improving spatial learning performance (as measured by the average number of reversals) between days 7 and 12 (Fig. 3D). In addition, no differences between any groups were found in the number of Nissl-stained cells in CN tissue adjacent to the lesion (or the corresponding area in the sham control rats). There were also no differences for any of the groups in the amount of HRP transported from the injection site (near the area of the lesion in the CN) to the SN, as indicated by the number of HRP-labeled cells in the SNc and the size of the HRP-labeled area of the substantia nigra pars reticulata.

These results indicate that a 20 mg/kg dose of AGF2 can counteract spatial learning deficits caused by bilateral damage to the caudate nucleus. This dose of AGF2 appears to be in the optimal range for promoting such recovery, since a higher dose (30 mg/kg) and a lower dose (10 mg/kg) were not as efficacious. Similarly, neither 30 mg/kg G_{M1} ganglioside nor 2 mg/kg d-amphetamine treatments were as effective as the 20 mg/kg dose of AGF2, although both of these treatments were shown to improve performance during the early (days 7–12) period of testing. The behavioral recovery following the 20 mg/kg dose of AGF2 occurred even sooner (i.e., before the end of the first week of testing) than the G_{M1} or amphetamine effects. This suggests that the increased effectiveness of the AGF2 could be caused by an enhanced penetration through the blood–brain barrier, its higher distribution volume, and/or its longer plasma half-life.[3] The lack of a synergistic effect of the combined G_{M1}-plus-amphetamine treatment may reflect disruption of normal biochemical processes of these substances or an overdose effect (e.g., by promoting excessive levels of TH or DA that were

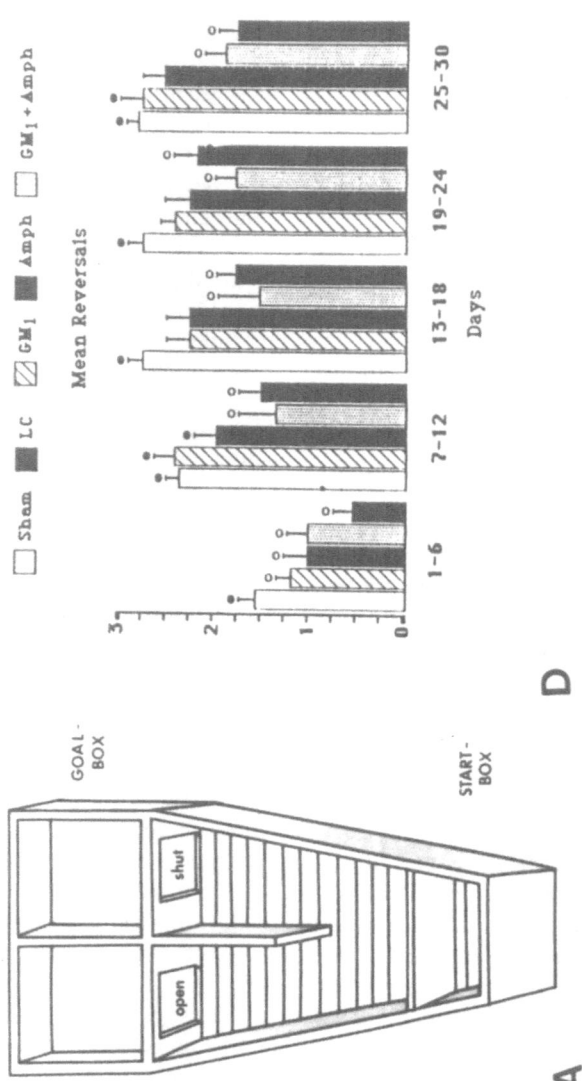

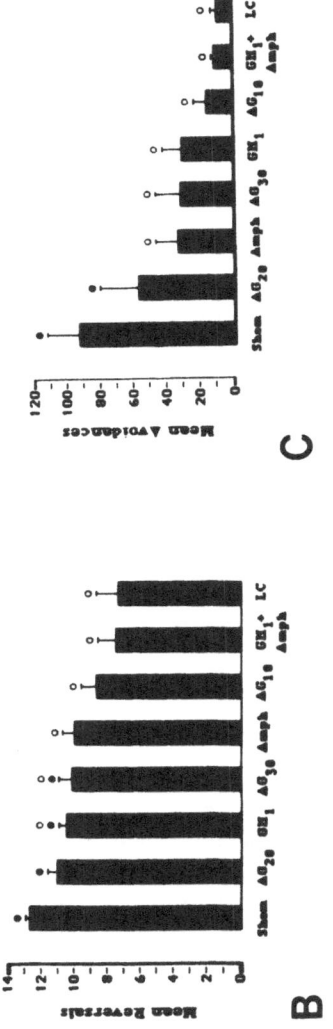

FIGURE 3. Rats with bilateral caudate nucleus lesions were tested for their ability to escape or avoid shock on a spatial reversal task (A). AGF2 at 20 mg/kg proved to be most effective in reducing the lesion-induced deficits on this task, as measured by the greater number of reversals (B) and avoidances (C) made by rats receiving this treatment. Time-course analysis indicated that both 30 mg/kg G_{M1} gangliosides and 2 mg/kg d-amphetamine treatments exerted beneficial effects on the rats' performance of this task within the first 2 weeks after surgery (D). (○) significantly different from Shams; (●) significantly different from LC.

disruptive to the animals). Tests using lower doses of this combination treatment may provide further insight into the nature of the behavioral recovery following both ganglioside and amphetamine treatments.

The absence of ganglioside effects on any of the histological measures may indicate that the treatments either had no appreciable consequences on structural morphology or that the treatment effects may have occurred at an earlier time period and were later masked by the slower spontaneous recovery of the LC group. This latter interpretation receives some support when the time course of behavioral recovery is considered; the behavioral effects of gangliosides and amphetamines occur early but are partially masked later by the slower improvement in performance of the LC rats (Fig. 3D). Whether or not this early behavioral recovery is mediated by neuronal sprouting or is biochemically induced cannot be ascertained at this time. Time-course analyses using these or other comparable histological measures would shed considerable light on the nature of the underlying mechanisms for behavioral recovery following ganglioside and amphetamine treatments.

Our recent data indicate that G_{M1} gangliosides and d-amphetamine treatments can accelerate behavioral recovery following bilateral CN lesions. Furthermore, AGF2 at the 20 mg/kg dose level exerts an earlier, more powerful, longer-lasting effect than G_{M1}, amphetamine, and either 10 mg/kg or 30 mg/kg doses of AGF2. Combined treatments of G_{M1} and amphetamine had no beneficial effect, but this may be because of the dose level used. Our histological results provided us with few clues as to what the underlying mechanism of this recovery may be, but the early onset of the behavioral recovery suggests that it is probably not mediated by structural, that is, anatomic changes but rather by more rapidly occurring changes in the chemistry of synaptic and dendritic processes that are affected by the lesion and subsequent ganglioside treatment.

5. GENERAL DISCUSSION AND CONCLUSIONS

In all but a few cases, our review of the literature has indicated that ganglioside treatments can ameliorate behavioral deficits caused by damage to pathways and related structures intimately connected with the hippocampus, cerebral cortex, and basal ganglia. Gangliosides have been shown to exert their beneficial effects on a variety of impaired behavioral functions, including motor asymmetries, hyperemotionality, hyperactivity, active avoidance, passive avoidance, spatial reversal learning, spatial alternation learning, and clinical signs of neurological functioning. Nonetheless, the evidence also indicates that ganglioside treatments may not be appropriate for all types of behavioral disruptions following CNS injury. They have been shown to be ineffective for improving rotational asymmetry following neurotoxic lesions[46] and extensive mechanical transections[11,16] of the nigrostriatal pathway, active avoidance learning after septal damage,[35] passive avoidance learning after lesions of the cholinergic forebrain nuclei,[8] and pattern and brightness discrimination after visual cortex lesions.[6]

Just why gangliosides are effective in some cases and not in others is unknown. However, an examination of those variables that affect the efficacy of ganglioside treatments and analyses of when gangliosides affect behavior have provided some insights into how gangliosides exert their functional effects. Some of the variables that we have reviewed include those involving lesion, treatment, and testing parameters (see Table I).

Of the lesion parameters, the type, location, and size of the lesion have all been implicated in affecting the behavioral outcomes of ganglioside treatments. Gangliosides have been shown to be therapeutically effective following electrolytic, aspiration, and mechanical lesions but are apparently ineffective after neurotoxic lesions.[46] Recent evidence, however, has indicated that ganglioside treatments may also work for these types of lesions.[45] Gangliosides have also been shown to be useful in overcoming deficits following damage to all structures and pathways for which their effects have been examined except for lesions of the visual cortex.[6] As was discussed in Section 3.2, this exception may involve disruptions of diurnal rhythms because of the "cortical blindness" caused by occipital injury, or it may be the result of the extent of damage. Lesion size may have a direct bearing on whether or not treatment will be successful. Besides the rather extensive lesions of the visual cortex,[6] extensive lesions of the nigrostriatal pathway also rendered ganglioside treatments ineffective.[11,16,47] Further investigations of how lesion size and location affect ganglioside-induced behavioral recovery would provide valuable information on how ganglioside treatments may be used most effectively and what the limitations of such treatments may be.

Of the treatment parameters investigated, the type and amount of gangliosides used and the time of treatment appear to have an appreciable effect on behavioral recovery; the route of administration does not seem to affect the recovery process. Of the molecular species of gangliosides that have been tested, G_{M1} alone is comparable to mixed gangliosides, and AGF2 has been shown to exert a more powerful and longer-lasting effect than G_{M1}.[7,14] This latter finding may be caused by the increased capacity of AGF2 to pass through the blood–brain barrier, its greater distribution volume, and its longer plasma half-life.[3] Our work with AGF2[14] indicates that the dose used may be an important variable for optimizing the beneficial effects of gangliosides. Further research is needed to determine dose levels that are most effective for different types, sizes, and locations of CNS injury.

The timing of treatment may also be an important factor for promoting behavioral recovery. It has been shown that optimal behavioral effects are observed when gangliosides are given within the first 2 hr after injury.[30] However, the first 2 hr does not represent a "critical window" of effective treatment, since Toffano and his colleagues[40,46,47] have found consistent behavioral improve-

TABLE I. Important Injury, Treatment, and Testing Parameters in Studies Designed to Test the Effects of Ganglioside Treatments on Behavioral Recovery following Brain Damage[a]

Study	Subject	Injury	Locus of injury	Treatment type, dose, and route	Treatment schedule	Start of treatment	Start of testing	Behavior tested	Effect	Reference
Toffano et al.	Rat	Mechanical	Partial NS	G_{M1}, 5 mg/kg, i.p.	Daily for 12 days	2 PO days	14 PO days	Rotation	+	47
Karpiak	Rat	Aspiration	Unilateral EC	Mixed, 50 mg/kg, i.m.	Daily	1 day preop	0 PO days	Spatial alternation	+	27
Agnati et al.	Rat	Mechanical	Partial NS	G_{M1}, 5 mg/kg, i.p.	Daily for 64 days	At surgery	8 PO days	Rotation	+	2
Toffano et al.	Rat	Mechanical	Partial NS	G_{M1}, 5 mg/kg, i.p.	Daily for 54 days	2 PO days	56 PO days	Rotation	+	45
	Rat	Neurotoxic	Partial NS	G_{M1}, 30 mg/kg, i.p.	Daily for 45 days	2 PO days	NA	Rotation	0	
Toffano et al.	Rat	Mechanical	Partial NS	G_{M1}, 5 mg/kg, i.p.	Daily for 8 days	2 PO days	8 PO days	Rotation	+	46
Sabel et al.	Rat	Electrolytic	Bilateral CN	G_{M1}, 30 mg/kg, i.p.	Daily for 14 days	At surgery	10 PO days	Spatial reversal	+	38
Fass and Ramirez	Rat	Electrolytic	Bilateral EC	Mixed, 30 mg/kg, i.m.	Daily for 5 days and every other day for 10 more days	1 day preop	2 PO days	Open field activity	+	18

Study	Species	Lesion	Region	Treatment	Schedule	Start	Test	Behavioral test	Result	Ref.
Bassi et al.	Human	Ischemia	Cerebral cortex	G_{M1}, 20 mg, i.m.	2 times daily for 6 weeks	15 days after injury	15 days after injury	Neurological symptoms	+	4
Dunbar et al.	Rat	Aspiration	Mediofrontal cortex	G_{M1}, 30 mg/kg, i.p.	Daily for 14 days	At surgery	21 PO days	Spatial alternation	+	15
Savoini et al.	Rat	Mechanical	Partial NS	G_{M1}, NA	NA	2 PO days	7 PO days	Rotation	+	39
Sabel et al.	Rat	Mechanical	Partial NS	G_{M1}, 30 mg/kg, i.p.	Daily for 14 days	At surgery	2 PO days	Rotation and open field activity	+	37
Casamenti et al.	Rat	Electrolytic	Nucleus basalis	G_{M1}, 30 mg/kg, i.p.	Daily for 22 days	At surgery	10 PO days	Active avoidance	+	8
							20 PO days	Passive avoidance	0	
Battistin et al.	Human	Ischemia	Cerebral cortex	G_{M1}, 20 mg, i.m.	2 times daily for 6 weeks	10 days after injury	10 days after injury	Neurological symptoms	+	5
Li et al.	Rat	Mechanical	Partial NS	G_{M1}, 20 mg/kg, i.p.	Daily	At surgery	2 PO days	Rotation	+	30
Cahn et al.	Rat	Ischemia	Cerebral cortex	G_{M1} or AGF2, 1, 2.5, 5, 10, or 30 mg/kg, i.p.	2 times daily for 3 days	At surgery	1 PO day	Passive avoidance	+	7
Butler et al.	Rat	Aspiration	Visual cortex	G_{M1}, 30 mg/kg, i.p.	Daily for 18 days	At surgery	15 PO days	Brightness, Pattern discrimination	− / 0	6
Poplawski and Issacson	Rat	Electrolytic	Septum	G_{M1}, 30 mg/kg, i.p.	Daily for 3 days	2 days preop	1 PO day	Hyperemotionality	+	35
							40 PO days	Active avoidance	0	

a Abbreviations: NS, nigrostriatal pathway; EC, entorhinal cortex; CN, caudate nucleus; i.p., intraperitoneal; i.m., intramuscular; PO, postoperative; NA, information not available; Mixed, 16% G_{D1b}, 19% G_{T1}, 21% G_{M1}, and 39% G_{D1a} gangliosides.

ment when the treatment was started 2 days after the lesion, and ganglioside treatments improved the clinical signs of stroke patients even though the treatments were started 10–15 days after the cerebrovascular accidents.[4,5]

Of the testing parameters affecting the influence of gangliosides on behavioral recovery, the latencies between surgery, treatment, and the onset of behavioral testing may represent the most important variables. Knowing to what extent testing experience interacts with the treatment effect, for example, may have significant consequences for the most efficacious use of ganglioside treatments. Although we have shown that gangliosides can reduce behavioral deficits even when testing was started several days after the termination of treatment,[15] it is interesting to note that in the only other study in which this was done, a disruption of behavioral recovery was observed.[6] As discussed in Section 3.2, it was hypothesized that this disruption was caused by surgically induced "cortical blindness" or a lack of an interaction between the treatment and visual stimulation, a variable that had previously been shown to be an important factor for ganglioside-induced recovery.[47] Similarly, it has been shown that an interaction between sensorimotor experience and amphetamine treatment is necessary for amphetamine-induced behavioral recovery to occur following motor cortex injury[20] and visual cortex lesions.[21] Given our recent findings that amphetamine and G_{M1} gangliosides exert similar behavioral effects following CN lesions,[12–14] the extent to which sensory and motor stimulation may affect ganglioside-induced behavioral recovery is an interesting and important question that deserves more attention.

Finally, analyses of when gangliosides exert their behavioral effects have given us some clues into how they may be influencing the recovery process. Although the exact processes by which gangliosides work is still unknown, the early onset of behavioral improvements noticed in nearly all studies showing beneficial consequences of treatment suggests that the underlying basis for behavioral recovery has little to do with ganglioside-enhanced sprouting *per se*. Even though there is considerable indirect proof that gangliosides promote neuronal sprouting in the CNS, the evidence relating these indices of sprouting to behavioral recovery is far from conclusive. In fact, most of the time-course studies we have reviewed have revealed that gangliosides affect behavioral performance prior to the time considered necessary for functional reinnervation to occur. Therefore, we favor the hypothesis that gangliosides promote behavioral recovery through rapidly occurring biochemical alterations. These processes could involve enhanced neurotransmitter release or uptake (e.g., refs. 10, 34, 36), increased enzymatic activity (e.g., refs. 19, 26, 28), or some other biochemical influence that protects neuronal tissue during the acute phase of injury. The measurable physiological consequences of such early molecular events could include the obseved reductions in cerebral edema[28] and neuronal degeneration[2,38] after CNS injury.

Another intriguing but unexplored possibility is that gangliosides may promote recovery by stimulating other, undamaged areas of the brain; this possibility invokes such concepts of recovery as diaschisis and vicariation (for a review of these concepts, see ref. 24). Diaschisis as an explanation for behavioral recovery has had a recent rejuvenation in the guise of "remote functional deficits" being restored after brain damage.[22,41] It may be that gangliosides exert their effects by accelerating recovery from "neural shock" in areas of the brain undamaged by the lesion. Gangliosides may also activate areas of the brain associated with the damaged area, such as contralateral homologous structures or adjacent tissue, that may be capable of compensating for the loss of functioning in the damaged structure. Although these possibilities are very speculative, they would provide an explanation for studies that have shown a ganglioside-induced reduction in behavioral deficits despite an absence of evidence for neuronal sparing[14,39] or morphological changes. Tests using 2-DG or cytochrome oxidase techniques, such as used by Feeney and colleagues,[23,43] would expose the merits of these hypotheses.

In conclusion, although gangliosides are not a panacea for all types of CNS injury, they have been shown to be an effective treatment for a variety of behavioral deficits following damage to many different areas of the brain. It is still not known exactly how gangliosides exert their influence, but since the behavioral effects occur early and seem to parallel some of the effects of amphetamine, it probably does not involve the enhancement of neuronal sprouting. Further behavioral work is needed to gain a better understanding of the possible mechanisms of ganglioside-facilitated recovery and to test the limitations of this form of therapy before gangliosides can achieve their full potential as an effective pharmacological treatment for CNS injury.

References

1. Agid, Y., Javoy, F., and Glowinski, J., 1973, Hyper-reactivity of remaining dopaminergic neurons after partial destruction of the nigrostriatal dopaminergic system in the rat, *Nature* **245**:150–151.
2. Agnati, L. F., Fuxe, K., Calza, L., Benfenati, F., Cavicchioli, L., Toffano, G., and Goldstein, M., 1983, Gangliosides increase the survival of lesioned nigral dopamine neurons and favour the recovery of dopaminergic synaptic function in striatum of rats by collateral sprouting, *Acta Physiol. Scand.* **119**:347–363.
3. Aldinio, C., Valenti, G., Savoini, G., Kirschner, G., Agnati, L., and Toffano, G., 1984, Monosialoganglioside internal ester stimulates the dopaminergic reinnervation of the striatum after unilateral hemitransection in the rat, *Int. J. Dev. Neurosci.* **2**:267–275.
4. Bassi, S., Albizzati, M. G., Sbacchi, M., Frattola, L., and Massarotti, M., 1984, Double-blind evaluation of monosialoganglioside (G_{M1}) therapy in stroke, *J. Neurosci. Res.* **12**:493–498.
5. Battistin, L., Cesari, A., Galligioni, F., Marin, G., Massarotti, M., Paccagnella, D., Pellegrini, A., Testa, G., and Tonin, P., 1985, Effects of G_{M1} ganglioside in cerebrovascular diseases: A double-blind trial in 40 cases, *Eur. Neurol.* **24**:343–351.
6. Butler, W. M., Griesbach, E., Labbe, R., and Stein, D. G., 1987, Gangliosides fail to enhance behavioral recovery after bilateral ablation of the visual cortex, *J. Neurosci. Res.* **17**:404–409.

7. Cahn, J., Borzeix, M.-G., and Toffano, G., 1986, Effect of G_{M1} ganglioside and of its inner ester derivative in a model of transient cerebral ischemia in the rat, in: *Gangliosides and Neuronal Plasticity* (G. Tettamanti, R. Ledeen, K. Sandhoff, Y. Nagai, and G. Toffano, eds.), Liviana Press, Padua, pp. 435–443.
8. Casamenti, F., Bracco, L., Bartloini, L., and Pepeu, G., 1985, Effects of ganglioside treatment in rats with a lesion of the cholinergic forebrain nuclei, *Brain Res.* **338**:45–52.
9. Cuello, A. C., Stephens, P. H., Tagari, P. C., Sofroniew, M. V., and Pearson, R. C. A., 1986, Retrograde changes in the nucleus basalis of the rat, caused by cortical damage, are prevented by exogenous ganglioside G_{M1}, *Brain Res.* **376**:373–377.
10. Cumar, F. A., Maggio, B., and Caputto, R., 1978, Dopamine release from nerve endings induced by polysialogangliosides, *Biochem. Biophys. Res. Commun.* **84**:65–69.
11. Dunbar, G. L., Butler, W. M., Fass, B., and Stein, D. G., 1986, Behavioral and neurochemical alterations induced by exogenous gangliosides in brain-damaged animals: Problems and perspectives, in: *Gangliosides and Neuronal Plasticity* (G. Tettamanti, R. Ledeen, K. Sandhoff, Y. Nagai, and G. Toffano, eds.), Liviana Press, Padua, pp. 365–380.
12. Dunbar, G. L., DeAngelis, M., Hecht, S., Merbaum, S., and Stein, D. G., 1986, Systemic injections of G_{M1} gangliosides and *d*-amphetamine reduce spatial learning deficits caused by bilateral damage to the caudate nucleus, *Soc. Neurosci. Abstr.* **12**:1283.
13. Dunbar, G. L., Hecht, S. A., Merbaum, S. L., DeAngelis, M. M., and Stein, D. G., 1987, Use of gangliosides and amphetamine to promote behavioral recovery following bilateral caudate nucleus lesions, in: *A New Therapeutic Tool in CNS Pathology* (R. Malamed and A. Portera-Sanchez, eds.), Liviana Press, Padua (in press).
14. Dunbar, G. L., Hecht, S. A., Merbaum, S. L., DeAngelis, M. M., and Stein, D. G., Use of G_{M1} gangliosides, AGF2, and *d*-amphetamine as a pharmacological treatment for reducing learning deficits in rats with bilateral caudate nucleus lesions, (in press).
15. Dunbar, G. L., Sabel, B. A., Firl, A. C., and Stein, D. G., 1984, G_{M1} gangliosides reduce spatial alteration deficits following bilateral lesions of the mediofrontal cortex, *Soc. Neurosci. Abstr.* **10**:1051.
16. Dunbar, G. L., Sapozhnikov, P., and Stein, D. G., 1987, G_{M1} gangliosides are ineffective in reducing amphetamine-induced rotational asymmetry, but protect rats from aphagia and adipsia following complete nigrostriatal transections, *Soc. Neurosci. Abstr.* **13**:1608.
17. Dunkel, I. J., Jones, L. S., and Davis, J. N., 1984, G_{M1} ganglioside administration does not induce sprouting in dopaminergic nigrostriatal neurons following a unilateral electrolytic substantia nigral lesion, *Soc. Neurosci. Abstr.* **10**:1020.
18. Fass, B., and Ramirez, J., 1984, Effects of ganglioside treatments on lesion-induced behavioral impairments and sprouting in the CNS, *J. Neurosci. Res.* **12**:445–458.
19. Fass, B., and Stein, D. G., 1987, Effects of fimbria–fornix transection and ganglioside treatments on histochemical staining for glucose-6-phosphate dehydrogenase in the lateral septum, *Synapse* **1**:70–81.
20. Feeney, D. M., Gonzales, A., and Law, W. A., 1982, Amphetamine, haloperidol, and experience interact to affect rate of recovery after motor cortex injury, *Science* **217**:855–857.
21. Feeney, D. M., and Hovda, D. A., 1985, Reinstatement of binocular depth perception by amphetamine and visual experience after visual cortex ablation, *Brain Res.* **342**:352–356.
22. Feeney, D. M., and Sutton, R. L., 1987, Pharmacotherapy for recovery of function after brain injury, *C.R.C. Crit. Rev. Clin. Neurobiol.* **3**:135–197.
23. Feeney, D. M., Sutton, R. L., Boyeson, M. G., and Dail, W. G., 1985, The locus coeruleus and cerebral metabolism: Recovery of function after cortical injury, *Physiol. Psychol.* **13**:197–205.
24. Finger, S., and Stein, D. G., 1982, *Brain Damage and Recovery: Research and Clinical Perspectives*, Academic Press, New York.
25. Heywood, R., Chesterman, H., Hunter, B., Palmer, A. K., Majeed, S. K., and Prentice, D. E., 1983, The toxicology of a ganglioside extract (cronassial), *Toxicol. Lett.* **15**:275–282.

26. Janigro, D., DiGregorio, F., Vyskocil, F., and Gorio, A., 1984, Gangliosides' dual mode of action, *J. Neurosci. Res.* **12**:499–509.

27. Karpiak, S. E., 1983, Ganglioside treatment improves recovery of alternation behavior after unilateral entorhinal cortex lesion, *Exp. Neurol.* **81**:330–339.

28. Karpiak, S. E., and Mahadik, S. P., 1984, Reduction of cerebral edema with G_{M1} ganglioside, *J. Neurosci. Res.* **12**:485–492.

29. Lang, W., 1981, Pharmacokinetic studies with [^{3}H] labeled exogenous gangliosides injected intramuscularly into rats, in: *Gangliosides in Neurological and Neuromuscular Function, Development, and Repair* (M. M. Rapport and A. Gorio, eds.), Raven Press, New York, pp. 241–251.

30. Li, Y. S., Mahadik, S. P., Rapport, M. M., and Karpiak, S. E., 1986, Acute effects of G_{M1} ganglioside: Reduction in both behavioral asymmetry and loss of Na^+,K^+-ATPase after nigrostiatal transection, *Brain Res.* **377**:292–297.

31. Oderfeld-Nowak, B., Wojcik, M., Ulas, J., and Potempska, A., 1981, Effects of chronic ganglioside treatment on recovery processes in hippocampus after brain lesions in rats, in: *Gangliosides in Neurological and Neuromuscular Function, Development, and Repair* (M. M. Rapport and A. Gorio, eds.), Raven Press, New York, pp. 197–209.

32. Onn, S.-P., Berger, T. W., Stricker, E. M., and Zigmond, M. J., 1986, Effects of intraventricular 6-hydroxydopamine on the dopaminergic innervation of striatum: Histochemical and neurochemical analysis, *Brain Res.* **376**:8–19.

33. Orlando, P., Cocciante, G., Ippolito, G., Massari, P., Roberti, S., and Tettamanti, G., 1979, The fate of tritium labeled G_{M1} ganglioside injected in mice, *Pharmacol. Res. Commun.* **11**:759–773.

34. Pedata, F., Giovanelli, L., and Pepeu, G., 1984, G_{M1} ganglioside facilitates the recovery of high affinity choline uptake in the cerebral cortex of rats with a lesion of the nucleus basalis magnocellularis, *J. Neurosci. Res.* **12**:421–427.

35. Poplawsky, A., and Isaacson, R. L., 1987, The G_{M1} ganglioside hastens the reduction of hyperemotionality after septal lesions, *Behav. Neural Biol.* **48**:150–158.

36. Raiteri, M., Versace, P., and Marchi, M., 1985, G_{M1} monosialoganglioside inner ester induces early recovery of striatal dopamine uptake in rats with unilateral nigrostriatal lesion, *Eur. J. Pharmacol.* **118**:347–350.

37. Sabel, B. A., Dunbar, G. L., Butler, W. M., and Stein, D. G., 1985, G_{M1} gangliosides stimulate neuronal reorganization and reduce rotational asymmetry after hemitransections of the nigrostriatal pathway, *Exp. Brain Res.* **60**:27–37.

38. Sabel, B. A., DelMastro, R., Dunbar, G. L., and Stein, D. G., 1987, G_{M1} gangliosides reduce anterograde degeneration in brain damaged rats, *Neurosci. Lett.* **77**:360–366.

39. Sabel, B. A., Slavin, M. D., and Stein, D. G., 1984, G_{M1} ganglioside treatment facilitates behavioral recovery from bilateral brain damage, *Science* **225**:340–342.

40. Savoini, G., Fuxe, K., Agnati, L. F., Calza, L., Morani, F., Lombardi, M. G., Goldstein, M., and Toffano, G., 1985, Effect of G_{M1} ganglioside on recovery of dopaminergic nigro-striatal neurons after lesion, in: *Central Nervous System Plasticity and Repair* (A. Bignami, F. E. Bloom, C. L. Bolis, and A. Adeloye, eds.), Raven Press, New York, pp. 75–85.

41. Schallert, T., Hernandez, T. D., and Barth, T. M., 1986, Recovery of function after brain damage: Severe and chronic disruption by diazepan, *Brain Res.* **379**:104–111.

42. Stewart, O., Loesche, J., and Horton, W. C., 1977, Behavioral correlates of denervation and reinnervation of the hippocampal formation of the rat: Open field activity and cue utilization following bilateral entorhinal cortex lesions, *Brain Res. Bull.* **2**:41–48.

43. Sutton, R. L., Chen, M. J., Hovda, D. A., and Feeney, D. M., 1986, Effects of amphetamine on cerebral metabolism following brain damage as revealed by quantitative cytochrome oxidase histochemistry, *Soc. Neurosci. Abstr.* **12**:1404.

44. Tettamanti, G., Venerando, B., Roberti, S., Chigorno, V., Sonnino, S., Ghidoni, R., Orlando, P., and Massari, P., 1981, The fate of exogenously administered gangliosides, in: *Gangliosides*

in *Neurological and Neuromuscular Function, Development, and Repair* (M. M. Rapport and A. Gorio, eds.), Raven Press, New York, pp. 225–240.

45. Tilson, H. A., Harry, G. J., Nanry, K., Hudson, P., and Hong, J. S., 1986, Ganglioside interactions with the dopaminergic system in rats, *Soc. Neurosci. Abstr.* **12:**1103.

46. Toffano, G., Agnati, L. F., Fuxe, K., Aldinio, C., Consolazione, A., Valenti, G., and Savoini, G., 1984, Effect of G_{M1} ganglioside treatment on the recovery of dopaminergic nigrostriatal neurons after different types of lesion, *Acta Physiol. Scand.* **122:**313–321.

47. Toffano, G., Savoini, G., Aporti, F., Calzolari, S., Consolazione, A., Maura, G., Marchi, M., Raiteri, M., and Agnati, L. F., 1984, The functional recovery of damaged brain: The effect of G_{M1} monosialoganglioside, *J. Neurosci. Res.* **12:**397–408.

48. Toffano, G., Savoini, G. E., Moroni, F., Lombardi, G., Calza, L., and Agnati, L. F., 1983, G_{M1} gangliosides stimulate the regeneration of dopaminergic neurons in the central nervous system, *Brain Res.* **261:**163–166.

49. Toffano, G., Savoini, G. E., Moroni, F., Lombardi, G., Calza, L., and Agnati, L. F., 1984, Chronic G_{M1} ganglioside treatment reduces dopamine cell body degeneration in the substantia nigra after unilateral hemitransection in rat, *Brain Res.* **296:**233–239.

50. Ungerstedt, U., 1971, Striatal dopamine release after amphetamine or nerve degeneration revealed by rotational behaviour, *Acta Physiol. Scand.* [*Suppl.*] **367:**49–68.

11

ACUTE GANGLIOSIDE EFFECTS LIMIT CNS INJURY
FUNCTIONAL AND BIOCHEMICAL CONSEQUENCES

STEPHEN E. KARPIAK, YU S. LI, AND SAHEBARAO P. MAHADIK

ABSTRACT. There are many reports that ganglioside treatment of animals following CNS injury results in facilitated recovery. One mechanism by which gangliosides promote recovery may be their acute effect ("protection") on early injury processes. We have found that within 48 hr after CNS injury (e.g., lesions, ablations, denervation, ischemia), there are reduced (1) behavioral deficits, (2) edema, (3) losses of membrane Na^+,K^+-ATPase activity, and (4) mortality. The data support the hypothesis that ganglioside administration may be preserving membrane structure, thereby limiting the extent of CNS damage at the time of injury and providing optimal conditions for subsequent CNS recovery and repair (i.e., plasticity).

1. LONG-TERM GANGLIOSIDE EFFECTS: INCREASED PLASTICITY

Recent research efforts have focused on studying the ability of ganglioside treatment to facilitate recovery after central nervous system damage. These experiments gained impetus from earlier, and ongoing, *in vitro* and peripheral nervous system studies. The *in vitro* studies had shown that when gangliosides were added to either neuronal cell line cultures or to neural tissue cultures, increased neuritic outgrowth resulted.[9,32] Parallel studies examined the effects of ganglioside treatment in animals with peripheral nerve damage (e.g., sciatic nerve

STEPHEN E. KARPIAK, YU S. LI, AND SAHEBARAO P. MAHADIK • Division of Neuroscience, New York State Psychiatric Institute, and Departments of Psychiatry and Biochemistry and Molecular Biophysics, College of Physicians and Surgeons, Columbia University, New York, New York 10032.

crush[10] or diabetic neuropathy[27]). In either paradigm, it was demonstrated that systemic ganglioside injections resulted in facilitated peripheral nerve regeneration and muscle reinnervation.

Based on these *in vitro* and PNS observations, studies were begun to assess the effects of ganglioside treatment on recovery processes following CNS injury. It was hypothesized that any facilitated recovery seen as a result of ganglioside treatment might be occurring through an increase in neuronal sprouting or, more generally, neuronal plasticity. The earliest *in vivo* mammalian studies, using biochemical and histochemical indices, reported that after brain lesions in rats that were subsequently treated daily with gangliosides, there was evidence for facilitated neuronal sprouting.[36,37] These conclusions were based on assays of rat CNS tissue 2–4 weeks after the CNS damage. Since these earliest observations, other data have been reported supporting hypotheses that ganglioside treatment may promote/facilitate neuronal sprouting following CNS damage.[1,6,11,13,34,39] These reported effects were "long term," occurring no sooner than 1–2 weeks after damage.

2. ACUTE GANGLIOSIDE EFFECTS

2.1. UNILATERAL ENTORHINAL CORTICAL LESIONS

In order to assess whether ganglioside-enhanced CNS regeneration in response to injury was paralleled by facilitated functional recovery, we first studied a well-established model wherein unilateral entorhinal cortical (EC) lesions result in a denervation of the granule cells of the dentate gyrus.[24] Rats trained on an alternation behavior lose the behavior after the EC lesion but regain the behavior as the denervated zone of the dentate gyrus is reinnervated by sprouting of cholinergic collaterals. Our studies showed that ganglioside treatment in rats with unilateral EC lesions did result in facilitated recovery of behavior.[14] However, the study provided two clear indications that the improved recovery was probably not the direct result of facilitated sprouting.

First, the mortality 24 hr after the ablation of the EC was 20% for controls and only 11% for ganglioside-treated animals.[20] Secondly, ganglioside-treated rats showed within 24 hr after the EC lesions only 50% of the behavioral loss as compared to controls.[14–17,20] These two short-term effects suggested that the ganglioside treatments were exerting a significant acute effect that was independent of any sprouting phenomenon. We concluded that the overall facilitated recovery was probably related to the reduced functional deficit seen at 24 hr after the EC lesion. We hypothesized that this acute effect reflected a reduction in the extent of CNS damage (i.e., neuronal process degeneration and cell loss) occurring at the time of injury (EC ablation).[14,17]

In a histochemical study,[8] quantitative analyses of the dentate 1–15 days after a unilateral EC lesion in rats treated with gangliosides indicated that there was no increase in cholinergic collateral sprouting. In fact, they found a decrease. Although increases in cholinergic enzymes have been found following unilateral EC lesions in rats treated with gangliosides,[39] these changes were long term, occurring 15–30 days post-lesion, and do not parallel any of the facilitated functional recoveries reported.

2.2. BILATERAL ENTORHINAL CORTICAL LESIONS

In order to evaluate whether or not ganglioside treatment affects functional recovery independent of sprouting, we studied the behavior of animals with bilateral EC lesions.[29,30] It is believed that functional recovery seen after bilateral EC lesions is not dependent on sprouting, since contralateral EC inputs are eliminated, and the time course of recovery does not parallel that of sprouting. Fass and Ramirez[8] first reported that the typical hyperactivity seen in rats following bilateral EC lesions was reduced in ganglioside-treated rats. This reduction in hyperactivity was seen as soon as 48 hr after the EC lesions, indicative of an acute ganglioside effect cleary independent of sprouting.

In a more extensive study, Ramirez et al.[29,30] studied rats' functional recovery of a previously learned alternation behavior. In this study, rats exhibit a severe impairment on the learned alternation behavior immediately (48 hr) following the bilateral EC lesions. However, ganglioside-treated rats commit significantly fewer choice errors and perseverative errors and reach criterion sooner. These findings show that ganglioside injections improve the extent but not rate of functional recovery in a system in which sprouting is precluded. Again, close examination of the data (Figs. 1 and 2) shows that the facilitatory effects of the ganglioside injections are evident during the acute (24–48 hr) recovery period, lending support to the hypothesis that ganglioside injections maybe "limiting" the extent of injury resulting from the lesions.

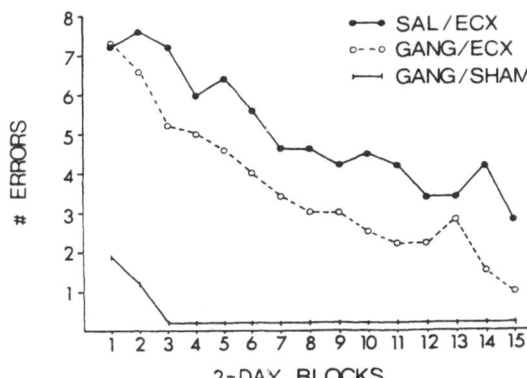

FIGURE 1. Time course of changes in total number of errors after bilateral entorhinal cortical lesions. Data are averaged over 2-day blocks.

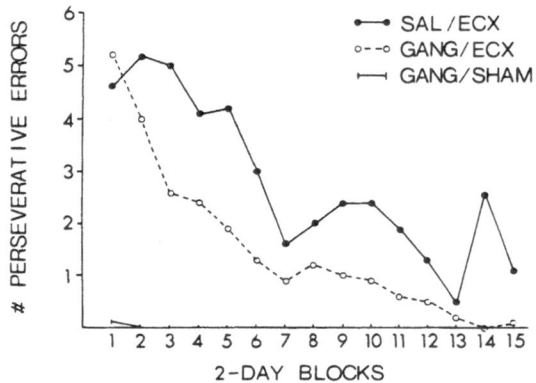

FIGURE 2. Time course of changes in total number of perseverative errors after bilateral entorhinal cortical lesions. Data are averaged over 2-day blocks.

2.3. NIGROSTRIATAL TRANSECTION: REDUCED ASYMMETRY

Considerable data have been obtained by studying the effects of ganglioside treatment in rats that have undergone unilateral partial hemitransection of the nigrostriatal pathway. It has been reported that as early as 4–5 days after the transection, striatal dopaminergic uptake, which is substantially reduced after the transection, is maintained at near-normal levels in G_{M1} ganglioside-treated rats.[37] At 8 days post-transection, G_{M1}-treated rats show decreased apomorphine-induced rotational behavior. Further, no difference in substantia nigra EEG activity (left versus right power ratio) was seen in G_{M1}-treated rats. In saline controls a marked difference in EEG activity exists between the transected and untransected sides of the brain.[37] These, as well as several histochemical studies, provide the strongest evidence that there may be regeneration of the ipsilateral and contralateral nigrostriatal pathways in ganglioside-treated rats after nigrostriatal transection.

An even more short-term, acute ganglioside effect has been observed in this lesion paradigm. It was reported that 48 hr after a partial transection of the nigrostriatal pathway, amphetamine-induced asymmetric rotational behavior was significantly reduced in rats treated with G_{M1} ganglioside.[33] This observation was replicated in our laboratories.[23] Dopamine-agonist-induced rotation in animals with unilateral nigrostriatal lesions has long been related to the imbalance in dopaminergic activity between the lesioned and nonlesioned sides of the brain and is accepted as a quantitative index of the asymmetry.[38]

Since ganglioside injections have an acute effect on the CNS following injury, the time interval between the injury and ganglioside administration is probably critical. Given the initial observation that asymmetric rotation is reduced as early as 48 hr after hemitransection,[33] an experiment was designed to assess when ganglioside treatment produces optimal functional recovery after injury (i.e., reduces asymmetry). Our study showed that a maximal reduction in rotational behavior could be achieved by injecting rats with G_{M1} ganglioside within 0–2 hr after the lesion.[23]

Rats that received their first G_{M1} injections at 4, 8, or 12 hr after surgery (Fig. 3) showed small reductions in rotation that were not statistically significant. Our data suggest that a critical period exists when adequate levels of ganglioside should be present to facilitate recovery. Since animals injected 4 hr or more after injury show no significant reduction in asymmetric rotation, the effectiveness of gangliosides may be optimal when they are associated with early rather than late injury processes.

3. G_{M1} GANGLIOSIDE REDUCES EDEMA: PROTECTION OF MEMBRANE NA^+,K^+-ATPASE

Since we had hypothesized that gangliosides may well be limiting the extent of CNS damage at the time of injury, we have begun to examine injury-associated parameters in order to determine whether or not this is the case. With our first experiments,[19] we studied the effects of G_{M1} treatment on cerebral edema in rats following an intracerebral mechanical lesion. We hypothesized that if gangliosides reduced the extent of damage (e.g., edema, cell loss, fiber degeneration), then the potential for recovery was increased. This view seemed also to coincide with the observation that there is increased cell survival following damage in ganglioside-treated animals.[36,37]

We found that 48 hr after a cortical lesion, rats treated with G_{M1} ganglioside showed a 33% reduction in edema at the site of injury. There were no effects on CNS water content outside the lesion area.[19,20] Subsequently, we have examined the effects of G_{M1} ganglioside on levels of plasma membrane Na^+,K^+-ATPase and tissue potassium. Plasma membrane Na^+,K^+-ATPase and intracellular potassium are both markedly reduced in edemic tissue, indicating membrane failure and disruption of plasma membrane ionic balances.[20] In addition to the func-

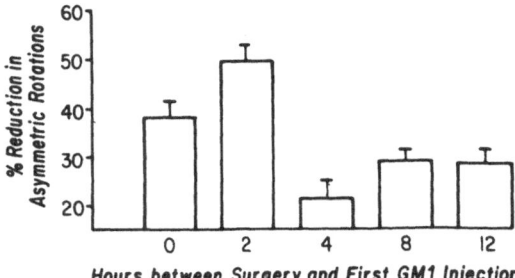

FIGURE 3. Percentage reduction in asymmetric rotations (as compared to controls) in rats treated with G_{M1} ganglioside. Rats were tested 48 hr after unilateral hemitransection of the nigrostriatal pathway.

tional significance of Na^+,K^+-ATPase, this enzyme is highly enriched in synaptic plasma membranes and is therefore a good marker for synaptic membrane integrity. At 48 hr after a cortical lesion, we found a 56% reduction in Na^+,K^+-ATPase activity and a 55% reduction in intracellular potassium. In contrast, G_{M1} ganglioside-treated rats showed only a 31% reduction in Na^+,K^+-ATPase activity and a 28% reduction in potassium.[20] No changes were found in blood–brain barrier permeability (determined with iodinated albumin) following ganglioside treatment.

3.1. MEMBRANE Na^+,K^+-ATPASE

There is no clear evidence to indicate what short-term process is being affected by the gangliosides. However, our analyses of edema, and particularly membrane-associated Na^+,K^+-ATPase activity, may provide some clues regarding the mechanism(s) by which gangliosides are acutely affecting pathophysiological processes associated with CNS injury. It has been established that membrane Na^+,K^+-ATPase, the so-called Na^+/K^+ pump, plays a fundamental role in maintaining membrane homeostasis and excitability,[35] which are essential for normal cell function. Its significance in repair of neuronal and glial cell damage is not yet clear. Evidence has shown that CNS injury begins with membrane damage and involves the loss of Na^+,K^+-ATPase activity.[31] Plasma membrane disorganization probably results in the loss of the enzyme's activity. Since the loss of activity of this enzyme occurs very early after injury, it is most likely involved in the acute phase of the injury process. The loss of this enzyme activity probably reflects a series of biochemical changes (e.g., lipid hydrolysis, phospholipase activation, levels and membrane action of arachidonic acid, ionic permeation) that lead to membrane failure following injury. With ganglioside injections, even in a short-term protocol, the maintenance of higher levels of Na^+,K^+-ATPase may minimize neuronal and glial membrane dysfunction and subsequent degeneration, thus contributing to facilitated recovery.

3.2. PROTECTION OF STRIATAL Na^+,K^+-ATPASE AFTER HEMITRANSECTION

Having seen that the loss of membrane Na^+,K^+-ATPase is reduced with ganglioside treatment after cerebral cortical lesions, we began to study the levels of this enzyme in the striatum of rats that had undergone unilateral partial hemitransections of the nigrostriatal pathway. Since we had seen that G_{M1} reduces (at 48 hr post-transection) asymmetric rotation, and since Na^+,K^+-ATPase levels are indicative of membrane integrity, we predicted that the activity of this enzyme in the striatum following partial denervation (hemitransection) might also be spared, "protected" by ganglioside treatment.

Rats were hemitransected and injected with G_{M1} ganglioside (20 mg/kg, i.p.) at 0.5 and 24 hr post-surgery. At 48 hr the brains were removed for ATPase analysis.

The Na^+,K^+-ATPase was assayed in a crude total membrane preparation using our standard procedure modified from published reports.[2,3] Animals were anesthetized (ether) and perfused with phosphate-buffered saline, and their left and right striata were dissected out. A membrane fraction was prepared by homogenizing specimens in 5 ml of ice-cold buffer (40 mM Tris-HCl, pH 7.5; 10 mM $MgCl_2$; 10 mM EDTA) and centrifuging for 30 min at 100,000 g. The resulting pellet was suspended in the homogenizing buffer. Five hundred microliters of reaction mixture contained 40 mM Tris-HCl, pH 7.5, 150 mM NaCl, 40 mM KCl, 10 mM $MgCl_2$, 2 mM EDTA, 2 mM EGTA, 4 mM ATP, and 100–200 μg of protein. The inorganic phosphate released at 37°C for 30 min was determined by the method of Eibl and Lands.[7] The Na^+,K^+-ATPase activity was then estimated as the difference between the activities in the absence and presence of 5 mM ouabain.

By comparing the striatal Na^+,K^+-ATPase from the transected side with that from the untransected side, we found a 35.8% activity reduction in denervated striata from saline controls, whereas G_{M1}-treated rats showed only a 6.8% decrease in activity ($P < 0.025$; Fig. 4).[18,23] The results demonstrate an acute effect of G_{M1} on this enzyme indicative of either a protective or restorative effect on the axonal and dendritic degeneration that occurs after the transection.

The amphetamine-induced rotational behavior is a reflection of the imbalance in dopamine transmission following unilateral nigrostriatal pathway interruption. The maintenance of striatal membrane Na^+, K^+-ATPase on the transected side in G_{M1}-treated rats may diminish this imbalance. This compensatory effect of G_{M1} on Na^+,K^+-ATPase may be the mechanism by which a balance in dopaminergic function is restored, resulting in a reduction in asymmetric rotation. However, direct measurement of striatal dopaminergic turnover is needed to support this hypothesis.

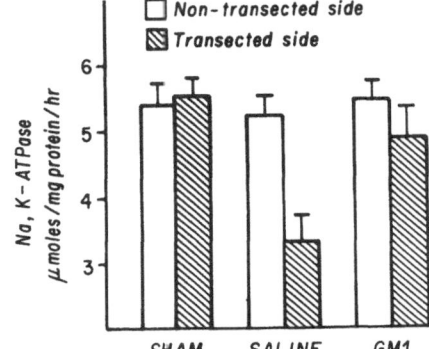

FIGURE 4. Striatal membrane Na^+,K^+-ATPase activity 48 hr after unilateral hemitransection of the nigrostriatal pathway: reduction of enzyme loss by G_{M1} ganglioside treatment.

4. GANGLIOSIDE TREATMENT REDUCES MORTALITY FROM ISCHEMIA

The following study was undertaken to extend examination of the acute effects of ganglioside treatment on injured CNS tissue. We have examined the effects of G_{M1} ganglioside and AGF2 (a G_{M1} derivative) on a paradigm of global ischemia in the Mongolian gerbil.[17,18] Our choice to study ischemia was based on the fact that no previous reports had examined the effects of ganglioside on "closed-head" injury, and a clinical report showed that ganglioside treatment improved functional recovery following stroke.[4] In addition, many of the molecular events (mechanisms) involved in the pathophysiology of ischemia are known. Consequently, we would be in a more advantageous position to study the mechanism(s) by which gangliosides affect injury processes.

4.1. GLOBAL ISCHEMIA MODEL

The Mongolian gerbil has been used as an experimental model to study cerebral ischemia since most gerbils have an incomplete circle of Willis. This results in little or no vascular communication between the hemispheres.[22] Consequently, following a partial or complete litigation (occlusion) of the carotid artery, ischemia is primarily lateralized to one cerebral hemisphere. This phenomenon allows for comparisons between the occluded and nonoccluded sides of the brain, with the animal serving as its own control.

Male gerbils (80–90 g) were anesthetized (i.m.) with a mixture of ketamine

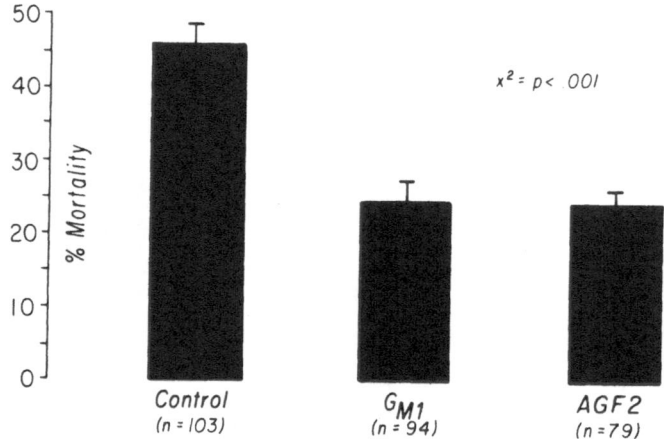

FIGURE 5. Mortality in gerbils 48 hr after unilateral permanent occlusion of carotid artery.

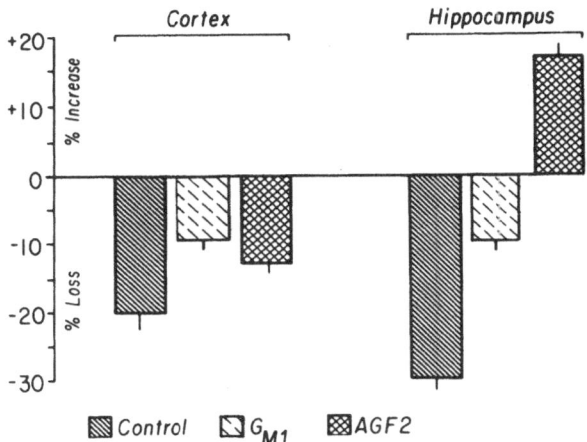

FIGURE 6. Membrane Na$^+$,K$^+$-ATPase activity in cortex and hippocampus of gerbils 48 hr after unilateral permanent occlusion of carotid artery. Percentages are based on comparison of the occluded versus nonoccluded sides of the brain.

(Vetalar, 87.5 mg/kg) and xylazine (Rompun, 7.5 mg/kg). An incision was made on the ventral surface of the neck, the salivary glands were moved laterally, and the right carotid sheath was exposed. Both the vagus and sympathetic nerves were separated from the right common carotid artery, which was then permanently ligated using No. 0 silk thread. Gerbils received ganglioside injections (20 mg/kg i.m.; Fidia Research Laboratories) 0.5 and 24 hr after surgery. There were three groups, receiving, respectively, saline controls, monosialoganglioside (G_{M1}), and AGF2 ganglioside derivative. AGF2, an internal ester of G_{M1}, has been reported to have a longer half-life in serum than G_{M1} because of slow hydrolysis,[1,28] and because it is a less polar compound, larger quantities may cross the blood–brain barrier.

4.2. REDUCED MORTALITY FOLLOWING GANGLIOSIDE INJECTIONS

Forty-eight hours after permanent unilateral ligation of the common carotid, saline-injected gerbils had a 49% mortality (Fig. 5). G_{M1}- and AGF2-injected gerbils showed almost identical mortalities of 27% and 26%, respectively. Ganglioside treatments reduced mortality by 49%.

By comparing levels of membrane Na$^+$,K$^+$-ATPase activity in the occluded side of the brain with that in the nonoccluded side of the brain in saline-injected controls, we found significant decreases in enzyme activity (Fig. 6): a 19.8% decrease ($P < 0.01$) in the cortex and a 34.7% decrease ($P < 0.01$) in hippocampus. No statistical differences in enzyme activity between the occluded and nonoccluded sides of the brain were found in either G_{M1}- or AGF2-treated rats.

Ganglioside (G_{M1} or AGF2) treatment results in a 48% decrease in mortality at 48 hr after the induction of ischemia in gerbils by permanent unilateral ligation of the common carotid artery. We had previously found that after cortical aspiration, G_{M1} ganglioside treatment results in reduced mortality.[16] This reduction in mortality, particularly in the ischemia model, supports the view that gangliosides pharmacologically affect the acute phase following CNS injury. If the extent of injury and, therefore, any associated functional deficits can be reduced during the acute phase following CNS damage, the potential for subsequent recovery should be maximized.

5. MECHANISM: MEMBRANE PROTECTION

The mechanisms by which ganglioside treatments result in reduced mortality and improved functional recovery are not yet known. Analysis of membrane Na^+,K^+-ATPase activity in the ischemia study as well as in the striatum following denervation indicates that the possible "locus" of action may be on the stability of plasma membranes. We had found that ganglioside treatment of rats with open-head CNS injury leads to a reduction in edema and in a reduction in losses of membrane Na^+,K^+-ATPase and intracellular K^+ activity at the locus of injury.[17] Using hippocampal slices, Bianchi et al.[5] report similar protection of ATPase activity either by in vitro or in vivo administration of G_{M1} ganglioside. Consequently, attention has been focused on a possible membrane mechanism by which gangliosides may be pharmacologically active. This mechanism is further emphasized since exogenous gangliosides have been shown to insert functionally into membranes[26] and to modulate ATPase activity in vitro and in vivo.[21,25] Ganglioside protection from the loss of Na^+,K^+-ATPase activity may be indicative of protection of membrane structure and function.

Stabilizing membrane structure and therefore "normal" ionic gradients may well minimize membrane failure and subsequent deterioration. Protection from the loss of activity of the Na^+,K^+-ATPase enzyme probably reflects effects on one or a series of membrane biochemical changes (e.g., lipid hydrolysis, phospholipase activation, production and membrane action of arachidonic acid, ionic imbalance), including Ca^{2+}-ATPase, intracellular Ca^{2+}, and pH, which occur as a result of injury and lead to membrane failure. A number of in vitro and in vivo studies have shown that G_{M1} treatments protect neuronal as well as neuromuscular resistance to hypoxia and ionic disturbances, improve conduction velocity and axonal morphology in neuropathy, prevent ultrastructural deterioration of mitochondria, and reduce retrograde axonal degeneration in the CNS after injury.[5] These data, together with evidence for gangliosides' ability to reduce cerebral edema and mortality after severe CNS injury, strengthen the hypothesis that gangliosides may be preserving membrane structure by preventing the "deterioration of the membrane microenvironment."[5,12] This acute ganglioside effect on early injury processes may well provide an optimal environment that is conducive for subsequent injury-induced neuronal plasticity.

ACKNOWLEDGMENTS. The authors wish to acknowledge the technical assistance of F. Vilim and P. Aceto. Supported in part by NSF (BNS8500296).

REFERENCES

1. Aldinio, C., Valenti, G., Savoini, G. E., Kirschner, G., Agnati, L. F., and Toffano, G., 1984, Monosialoganglioside internal ester stimulates the dopaminergic reinnervation of the striatum after unilateral hemitransection in rat, *Int. J. Dev. Neurosci.* **2**:267–275.
2. Atterwill, C. K., Cunningham, V. J., and Balazs, R., 1984, Characterization of Na,K-ATPase in cultures and separated neuronal and glial cells from rat cerebellum, *J. Neurochem.* **43**:8–18.
3. Averet, N., Rigoulet, M., and Cohadon, F., 1984, Modification of synaptosomal Na,K-ATPase activity during vasogenic brain edema in the rabbit, *J. Neurochem.* **42**:275–277.
4. Bassi, S., Albizzati, M. G., Sbacchi, M., Frattola, L., and Massarotti, M., 1984, Double-blind evaluation of monosialoganglioside (G$_{M1}$) therapy in stroke, *J. Neurosci. Res.* **12**:493–498.
5. Bianchi, R., Janigro, D., Milan, F., Giudici, G., and Corio, A., 1986, *In vivo* treatment with G$_{M1}$ prevents the rapid decay of ATPase activities and mitochondrial damage in hippocampal slices, *Brain Res.* **364**:400–404.
6. Doherty, P., Dickson, J. G., Flanigan, T. P., and Walsh, F. S., 1985, Ganglioside G$_{M1}$ does not initiate, but enhances neurite regeneration of nerve growth factor-dependent sensory neurons, *J. Neurochem.* **44**:1259–1265.
7. Eibl, H., and Lands, W., 1969, A new sensitive determination of phosphate, *Anal. Biochem.* **30**:51–57.
8. Fass, B., and Ramirez, J., 1984, Effects of ganglioside treatments on lesion-induced behavioral impairment and sprouting in the CNS, *J. Neurosci. Res.* **12**:445–458.
9. Ferrari, G., Fabris, M., and Gorio, A., 1983, Gangliosides enhance neurite outgrowth in PC12 cells, *Dev. Brain Res.* **8**:215–221.
10. Gorio, A., Marini, P., and Zanoni, R., 1983, Muscle reinnervation III. Motor neuron sprouting capacity, enhancement by exogenous gangliosides, *Neuroscience* **8**:417–429.
11. Gradkowska, M., Skup, M., Kiedrowski, L., Calzolari, S., and Oderfeld-Nowak, B., 1986, The effect of G$_{M1}$ ganglioside on cholinergic and serotoninergic systems in the rat hippocampus following partial denervation is dependent on the degree of fiber degeneration, *Brain Res.* **375**:417–425.
12. Janigro, D., DiGregorio, F., Vyskocil, F., and Gorio, A., 1984, Gangliosides' dual mode of action: A working hypothesis, *J. Neurosci. Res.* **12**:499–509.
13. Johnsson, G., Gorio, A., Hallman, H., Janigro, D., Kojima, H., Luthman, J., and Zanoni, R., 1984, Effects of G$_{M1}$ ganglioside on developing and mature serotonin and noradrenaline neurons lesioned by selective neurotoxins, *J. Neurosci. Res.* **12**:459–475.
14. Karpiak, S. E., 1983, Ganglioside treatment improves recovery of alternation behavior after unilateral entorhinal cortical lesion, *Exp. Neurol.* **81**:330–339.
15. Karpiak, S. E., 1984, Exogenous gangliosides enhance recovery from CNS injury, in: *Ganglioside Structure, Function, and Biomedical Potential* (R. Ledeen, R. Yu, M. M. Rapport, and Y. Susuki, eds.), Plenum Press, New York, pp. 489–497.

16. Karpiak, S. E., 1985, Treating brain injury with gangliosides: A reply, *Int., Psychiatry* **3**:199–210.
17. Karpiak, S. E., Li, Y. S., Aceto, P., and Mahadik, S. P., 1986, Acute effects of gangliosides on CNS injury, in: *Neuronal Plasticity and Gnagliosides* (G. Tettamanti, R. Ledeen, Y. Nagai, S. Sandhoff, and G. Toffano, eds.), Springer-Verlag, Berlin pp. 407–414.
18. Karpiak, S. E., Li, Y. S., and Mahadik, S. P., 1987, Gnagliosides [G_{M1} & AGF2] reduce mortality due to ischemia: Protection of membrane function, *Stroke* **18**:184–187.
19. Karpiak, S. E., and Mahadik, S. P., 1984, Reduction of cerebral edema with G_{M1} ganglioside, *J. Neurosci. Res.* **12**:485–492.
20. Karpiak, S., and Mahadik, S. P., 1984, G_{M1} ganglioside limits CNS pathology, in: *Cellular and Pathological Aspects of Glycoconjugate Metabolism* (H. Dreyfus, R. Massarelli, L. Freysz, and G. Rebel, eds.), INSERM, Paris, Vol. 126, pp. 585–598.
21. Leon, A., Facci, L., Benvegnu, D., and Toffano, G., 1981, Activation of Na,K-ATPase by nanomolar concentrations of G_{M1} ganglioside, *J. Neurochem.* **37**:350–357.
22. Levine, S., and Sohn, D., 1969, Cerebral ischemia in infant and adult gerbils. Relation to incomplete circle of Willis, *Arch. Pathol.* **87**:315–317.
23. Li, Y. S., Mahadik, S. P., Rapport, M. M., and Karpiak, S. E., 1986, Acute effects of G_{M1} ganglioside: Reduction in both behavioral asymmetry and loss of Na,K-ATPase after nigrostriatal transection, *Brain Res.* **377**:292–297.
24. Loesche, J., and Steward, O., 1977, Behavioral correlates of denervation and reinnervation of the hippocampal formation of the rat: Recovery of alternation performance following unilateral entorhinal cortex lesions, *Brain Res. Bull.* **2**:31–39.
25. Mahadik, S. P., Korenovsky, A., and Karpiak, S. E., 1985, G_{M1} alters Na,K-ATPase levels in rat CNS regions, *Trans. Am. Soc. Neurochem.* **16**:231.
26. Moss, J., Fishman, P. H., Manganiello, V. C., Vaughan, M., and Brady, R. D., 1976, Functional incorporation of ganglioside in to intact cells: Induction of choleragen responsiveness, *Proc. Natl. Acad. Sci. U.S.A.* **73**:1034–1037.
27. Norido, F., Canella, R., Zanoni, R., and Gorio, A., 1984, Development of diabetic neuropathy in the C57BL/KS mouse and its treatment with gangliosides, *Exp. Neurol.* **83**:221–232.
28. Raiteri, M., Versace, P., and Marchi, M., 1985, G_{M1} monosialoganglioside inner ester induces early recovery of striatal dopamine uptake in rats with unilateral nigrostriatal lesions, *Eur. J. Pharmacol.* **118**:347–350.
29. Ramirez, J. J., Karpiak, S., Kilfoil, T., Henschel, B., and Grones, W., 1985, Ganglioside administration reduces behavioral deficits after bilateral entorhinal cortex lesions, *Soc. Neurosci. Abstr.* **11**:251.
30. Ramirez, J. J., Fass, B., Kilfoil, T., Henschel, B., Grones, W., and Karpiak, S. E., 1987, Ganglioside-induced enhancement of behavioral recovery after bilateral lesions of the entorhinal cortex, *Brain Res.* **414**:85–90.
31. Rigoulet, M., Guerin, B., Cohalon, F., and Vandendreissche, M., 1979, Unilateral brain injury in the rabbit: Reversible and irreversible damage of the membrane ATPase, *J. Neurochem.* **32**:35–43.
32. Roisen, F. J., Bartfeld, H., Nagele, R., and Yorke, G., 1981, Ganglioside stimulation of axonal sprouting *in vitro, Science* **214**:577–578.
33. Sabel, B. A., Dunbar, G. L., and Stein, D. G., 1984, Gangliosides minimize behavioral deficits and enhance structural repair after brain injury, *J. Neurosci. Res.* **12**:429–443.
34. Sparrow, J. R., and Grafstein, B., 1982, Sciatic nerve regeneration in ganglioside-treated rats, *Exp. Neurol.* **77**:230–235.
35. Stahl, W. L., 1984, Na,K-ATPase: Structure, function and conformations, *Ann. Neurol.* **16**:S121–S127.
36. Toffano, G., Savoini, G., Moroni, F., Lombardi, G., Calza, L., and Agnati, L. F., 1983, G_{M1}

ganglioside stimulates the regeneration of dopaminergic neurons in the central nervous system, *Brain Res.* **261**:163–166.

37. Toffano, G., Savoini, G., Aporti, F., Calzolari, S., Consolazione, A., Maura, G., Marchi, M., Raiteri, M., and Agnati, L. F., 1984, The functional recovery of damaged brain: The effect of G_{MI} monosialoganglioside, *J. Neurosci. Res.* **12**:397–408.

38. Ungerstedt, U., 1971, Striatal dopamine release after amphetamine or nerve degeneration revealed by rotational behavior, *Acta Physiol. Scand.* **82**:49–68.

39. Wojcik, M., Ulas, J., and Oderfeld-Nowak, B., 1982, The stimulating effect of ganglioside injections on the recovery of choline acetyltransferase activities in the hippocampus of the rat after septal lesions, *Neuroscience* **7**:494–506.

12

A Rationale for the Use of Melanocortins in Neural Injury

Paul De Koning and Willem Hendrik Gispen

ABSTRACT. Peptides derived from ACTH/MSH (melanocortins) exert trophic influences on central and peripheral nervous tissue. The influence of melanocortins during ontogeny, following neural damage, and in certain neurological diseases are reviewed, and possible clinical indications for melanocortin therapy are given. The capacity and possible pathophysiological mechanism for melanocortins to enhance functional recovery following peripheral nerve damage as measured by functional, histological, and electrophysiological test methods are discussed extensively. Structure–activity studies have shown that the neurotrophic potency is not related to corticotropic or immunosuppressant activity but resides in the $ACTH_{4-10}$ sequence present in α- and β-MSH and ACTH. The stable $ACTH_{4-9}$ analogue Org.2766 is also active. The peptides are only effective if they are given during the first few days after injury, suggesting that they may be stimulating the initial sprouting response. We present evidence that MSH-like peptides may be formed locally in response to injury and thus play a biologically significant role in the regulation of nerve regeneration.

Evidence is accumulating to suggest that Org.2766 and α-MSH may exert their neurotrophic influences in the central nervous system as well. Chronic treatment of aging rats counteracts degenerative processes occurring in the hippocampus of senile rats. Furthermore, subchronic treatment of rats bearing lesions either in the n. parafascicularis or in the septal complex facilitated recovery of function as tested in several behavioral test systems.

1. Introduction

Little progress has been made in the treatment of peripheral and central neural disorders. There are only a few neurological diseases the molecular mechanisms of which are understood and for which, on the basis of this understanding, adequate therapy has been devised. As to neural damage we are at the stage of beginning to understand some of the complexity of the processes that are active

PAUL DE KONING AND WILLEM HENDRIK GISPEN • Division of Molecular Neurobiology, Rudolf Magnus Institute for Pharmacology, and Institute of Molecular Biology and Medical Biotechnology, University of Utrecht, 3584 CH Utrecht, The Netherlands.

in and around the site of lesion. Enormous efforts are being made to identify the nature and to study the expression of intrinsic as well as extrinsic factors that promote neurite outgrowth in brain and peripheral nerve. The recent demonstration of a family of growth-associated proteins provides evidence for intrinsic mechanisms regulating axonal growth.[78] The proteins appear in axons that do regenerate but are not expressed in neurons that fail to regenerate their axons. Among the factors with an extrinsic neurotrophic effect on regenerating peripheral nerve tissue are nerve growth factor, adenosine 3',5'-monophosphate, gangliosides, TRH, and melanocortins (reviewed in ref. 12). This chapter deals with the neurotrophic effects of melanocortins, that is, peptides derived from ACTH and MSH and their synthetic analogues.

It was David De Wied who provided the experimental basis for the notion that the central nervous system could be considered a target for circulating pituitary peptide hormones. He demonstrated[26] that pituitary hormones like ACTH exert modulatory influences on adaptive behavior by a direct effect on certain brain centers. The observation that ACTH and congeners are endogenous to certain neuronal circuits in which they are formed by selective processing of a 31-kDa precursor peptide, proopiomelanocortin, justifies their being viewed as hormones as well as neuropeptides, having neurotransmitter as well as neuromodulatory properties. Since neural tissue may be considered a target tissue for ACTH, the peptide may exert a trophic influence similar to that seen in its peripheral target tissue (adrenal).

Indeed, evidence has suggested that removal of pituitary trophic hormones reduced the rate of macromolecular biosynthesis in certain regions of the rat brain, and replacement therapy with ACTH fragments restored this lower synthesis rate to normal.[31] At the same time various groups of researchers reported evidence that melanocortins, and fragments thereof, affected development and maturation of fetal brain tissue and motor systems. Moreover, it became increasingly evident that neuropeptides regulate the excitability of neurons at many levels of the central nervous system, including the reticular formation and the spinal cord. The connection between the studies on the influence of neuropeptide administration on behavioral responses and the peptide effects on the neuromuscular system is that the evoked behavioral responses make use of the same motor pathways. Taken together, these observations led us to investigate the possible beneficial role of ACTH and congeners in repair of neural damage and in certain neurological diseases.

The availability of ACTH analogues such as $ACTH_{4-10}$ and Org.2766 makes it possible to distinguish between the actions of corticoids and corticotropin in itself, since these analogues are devoid of the classical adrenocortical secretional activity but possess both neurotropic and myotropic actions like those of the parent molecules ACTH and MSH. Furthermore, steroid and peptide hormones are sometimes known to have antagonistic effects on behavior and muscle.[27,42,65] This differentiation also obviated the need to perform experiments in hypophysectomized or adrenalectomized animals or *in vitro* experiments on nerve–muscle preparations.

2. TROPHIC INFLUENCES OF MELANOCORTINS IN DEVELOPMENT

Both experimental brain lesion studies and experiments employing brain tissue extracts pointed to a fetal growth-promoting factor of hypothalamic origin. In a screening model for intrauterine fetal growth, a variety of peptides derived from proopiomelanocortin were tested, including $ACTH_{1-24}$, α-MSH, $ACTH_{4-10}$, and a potentiated $ACTH_{4-9}$ analogue, Org.2766 (Fig. 1). Of these peptides, only α-MSH increased intrauterinic growth.[90] Injection of purified anti-α-MSH antibodies directly into the intact fetus inhibited the growth of the fetus and of its brain, suggesting a physiological role for α-MSH in fetal development.[89,91,92] The unique trophic effect of α-MSH on body growth was not detected when the peptide was given in the first 2 weeks of postnatal life, which might indicate that the peptide acts via the placenta.[90] This primary activity differs from known CNS and PNS effects of peptides in either perinatal or adult rats and underscores the notion that there is a multiplicity of information encoded in the "open" ACTH molecule that, in combination with the heterogeneity of neural tissue, will make it difficult to unravel the complex molecular mechanism of action of ACTH in the nervous system.[28]

Another line of research dealt with eye opening as an index of brain maturation and the effects of ACTH and congeners injected in neonates.[95] The authors based their work on the notion that perinatal activation and hormone treatment of young rats may affect behavior seen in adulthood.[72] Injection on the third postnatal day of life of either $ACTH_{1-39}$, $ACTH_{1-24}$, $ACTH_{1-18}$, or $ACTH_{1-16}$ accelerated the eye opening of both male and female pups by approximately 1–2 days. The peptides $ACTH_{4-10}$, $ACTH_{1-10}$, Org.2766, and α-MSH were not effective in this respect.[95] It is tempting to assume that this is a reflection of an "extra target" effect of ACTH directly on the developing central nervous system.

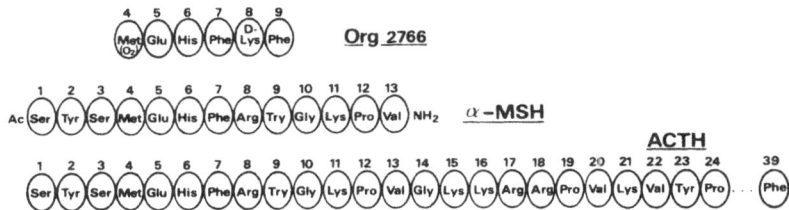

FIGURE 1. Primary peptide structures of ACTH, α-MSH, and the $ACTH_{4-9}$ analogue Org.2766.

Treatment with $ACTH_{4-10}$ or Org.2766 in neonates increases the complexity of postsynaptic folds and the rate at which they invaginate into the muscle fiber and also enhances the maturation of neuromuscular function.[39,84] In this respect, it was suggested that melanocortins like β-endorphin may influence neuromuscular maturation and function by an effect on end-plate acetylcholinesterase that increases the amount of acetylcholine in the cleft.[46,84,94]

This section on the developmental influences of ACTH precedes those on the effects of melanocortins on CNS and PNS plasticity since it has long been recognized that postlesion mechanisms are often reminiscent of those processes playing a role in the ontogeny of the nervous system.[97]

3. MELANOCORTINS AND CNS PLASTICITY

Behavioral studies in adult animals and humans and studies on the development and maturation of the central nervous system in rats show that melanocortins are able to influence central nervous system structures in a direct fashion, circumventing peripheral target tissues.[28] The mechanism by which such effects are brought about is not clear. It may be that enhancement of glucose uptake and protein synthesis is part of the trophic repertoire of the peptide responsible for the enhanced growth and maturation.[32]

In recent tissue culture studies, trophic effects of ACTH on cultured embryonic chick brain cortical cells have been reported,[19] but we have been unable to demonstrate such effects in a variety of tissue culture systems (P. M. Edwards, unpublished data). In a series of experiments, Azmitia[3,4] showed that in the absence of hippocampal cells, melanocortins exert a trophic response on cultured fetal rat mesencephalic cells. In the presence of the fetal hippocampal target cells, apparently optimal delivery of a hippocampal-borne trophic factor is ensured, leaving little role for exogenously added neuropeptides. Curiously, in addition to $ACTH_{4-10}$, Org.2766, α-MSH, and $ACTH_{1-39}$, $ACTH_{11-24}$ also exerted trophic influences on the isolated mesencephalic serotonergic cells. In the peripheral nervous system following injury, the latter peptide was without trophic effect in a wide dose range tested.[8]

Early studies of the effect of melanocortins on recovery from CNS lesions gave conflicting results (for review see ref. 6). Peptides with full endocrine activity were used, since the rationale behind the treatment was reduction of reactive scar tissue believed to limit CNS regeneration. However, the studies on the peripheral nervous system by Strand's group and our own have shown that the immunosuppressant and corticotropic activities are not involved in the trophic response and may have disturbed the final outcome of previous CNS studies.

Presently, several reports have been published that suggest that the effects of damage in the central nervous system may be reduced by treatment with melanocortins. Flohr and Luneburg[38] showed that systemic treatment with $ACTH_{4-10}$ improved the acquisition and maintenance of the compensated state following unilateral labyrinthectomy in *Rana temporaria*.

Isaacson and Poplawsky[50,51] used the disappearance of hyperemotionality of rats, induced by septal area lesions, as an index of functional recovery from brain damage. The peptides $ACTH_{4-10}$ and Org.2766, given subcutaneously for 4 consecutive days beginning immediately after surgery, resulted in a smaller than usual lesion-induced increase in emotionality scores. The Org.2766 treatment also facilitated the return to normal values over subsequent days after surgery. However, the effect of $ACTH_{4-10}$ on emotionality was found only on the first testing day, which was also the last day on which $ACTH_{4-10}$ was given. Reduced emotionality was not found on subsequent test days. This may only indicate that the ACTH fragment was not given for a sufficient number of days, since it was found that in order to find facilitation of recovery in the PNS, a series of treatments lasting at least 6 and preferably 8 days after nerve crush must be given.[34] Weeks after the daily tests for emotionality, the animals were trained on the two-way active avoidance task.[50,51] The typical increase in avoidance performance seen in animals with septal lesions was observed in previously Org.2766- or $ACTH_{4-10}$-treated animals. Only the prior Org.2766 treatment reduced the number of intertrial responses that are typical of the septal lesion.

The beneficial effects of melanocortins following CNS lesions also became apparent from studies employing lesions of the parafascicular nucleus in the rat.[67] Animals that had been treated daily with α-MSH or Org.2766 for 2 weeks starting on the third day following surgery acquired a reversal learning task in a T maze with fewer errors than did the saline-treated controls; α-MSH seemed to be more potent than Org.2766 in reducing the reversal learning deficit. This observation was corroborated by the fact that at the end of the treatment period, the abnormal grasping response that results from a parafascicular lesion was slightly ameliorated in α-MSH- but not in Org.2766-treated animals. Since acute treatment with Org.2766 or α-MSH does not influence reversal performance in the animals with lesions, it was concluded that the beneficial effect of the neuropeptide treatment could be explained in terms of facilitation of recovery of cognitive functions in rats with bilateral lesions in the nucleus parafascicularis. Recently, Wolterink and Van Ree[103] reported that daily intraaccumbal, subcutaneous, or oral administration of Org.2766 accelerated the functional recovery of impaired motor activity following bilateral destruction of the n. accumbens of the rat by local application of 6-hydroxydopamine. The reduced motor activity of such rats was notable at postlesion day 7 but not at day 21, suggesting a functional recovery of the behavioral impairment. The authors suggest that central dopamine systems are involved in the spontaneous and peptide-facilitated recovery of impaired motor activity induced by these accumbal lesions.

Other experiments indicated that ACTH administration reduced the effect of amygdala damage in the performance of a two-way active avoidance task,[17] and a reduction by Org.2766 of attentional and "working memory" deficits produced by hippocampal lesions was also observed.[45]

Whether the facilitation of function by melanocortins after central nervous system damage depends on an enhancement of cellular responses involved in the repair mechanisms, as found in the peripheral system, remains to be determined. Nevertheless, these data may serve as a first indication that melanocortins have a beneficial role as trophic factors in the central nervous system after damage.

Like the importance of developmental mechanisms to the understanding of postlesion plasticity in the central nervous system, changes in the CNS related to age are also of significance. Gage et al.[40] approached this issue by stating that "aging can result in naturally occurring brain damage, with anatomical, biochemical and functional changes which appear to be substantial yet selective." Furthermore, several authors stress the importance of trophic factors in brain aging and disease (see, for instance, ref. 2). Thus, it seems appropriate to discuss briefly the interesting findings of Landfield et al.,[60] who showed that chronic treatment with Org.2766 resulted in diminished signs of hippocampal aging.

In a series of experiments, Landfield and his associates[60] have tested the hypothesis that changes in neural–endocrine interactions may be of specific relevance to changes in brain regions that contain cytoplasmic and nuclear receptors for the glucocorticoids. From this work it has become clear that certain changes, such as an enhancement of astrocyte size and number as well as their dispersion in the hippocampus, are related to circulating corticosterone levels. In adult rats maintained on high doses of corticosteroids for 6 to 7 months, there was evidence of enhanced glial reactivity in comparison to age-matched controls without such treatment. The changes are thought to be the consequence of increased intracellular calcium levels induced by the glucocorticoids.[61] Conversely, in adrenalectomized rats maintained on a low dose of corticosteroids, there was less glial pathology than observed in the intact animals. It was argued that enhanced levels of ACTH induced by the low level of corticosteroids were counteracting the usual changes found in the hippocampus with age. Following 9 months of treatment with Org.2766, an $ACTH_{4-9}$ analogue without peripheral adrenocorticotrophic effects, fewer of the usual effects of aging were found in the brains of animals that were 27 months old at the time of examination. The peptide-treated animals had an increased density of neural cells and fewer reactive astrocytes. In addition, the neuropeptide-treated animals displayed latency times in a reversal learning task that were similar to those of younger controls and less like the age-matched cohorts.[59] The mechanism by which these effects of the ACTH-related neuropeptides are brought about is largely unknown. It is possible that a changed fluidity of synaptosomal membranes may be responsible, at least in part, for the altered neural activities occurring within the hippocampus following neuropeptide administration.[47,49] ACTH and related peptides may increase lipid fluidity of brain membranes, in particular the synaptic plasma membranes derived from the hippocampus of older rats.[48,96] Clearly, additional *in vivo* data on neuronal membrane properties and on the mechanisms through which ACTH treatment may counteract losses in neuroplasticity of aging are needed and represent an important area for future research.

4. REGENERATION IN THE PERIPHERAL NERVOUS SYSTEM

The neuron is a very specialized and differentiated cell and has proven to be the most vulnerable cell in the mammalian central and peripheral nervous system. In general, it is assumed that damage to cell bodies of neurons results in irreversible degeneration and cell death. On the other hand, if the damage is restricted to the neuronal processes (dendrites and axons), regeneration with resulting reinnervation of the target is, in principle, possible. For reasons still not completely understood, it appears that neurons in the peripheral nervous system show better axonal regeneration than neurons in the central nervous system. The milieu surrounding the damaged axon is important in this respect, for if a motor axon is damaged within the vertebral column, hardly any outgrowth of newly formed sprouts is seen, as is typical of central nervous system neurons. If the same sort of lesion is placed distally outside the vertebral column, axonal regeneration and eventual target muscle reinnervation are evident. Ramon y Cajal demonstrated that postlesion brain neuron axonal regeneration could be facilitated by the implantation of pieces of sciatic nerve.[69]

It is well known that the outgrowth and elongation of regenerating axons are guided by a variety of humoral and structural factors that are from neuronal, glial, and target cell origin (reviewed in ref. 98). Recently, a small family of proteins was discovered whose synthesis increased dramatically (100-fold) following axotomy.[5,78,102] These proteins, termed growth-associated proteins (GAPs; designated GAP50, GAP43, and GAP24 to indicate their respective molecular weights in thousands), have been considered to play a crucial role in the capacity of axons to grow, since their genes are expressed in injured nerves that do regenerate (e.g., toad optic nerve, rabbit hypoglossal nerve) and not in nerves that do not successfully reform their axons (e.g., rabbit optic nerves).

The nature of the contribution of GAPs to the process of axonal regeneration is unknown.[77] A possible clue to the role of one of the GAPs, GAP43, arose from collaborative studies between the research groups of Skene and Willard, Routtenberg, Pfenninger, Benowitz, and Gispen. The conclusion from these cross-laboratory investigations is that GAP43 is identical to B-50 (Gispen lab), protein F1 (Routtenberg lab), and pp46 (Pfenninger lab). Of these proteins B-50 is the best characterized molecule in terms of chemical properties, subcellular localization, and function.[21,104] This acidic neuron-specific phosphoprotein (48 kDa, IEP 4.5) is localized in the presynaptic plasma membrane. In growth cone particles isolated from fetal rat brain, B-50 is a major phosphoprotein.[20] The kinase responsible for the phosphorylation of B-50 is identical to the Ca^{2+}-dependent protein kinase C.

In the adult rat brain, B-50 is supposed to modulate the activity of phosphatidylinositol (PIP) kinase: an increase in the degree of phosphorylation of B-50 inhibits PIP kinase, whereas a decrease in the degree of phosphorylation of B-50 leads to a stimulation of PIP kinase.[52] This implies that the phosphorylation state of B-50 determines the amount of phosphatidylinositol-4,5-biphosphate (PIP$_2$) available for receptor-mediated hydrolysis into diacylglycerol (DG) and inositol triphosphate (IP$_3$).[41] The IP$_3$ is thought to act as a signal for the mobilization of calcium from endoplasmic reticulum stores, whereas DG is known to stimulate protein kinase C.[53] The activation of protein kinase C by DG and Ca^{2+} results in an enhanced B-50 phosphorylation, and this in turn diminishes the amount of PIP$_2$. In this way B-50, alias GAP43, may be involved in a feedback mechanism operative in transmembrane signal transduction.[41] These results invite the speculation that the phosphorylation state of B-50/GAP43 may determine the degree of sensitivity of the regenerating axon to extrinsic neurotrophic or neurite-promoting factors. The observation that tumor-promoting compounds such as phorbol-12,13-dibutyrate (PDB) (1) exhibit profound neurotrophic effects on primary cultured embryonic neurons[63] and (2) stimulate the phosphorylation of B-50 through activation of protein kinase C constitutes provoking, although circumstantial, evidence for such a role of B-50/GAP43 in axonal growth.

5. MELANOCORTINS AND PNS PLASTICITY

5.1. RECOVERY OF FUNCTION FOLLOWING A CRUSH LESION

Nontransecting nerve damage, such as a crush lesion, results in Wallerian degeneration during which the endoneural tubes remain intact, permitting a rapid and appropriate reinnervation process. The speed by which the regenerating sprouts grow into the distal portion of the damaged nerve is approximately that of the slow axonal transport (3–4 mm per day). However, this speed of outgrowth depends largely on the severity of the lesion and the animal species used for the studies on regeneration of the peripheral nervous system. In humans, the regenerative capacity seems less than that in rodents, dogs, and cats.

5.1.1. RETURN OF SENSORY FUNCTION

Return of sensory function following a crush lesion of the sciatic or tibial nerve can be accurately followed by applying a small electric current locally to the foot sole. A normal rat invariably retracts its paw instantaneously when the

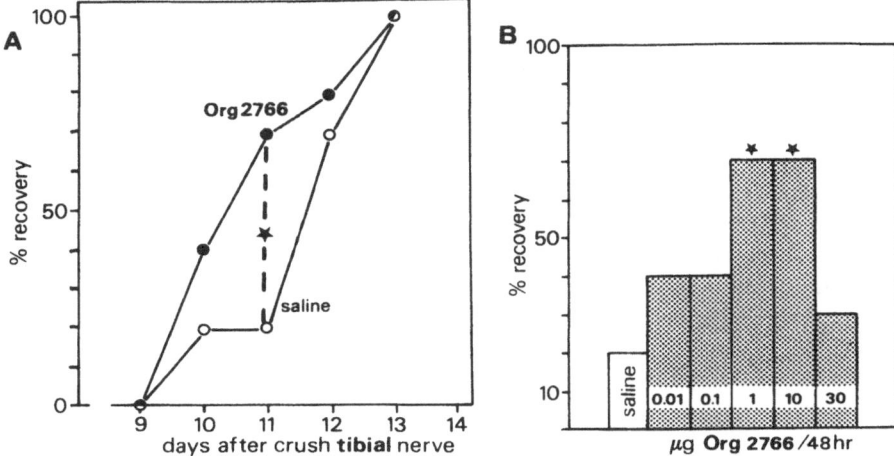

FIGURE 2. A: Sensory recovery. Return of sensory function in the foot sole following a crush lesion of the tibial nerve as measured with the local electric foot sole stimulation test (see ref. 22). Indicated is the recovery of animals that received 1 μg Org.2766/48 hr s.c. (solid points) or saline (open points). *Chi square $P < 0.05$. B: Dose–response curve. Indicated are the percentages of animals that show full sensory recovery on day 11 following a crush lesion of the tibial nerve as measured with the abovementioned test. Each group of ten rats received a different dosage of Org.2766, which is indicated in the bars. Injections every 48 hr s.c. *Chi square $P < 0.05$. (From DeKoning et al.[22])

skin of the foot sole closes the electric circuit between the stimulation poles.[22] In this way the ingrowth of the regenerating sciatic nerve in the foot sole can be monitored. By use of a standardized crush procedure and this local electric foot sole stimulation test, it was shown that subcutaneous administration of Org.2766 every 48 hr beginning immediately following the surgery resulted in an enhanced recovery of sensory function in the rat foot sole (Fig. 2A). This facilitation of the recovery process is highly dose dependent (Fig. 2B). The dose–response relationship has a so-called inverted-U shape or bell shape with low (0.01 and 0.1 μg) and high (30 μg) doses being inactive; the intermediate doses (1 and 10 μg) effectively enhance recovery. As discussed elsewhere,[28] such peculiar relationships have been reported for a variety of neural effects of melanocortins. At present, such observations remain largely unexplained but underscore the necessity to test a wide range of dosages in the assessment of the neurotrophic efficacy of peptides.

This recent study by our group confirms and extends earlier observations on the enhancement of sensorimotor function following crush lesion of the sciatic nerve by melanocortins as assessed by a less sensitive hot air reflex withdrawal test.[8,10] The first systematic study of the effect of ACTH on peripheral nerve regeneration, excluding an action mediated through the adrenal cortex, is that by

Strand and Kung.[83] These authors showed that treatment of adrenalectomized rats with $ACTH_{1-39}$ enhanced return of sensorimotor function following sciatic nerve crush. Detailed structure–activity studies revealed that the active site in the "open" ACTH/MSH molecule resembles that involved in the melanotropic rather than the corticotropic action of these peptides, for in addition to $ACTH_{1-24}$ and $ACTH_{1-16}$, the peptides α-MSH, $ACTH_{1-10}$, $ACTH_{4-10}$, and $ACTH_{6-10}$ enhanced sensory recovery, whereas $ACTH_{4-7}$ was inactive (Fig. 1).[8,11] However, the effectiveness of the analogue Org.2766 is puzzling in this respect, for this $ACTH_{4-9}$ analogue is protected against breakdown mainly because of changes in the amino acids at positions 8 and 9, which in the parent melanocortin molecule are active in the melanotropic properties.[44] Despite this fact, Org.2766 is as effective as $ACTH_{4-10}$ and α-MSH (Ac-Ser^1-$ACTH_{1-13}$-NH_2) in facilitating return of sensorimotor function after peripheral nerve damage.

5.1.2. RETURN OF MOTOR FUNCTION

Recovery from peripheral nerve damage can be described in terms of speed and quality. The sensory test described above primarily assesses the speed by which proper sensory function reappears following a crush lesion of the sciatic

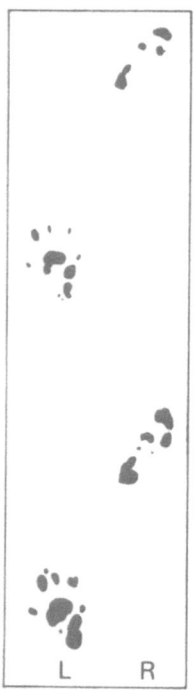

FIGURE 3. Walking pattern of a rat in which the right sciatic nerve had been crushed 11 days previously. The footprints on the crushed side differ markedly from those on the noncrushed side (L).

nerve. Recently, De Medinacelli et al.[25] described an elegant and simple test that allows the analysis of the walking pattern of a rat. Since the walking pattern is the result of the coordinated use of different muscle groups, the test gives information about the qualitative aspects of nerve function. Several parameters can be measured from these walking patterns, such as footprint length, toe spreading, step distance, etc. (Fig. 3). By means of a formula into which the numerical values of these parameters are incorporated, the motor function of the crushed sciatic nerve is calculated relative to the function of the sciatic nerve on the noncrushed side. This sciatic functional index (SFI) is set at −100% immediately following unilateral crushing of the sciatic nerve. As a result of reinnervation of different muscle groups, e.g., calf muscles or small muscles of the foot, normalization of the different parameters occurs, resulting in an increase in the SFI, which, following a crush lesion, eventually becomes 0%, indicating complete normalization of the walking pattern. Recently, De Koning et al.[23] showed that treatment with either α-MSH or Org.2766 in dosages also used in the sensory function test resulted in an enhanced normalization of the walking pattern. Thus, in addition to an effect on sensory modalities, the peptide treatment enhanced return of normal motor function following peripheral nerve damage in the rat.

5.2. ROUTE OF ADMINISTRATION

In most studies of the effects of melanocortins on peripheral nerve regeneration, subcutaneous injections of peptides dissolved in saline or complexes with zinc phosphate have been used.[8] The trophic influence of Org.2766 was also seen after subcutaneous administration of biodegradable microspheres containing absorbed Org.2766, which resulted in prolonged release of the peptide (C. E. E. M. Van der Zee, unpublished data). Oral administration of Org.2766 in the drinking water proved to be ineffective in facilitating sensory recovery after a peripheral nerve crush (C. E. E. M. Van der Zee, unpublished data). However, it has been reported that oral administration of Org.2766 via bolus injection into the stomach enhanced the normalization of impaired motor activity that resulted from bilateral destruction of the n. accumbens in the rat.[103] In view of the hypothesis that is discussed in Section 7, the results of studies employing local application of melanocortins are of profound interest. Local application of α-MSH in Accurel® polypropylene tubes or of Org.2766 in a biodegradable matrix around a crushed or transected nerve resulted in an enhanced functional recovery[35] (C. E. E. M. Van der Zee, unpublished data).

5.3. ELECTROPHYSIOLOGY

The early studies by Torda and Wolff[94] showed an increased ability of the brain to synthesize acetylcholine in both control and hypophysectomized rats following ACTH administration. Furthermore, administration of ACTH and ACTH$_{4-10}$ to hypophysectomized rats induced an ability to maintain the amplitude of muscle action potential and contraction strength unaltered during indirect muscle stimulation and to reduce fatigue upon repetitive stimulation.[43,86] An increase in muscle action potential amplitude is also observed following adrenalectomy, and even more in stressed adrenalectomized rats.[35,62,86] These observations clearly indicated an extraadrenal influence of ACTH.

In an isolated nerve–muscle preparation, Birnberger et al.[13] noted a decrease of the amplitude of end-plate potentials (EPPs) following the addition of ACTH to the perfusion medium; ACTH$_{4-10}$ was without effect on the EPP. Since the resting membrane potential was not affected, the observed effect of ACTH could occur through presynaptic suppression of acetylcholine release or interference of the peptide with postsynaptic processes at the receptor site.

A further insight into the localization of the action of ACTH and fragments was gained by studying the contraction time, half-relaxation time, twitch duration, and miniature end-plate potentials (MEPPs) in an in situ nerve–muscle preparation; MEPPs are fluctuations in EPP of unstimulated muscle fibers produced by spontaneous liberation of quanta of acetylcholine from presynaptic terminals.[53] ACTH and ACTH$_{4-10}$ augmented the frequency of MEPPs while leaving the magnitude of MEPPs, contraction time, half-relaxation time, and twitch duration unaffected, pointing to a presynaptic action of the peptides.[43] The effectiveness of ACTH$_{4-10}$ in increasing muscle contraction strength and decreasing fatigue is lost on direct muscle stimulation or when the muscle is stimulated through the distal stump of the motor nerve cut just prior to the beginning of the experiment.[43]

The influence on the central excitatory state of α motor neurons or higher excitatory brain centers in the brainstem may also be of relevance to the observed effects. Krivoy and Zimmerman[54,55] reported a neuromodulatory effect of β-MSH on α motor neurons: β-MSH selectively facilitates the postdetonation recovery of α motor neurons, thus shortening the time interval required before the next spike potential can be evoked. The synaptic delay time, rise time of the excitatory postsynaptic potentials (EPSPs), and resting membrane potentials of the α motor neurons are not affected, nor does β-MSH provoke spontaneous discharge of α motor neurons; β-MSH, however, does increase the probability that α motor neurons react to an orthodromic stimulation.[56] This action of β-MSH is rather selective on motor neurons, as Renshaw cells are not influenced. This excludes the possibility that suppression of recurrent inhibition is responsible for the observed facilitatory effect of β-MSH. Neither was there a spread of activity to other spinal segments, nor did convulsions occur on local administration of β-MSH.

Neuropeptides are effective in raising a depressed excitatory state of neuron function (following hypophysectomy or adrenalectomy) to normal. This is also illustrated by their beneficial influence on regenerating nerves and the observations that the neuromuscular system of immature rats is even more sensitive than that of hypophysectomized adult rats to the ameliorative action of ACTH/ MSH$_{4-10}$. In acute experiments following ACTH$_{4-10}$ administration to 9- to 15-day-old rats, the muscle contraction amplitude was increased and the onset of fatigue delayed during continuous supermaximal indirect stimulation. Moreover, the half-relaxation time is markedly shortened in these young animals, indicating a myotropic as well as a neurotropic action, which is not observed in adult rats.[79]

Chronic daily administration of either ACTH$_{4-10}$ or Org.2766 (an ACTH$_{4-9}$ analogue) starting at the day of birth also markedly increases muscle twitch and tetanic tension in infant rats. They also show an increased grasping ability and prolonged spontaneous motor activity when exposed to stress.[1,71] During the first 2 weeks of maturation, numerous changes occur in skeletal muscles and the nerve fibers that innervate them. The adult condition of single-fiber innervation is attained because of a progressive atrophy of superfluous nerve branches to individual muscle fibers.[15] Acetylcholine receptors become concentrated at the junctional region instead of being present along the entire length of the fetal muscle fiber.[29] The complex sarcoplasmic reticulum and T-tubule system develops and, together with the maturation of the Ca^{2+} uptake mechanism, is responsible for observed changes in the contraction–relaxation cycle.[73] Because of a concentration of cholinesterase at the neuromuscular junction, the rise time and decay period of MEPPs are decreased, and the MEPPs are increased in frequency.[29] End-plate potentials become single units, and the mean resting potential is increased, probably as a result of a shift in transmembrane concentrations of Na^+ and K^+ ions.

If ACTH/MSH$_{4-10}$ should promote Ca^{2+} uptake into nerve terminals, the release of acetylcholine would be stimulated. Immature muscle fibers with an excess of nonjunctional membrane receptors and still low levels of acetylcholinesterase, when exposed to an increased available amount of acetylcholine, could show enhanced muscle contraction amplitudes and delayed fatigue. Modulation of Ca^{2+} uptake by ACTH/MSH$_{4-10}$ in muscle might be responsible for the observed shortening of half-relaxation time in these young animals.[79] ACTH is reported to be present in spinal cord neurons in culture only at immature stages and restricted in its distribution to peripheral nerve axons.[46] It is not established whether ACTH, like β-LPH, selectively inhibits motor end-plate acetylcholinesterase, thereby augmenting acetylcholine activity. Treatment with ACTH$_{4-10}$ or Org.2766 accelerates the maturation of the end plate in infant rats. This is visualized by the scanning electron microscope as an increased complexity of postjunctional folds and an enhanced rate of invagination into the muscle fiber at earlier stages of development.[39] The undeveloped neuromuscular system of the immature rat and the depressed neuromuscular system of hypophysectomized rats, both susceptible to the ameliorative action of ACTH, share the slow-type muscle response.

Following denervation of muscle, the early stages of reinnervation are characterized by polyneural innervation. This superfluous innervation is eliminated during subsequent regeneration, and the mature ratio with one nerve fiber to one muscle fiber is reestablished.[93] However, the regenerated motor unit is usually larger, and the territory it occupies is more compact.[58] Administration of $ACTH_{4-10}$ starting on the day of crush denervation of the extensor digitorum longus muscle results in the formation of more and smaller motor units.[70] Low-frequency stimulation of these regenerated motor units results in a higher activity index (mean contraction amplitude after 1 min of stimulation) in the $ACTH_{4-10}$-treated animals as well as in a higher amplitude of tetanic tension at high-frequency stimulation and an improved ability to maintain this tetanic tension at above optimum frequency stimulation.[70,71] Smaller, accurately controlled motor units are better capable of performing a fine motor act. The maintenance of a high level of activity for prolonged periods of time is also dependent on the small motor unit population.[18]

The muscle twitch tension of the extensor digitorum longus muscle did not differ between the $ACTH_{4-10}$- and saline-treated rats. This reflects that, "in total," as many muscle fibers are reinnervated in both groups. These muscle fibers are capable of responding once in a single maximal effort, but in maintaining maximal tension an orderly coordinated recruitment and firing rate of motor units is needed. These conditions are better achieved under ACTH treatment. Human studies also indicate a disturbed pattern of motor unit recruitment following regeneration.[64] In line with the formation of more and smaller motor units as a result of $ACTH_{4-10}$ treatment following crush denervation is the observation that $ACTH_{4-10}$ treatment following crush lesion of the sciatic nerve results in the outgrowth of more and, on the average, smaller nerve fibers.[9] The peptide treatment also prevented the postrecovery decrease in sciatic nerve fibers.

A long-lasting beneficial effect of short-term ACTH/MSH treatment following a crush lesion of the sciatic nerve is convincingly demonstrated by the longitudinal follow-up of nerve conduction in the regenerated nerve. Rats that had been treated with Org.2766 during the first 8 days following a crush lesion of the sciatic nerve show complete recovery of motor and sensory nerve conduction velocity 90 and 110 days following the surgery, respectively. A 20 to 35% reduction in conduction velocity remains in the saline-treated rats even 200 days following the crush.[23]

Thus, at the neurophysiological level a beneficial effect of ACTH/MSH on nerve regeneration is evident.

5.4. HISTOLOGY

In the study by Strand and Kung,[83] it is suggested that more rapid outgrowth of the regenerating axons in ACTH-treated, adrenalectomized rats is in part responsible for the enhanced return of function. Furthermore, it was observed that the peptide treatment increased the number of large end plates, which was accompanied by an increase in the frequency of preterminal branching in end plates. This latter finding was also reported by Shapiro *et al.*[75] Also, studies from our own group suggest that enhanced return of function is caused by an action of the peptide on axonal outgrowth. However, our data seem to indicate that melanocortins facilitate the induction of sprouting (time of start and/or number) rather than the rate of outgrowth. This has been assessed in a number of studies using quantitative light microscopic, electron microscopic, and immunohistochemical techniques.

Treatment with $ACTH_{4-10}$ and α-MSH results in an increase in the number of regenerating myelinated fibers as visualized in the light microscope with paraphenylenediamine. The effect of these peptides was most marked during the earliest stages of regeneration, when the first myelinated fibers were detectable (8 days following the crush), and declined thereafter.[10,99] In an electron microscopic study using a small number of animals ($n = 3$), axon counts suggested that, in addition to an increased number of myelinated axons, the number of unmyelinated fibers was also enhanced. The peptide treatment did not affect the degree of myelination; the number of myelin lamellae was not enhanced in peptide-treated animals.[9]

In order to examine the effects of melanocortins during the very early stages of nerve regeneration in more detail, we employed immunochemical labeling of axons with affinity-purified neurofilament-binding antibodies. The neuron-specific localization of the neurofilament proteins and the rapid degradation of the neurofilament proteins distal to the crush enable the visualization of newly formed sprouts using the fluorescence microscope at early times following the lesion.[101] With this technique it has now been demonstrated[101] that Org.2766 increases the number of outgrowing fibers as early as 48 hr following a crush lesion. The percentage difference between the axon counts in control and peptide-treated rats remained fairly constant in time when measured at greater distances from the site of the lesion. This implies that melanocortins have no effect on the growth rate of the newly formed sprouts. In addition to these early effects of melanocortins on sprout formation, the peptide treatment also prevented the postrecovery decrease in sciatic nerve fibers.[10] This is the degeneration of nerve fibers that failed to make contact with appropriate target cells or lost their connection during elimination of polyinnervation of muscle cells. This late effect of melanocortins may indicate an effect on synaptogenesis.

6. NEUROTROPHIC EFFECT AND PATHOPHYSIOLOGICAL MECHANISM

As discussed in Section 1, one may argue that the facilitation of recovery following nerve damage is the result of the trophic influence that circulating melanocortins exert on neural tissue in general. In fetal life, α-MSH but not

ACTH seems to facilitate fetal and brain growth in general.[91] Thus, on the one hand, the question arises whether or not the peptide treatment mimics or amplifies the effect of natural circulating melanocortins. On the other hand, it becomes clear that neurotrophic factors both are formed and operate in the vicinity of the lesion (for a review see ref. 97). In fact, Politis and Spencer[68] developed an *in vivo* bioassay for neurotrophic activity based on their finding that the repair of damaged peripheral nerve is facilitated by the implantation of a piece of degenerating nerve tissue in the vicinity of the lesion. They suggested that a trophic humoral factor is released from the degenerating tissue and that this factor enhances the repair process. Such studies led us to investigate whether there was a connection between the ability of α-MSH and that of degenerating nerve tissue to stimulate sprouting. This seemed all the more compelling in view of the report by Dräger *et al.*[30] that neurofilament protein (150 kDa) contains an immunologically recognized α-MSH-like portion. This protein has been shown to break down in the early stages of the degenerative process.[7,80] We therefore investigated the possible presence of an α-MSH-like principle in the degenerating nerve during the period of 150-kDa neurofilament breakdown.

First, we were able to confirm the observation by Dräger *et al.* that the NF150 protein is specifically recognized by antisera against α-MSH.[30,33,34,100] Although Shaw *et al.*[76] demonstrated that the antibody used by Dräger *et al.*[30] recognized an epitope that was identical to Ac-Ser-Tyr-Ser (α-MSH$_{1-3}$), Verhaagen *et al.*[100] showed that anti-α-MSH antibodies recognizing the ACTH$_{4-10}$ amino acid sequence also react with NF150. Our subsequent efforts to demonstrate such a principle by means of a radioimmunoassay for α-MSH were unsuccessful (J. Verhaagen, unpublished data). A number of explanations can be given making it plausible that the amount of α-MSH-like material being formed in the degenerating nerve would escape detection by a radioimmunoassay. In contrast to this unsuccessful immunochemical approach are the results of the bioassay for α-MSH-like activity in degenerating nerve. Edwards *et al.*[34] showed that only extracts of degenerating and not of nondegenerating intact rat sciatic nerves facilitated melanosome dispersion in melanophores of tail fin pieces obtained from *Xenopus laevis* tadpoles. Thus, degenerating nerves contain a factor that has biological activity much the same as α-MSH.

Furthermore, if exogenous α-MSH were to mimic the effect of an endogenous factor released from the degenerating nerve during a period shortly following the nerve damage, then the pharmacological treatment should only be effective during a period immediately following the crush lesion. Indeed, the evidence obtained points to a critical period within the first week or so after crush in which the repair process can be enhanced by treatment with α-MSH.[34]

Hence, the hypothesis was proposed that the neurotrophic peptide given as a pharmacologically active factor was to mimic or amplify a natural aspect of the physiological repair mechanism following peripheral nerve damage. It is suggested that the selective proteolytic cleavage of the 150-kDa neurofilament pro-

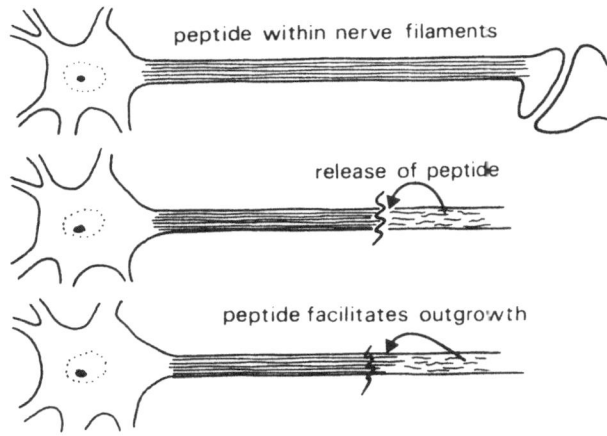

peptide within nerve filaments

release of peptide

peptide facilitates outgrowth

FIGURE 4. Influence of a locally produced neurite outgrowth-promoting factor. Artist impression of the hypothesis proposed by Edwards *et al.*[35] that breakdown of neurofilament results in the local formation of an MSH-like factor that promotes axonal regeneration.

tein, which is a well-known event in peripheral axon degeneration, plays an important role in the local delivery of a neurotrophic α-MSH-like peptide (Fig. 4).[34,74]

7. LOCAL APPLICATION OF α-MSH AND THE REPAIR OF TRANSECTED RAT SCIATIC NERVE

If our hypothesis on the mode of action of melanocortins in peripheral nerve regeneration is correct, then local application of α-MSH should be about as effective as the subcutaneous route of administration used in our studies so far. Recently, we completed a study in which we used microporous Accurel® polypropylene tubes to enclose the repair sites of transected and sutured rat sciatic nerves (Fig. 5).[14,35] Microporous Accurel® polypropylene tubes can adsorb high quantities of peptide hormones, and this feature was used to deliver α-MSH at the repair site.[57] The total load of α-MSH was 2–3 μg/5-mm tube. *In vitro* studies had indicated that the release rate from the luminal surface was maximally 1 μg/4 hr measured in the first release volume and thereafter declined rapidly.[57] The Accurel® polypropylene tube was surrounded by an impermeable polythene sleeve to minimize leakage of α-MSH from the repair site. Diffusion could now occur only at the end of the tube. Any observed enhancement of recovery of nerves so treated should result from a local action of the peptide at the repair site.

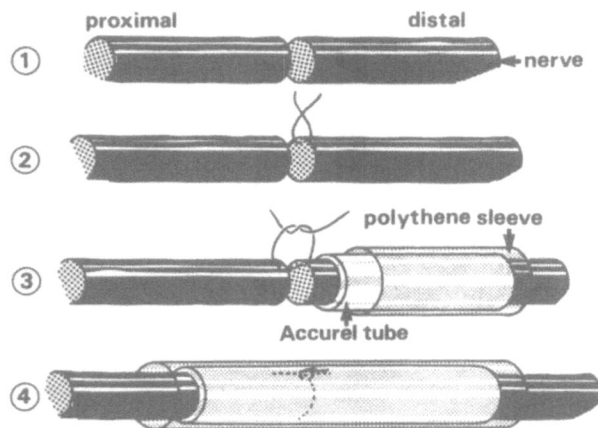

FIGURE 5. Local delivery of α-MSH. Diagram to show procedure for placing Accurel® poly-propylene tubes around transected rat sciatic nerve. (From Edwards *et al.*[35])

Indeed, compared to transected nerves that had only been sutured, a marked reduction of the recovery period is observed when α-MSH is applied locally to the repair site by means of the Accurel® polypropylene tube (Fig. 6). The tubes alone also had a significant but smaller effect on the regeneration of the trans-ected nerve, possibly as a result of the maintenance of a beneficial milieu around

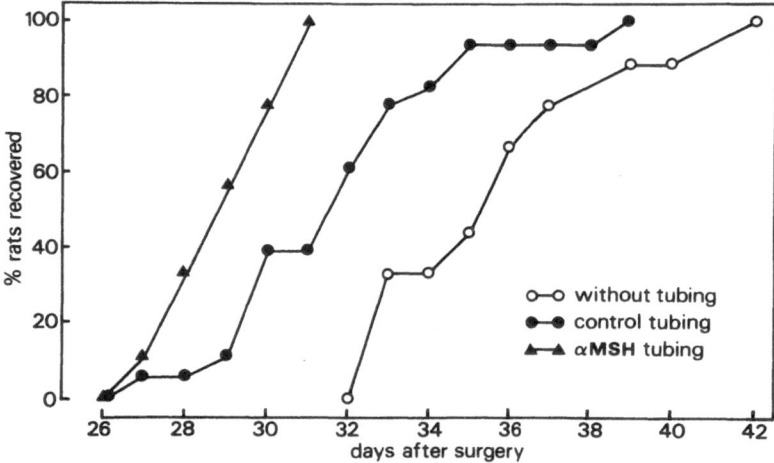

FIGURE 6. Recovery of sensory function of the foot sole following transection and subsequent stitching together of the proximal and distal stump of the rat sciatic nerve, as measured with the local electric foot sole stimulation test (see ref. 22). The repair site was either left without tube, surrounded by an Accurel® polypropylene tube preloaded with α-MSH, or surrounded by a control Accurel® polypropylene tube. (From Edwards *et al.*[35])

the repair site. The results are in keeping with the notion that exogenous α-MSH mimics a natural, locally produced signal in the pathophysiology of nerve repair mechanisms. Furthermore, the data suggest a potential means of improving the outcome of surgical nerve repair in the clinic.[35] Recently, C. E. E. M. Van der Zee (unpublished data) demonstrated that local application of 10 μg Org.2766 in a biodegradable matrix around a crush lesion facilitated nerve regeneration. Placement of the matrix with Org.2766 around the contralateral undamaged nerve had no effect on the recovery of the damaged nerve. One single injection of 10 μg Org.2766 subcutaneously in the neck immediately following the surgery was also ineffective in facilitating recovery. These latter observations underscore the importance of local production and action of neurotrophic peptides following peripheral nerve damage.

8. CLINICAL PERSPECTIVES

Natural $ACTH_{1-39}$ and synthetic $ACTH_{1-24}$ have been widely used in a variety of neurological diseases such as multiple sclerosis, myasthenia gravis, lesions and compressions of peripheral nerves, and neuropathies. These diseases are characterized by inflammation, sometimes of autoimmune origin, and de-myelination. The reported outcomes of these studies are contradictory, and the slight ameliorative action of ACTH that was sometimes found might very well be attributed to the corticotropic action of ACTH. Indeed, long-term glucocorticoid therapy has taken the place of ACTH in the management of multiple sclerosis and myasthenia gravis.[62] The one disadvantage that glucocorticoid therapy has over $ACTH_{1-39}$ administration is the steroid-induced myopathy, which, however, can rapidly be reversed by ACTH administration and which can partly be prevented by administering glucocorticoids on alternating days.

The introduction of the noncorticotrophic ACTH fragments such as $ACTH_{4-10}$, $ACTH_{4-9}$, MSH, and their analogues (e.g., Org.2766, a tri-substituted degradation-resistant $ACTH_{4-9}$ analogue) permits investigation of the possible beneficial effects of these neurotrophic peptides in different neurological diseases. The advantage of these ACTH fragments is that their use in humans and animals, for reasons other than those discussed in this chapter, has shown no toxic side effect whatsoever.[28] On the basis of the results discussed here, two main groups of neurological disorders theoretically warrant further investigation. The first group includes diseases characterized by a pathologically depressed state of motor neuron function, such as amyotrophic lateral sclerosis, spinal muscular atrophy, and some polyneuropathies. The second group comprises diseases in which peripheral sprouting is the main characteristic, e.g., peripheral nerve lesions. The latter possible indication for neuropeptide therapy is discussed first.

Based on the hypothesis that the beneficial effects of neuropeptide treatment following peripheral nerve damage occur because these neuropeptides mimic the actions of a locally produced MSH-like factor formed during nerve degeneration, local application of neuropeptides (MSH and Org.2766) has proved to be very effective in enhancing functional recovery. The observation that this ameliorative effect can be produced by local application of Org.2766 in a biodegradable matrix opens new perspectives. This matrix in itself will not hamper regeneration, can be easily applied, need not be removed after successful regeneration, and is not toxic to animals or humans. However, an enhancement of this functional recovery is not the only or most important reason for neuropeptide administration. Histological, but especially electrophysiological, studies have shown the beneficial effect of short-term neuropeptide treatment following peripheral nerve damage to be long lasting.

The function and organization of the regenerated neuromuscular system in neuropeptide-treated animals resemble the normal state much more than that of nontreated animals.[23,70] This might indicate a better regenerative capacity following repeated nerve damage and a better capacity to compensate for neuronal degeneration as a result of aging.[16] We have recently obtained evidence for this suggestion. Without renewed therapy, following a second crush lesion in the same sciatic nerve, animals that had been treated with Org.2766 following the first crush lesion again showed an enhanced recovery compared to animals that had been treated with saline following the first crush (time interval between two lesions 54 days). The recovery of the previously Org.2766-treated animals was similar to that of age-matched controls in which the sciatic nerve was crushed for the first time. The results did not show a conditioning effect of the first crush and underscore the suggestion of more complete regeneration under Org.2766 therapy.

The other possible indication for neuropeptide treatment is a neurological disease in which a depressed state of motor neuron function can be assumed. One of the complaints of patients with these neuromuscular diseases is that they tire easily. In view of animal studies in which $ACTH_{1-39}$, $ACTH_{1-24}$, and $ACTH_{4-10}$ significantly decreased neuromuscular fatigue, Strand et al. have administered $ACTH_{4-10}$ to patients with various neuromuscular diseases.[87,88] The possible beneficial effect was assessed by measuring the fall in muscle action potential (MAP) of the opponens pollices muscle on repeated supramaximal stimulation of the median nerve. In one patient with a progressive spinal muscular atrophy of the Kugelberg–Welander type (age 24 years), control measurements showed a decrease of the evoked MAPs to 55% on the fifth MAP; subsequent infusion of 3 mg $ACTH_{4-10}$ resulted in no decrement as assessed at several times following the infusion. This beneficial effect lasted for over 10 days after a single 6-mg infusion. Responses in patients with other disorders were less favorable (myasthenia gravis) or absent (muscular dystrophy). This can be explained on the basis of animal studies that show the action of neuropeptides to be at the level of the central or peripheral motorneuron and not on the postsynaptic component of the neuromuscular junction or on the muscle itself (at least in adult animals).[43] The results also underscore the necessity to test a wide range of doses. It is very hard to interpret the results of one acute infusion other than in terms of changes in neuronal excitability, which is also suggested for the infusion of TRH and analogues in patients with ALS.[37]

Future investigation into the effects of chronic treatment with $ACTH_{4-10}$/ Org.2766 is warranted in patients with a depressed state of motor neuron function. The mediation of both short-term functional effects and long-term trophic influences by a single agent is observed in the effects of many peptide hormones on their peripheral target cells. $ACTH_{4-10}$ and Org.2766 are known to enhance peripheral sprouting but also increase the frequency of preterminal branching in end plates during either ontogeny or nerve regeneration.[1,75] Chronic treatment of patients with neuromuscular diseases with $ACTH_{4-10}$ or Org.2766 might enhance collateral sprouting, which is the compensatory mechanism of the nervous system to motor neuron degeneration. We are presently doing a pilot study in which the effects of Org.2766 administration to patients with ALS will be investigated. The possible acute and chronic effects will be investigated by means of single-fiber and macro-EMGs. Single-fiber EMG can register acute effects through jitter measurements and chronic effects through fiber density measurements. This latter parameter, together with the results of macro-EMG measurements, provides information on reshuffling of the motor unit as a result of degeneration and compensatory regeneration.[81]

With respect to neuropathies, it should be noted that we have recently been able to show that in an animal model for cisplatin neurotoxicity, concurrent treatment with Org.2766 greatly protected the animals from the neurotoxic side effects of the cytostatic treatment.[24] A pilot study is now in progress in which the possible protective properties of Org.2766 against the neurotoxic side effect of cisplatin therapy in patients with ovarian cancer is being investigated. In order to be able to record even small disturbances in nerve function, we have set up a number of quantitative methods to measure somatosensory function in cisplatin-treated patients.[36]

In conclusion, it seems unlikely that there will be a single effective drug in the therapy of nerve injury and neurodegenerative disorders. However, the results of animal and human neuropeptide treatment discussed here warrant future investigation of these neurotrophic substances in clinical neurological practice.

REFERENCES

1. Acker, G. R., Frischer, R., and Strand, F. L., 1985, ACTH peptide neuromodulation in the developing neuromuscular system as seen through three different perspectives, Ann. N.Y. Acad. Sci. USA 435:370–375.
2. Appel, S. H., Ojika, K., Tomozawa, Y., and Bostnick, R., 1985, Trophic factors in brain aging and disease, in: Senile Dementia of the Alzheimer Type (J. Traber and W. H. Gispen, eds.), Springer-Verlag, Berlin, pp. 581–584.
3. Azmitia, E. C., 1986, Neuropeptide stimulation of serotonergic neuronal maturation in tissue culture: Modulation by hippocampal cells, Symp. Neuropeptides Brain Function, Utrecht, Abstr. S28.

4. Azmitia, E. C., and de Kloet, E. R., 1987, Neuropeptide stimulation of serotonergic neuronal maturation in tissue culture: Modulation by hippocampal cells, *Prog. Brain Res.* **72**:311–318.
5. Benowitz, L., Shaskoua, V., and Yoon, M. G., 1981, Specific changes in rapidly transported proteins during regeneration of the gold fish optic nerve, *J. Neurosci.* **1**:300–307.
6. Berry, M., Knowles, J., Willis, P., Riches, A. C., Morgans, G. P., and Steers, D., 1979, A reappraisal of the effect of ACTH on the response of the central nervous system to injury, *J. Anat.* **128**:859–871.
7. Bignami, A., Dahl, D., Nguyen, B. T., and Croby, C. J., 1981, The fate of axonal debris in Wallerian degeneration of rat optic and sciatic nerves. Electron microscopy and immunofluorescence studies with neurofilament antisera, *J. Neuropathol. Exp. Neurol.* **40**:537–550.
8. Bijlsma, W. A., Jennekens, F. G. I., Schotman, P., and Gispen, W. H., 1981, Effects of corticotrophin (ACTH) on recovery of sensori-motor function in the rat: Structure–activity study, *Eur. J. Pharmacol.* **76**:73–79.
9. Bijlsma, W. A., van Asselt, E., Veldman, H., Jennekens, F. G. I., Schotman, P., and Gispen, W. H., 1983, Ultrastructural study of the effect of ACTH(4–10) in nerve regeneration: Axons become larger in number and smaller in diameter, *Acta Neuropathol. (Berl.)* **62**:24–30.
10. Bijlsma, W. A., Jennekens, F. G. I., Schotman, P., and Gispen, W. H., 1983, Stimulation by ACTH(4–10) of nerve fiber regeneration following sciatic nerve crush, *Muscle Nerve* **6**:104–112.
11. Bijlsma, W. A., Schotman, P., Jennekens, F. G. I., Gispen, W. H., and de Wied, D., 1983, The enhanced recovery of sensorimotor function in rats is related to the melanotropic moiety of ACTH/MSH neuropeptides, *Eur. J. Pharmacol.* **92**:231–236.
12. Bijlsma, W. A., Jennekens, F. G. I., Schotman, P., and Gispen, W. H., 1984, Neurotrophic factors and regeneration in the peripheral nervous system, *Psychoneuroendocrinology* **9**:199–215.
13. Birnberger, K. L., Rudel, R., and Struppler, A., 1977, ACTH and neuromuscular transmission: Electrophysiological *in vitro* investigation of the effects of corticotropin and an ACTH fragment on neuromuscular transmission, *Ann. Neurol.* **1**:270–275.
14. Boer, G. J., Kruisbrink, J., and van Pelt-Heerschap, H., 1983, Long-term and constant release of vasopressin from Accurel® tubing: Implantation in the Brattleboro rat, *J. Endocrinol.* **98**:147–152.
15. Brown, M. C., Jansen, J. K. S., and Van Essen, D., 1976, Polyneural innervation of skeletal muscle in newborn rats and its elimination during maturation, *J. Physiol. (Lond.)* **261**:387–422.
16. Brown, W. F., 1973, Functional compensation of human motor units in health and disease, *J. Neurol. Sci.* **20**:199–209.
17. Bush, D. F., Lovely, R. H., and Pagano, R. R., 1973, Injection of ACTH induces recovery from shuttle-box avoidance deficits in rats with amygdaloid lesions, *J. Comp. Physiol. Psychol.* **83**:168–172.
18. Close, R., 1967, Properties of motor units in fast and slow skeletal muscles of the rat, *J. Physiol. (Lond.)* **193**:45–55.
19. Daval, J. L., Louis, J. C., Gerard, M. J., and Vincendon, G., 1983, Influence of adrenocorticotropic hormone on the growth of isolated neurons in culture, *Neurosci. Lett.* **36**:299–304.
20. De Graan, P. N. E., Van Hooff, C. O. M., Tilly, B. C., Oestreicher, A. B., Schotman, P., and Gispen, W. H., 1985, Phosphoprotein B-50 in nerve growth cones from fetal rat brain, *Neurosci. Lett.* **61**:235–241.
21. De Graan, P. N. E., Oestreicher, A. B., Schrama, L. H., and Gispen, W. H., 1986, Phosphoprotein B-50, localization and function, *Prog. Brain Res.* **69**:37–50.
22. De Koning, P., Brakkee, J. H., and Gispen, W. H., 1986, Methods for producing a reproducible crush in the sciatic and tibial nerve of the rat and rapid and precise testing of return of sensory function. Beneficial effects of melanocortins, *J. Neurol. Sci.* **74**:237–246.
23. De Koning, P., and Gispen, W. H., 1987, Org.2766 improves functional and electrophysiological aspects of regeneration of sciatic nerve in the rat, *Peptides* **8**:415–422.

24. De Koning, P., Neijt, J. P., Jennekens, F. G. I., and Gispen, W. H., 1987, Org.2766 protects from cisplatin neurotoxicity in rats, *Exp. Neurol.* **97**:746–750.

25. De Medinacelli, L., Freed, W. J., and Wyatt, R. J., 1982, An index of the functional condition of rat sciatic nerve based on measurements made from walking trades, *Exp. Neurol.* **77**:634–643.

26. De Wied, D., 1969, Effects of peptide hormones on behavior, in: *Frontiers in Neuroendocrinology* (W. F. Ganong and L. Martini, eds.), Oxford University Press, New York, pp. 97–140.

27. De Wied, D., 1974, Pituitary–adrenal system and behavior, in: *The Neurosciences* (F. D. Schmitt and F. G. Worden, eds.), MIT Press, Cambridge, pp. 653–666.

28. De Wied, D., and Jolles, J., 1982, Neuropeptides derived from pro-opiocortin: Behavioral, physiological and neurochemical effects, *Physiol. Rev.* **62**:976–1059.

29. Diamond, J., and Miledi, R., 1962, A study of fetal and newborn rat muscle fibers, *J. Physiol. (Lond.)* **162**:393–408.

30. Dräger, U. C., Edwards, D. L., and Kleinschmidt, J., 1983, Neurofilaments contain α-melanocyte-stimulating hormone (αMSH)-like immunoreactivity, *Proc. Natl. Acad. Sci. USA* **80**:6408–6412.

31. Dunn, A. J., and Schotman, P., 1981, Effects of ACTH and related peptides on cerebral RNA and protein synthesis, *Pharmacol. Ther.* **12**:353–372.

32. Dunn, A. J., and Schotman, P., 1986, Effects of ACTH and related peptides on cerebral RNA and protein synthesis, in: *Neuropeptides and Behavior,* Volume 1 (D. De Wied, W. H. Gispen, and T. B. Van Wimersma Greidanus, eds.), Pergamon Press, Oxford, pp. 165–188.

33. Edwards, P. M., and Gispen, W. H., 1985, Melanocortin peptides and neural plasticity, in: *Senile Dementia of Alzheimer Type* (J. Traber and W. H. Gispen, eds.), Springer-Verlag, Berlin, pp. 231–240.

34. Edwards, P. M., van der Zee, C. E. E. M., Verhaagen, J., Schotman, P., Jennekens, F. G. I., and Gispen, W. H., 1984, Evidence that the neurotrophic actions of α-MSH may derive from its ability to mimic the actions of a peptide formed in degenerating nerve stumps, *J. Neurol. Sci.* **64**:333–340.

35. Edwards, P. M., Kuiters, R. R. F., Boer, G. J., and Gispen, W. H., 1986, Recovery from peripheral nerve transection is accelerated by local application of α-MSH by means of Accurel® polypropylene tubes, *J. Neurol. Sci.* **74**:171–176.

36. Elderson, A., Neijt, J. P., De Koning, P., and Gispen, W. H., 1986, A new and sensitive procedure to monitor cisplatin neurotoxicity, in: *5th NCI/EORTC Symposium on New Drugs in Cancer Therapy,* EORTC, Amsterdam, *Abstr.* 1.31.

37. Engel, W. K., Siddeque, T., and Nicoloff, J. T., 1983, Effect on weakness and spasticity in amyotrophic lateral sclerosis of thyrotropin releasing hormone, *Lancet* **2**:73–75.

38. Flohr, H., and Luneburg, U., 1982, Effects of $ACTH_{4-10}$ on vestibular compensation, *Brain Res.* **248**:169–173.

39. Frisher, R. E., El-Kawa, N., and Strand, F. L., 1985, ACTH peptides as organizers of neuronal patterns in development: Maturation of the rat neuromuscular junction as seen by scanning electron microscopy, *Peptides* **6**:13–19.

40. Gage, F. H., Björklund, A., Stenen, U., and Dunnett, S. B., 1983, Intracerebral grafting in the aging brain, in: *Aging of the Brain* (W. H. Gispen and J. Traber, eds.), Elsevier, Amsterdam, pp. 125–137.

41. Gispen, W. H., 1986, Phosphoprotein B-50 and phosphoinositides in brain synaptic plasma membranes: A possible feedback relationship, *Trans. Biochem. Soc. UK* **14**:163–165.

42. Gispen, W. H., and Zwiers, H., 1985, Behavioral and neurochemical effects of ACTH, in: *Handbook of Neurochemistry,* Volume 8 (A. Lajtha, ed.), Plenum Press, New York, pp. 375–412.

43. Gonzalez, E. R., and Strand, F. L., 1981, Neurotrophic action of $MSH/ACTH_{4-10}$ on neuromuscular function in hypophysectomized rats, *Peptides* **2**:107–113.

44. Greven, H. M., and de Wied, D., 1973, The influence of peptides derived from corticotrophin (ACTH) on performance: Structure–activity studies, *Prog. Brain Res.* **39**:430–442.

45. Hannigan, J. H., and Isaacson, R. L., 1984, The effects of Org.2766 on the performance of sham, neocortical and hippocampal lesioned rats in a food search task, *Pharm. Biochem. Behav.* **23**: 1019–1027.
46. Haynes, L. W., and Smith, M. E., 1984, The actions of proopiomelanocortin peptides at the developing neuromuscular junction, *Trends Pharmacol. Sci.* **5**:165–168.
47. Hershkowitz, M., 1983, Mechanisms of brain aging. The role of membrane fluidity, in: *Aging of the Brain* (W. H. Gispen and J. Traber, eds.), Elsevier, Amsterdam, pp. 85–100.
48. Hershkowitz, M., Heron, D., Samuel, D., and Shinitzky, M., 1982, The modulation of protein phosphorylation and receptor binding in synaptic membranes by changes in lipid fluidity: Implications for aging, *Prog. Brain Res.* **56**:419–434.
49. Hershkowitz, M., Zwiers, H., and Gispen, W. H., 1982, The effect of ACTH on rat brain synaptic plasma membrane lipid fluidity, *Biochim. Biophys. Acta* **692**:495–497.
50. Isaacson, R. L., and Poplawsky, A., 1983, An ACTH$_{4-9}$ analog (Org.2766) speeds recovery from septal hyperemotionality in the rat, *Behav. Neural Biol.* **39**:52–59.
51. Isaacson, R. L., and Poplawsky, A., 1985, ACTH$_{4-10}$ produces a transient decrease in septal hyperemotionality, *Behav. Neural Biol.* **43**:109–113.
52. Jolles, J., Zwiers, H., Van Dongen, C. J., Schotman, P., Wirtz, K. W. A., and Gispen, W. H., 1980, Modulation of brain polyphosphoinositide metabolism by ACTH-sensitive protein phosphorylation, *Nature* **286**:623–625.
53. Katz, B., 1966, *Nerve, Muscle and Synapse*, McGraw-Hill, New York.
54. Krivoy, W. A., and Zimmermann, E., 1976, Actions of β-melanocyte stimulating hormone (β-MSH) and the melatonin (*M*) on single units of cat spinal cord, *Fed. Proc.* **35**:646.
55. Krivoy, W. A., and Zimmerman, E., 1977, An effect of β-melanocyte-stimulating hormone (β-MSH) on motoneurons of cat spinal cord, *Eur. J. Pharmacol.* **46**:315–322.
56. Krivoy, W. A., Coven, J. A., and Stewart, J. M., 1985, Modulation of spinal synaptic transmission by beta-melanocyte stimulating hormone (beta-MSH), *Psychoneuroendocrinology* **10**:103–108.
57. Kruisbrink, J., and Boer, G. J., 1984, Controlled long-term release of small peptide hormones using a new microporous polypropylene polymer; its application for vasopressin in the Brattleboro rat and potential perinatal use, *J. Pharmacol. Sci.* **73**:1713–1718.
58. Kugelberg, E., 1981, The motor unit: Morphology and function, in: *Motor Unit Types, Recruitment and Plasticity in Health and Disease* (J. E. Desmedt, ed.), S. Karger, Basel, pp. 1–16.
59. Landfield, P. W., 1983, Mechanisms of altered neural function during aging, *Dev. Neurol.* **7**:51–71.
60. Landfield, P. W., Baskin, R. K., and Pitler, T. A., 1981, Brain aging correlates: Retardation by hormonal pharmacological treatments, *Science* **214**:581–584.
61. Landfield, P. W., Pitler, T. A., and Applegate, M. D., 1986, The aged hippocampus: A model system for studies on mechanisms of behavioral plasticity and brain aging, in: *The Hippocampus*, Vol. 3 (R. L. Isaacson and K. H. Pribram, eds.), Plenum Press, New York, pp. 323–368.
62. Liversedge, L. A., 1977, Treatment and management of multiple sclerosis, *Br. Med. Bull.* **33**:78–83.
63. Montz, H. P. M., Davis, G. E., Skaper, S. O., Manthorpe, M., and Varon, S., 1985, Tumor-promoting phorbol diesters mimics two distinct neuronotrophic factors, *Brain Res.* **355**:150–154.
64. Milner-Brown, H. S., Stein, R. B., Lee, R. G., and Brown, W. F., 1981, Motor unit recruitment in patients with neuromuscular disorders, in: *Motor Unit Types, Recruitment and Plasticity in Health and Disease* (J. E. Desmedt, ed.), S. Karger, Basel, pp. 305–318.
65. Namba, T., Shapiro, M. S., Arimori, S., and Grob, D., 1967, Effects of corticotropin in patients with generalized myasthenia gravis, *J. Clin. Invest.* **46**:1100.
66. Nishizuka, Y., 1984, Turnover of inositol phospholipids and signal transduction, *Science* **225**:1365–1370.

67. Nyakas, C., Veldhuis, H. D., and De Wied, D., 1985, Beneficial effect of chronic treatment with Org.2766 and α-MSH on impaired reversal learning of rats with bilateral lesions of the parafascicular area, *Brain. Res. Bull.* **15**:257–265.

68. Politis, M. J., and Spencer, P. S., 1983, An *in vivo* assay of neurotrophic activity, *Brain Res.* **278**:229–231.

69. Ramon y Cajal, S., 1928, *Degeneration and Regeneration of the Nervous System*, Hafner, New York.

70. Saint-Côme, C., and Strand, F. L., 1985, ACTH/MSH$_{4-10}$ improves motor unit reorganization during peripheral nerve regeneration in the rat, *Peptides* **6**:77–83.

71. Saint-Côme, C., Acker, G. R., and Strand, F. L., 1982, Peptide influences on the development and regeneration of motor performance, *Peptides* **3**:439–442.

72. Sandman, C. A., and O'Halloran, J. P., 1986, Pro-opiomelanocortin, learning, memory and attention, in: *Neuropeptides and Behavior*, Volume 1 (D. de Wied, W. H. Gispen, and T. B. van Wimersma Greidanus, eds.), Pergamon Press, Oxford, pp. 397–420.

73. Schiaffino, S., and Margreth, A., 1969, Coordinated development of the sarcoplasmic reticulum and T-system during postnatal differentiation of rat skeletal muscle, *J. Cell. Biol.* **41**:855–875.

74. Schlaepfer, W. W., Lee, C., Trojanowski, J. Q., and Lee, V. M. Y., 1984, Persistence of immunoreactive neurofilament protein breakdown products in transected rat sciatic nerve, *J. Neurochem.* **43**:857–864.

75. Shapiro, M. S., Namba, T., and Grob, D., 1968, The effect of corticotropin on the neuromuscular junction. Morphological studies in rabbits, *Neurology (Minneap.)* **18**:1018–1022.

76. Shaw, G., Fisher, S., and Weber, K., 1985, α-MSH and neurofilament M-protein share a continuous epitope but not extended sequences: An explanation for neurofibrillary staining with α-MSH antibodies, *FEBS Lett.* **181**:343–346.

77. Skene, J. H. P., 1984, Growth-associated proteins and the curious dichotomies of nerve regeneration, *Cell* **37**:697–700.

78. Skene, J. H. P., and Willard, M., 1981, Changes in axonally transported proteins during axon regeneration in toad retinal ganglion cells, *J. Cell Biol.* **89**:86–95.

79. Smith, C. M., and Strand, F. L., 1981, Neuromuscular response of the immature rat to ACTH/MSH$_{4-10}$, *Peptides* **2**:197–206.

80. Soifer, D., Igbal, K., Czosnek, H., De Martini, J., Sturman, J. A., and Wisniewski, H. M., 1981, The loss of neuron-specific proteins during the course of Wallerian degeneration of optic and sciatic nerve, *J. Neurosci.* **5**:461–470.

81. Stålberg, E., 1984, Electrophysiological studies of reinnervation in ALS, in: *Human Motor Neuron Diseases* (L. P. Rowland, ed.), Raven Press, New York, pp. 47–59.

82. Strand, F. L., 1969, Correlation of stress, blood ACTH levels and action potential characteristics in the intact rat, *Fed. Proc.* **28**:438.

83. Strand, F. L., and Kung, T. T., 1980, ACTH accelerates recovery of neuromuscular function following crushing of peripheral nerve, *Peptides* **1**:135–138.

84. Strand, F. L., and Smith, C. M., 1986, LPH, ACTH, MSH and motor systems, in: *Neuropeptides and Behavior*, Volume 1 (D. de Wied, W. H. Gispen, and T. B. van Wimersma Greidanus, eds.), Pergamon Press, Oxford, pp. 245–272.

85. Strand, F. L., Friedebold, G., and Stoboy, H., 1962, Electrical characteristics of rat skeletal muscle following adrenalectomy, *Acta Physiol. Pharmacol. Neerl.* **11**:213–234.

86. Strand, F. L., Stoboy, H., and Cayer, A., 1973/74, A possible direct action of ACTH on nerve and muscle, *Neuroendocrinology* **13**:1–20.

87. Strand, F. L., Cayer, A., Gonzalez, E., and Stoboy, H., 1976, Peptide enhancement of neuromuscular function: Animal and clinical studies, *Pharmacol. Biochem. Behav.* **5**:179–187.

88. Strand, F. L., Stoboy, H., Friedebold, G., Krivoy, W. A., Heyck, H., and Van Riezen, H.,

1977, Changes in muscle action potentials in patients with diseases of motor units following the infusion of a peptide fragment of ACTH, *Arzneim. Forsch. Drug Res.* **27**:681–683.

89. Swaab, D. F., and Boer, G. J., 1978, The fetal brain and intrauterine growth, *Postgrad. Med. J.* **54**:63–73.

90. Swaab, D. F., and Honnebier, W. J., 1974, The role of the fetal hypothalamus in development of the feto-placental unit and in parturition, *Prog. Brain Res.* **41**:275–280.

91. Swaab, D. F., and Martin, J. T., 1981, Functions of α-melanotropin and other opiomelanocortin peptides in labour, intrauterine growth and brain development: Peptides of the pars intermedia, *CIBA Found. Symp.* **81**:196–217.

92. Swaab, D. F., Visser, M., and Tilders, F. J. H., 1976, Stimulation of intrauterine growth in rat by α-melanocyte-stimulating hormone, *J. Endocrinol.* **70**:445–455.

93. Thompson, W., and Jensen, J. K. S., 1977, The extent of sprouting of remaining motor units in partly denervated immature and adult rat soleus muscle, *Soc. Neurosci. Abstr.* **2**:523–535.

94. Torda, C., and Wolff, H., 1952, Effect of pituitary hormones, cortisone and adrenalectomy on some aspects of neuromuscular systems and acetylcholine synthesis, *Am. J. Physiol.* **169**:140–149.

95. Van der Helm-Hylkema, H., and de Wied, D., 1976, Effect of neonatally injected ACTH and ACTH analogs on eye-opening of the rat, *Life Sci.* **18**:1099–1104.

96. Van Dongen, C. J., Hershkowitz, M., Zwiers, H., De Laat, S., and Gispen, W. H., 1983, Lipid fluidity and phosphoinositide metabolism in brain membranes of aged rats: Effects of $ACTH_{1–24}$, in: *Aging of the Brain* (W. H. Gispen and J. Traber, eds.), Elsevier, Amsterdam, pp. 101–114.

97. Varon, S., 1985, Factors promoting the growth of the nervous system, *Discussions in Neurosciences, FESN*, Geneva, Vol. II, no. 3.

98. Verhaagen, J., and Gispen, W. H., 1987, Peripheral nerve regeneration, neurotrophic factors and neuropeptides, in: *Recovery of Function in the Nervous System* (F. Cohadron and J. Lobo-Antunes, eds.), Livioma Press, Padova (in press).

99. Verhaagen, J., Edwards, P. M., Jennekens, F. G. I., Schotman, P., and Gispen, W. H., 1986, α-Melanocyte-stimulating hormone stimulates the outgrowth of myelinated nerve fibers after peripheral nerve crush, *Exp. Neurol.* **92**:451–454.

100. Verhaagen, J., Edwards, P. M., Schotman, P., Jennekens, F. G. I., and Gispen, W. H., 1986, Characterization of epitopes shared by α-melanocyte-stimulating hormone (α-MSH) and the 150 kD neurofilament protein (NF150): Relationship to neurotrophic sequences, *J. Neurosci. Res.* **16**:589–600.

101. Verhaagen, J., Edwards, P. M., Jennekens, F. G. I., Schotman, P., and Gispen, W. H., 1987, Early effect of an ACTH(4–9) analog (Org.2766) on regenerative sprouting demonstrated by the use of neurofilament-binding antibodies isolated from a serum raised by α-MSH immunization, *Brain Res.* **404**:142–150.

102. Willard, M., and Skene, J. H. P., 1982, Molecular events in axonal regeneration, in: *Repair and Regeneration of the Nervous System* (A. Nicholls, ed.), Springer-Verlag, Berlin, Heidelberg, pp. 71–89.

103. Wolterink, G., and van Ree, J. M., 1986, Org.2766 accelerates functional recovery of impaired motor activity due to lesions in the nucleus accumbens of rats, in: *Symposium on Neuropeptides and Brain Function*, Utrecht, *Abstr.* P41.

104. Zwiers, H., Schotman, P., and Gispen, W. H., 1980, Purification and some characteristics of an ACTH-sensitive protein kinase and its substrate protein in rat brain membranes, *J. Neurochem.* **34**:1689–1699.

13

DEVELOPMENTAL NEUROBIOLOGY AND THE PHYSIOPATHOLOGY OF BRAIN INJURY

GUSTAVE MOONEN, PAUL DELREE, PIERRE LEPRINCE, JEAN-MICHEL RIGO, BERNARD ROGISTER, AND PHILIPPE P. LEFEBVRE

ABSTRACT. Neuroontogenesis results from the integration of various elementary events such as cell proliferation, migration, and death, synaptogenesis, and synaptolysis. This chapter describes those aspects of the mechanisms involved in nervous system development that might potentially help to improve the management of nervous system injury. Some of these aspects are (1) the neuronal proliferation that has been shown to persist in some instances in the brain of adult birds and mammals and (2) the neuronal migration that involves complex cellular and molecular interactions between neurons and guiding glial cells. Some of these interactions would also play a role in the control of axonal elongation. Also involved are (3) the neuronotrophic influences of various origins that are thought to regulate neuronal cell survival, including the well-demonstrated model of nerve growth factor. Neuronal survival could, however, result from a delicate balance between these neuronotrophic influences and recently described endogenous neuronotoxic activities, which are in some cases related to the putative excitatory neurotransmitters glutamate and aspartate. Finally, there is (4) the role of astrocytic cells in the release of neuronotrophic and neuronotoxic activities and the control by growth (mitogenic) factors of the proliferation of developing astrocytes and oligodendrocytes that play a major role in brain reaction to injury.

Understanding the regulation of these developmental events might potentially expand research into new therapeutic areas and generate new concepts concerning neuronal replacement, prevention of secondary neuronal cell death, stimulation of neuronal regeneration, and control of glial cell proliferation in the injured nervous system.

GUSTAVE MOONEN, PAUL DELREE, PIERRE LEPRINCE, JEAN-MICHEL RIGO, BERNARD ROGISTER, AND PHILIPPE P. LEFEBVRE • Department of Human Physiology and Physiopathology, University of Liège, Institute L. Frédéricq, B-4020 Liège, Belgium.

1. INTRODUCTION

Neuroontogenesis involves a harmonious integration (in both time and space) of various elementary events (Fig. 1). Each of these steps results from the expression of intrinsic neuronal and glial properties modulated by environmental factors. The molecular basis of the intercellular interactions that take place during several of these elementary events is beginning to be understood. It is the purpose of the present review to discuss how data gathered through developmental studies might help the understanding of brain reaction to injury and hence better define the cellular and molecular targets for a pharmacological approach.

Nervous system reaction to injury can be considered one possible expression of neuroplasticity (i.e., ability to change). If it leads to functional recovery, one can talk of adaptative plasticity. If, on the other hand, it results in an impairment of regeneration, one can talk of maladaptative plasticity. The two can be associated: after traumatic damage to cortical areas, for instance, functional recovery (adaptative plasticity) and posttraumatic epilepsy (maladaptative plasticity) can both occur.

2. NEURONAL PROLIFERATION

Neuronal proliferation occurs in restricted areas of the developing central nervous system. In most instances, the germinal layers are located in periventricular areas; the external granular layer of the cerebellum, which is subpial, is an important exception.

The regulation of the final neuronal number in a developing nervous system is, at least theoretically, controlled at two different levels (Fig. 2). The first is the regulation of neuronal proliferation, and the second is the regulation of neuronal stabilization, which can be defined as the process during which redundant neurons are eliminated. Those two processes result in a matching between neuronal

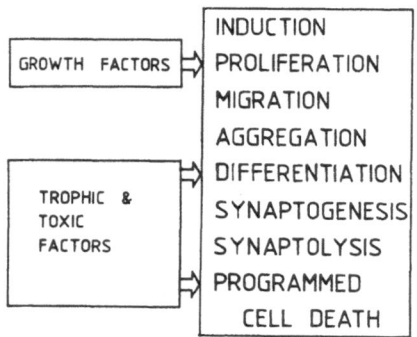

FIGURE 1. Sequence of elementary events during nervous system ontogenesis. Target events for growth (mitogenic) and neuronotrophic and neuronotoxic factors are indicated.

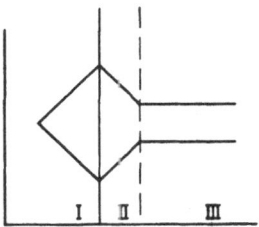

I Neuronal proliferation :
  - Neuronal Mitogen Factors (?)

II Neuronal stabilization :
  - Neuronotrophic Factors
  - Neuronotoxic Factors (?)

III Neuronal maintenance :
  - Neuronotrophic Factors

FIGURE 2. Schematic representation of the evolution of neuronal number at a given location of the developing nervous system as a function of time.

numbers and the size of target territories. So far, little is known about the molecular mechanisms involved in the regulation of neuronal proliferation.

In an extensive study of neuronal proliferation in rat cerebellum,[66] we were able to show *in vitro* that insulin was effective in maintaining neuronal proliferation of external granule neurons but had the characteristics of a progression factor (see Section 5). The optimal concentration of insulin was largely supraphysiological (Fig. 3), suggesting that the endogenous ligand of the receptor that binds insulin is not insulin itself but another peptide such as one of the somatomedins.

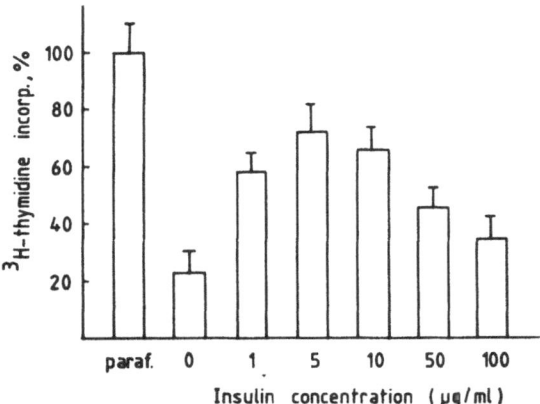

FIGURE 3. Incorporation of [³H]thymidine by 7-day-old rat paraflocculi maintained in suspension culture for 24 hr in the presence of increasing concentrations of insulin. At that particular stage of development, more than 90% of [³H]thymidine is incorporated in proliferating neuroblasts. Incorporation was performed for 60 min. at the end of the 24 hr of incubation and is expressed as percentage of the radioactivity incorporated in 60 min by freshly dissected parafloccculi (first column) (see also ref. 66).

None of the purified growth factors (such as EGF, FGF, PDGF), tissue extracts, neurotransmitters,[44,45] or conditioned media showed an activity that could be expected from a competence factor. It is possible that the proliferation of neurons, which are unique in the sense that after their last "differentiating" mitosis, they never proliferate again, is regulated by unique mechanisms involving proliferation inhibition factors rather than growth (mitogenic) factors. This last assumption, however, needs to be reconsidered in the light of recent works[2,7,29,42,70] showing that neuronogenesis can occur in the nervous system of adult birds and mammals and, in some of these instances, that the newly formed neurons are included in functional circuits.[77] However, an extensive study performed in primates could not, at least in uninjured brain, demonstrate neuronogenesis in adults.[82] Despite these last data, understanding of the mechanisms responsible for the control of developmental neuronal proliferation could generate new concepts in the field of neuronal replacement after nervous system injury.

3. NEURONAL MIGRATION

Developmental neuronal migration is a cell body translocation from the germinal zones to nuclei or layers in which neurons establish their final positions.[27] The characterization of the cellular and molecular events involved in that process is a central problem in developmental neurobiology, since this information might help to understand how cytoarchitectonic and functional organization are established as well as the pathogenesis of inborn errors of morphogenesis that primarily affect the migration process. Since the pioneering work of Rakic and co-workers,[81] it is presently believed that neuronal migration involves an intimate relationship between migratory neurons and a peculiar class of astrocytes, the radial glia. This hypothesis is based on electron microscopic and immunocytochemical data[25] and fits with the observation of a radial migration, since the guiding astrocytes have a radial orientation. However, it has to be pointed out that not every neuronal migration is radial. For instance, proliferative neuroblasts from the lateral lip of the rhombencephalon first migrate tangentially on the cerebellum anlage, where they organize into the external granular layer (EGL). Here, they proliferate again, and postmitotic neurons then migrate radially in an inward direction to the internal granular layer (IGL). At the molecular level, three categories of agents have been found or suggested to be involved in neuronal migration: plasminogen activator proteases, cell adhesion molecules, and extracellular matrix components.

3.1. PLASMINOGEN ACTIVATORS

The observation that neurons migrate inside a densely packed neuropile prompted us to consider the possible role of extracellular neutral proteolysis during neuronal migration. We focused on the plasminogen activator serine proteases because these enzymes are known to be involved in several phenomena that involve cell migration or tissue remodeling. We were able to show that two biochemically and immunologically different plasminogen activators, the urokinase type and the tissue type, were found in culture media conditioned by developing cerebral cortex or cerebellum.[63] Involvement of these proteases in neuronal migration was suggested by the demonstration that synthetic inbibitors of these proteases were able to block neuronal migration in two different *in vitro* assays: tridimensional suspension cultures of 7-day-old rat paraflocculi[62] and newborn rat cerebellum microexplants. This was recently confirmed using a plasminogen activator inhibitor secreted by a glioma cell line[33] and a modified version of our tridimensional assay.

Several questions still remain unanswered. Which of the two plasminogen activators released in the extracellular medium controls neuronal migration? At which steps of that process are the proteases acting, and which is the actual substrate for these proteases? Using medium conditioned by enriched granule cell cultures (these cultures contain more than 90% neurofilament-positive granulelike neurons), we recently showed that granule cells release mainly urokinase. This result suggests that urokinase might be the plasminogen activator involved in neuronal migration. If one considers, as a model, the inward migration of cerebellar granule cells, the following steps could be considered: detachment of postmitotic premigratory neurons from EGL, modulation of the migrating granule cell–radial glia interaction during the migration, and detachment of postmigratory neurons from radial glia, allowing them to settle in the internal granular layer. A modified fibrin overlay technique applied by Soreq and Miskin[99] on cerebellar slices shows that plasminogen activator activity is present at the inner part of EGL as well as in IGL, suggesting that proteolysis controls cell attachment during nonmigrating stages rather than modulating granule cell–radial glia process (Bergman fibers of the cerebellum) interaction during the migration.

3.2. CELL ADHESION MOLECULES

L1 antigen[89] is one member of a family of closely related molecules,[19,24,39,87] the neural cell adhesion molecules (nCAMs), that are involved in adhesion between neuronal cell bodies and between neurites as well as in nerve–muscle and neuron–glia interactions.[32] L1 was discovered using a monoclonal antibody that was obtained after immunization with a crude glycoprotein fraction of early postnatal mouse cerebellum. Immunohistological studies show that L1 antigen is located on postmitotic premigratoring and migrating neurons of developing cerebellum. In a culture assay, Fab fragments of poly- and monoclonal antibodies against L1 were able to block neuronal migration.[51]

3.3. EXTRACELLULAR MATRIX COMPONENTS

The number of identified extracellular matrix components[12,56] is growing, and these include collagen and related molecules, noncollagenous glycoproteins (laminin, fibronectin, entactin), glycosaminoglycans, and proteoglycans. Laminin is synthesized by Schwann cells[16,56] and promotes neuritic elongation[17,56,85] by both peripheral and central nervous system neurons. It was found, in an *in vitro* assay, to be able to promote migration of cerebellar granule cells.[92] As a matter of fact, in control conditions, granule cells were associated with GFAP-positive cells (which most likely represent radial glia processes), whereas on a laminin-coated substratum, granule cells detached from the glial processes and migrated directly on the substratum. No such effect was observed using various types of collagen or fibronectin despite the fact that fibronectin is also synthesized by astrocytes.[49,79] The effect of laminin is blocked by antilaminin antibodies, and laminin was demonstrated to be synthesized by astrocytes.[92]

An important question that has to be solved in the future is how plasminogen activators, neural cell adhesion molecules, and extracellular matrix glycoproteins interact to control neuronal migration. Figure 4 shows a tentative model of this interaction.

The first pathological implications of neuronal migration studies are obviously those inborn errors of morphogenesis in which migration is impaired.[40] It is worth pointing out that both migration deficits, such as in pachygyria or

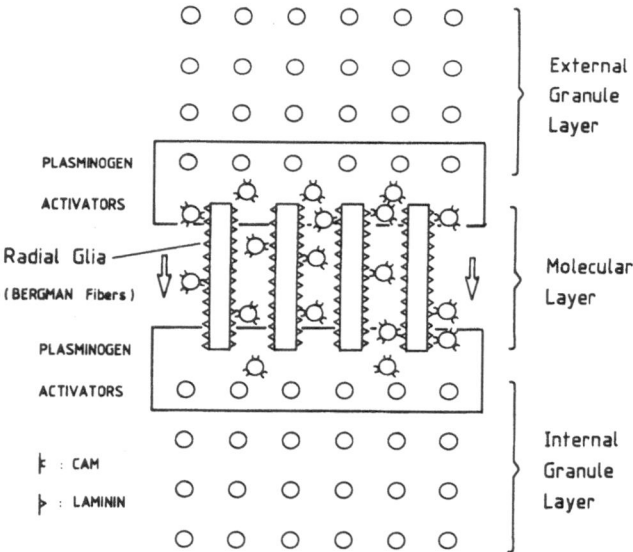

FIGURE 4. Possible sites of action of plasminogen activators, cell adhesion molecules (CAM), and laminin during the inward migration of cerebellar granule cells. Plasminogen activators could control the detachment of postmitotic premigratory neurons from the external granule layer and/or postmigratory neurons from the radial glial processes. The CAMs "link" migrating neurons and the glia, which are coated with laminin.

lissencephalia, and hypermigration with subpial neuronal heterotopies, such as in the fetal alcohol syndrome,[15] are found and that these diseases lead to severe mental retardation (when developmental neuronal migration is impaired).

Second, neural grafting techniques have become important tools in order to generate functional restoration in experimentally damaged brains and have even been tried in humans.[9,76] With the increasing use of stereotactic injection of neuronal and glial cell suspensions, induction or control of migration of grafted cells might become mandatory.

4. NEURONAL STABILIZATION

As mentioned earlier, neuronal stabilization is a process during which redundant neurons are eliminated. Indeed, predictable waves of neuronal death occur in the developing nervous system, allowing precise matching between neuronal populations and the size of target territories.[5,14,34] This was elegantly demonstrated by target grafting and removal techniques, as illustrated in Fig. 5. This also suggests the secretion by the target of a signal responsible for neuronal survival. That signal was shown to be chemical and is presently called a neuronotrophic factor. The best known neuronotrophic factor is the nerve growth factor (NGF). Indeed, the concepts deriving from the study of NGF have been guidelines for the whole field of neuronotrophic factors. Figure 6 summarizes the

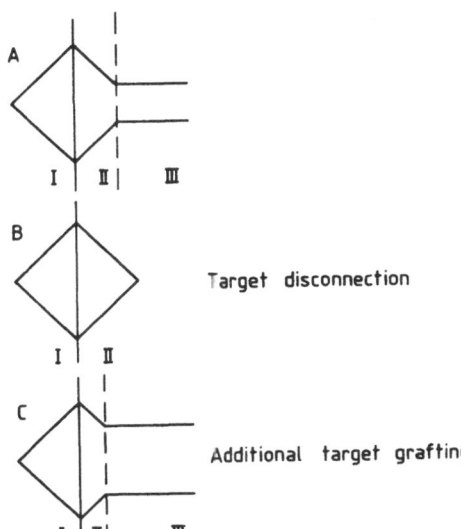

FIGURE 5. Schematic representation of experimental modulation of developmental neuronal death. (A) Normal situation (see Fig. 2). (B) After target removal, virtually all neurons that lack target-derived trophic support die. (C) Additional target grafting increases target-derived trophic support and rescues part of the neuronal population.

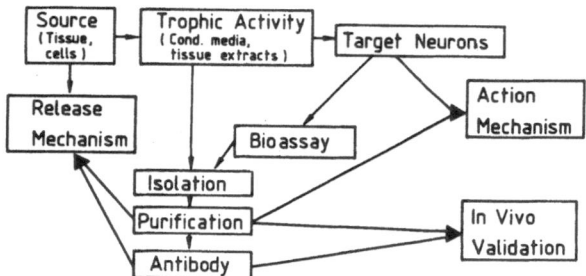

FIGURE 6. Experimental strategy used for characterization of neuronotrophic factors.

experimental strategy in that field. So far, three neuronotrophic factors have been purified.[4,5,10,103] Since several recent reviews have been devoted to neuronotrophic factors,[20,30,100-102] we focus on those aspects that are relevant to the topic of brain injuries.

4.1. NEURONOTROPHIC FACTORS

Potential neuronotrophic* effects on neurons are summarized in Fig. 7. According to their origin, they could be classified in the following way:

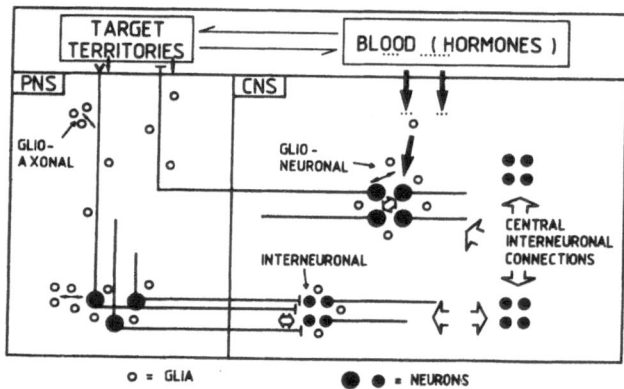

FIGURE 7. Potential neuronotrophic effects on neurons in peripheral and central nervous system.

---

*We use the term neuronotrophic rather than neurotrophic. Strictly speaking, the term factor should be used only when the molecule responsible for the neuronotrophic activity is purified and characterized. The expression neuronotrophic activity should be used when a biological effect on neuronal survival is present in a biological fluid but not yet characterized at the molecular level.

1. Retrograde transsynaptic represents the classical target-derived neuronotrophic interactions documented for several neuronal systems in
   developmental neurobiology.
2. Anterograde transsynaptic is much less thoroughly documented. Such
   effects are obvious in clinical situations, the more frequently cited example probably being neurogenic muscle atrophy, i e., the muscle atrophy
   that follows denervation.
3. Systemic represents trophic influences coming from the blood and includes hormonal effects on neuronal survival.
4. Glioneuronal. Increasing evidence has been obtained in the last decade
   not only for glial control of the metabolic environment of neurons ($K+_{ex}$
   regulation,[22] pyruvate release,[93] neurotransmitter metabolism,[38] etc.)
   but also for a glial origin of neuronotrophic activity.[3,52,67,86]

Those multiple trophic actions on neurons raise the concept of a trophic
input (Fig. 8) that represents the combined neuronotrophic effect of the various
individual trophic components addressing a given neuron. The concept of trophic
input generates another one, which is that of the trophic threshold, defined as that
threshold amount of trophic input that is needed for neuronal survival. The
trophic threshold could vary, being high during development and regeneration
and low during "regular neuronal maintenance" (Fig. 8). However, during
development, the target-derived trophic input plays a critical role in the survival

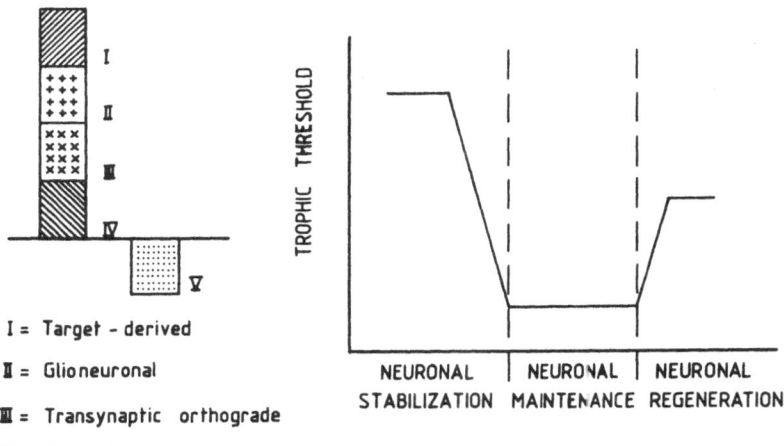

I = Target - derived

II = Glioneuronal

III = Transynaptic orthograde

IV = Systemic

V = Neuronotoxic

FIGURE 8. Left: Possible influences on neuronal survival classified as trophic (above the base line)
or toxic (below the base line). The trophic influences have been further subdivided according to their
origin. Right: Possible variation of the trophic threshold (minimal amount of trophic input needed for
neuronal survival) in developing or regenerating neurons as compared to normal adult neurons
(regular neuronal maintenance).

of several neuronal types. This means that suppressing this input by target removal or by injection of antibodies against the target-derived trophic factor induces the death of these neurons. This might be true *in vivo* because at a given developmental period, the target-derived trophic input represents the only, or the largely dominant, trophic input. Indeed, *in vitro* experiments have shown that the glial trophic input can be a surrogate for the target-derived one.[104] If this is also true for adult regenerating neurons, it means that supplying those neurons with any one of the trophic inputs might improve their survival (see also Section 5). To test this hypothesis, adult regenerating neurons have to be studied as illustrated in Fig. 9 (P. Delree, P. Leprince, B. Rogister, and G. Moonen, unpublished observation).

4.2. NEURONOTOXIC FACTORS

The simultaneous occurrence of constructive and destructive events is ubiquitous in developmental biology. In nervous system development, for instance, both neurogenesis and neuronal death, synaptogenesis and synaptolysis,[13,83] occur. In a previous study of neuronotrophic activity in developing cerebellum,[29] we were able to show the simultaneous release of both neuronotrophic and neuronotoxic activities, which could be separated by a simple physical method, the latter activity being associated with a low-molecular-weight fraction. We were recently able to demonstrate[46] that (1) the neuronotoxic activity is released by astrocytes but not by neurons, (2) the toxicity is directed to neurons but not to astrocytes, (3) astrocytes also release a high-molecular-weight neuronotrophic activity, (4) increasing extracellular K^+ concentration induces an enhanced release of neuronotoxic but not neuronotrophic activity, and (5) neurons can be desensitized to the neuronotoxic activity.

Those data might be important in understanding brain reaction to injury and the physiopathology of secondary neuronal cell death. Indeed, in several pathological conditions, an abrupt increase of brain extracellular K^+ is known to occur, inducing an astrocytic depolarization.[35,43,65,81,84,105] Such pathological conditions include status epilepticus,[53] ischemia, or hypoglycemia[2] and can lead to neuronal death.[72] In those conditions, an imbalance between astrocytic neuronotrophic and neuronotoxic activities could be generated as one step of a pathophysiological sequence leading to neuronal death. If the neuronotoxic factor can be identified and its mechanism of action understood, this could open new therapeutic prospects. It is also worth mentioning here that other endogenous neuronotoxins have been demonstrated that are members of the excitotoxin family[71,91] and could also participate in the physiopathology of neuronal death after brain injury. On the basis of its spectrum of neuronal targets, the astrocytic neuronotoxic factor does not seem to belong to this neuronotoxin group.

Excitotoxins, which are related to the putative excitatory neurotransmitters glutamate and aspartate, induce very peculiar neuronal lesions, axon-sparing lesions. Indeed, after local injection, dendritosomatic lesions are observed,

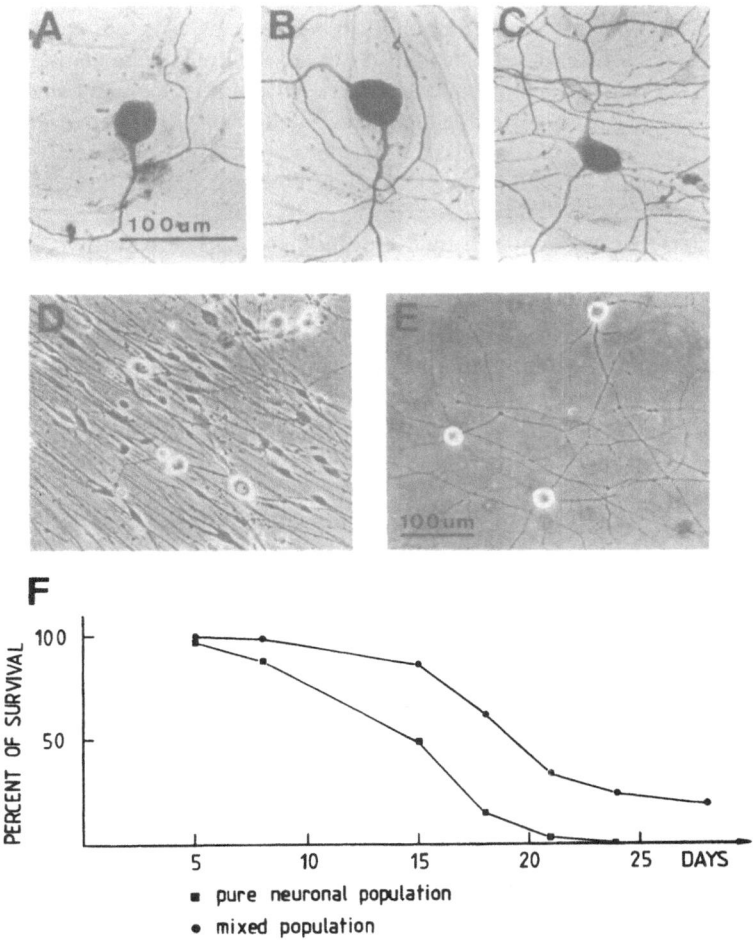

FIGURE 9. Dorsal root ganglion (DRG) neurons dissected from adult (3- to 6-month-old) rats and cultivated in serum-free medium on laminin substratum. A–C: Bright-field micrographs after immunohistochemical demonstration of neurofilament proteins of such neurons cultivated for 8 days: (A) unipolar, (B) bipolar, and (C) multipolar neurons. Note that a significant percentage of these neurons become multipolar in such *in vitro* regenerative conditions. D and E: Phase-contrast micrographs of living DRG neurons cultivated for 4 days in the presence of nonneuronal cells (D) or after elimination of nonneuronal cells by centrifugation on Percoll gradient (E). F: Evolution of the number of adult rat DRG neurons cultivated in the presence (●, illustrated by micrograph D) or the absence (■, illustrated by micrograph E) of nonneuronal (including Schwann) cells. A survival-promoting effect of the nonneuronal cells is obvious (P. Delree, P. Leprince, B. Rogister, and G. Moonen, unpublished observation).

whereas local axons and axonal terminals are spared. Kainic acid is unique in that respect since, aside from the lesions at the local site of injection, it also induces distant lesions that are thought to be mediated by glutamatergic projections and closely resemble the lesions observed in human status epilepticus.[26,42] Interestingly, folic acid and folate derivatives also produce the distant lesions but without inducing local lesion at the injection site.[73,74] In all these cases, distal lesions were suppressed by benzodiazepines[8,23] (which potentiate GABA effects) or (although it has only been tested in few experimental models) glutamate antagonists.[58,75,96,97] The excitotoxin hypothesis is also thought to be valid in ischemic lesions, as suggested by Meldrum's group. These authors also suggest that the neurotoxins induce alterations in the membrane functional or structural integrity, leading to massive inward Ca^{2+} fluxes, which would be the final mechanism leading to neuronal death[59,95] as has also been suggested in non-neuronal systems.[90] Indeed, in experimental ischemia (see M. S. Beattie *et al.*, Chapter 3), a decrease of extracellular Ca^{2+} is observed.[31,36] Part of that Ca^{2+} is likely to diffuse into neurons because of the concentration gradient.

4.3. INTERFERENCE BETWEEN NEURONOTROPHIC AND NEURONOTOXIC ACTIVITIES

From data reported in the two previous sections, it can be suggested that improved neuronal survival after nervous system injury could be achieved using two different strategies: (1) supplying injured neurons with an excess of neuronotrophic factor(s) and (2) antagonizing the neuronotoxic activity. Figure 10 (G. Moonen, P. Leprince, and P. P. Lefebvre, unpublished results) shows that when cultured neurons are supplied with additional neuronotrophic activity, the effect of the neuronotoxic activity is suppressed. On the other hand, if the neuronotoxic activity can be characterized at the molecular level, designing specific antagonists should improve neuronal survival. These two, not mutually exclusive, pharmacological approaches, when applied in the acute phase of brain injury, could result in neuronal sparing and hence in better conditions for functional recovery.

5. GROWTH (MITOGENIC) FACTORS

Unlike neurons (Section 1), glial cells are able to resume proliferation in adult mammals, including primates and humans. Although this was known for a long time for astrocytes, it has only recently been clearly documented for oligodendrocytes both *in vivo*[1,54] and *in vitro*.[88,107] Cellular proliferation is presently thought to be regulated at several levels. Progression factors have to be continu-

FIGURE 10. Survival of cerebellar granule cells (150,000 cells per 6-mm-diameter well) cultured for 24 hr in serum-free medium and treated for the next 24-hr period by (upper panel) Increasing dilution of a YM2 (cut-off 1000 Da) ultrafiltrate of medium conditioned by astrocytes (neuronotoxic activity) or (lower panel) increasing dilution of a YM2 (cut-off 1000 Da) ultrafiltrate of medium conditioned by astrocytes and supplemented at each dilution of the neurotoxic activity-containing medium with a constant amount of tenfold-concentrated PM10 (cut-off 10 kDa) retentate of the same conditioned medium (neuronotrophic activity). The neuronotoxic activity is almost completely suppressed by the addition of the neuronotrophic activity-containing medium. Results are expressed as percentage of survival measured in control unconditioned medium (C).

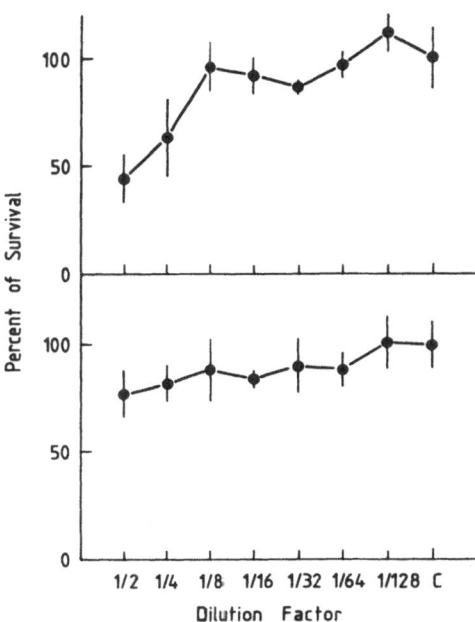

ously present and include several members of the insulin family, whereas competence factors act as triggers and need only to be present at a given period of the cell cycle.[11] Several growth factors able to induce proliferation of astrocytes and oligodendrocytes have recently been characterized.[21,47,48,50,60,98,106] This characterization results either from the study of the effect on glial cells of factors active in nonneuronal systems or from the isolation from brain extracts of factors able to induce glial proliferation. In one instance such a factor (AGF, astrocyte growth factor) isolated from beef brain turned out to be a known mitogen in other systems (FGF, fibroblast growth factor).[78] The cellular origin in brain of these factors is not completely known, although at least one of them is located in neurons in immunohistochemical preparations.[78] Hence, the possibility that injured neurons release astrocytic mitogens as part of the events leading to gliosis is open but remains to be experimentally proven. Cultured astrocytes can also be morphologically altered from a flat to a stellate shape by several agents, including cAMP derivatives,[64] brain extracts, or injured brain extracts (morphogens) (see M. Nieto-Sampedro, Chapter 15). Ultrastructural studies showed, as result of the action of some of these agents, an increased content of intermediate filaments, whereas measurements of the glial fibrillary acidic protein (the subunit of the astrocytic intermediate filament) showed an increased content of that astroglial-specific protein.[94] Postlesion gliosis is likely to result both from mitogenic and morphogenic stimuli. Therefore, pharmacological modulation of these two aspects of glial reaction to injury is becoming a possibility.

In a previous study of plasminogen activators in developing nervous system, we were able to characterize two of them, the tissue type and the urokinase type (Fig. 11). The last one was found to be mitogenic for astrocytes, as illustrated in Fig. 12. In the peripheral nervous system, urokinase is also mitogenic for Schwann cells but is released only by neurons. Schwann cells themselves release the tissue-type plasminogen activator, which has no proliferation stimulation effect.[6] When astrocytes are stimulated with AGF, their plasminogen activator release into the medium is stimulated (B. Rogister, P. Leprince, B. Pettman, G. Labourdette, M. Sensenbrenner, and G. Moonen, unpublished results). The same phenomenon is observed with Schwann cells, which, after stimulation by cholera toxin, a known mitogen for these cells, increase their secretion of tissue-type plasminogen activator.[6] The functional significance of that modulated plasminogen activator secretion is presently unknown. In light of the reported effect of plasminogen activators in neuronal migration (see Section 2), our current hypothesis is that these extracellular neutral serine proteases modulate cell adhesion and intercellular association. In that respect, it is worth

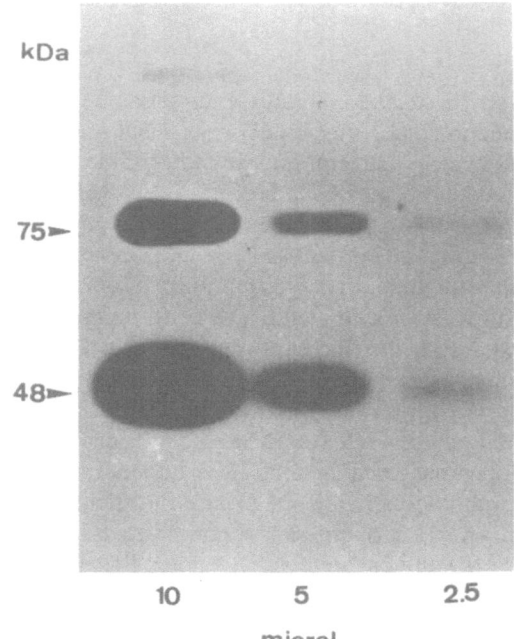

FIGURE 11. Zymographic analysis after SDS-PAGE of medium conditioned by 7-day-old cerebellar microexplants. The amounts of medium loaded on the gel are shown. The molecular weights of the observed plasminogen activators are shown (48,000 for rat urokinase and 75,000 for rat tissue-type activator).

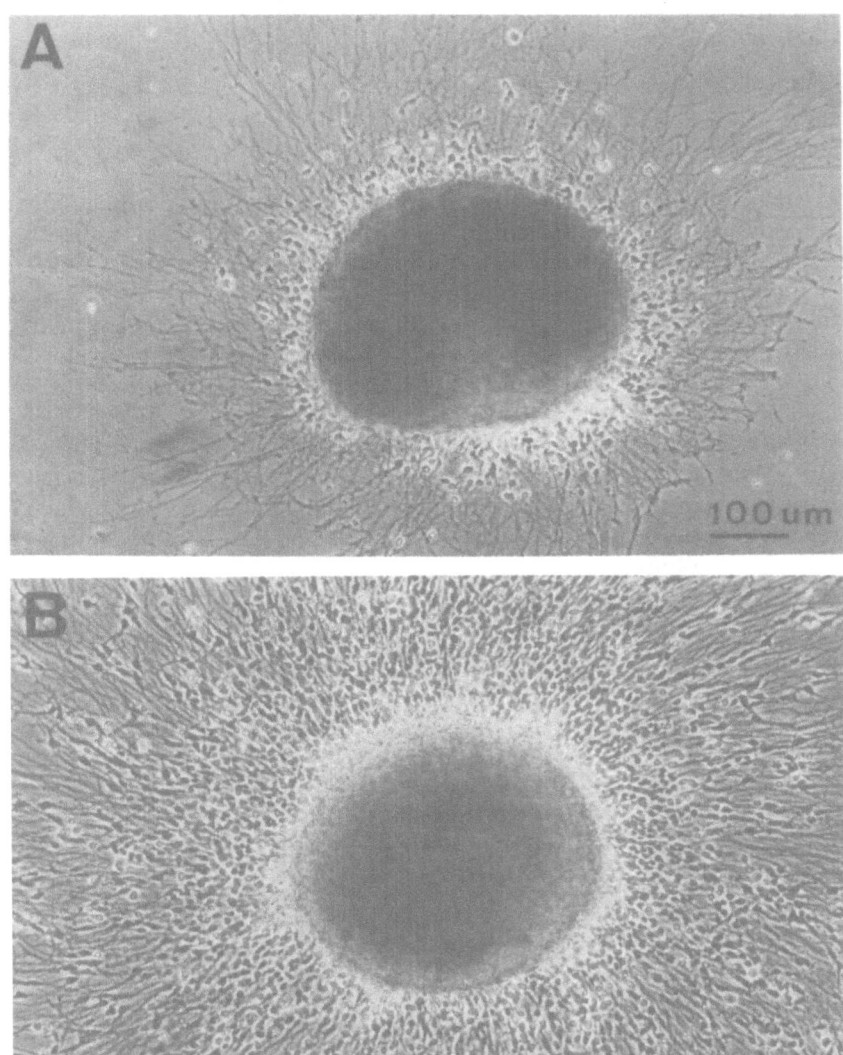

FIGURE 12. Phase-contrast micrographs of newborn rat cerebellum microexplants[28] cultured for 48 hr in Eagle's minimum essential medium supplemented with insulin (5 μg/ml) and in the absence (A) or the presence (B) of purified human urokinase (12 U/ml). The outgrowing cells are positive for GFAP in immunohistochemical preparations and can be identified as astrocytes. The proliferation-stimulating effect of urokinase was quantified by [³H]thymidine incorporation measurement (see ref. 63).

mentioning that video time-lapse studies have shown that when Schwann cells are stimulated to proliferate, they stop migrating.[18]

6. CONCLUSION

Many experimental and clinical observations demonstrate that functional restoration after nervous system injury is more effective in lower than higher vertebrates and in peripheral than in central mammalian nervous system. It is also more effective in developing than in adult mammalian central nervous system. Comparing regenerative (developing) and nonregenerative (adult) systems is one way to understand why adult mammalian central nervous system lacks effective regenerative capacity. Hence, the first contribution of developmental neurobiology to that field is a comparative one.

When Harrison (1907) explanted *in vitro* a fragment of neural tube of frog embryo and so created the tissue culture technique, he wanted to answer a specific question about the origin of nerve fibers, a question that had led Golgi and Ramon y Cajal into controversy. Tissue culture has since become a major tool in neurobiology, with an increasing sophistication of techniques (Fig. 13).

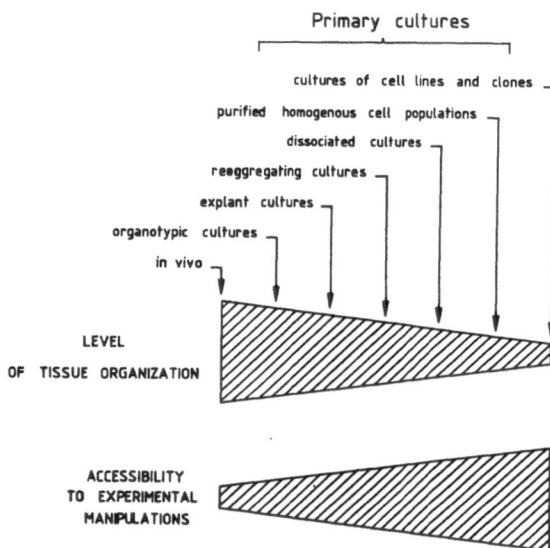

FIGURE 13. Methods for cultivating nervous tissue have been classified as a function of the level of tissue organization and the accessibility to experimental manipulation. For instance, tissue organization is higher when primary dissociated cultures contain several cell types as compared to culture techniques allowing the separation of homogeneous cell types. Cell lines or clones allow genetic studies or somatic hybridization that are not possible using primary (i.e., not subcultured) cultures.

The second contribution of developmental neurobiology to the understanding of nervous system reaction to injury is logistic, allowing, for instance, bioassay of mitogens, morphogens, neuronotrophic factors, etc. in fluids or tissue samples taken from injured brain.[55,68,69]

In our opinion, however, the main contribution of developmental neurobiology is at the conceptual level. Understanding cellular interactions during normal development will help us to generate new concepts and ultimately can lead to purification of molecules that may become important potential pharmacological agents that may eventually limit the effect of injury and improve functional restoration in injured human nervous system.

ACKNOWLEDGMENTS. G.M. and P.L. are, respectively, Maître de Recherches and Chargé de Recherches at the Fonds National de la Recherche Scientifique, Belgium. The authors acknowledge the support of the Fonds de la Recherche Scientifique Médicale, Belgium, and of the Fondation Médicale Reine Elisabeth, Belgium.

REFERENCES

1. Arenella, L., and Herndon, R. M., 1984, Mature oligodendrocytes: Division following experimental demyelination in adult animals, *Arch. Neurol.* **41**:1162–1165.
2. Astrup, J., and Norberg, K., 1976, Potassium activity in cerebral cortex in rat during progressive severe hypoglycemia, *Brain Res.* **103**:418–423.
3. Banker, G., 1980, Trophic interactions between astroglial cells and hippocampal neurons in culture, *Science* **209**:809–810.
4. Barbin, G., Manthorpe, M., and Varon, S., 1984, Purification of the chick eye ciliary neuronotrophic factor (CNTF), *J. Neurochem.* **43**:1468–1478.
5. Barde, Y. A., Edgar, D., and Thoenen, H., 1982, Purification of a new neuronotrophic factor from mammalian brain, *Eur. Mol. Biol. Org. J.* **1**:549–553.
6. Baron-Van Evercooren, A., Leprince, P., Rogister, B., Lefebvre, P. P., Delree, P., Selak, I., and Moonen, G., 1986, Plasminogen activators in developing peripheral nervous system, cellular origin and mitogenic effect, *Dev. Brain Res.* **36**:101–103.
7. Bayer, S. A., 1985, Neuron production in the hippocampus and olfactory bulb of the adult rat brain: Addition or replacement? *Ann. N.Y. Acad. Sci.* **457**:163–172.
8. Ben-Ari, Y., Tremblay, E., Ottersen, O. P., and Naquet, R., 1979, Evidence suggesting secondary epileptogenic lesions after kainic acid: Pretreatment with diazepam reduces distant, not local brain damage, *Brain Res.* **165**:362–365.
9. Björklund, A., and Gage. F. H., 1985, Neural grafting in animal models of neurodegenerative diseases, *N.Y. Acad. Sci.* **457**:53–81.
10. Bocchini, V., and Angeletti, P. U., 1969, The nerve growth factor: Purification as a 30,000 molecular weight protein, *Proc. Natl. Acad. Sci. U.S.A.* **64**:787–794.
11. Brashaw, A., and Rubin, J. S., 1980, Polypeptide growth factors: Some structural and mechanistic considerations, *J. Supramol. Struct.* **14**:183–199.
12. Carbonetto, S., 1984, The extracellular matrix of the nervous system, *Trends Neurosci.* **10**:382–387.
13. Changeux, J. P., and Danchin, A., 1976, Selective stabilization of developing synapses as a mechanism for the specification of neuronal networks, *Nature* **264**:705–712.

14. Clarke, P. G. H., 1985, Neuronal death in the development of the vertebrate nervous system, *Trends Neurosci.* **8:**345–349.
15. Clarren, S. K., Alvord, E. C., and Sumi, S. M., 1978, Brain malformations related to prenatal exposure to ethanol, *J. Pediatr.* **92:**64–72.
16. Davis, G. E., Manthorpe, M., Engvall, E., and Varon, S., 1985, Isolation and characterization of rat schwannoma neurite-promoting factor: Evidence that the factor contains laminin, *J. Neurosci.* **5:**2662–2671.
17. Davis, G. E., Varon, S., Engvall, E., and Manthorpe, M., 1985, Substratum-binding neurite-promoting factors: Relationship to laminin, *Trends Neurosci.* **12:**528–532.
18. Dubois-Dalcq, M., Rentier, B., Baron-Van Evercooren, A., and Burge, B., 1981, Structure and behaviour of rat primary and secondary Schwann cells *in vivo*, *Exp. Cell Res.* **131:**283–297.
19. Edelman, G. M., Hoffman, S., Chuong, C.-M., Thiery, J.-P., Brackenbury, R., Gallin, W. J., Grumet, M., Greenberg, M. E., Hemperly, J. J., Cohen, C., and Cunningham, B. A., 1983, Structure and modulation of neural cell adhesion molecules in early and late embryogenesis, *Cold Spring Harbor Symp. Quant. Biol.* **48:**515–526.
20. Edgar, D., and Barde, Y.-A., 1983, Neuronal growth factors, *Trends Neurosci.* **6:**260–262.
21. Fischer, G., 1984, Growth requirements of immature astrocytes in serum-free hormonally defined medium, *J. Neurosci. Res.* **12:**543–552.
22. Franck, G., Grisar, T., and Moonen, G., 1983, Glial and neuronal Na$^+$, K$^+$ pump, *Adv. Cell. Neurobiol.* **4:**133–159.
23. Fuller, T. A., and Olney, J. W., 1981, Only certain anticonvulsants protect against kainate neurotoxicity, *Neurobehav. Toxicol. Teratol.* **3:**355–361.
24. Fushiki, S., and Schachner, M., 1986, Immunocytological localization of cell adhesion molecules L$_1$ and N-CAM and the shared carbohydrate epitope L$_2$ during the development of the mouse neocortex, *Dev. Brain Res.* **24:**153–157.
25. Gadisseux, J. F., and Evrard, R., 1985, Glial-neuronal relationship in the developing central nervous system, *Dev. Neurosci.* **7:**12–32.
26. Gibbs, W., Neale, E. A., and Moonen, G., 1982, Kainic acid sensitivity of mammalian Purkinje cells in monolayer cultures, *Dev. Brain Res.* **4:**103–108.
27. Goldman, S. A., and Nottebohm, F., 1983, Neuronal production, migration and differentiation in a vocal control nucleus of adult female canary brain, *Proc. Natl. Acad. Sci. U.S.A.* **80:**2390–2394.
28. Grau-Wagemans, M.-P., Selak, I., Lefebvre, P. P., and Moonen, G., 1984, Cerebellar macroneurons in serum-free cultures: Evidence for intrinsic neuronotrophic and neuronotoxic activities, *Dev. Brain Res.* **15:**11–19.
29. Graziadei, P. P. C., and Monti Graziadei, G. A., 1985, Neurogenesis and plasticity of the olfactory sensory neurons, *Ann. N.Y. Acad. Sci.* **457:**127–142.
30. Greene, L. A., and Shooter, E. M., 1980, The nerve growth factor: biochemistry, synthesis and mechanism of action, *Annu. Rev. Neurosci.* **3:**352–402.
31. Griffiths, T., Evans, M. C., and Meldrum, B. S., 1982, Intracellular sites of early calcium accumulation in the rat hippocampus during status epilepticus, *Neurosci. Lett.* **30:**329–334.
32. Grumet, M., and Edelman, G. M., 1984, Heterotypic binding between neuronal membrane vesicles and glial cells is mediated by a specific cell adhesion molecule, *J. Cell Biol.* **98:**1746–1756.
33. Guenther, J., Nick, H., and Monard, D., 1985, A glia-derived neurite promoting factor with protease inhibitory activity, *EMBO J.* **4:**1963–1966.
34. Hamburger, V., and Oppenheim, R. W., 1982, Naturally occuring neuronal death in vertebrates, *Neurosci. Comm.* **1:**39–55.
35. Hansen, A. J., 1977, Extracellular potassium concentration in juvenile and adult rat brain cortex during anoxia, *Acta Physiol. Scand.* **99:**412–420.

36. Harris, R. J., Symon, L., Bransdon, N. M., and Bayhan, M., 1981, Changes in extracellular calcium activity in cerebral ischemia, *J. Cereb. Blood Flow Metab.* **1**:203–210.
37. Heinemann, U., Konnerth, A., Pumain, R., and Wadman, W. J., 1986, Extracellular calcium and potassium concentration changes in chronic epileptic brain tissue, in: *Advances in Neurology*, Volume 44 (A. V. Delgado-Escueta, A. A. Ward, Jr., D. M. Woodbury, and R. J. Porter, eds.), Raven Press, New York, pp. 641–661.
38. Henn, F. A., Goldstein, M., and Hamberger, A., 1974, Uptake of the neurotransmitter candidate glutamate by glia, *Nature* **249**:663–664.
39. Hirn, M., Deagostini-Bazin, H., Gennarini, G., Santoni, M. J., He, H.-T., Hirsch, M. R., and Goridis, C., 1985, Structural and functional studies on N-CAM neural cell adhesion molecules, *J. Physiol. (Paris)* **80**:247–254.
40. Holmes, C. B., 1974, Inborn errors of morphogenesis. A review of localized hereditary malformations, *N. Engl. J. Med.* **291**:763–773.
41. Kaplan, M. S., and Hinds, J. W., 1977, Neurogenesis in the adult rat: Electron microscopic analysis of light radioautographs, *Science* **197**:1092–1094.
42. Köhler, C., 1983, Neuronal degeneration after intracerebral injections of excitotoxins. A histological analysis of kainic acid, ibotenic acid and quinolinic acid lesions in the rat brain, in: *Excitotoxins* (K. Fuxe, P. Roberts, and R. Schwarcz, eds.), Macmillan, London, pp. 99–111.
43. Kuffler, S. W., and Nicholls, J. G., 1966, The physiology of glia cells, *Ergeb. Physiol.* **57**:1–90.
44. Lauder, J. M., 1983, Hormonal and humoral influences in brain development, *Psychoneuroendocrinology* **8**:121–155.
45. Lauder, J. M., and Krebs, H., 1978, Serotonin and early neurogenesis, in: *Maturation of Neurotransmission* (A. Vernadakis, E. Giacobini, and G. Filogamo, eds.), S. Karger, Basel, pp. 171–180.
46. Lefebvre, P. P., Rogister, B., Delree, P., Leprince, P., Selak, I., and Moonen, G., 1986, Potassium-induced release of neuronotoxic activity by astrocytes *Brain Res.* **413**:120–128.
47. Lemke, G. E., and Brockes, J. P., 1984, Identification and purification of glial growth factor, *J. Neurosci.* **4**:75–83.
48. Leutz, A., and Schachner, M., 1981, Epidermal growth factor stimulates DNA-synthesis of astrocytes in primary cerebellar cultures, *Cell Tissue Res.* **220**:393–404.
49. Liesi, P., Kirkwood, T., and Vaheri, A., 1986, Fibronectin is expressed by astrocytes cultured from embryonic and early postnatal rat brain, *Exp. Cell Res.* **163**:175–185.
50. Lim, R., and Miller, J. F., 1984, An improved procedure for the isolation of glia maturation factor, *J. Cell. Physiol.* **119**:255–259.
51. Lindner, J., Rathjen, F. G., and Schachner, M., 1983, L₁ mono- and polyclonal antibodies modify cell migration in early postnatal mouse cerebellum, *Nature* **305**:427–430.
52. Lindsay, R. M., Barber, P. C., Sherwood, M. R., Zimmer, J., and Raisman, G., 1982, Astrocyte cultures from adult rat brain. Derivation, characterization and neurotrophic properties of pure astroglial cells from corpus callosum, *Brain Res.* **243**:329–343.
53. Lothman, E., Lamanna, J., Cordingley, G., Rosenthal, M., and Somjen, G., 1974, Levels of potassium in the cerebral cortex during electrical stimulation, seizures and spreading depression, *Soc. Neurosci. Abstr.* **4**:315.
54. Ludwin, S., 1985, Reaction of oligodendrocytes and astrocytes to trauma and implantation. A combined autoradiographic and immunohistochemical study, *Lab. Invest.* **52**:29–30.
55. Lundborg, G., Longo, F. M., and Varon, S., 1982, Nerve regeneration model and trophic factors *in vivo*, *Brain Res.* **232**:157–161.
56. Manthorpe, M., Engvall, E., Ruoslahti, E., Longo, F. M., Davis, G. E., and Varon, S., 1983, Laminin promotes neurite regeneration from cultured peripheral and central neurons, *J. Cell Biol.* **97**:1882–1890.
57. McGarvey, M. L., Baron-Van Evercooren, A., Kleinman, A. K., and Dubois-Dalcq, M.,

1984, Synthesis and effects of basement membrane component in cultured rat Schwann Cells, in: *The Role of Extracellular Matrix in Development* (R. L. Trelstad, ed.), Alan R. Liss, New York, pp. 123–143.

58. Meldrum, B. S., 1985, Possible therapeutic applications of antagonists of excitatory amino acid neurotransmitters, *Clin. Sci.* **68:**113–122.

59. Meldrum, B. S., 1986, Cell damage in epilepsy and the role of calcium in cytotoxicity, in: *Advances in Neurology,* Volume 44 (A. V. Delgado-Escueta, A. A. Ward, Jr., D. M. Woodbury, and R. J. Porter, eds.), Raven Press, New York, pp. 849–855.

60. Michler-Stuke, A., Wolff, J. R., and Bottenstein, J. E., 1984, Factors influencing astrocyte growth and development in defined media, *Int. J. Dev. Neurosci.* **2:**575–584.

61. Moonen, G., and Franck, G., 1977, Potassium effect on Na^+,K^+-ATPase activity of cultured newborn rat astroblasts during differentiation, *Neurosci. Lett.* **4:**263–267.

62. Moonen, G., Grau-Wagemans, M.-P., and Selak, I., 1982, Plasminogen activator–plasmin system and neuronal migration, *Nature* **298:**753–755.

63. Moonen, G., Grau-Wagemans, M.-P., Selak, I., Lefebvre, P. P., Rogister, B., Vassalli, J. D., and Belin, D., 1985, Plasminogen activator is a mitogen for astrocytes in developing cerebellum, *Dev. Brain Res.* **20:**41–48.

64. Moonen, G., Heinen. E., and Goessens, G., 1976, Comparative ultrastructural study of the effects of serum-free medium and dibutyryl-cyclic AMP on newborn rat astroblasts, *Cell Tissue Res.* **167:**221–227.

65. Moonen, G., and Nelson, P. G., 1978, Some physiological properties of astrocytes in primary cultures, in: *Dynamic Properties of Glia Cells* (E. Schoffeniels, G. Franck. D. B. Tower, and L. Hertz, eds.), Pergamon Press, New York, pp. 389–393.

66. Moonen, G., Selak, I., and Grau-Wagemans, M.-P., 1987, *In vitro* analysis of glial–neuronal communication during cerebellum ontogenesis, in: *Glial–Neuronal Communication in Development and Regeneration,* NATO ASI Series H, Volume 2 (H. H. Althaus and W. Seifert. eds.), Springer-Verlag, Berlin, pp. 324–337.

67. Muller, H. W., and Seifert, W., 1982, A neurotrophic factor (NTF) released from primary glial cultures supports survival and fiber outgrowth of cultured hippocampal neurons, *J. Neurosci. Res.* **8:**195–204.

68. Nieto-Sampedro, M., Lewis, E. R., Cotman, C. W., Manthorpe, M., Skaper, S. D., Barbin, G., Longo, F. M., and Varon, S., 1982, Brain injury causes a time-dependent increase in neuronotrophic activity at the lesion site, *Science* **217:**860–861.

69. Nieto-Sampedro, M., Manthorpe, M., Barbin, G., Varon, S., and Cotman, C. W., 1983, Injury-induced neuronotrophic activity in adult rat brain: Correlation with survival of delayed implants in the wound cavity, *J. Neurosci.* **3:**2219–2229.

70. Nottebohm, F., 1985, Neuronal replacement in adulthood, *Ann. N.Y. Acad. Sci.* **457:**143–161.

71. Olney, J. W., 1983, Excitotoxins: An overview, in: *Excitotoxins* (K. Fuxe, P. Roberts, and R. Schwarcz, eds.), Macmillan, London, pp. 82–96.

72. Olney, J. W., Collins, R. C., and Sloviter, R. S., 1986, Excitotoxic mechanisms of epileptic brain damage, in: *Advances in Neurology,* Volume 44 (A. D. Delgado-Escueta, A. A. Ward. Jr., D. M. Woodbury, and R. J. Porter, eds.), Raven Press, New York, pp. 857–877.

73. Olney, J. W., Fuller, T. A., Degubareff, T., and Labruyere, J., 1981, Intrastriatal folic acid mimics the distant but not local brain damaging properties of kainic acid, *Neurosci. Lett.* **25:**207–210.

74. Olney, J. W., Fuller, V. A., and Degubareff, T., 1981, Kainate-like neurotoxicity of folates, *Nature* **292:**165–167.

75. Olney, J. W., Labruyere, J., Collins, J. F., and Curry, K., 1981, D-Aminophosphonovalerate is 100-fold more powerful than D-α-amino adipate in blocking N-methylaspartate neurotoxicity, *Brain Res.* **221:**207–210.

76. Olson, L., Backlund, E. O., Freed, W., Herrera-Marschitz, M., Hoffer, B., Seiger, Å., and

Stromberg, I., 1985, Transplantation of monoamine-producing cell systems *in oculo* and intracranially: Experiments in search of a treatment for Parkinson's disease, *Ann. N.Y. Acad. Sci.* **457**:105–126.

77. Paton, J. A., and Nottebohm, F. N., 1984, Neurons generated in the adult brain are recruited into functional circuits, *Science* **225**:1046–1048.

78. Petteman, B., Labourdette, G., Weibel, M., and Sensenbrenner, M., 1986, The brain fibroblast growth factor (FGF) is localized in neurons, *Neurosci. Lett.* **68**:175–180.

79. Price, J., and Hynes, R. O., 1985, Astrocytes in culture synthesize and secrete a variant form of fibronectin, *J. Neurosci.* **8**:2205–2211.

80. Prince, D. A., Pedley, T. A., and Ransom, B. R., 1978, Flucfuations in ion concentrations during excitation and seizures, in: *Dynamic Properties of Glia Cells* (E. Schoffeniels, G. Franck, L. Hertz, and D. B. Tower, eds.), Pergamon Press, London, pp. 281–303.

81. Rakic, P., 1981, Neuronal glial interaction during brain development, *Trends Neurosci.* **4**:240–244.

82. Rakic, P., 1985, DNA synthesis and cell division in the adult primate brain, *Ann. N.Y. Acad. Sci.* **457**:193–212.

83. Rakic, P., Bourgeois, J. P., Eckenhoff, M. F., Zecevic, N., and Goldman-Rakic, P. S., 1986, Concurrent overproduction of synapses in diverse regions of the primate cerebral cortex, *Science* **232**:232–235.

84. Ransom, B. R., and Goldring, S., 1973, Ionic determinants of membrane potential of cells presumed to be glia in cerebral cortex of cat, *J. Neurophysiol.* **36**:885–886.

85. Rogers, S. L., Letourneau, P. C., Palm, S. L., McCarthy, J., and Farcht, L. T., 1983, Neurite extension by peripheral and central nervous system neurons in response to substratum-bound fibronectin and laminin, *Dev. Biol.* **98**:212–220.

86. Rudge, J. S., Manthorpe, M., and Varon, S., 1985, The output of neuronotrophic and neurite-promoting agents from rat brain astroglial cells: A microculture method for screening potential regulatory molecules, *Dev. Brain Res.* **19**:161–172.

87. Rutishauser, U., 1983, Molecular and biological properties of a neural cell adhesion molecule, *Cold Spring Harbor Symp. Quant. Biol.* **48**:501–514.

88. Saneto, R. P., and De Vellis, J., 1985, Effect of mitogens in various organs and cell culture conditioned media on rat oligodendrocytes, *Dev. Neurosci.* **7**:340–350.

89. Schachner, M., Faissner, A., Kruse, J., Lindner, J., Meier, D. H., Rathjen, F. G., and Wernecke, H., 1983, Cell-type specificity and developmental expression of neural cell-surface components involved in cell interactions and of structurally related molecules, *Cold Spring Harbor Symp. Quant. Biol.* **48**:557–568.

90. Schanne, F. A. X., Kane, A. B., Young, E. E., and Farber, J. L., 1979, Calcium dependence of toxic cell death: A common pathway, *Science* **206**:700–702.

91. Schwarcz, R., Whetsell, W. O., Jr., and Foster, A. C., 1983, The neurodegenerative properties of intracerebral quinolinic acid and its structural analog *cis*-2,3,-piperidine dicarboxylic acid, in: *Excitotoxins* (K. Fuxe, P. Roberts, R. Schwarcz, eds.), Macmillan, London, pp. 122–137.

92. Selak, I., Foidart, J. M., and Moonen, G., 1985, Laminin promotes cerebellar granule cells migration *in vitro* and is synthesized by cultured astrocytes, *Dev. Neurosci.* **7**:278–285.

93. Selak, I., Skaper, S. D., and Varon, S., 1985, Pyruvate participation in the low molecular weight trophic activity for CNS neurons in gliaconditioned media, *J. Neurosci.* **5**:23–28.

94. Sensenbrenner, M., Labourdette, G., Delaunoy, J. P., Pettman, B., Devillers, G., Moonen, G., and Bocq, E., 1980, Morphological and biochemical differentiation of glial cells in primary culture, in: *Tissue Culture in Neurobiology* (E. Giacobini, A. Vernadakis, and A. Shahar, eds.), Raven Press, New York, pp. 385–395.

95. Simon, R. P., Griffiths, T., Evans, M. C., Swan, J. H., and Meldrum, B. S., 1984, Calcium

overload in selectively vulnerable neurons of the hippocampus during and after ischemia: An E.M. study in the rat, *J. Cereb. Blood Flow Metab.* **4:**350–361.

96. Simon, R. P., Swan, J. H., Griffiths, T., and Meldrum, B. S., 1984, Pharmacologic blockade of excitatory amino acid neurotransmission attenuates the neuropathologic damage of ischemia, *Ann. Neurol.* **16:**112–124.

97. Simon, R. P., Swan, J. H., Griffiths, T., and Meldrum, B. S., 1984, N-Methyl-D-aspartate receptor blockade prevents ischemia brain damage, *Science* **226:**850–852.

98. Simpson, D. L., Morrison, R., De Vellis, J., and Herschman, H. R., 1982, Epidermal growth factor binding and mitogenic activity in purified populations of cells from the central nervous system, *J. Neurosci. Res.* **8:**453–462.

99. Soreq, H., and Miskin, R., 1983, Plasminogen activator in the developing rat cerebellum: Biosynthesis and localization in granular neurons, *Dev. Brain Res.* **11:**149–159.

100. Thoenen, H., and Barde, Y. A., 1980, Physiology of nerve growth factor, *Physiol. Rev.* **60:**1284–1335.

101. Varon, S., 1985, Factors promoting the growth of the nervous system, *Discussion in Neuroscience,* FSNS (Foundation for the Study of the Nervous System), Volume II, No. 3, pp. 1–62.

102. Varon, S., and Adler, R., 1980, Nerve growth factors and control of nerve growth, *Curr. Top. Dev. Biol.* **16:**207–252.

103. Varon, S., Nomura, J., and Shooter, E. M., 1967, The isolation of the mouse nerve growth factor protein in a high molecular weight form, *Biochemistry* **6:**2202–2209.

104. Varon, S., Raiborn, S., and Burnham, P. A., 1974, Comparative effects of nerve growth factor and ganglionic non-neuronal cells on purified mouse ganglionic neurons in culture. *J. Neurobiol.* **5:**355–371.

105. Vyskocil, F., Kriz, N., and Bures, J., 1972, Potassium selective microelectrodes used for measuring the extracellular brain potassium during spreading depression and anoxic depolarization, *Brain Res.* **39:**255–259.

106. Westermark, B., 1976, Density-dependent proliferation of human glia cells stimulated by epidermal growth factor, *Biochem. Biophys. Res.* **69:**304–310.

107. Wood, P. M., and Bunge, R. P., 1986, Evidence that axons are mitogenic for oligodendrocytes isolated from adult animals, *Nature* **320:**756–758.

14

GROWTH-ASSOCIATED TRIGGERING FACTORS AND CENTRAL NERVOUS SYSTEM RESPONSE TO INJURY

MICHAL SCHWARTZ, ADRIAN HAREL, CATHY STEIN-IZSAK, ARIE SOLOMON, VERED LAVIE, YOSEF BAWNIK, AND MICHAEL BELKIN

ABSTRACT. Mammalian central nervous system (CNS) neurons have negligible posttraumatic regenerative capacity, whereas nerves of lower vertebrates and of the peripheral nervous system of mammals regenerate spontaneously after injury.

The relationships between neurons and nonneuronal cells are vital for the neuron's maintenance and function. Trauma alters these relationships, causing nonneuronal cell proliferation, and in adult mammalian CNS creates an environment that is nonsupportive for regeneration. Introduction of a presumably supportive environment derived from a regenerating nerve to injured mammalian CNS induces a regenerationlike response. This effect is probably mediated by diffusible substances secreted by the nonneuronal cells.

We have applied diffusible substances obtained from either regenerating fish optic nerves or neonatal rabbit optic nerves around crushed adult rabbit optic nerve. This manipulation caused the adult nerve to show regenerative changes: increased protein synthesis in the retina, selective increase in synthesis of a few polypeptides in retina, sprouting from retina *in vitro*, increased viability of nerve fibers as shown by HRP staining, and the appearance of growth cones adjacent to glial limitans in the injured nerves. We termed these diffusible active factors "growth-associated triggering factors" (GATFs). One such factor was found to have molecular weight of less than 4000. The active preparation (media conditioned by regenerating fish optic nerve) causes, in addition to the phenomena described above, various other changes in the injured nerve itself: acceleration of nonneuronal cell proliferation, changes in the protein pattern, e.g., an increase in a 12-kDa polypeptide that might be a second mediator in the cascade of events leading to regeneration, increased laminin immunoreactive sites in the nerve, and the acquisition of GATF activity in media conditioned by the implanted injured nerves.

Comparison of mRNA derived from nonneuronal cells surrounding regenerating and non-

MICHAL SCHWARTZ, ADRIAN HAREL, CATHY STEIN-IZSAK, VERED LAVIE, AND YOSEF BAWNIK • Department of Neurobiology, The Weizmann Institute of Science, Rehovot, Israel.   ARIE SOLOMON AND MICHAEL BELKIN • Goldschleger Eye Institute, Tel Aviv University, Tel Hashomer, Israel.

regenerating fish optic nerves showed changes in the nonneuronal RNA-translated polypeptides. These mRNA preparations contain sequences homologous to the oncogenes *fos* and *myc*. The level of hybridization was found to increase during regeneration compared with that in the intact nerve. The significance of these oncogenes in the nonregenerating fish nerve and their increased expression during regeneration might be a mechanism whereby growth of nonneuronal cells is regulated.

It is suggested that nonneuronal cells have the capacity to contol neuronal regeneration ability provided that they undergo the required changes at the appropriate time. Any nonneuronal cell malfunction may lead to failure of regeneration. This brings an optimistic way to view regeneration, as it suggests that mammalian CNS glial cells have the capacity to support regeneration with appropriate modulation at the right time.

1. INTRODUCTION

The nervous system is a sophisticated communication network that senses, integrates, and transduces information between the external and internal milieus and within the latter. The integrity of the network, which is essential for its successful functioning, may be disrupted by an injury, with a consequent process of degeneration that leads to functional abnormalities that may be either reversible or irreversible. The functional activity may be rescued by early prevention of degeneration or by a process of regeneration. In order to prevent degeneration, the survival demands of the injured axon should be met prior to the period at which axonal disintegration commences; however, very little is known about the nature of these survival demands.

Whenever degeneration cannot be prevented, recovery of the injured neuron depends on its ability to regenerate. Neuronal regeneration means regrowth of injured axons followed by restoration of their synaptic connections and, finally, recovery of the original physiological functions. Different classes of neurons and neurons of different species differ in their ability to regenerate. Thus, for example, neurons of lower vertebrates ordinarily regenerate. This also holds for neurons of the peripheral nervous system (PNS) in mammals. Distinctively, most of the neurons of the central nervous system (CNS) in mammals seldom regenerate.[2,11,22,34]

Successful regeneration probably depends on a well-defined progression of the events that are involved in the various stages throughout the process. The cascade of events may be triggered by one or more signals that may be provided either by the axonal injury itself or by injury-induced changes in the neuronal environment. Induction of regeneration by the injury itself implies that regenerative and nonregenerative nerves differ in an intrinsic property that is essential for regeneration. Induction of regeneration by environmental factors implies that both the regenerative and nonregenerative nerves may be similar but that the environment of the nonregenerative nerves lacks constituents essential for regeneration (or contains inhibitory elements). Studies on regeneration have therefore focused on identifying the factors (neuronal or environmental) that allow the neurons to shift from a mature resting state into a growth state and thereby to accomplish the subsequent events needed for regeneration. In this chapter we discuss the literature related to the fate of the neuron in response to injury and how it is affected by the environment. In addition, our own results, which support the notion that environment-derived factors affect regeneration competence, are presented.

2. Background and Literature Survey

2.1. Regeneration-Associated Events in the Neuron

The neuronal cell body synthesizes and produces the materials required for growth of the nerve during development and during injury-induced regeneration as well as for axonal maintenance or maturation. Injury causes metabolic alterations that are reflected in morphological and biochemical changes in the cell body. Some of these changes have been correlated with regeneration and do not occur in nonregenerative systems. Most of the changes are presumably needed to equip the neurons with substances necessary for fiber construction, for recognition between fibers and supportive cells, and for target reconnection.

Neuronal substances required for axonal growth, maintenance, and function are synthesized in the cell body[36] and are transferred to the axon via axonal transport mechanisms. Axonal transport, therefore, should play a major role in the process of regeneration. Indeed, in addition to changes in synthesis, injury induces changes in type, amount, and rate of transport of neuronal substances, which include proteins, RNA, and polyamine-related compounds.[6,17,25,30,31,40,52,55,72] The transported RNA includes primarily t-RNA molecules, presumably participating in posttranslational modifications required for growth during regeneration[30,32] and for axonal maintenance. The polyamine-related compounds (i.e., putrescine, spermine, and spermidine) undergo increased axonal transport in regenerating optic nerves (examined in fish). In addition, there are changes in retrograde axonal transport of target- or environmental-derived substances.[20]

The anterogradely transported polypeptides that undergo changes after injury are the structural proteins, growth-associated proteins, and neurotransmitter-related proteins. Lipids were also shown to undergo changes in the course of regeneration.

2.1.1. Structural Proteins

In this category the only protein that has been intensively studied is tubulin.[24] During injury-induced regeneration there is an increase in tubulin synthesis in the fish optic nerve,[24,48] preferentially of the β subunit,[48] and a selective increase in the synthesis of two low-molecular-weight microtubule-associated proteins (τ factors).[48] The synthesis of other cytoskeleton-related proteins also increases. This includes actin, neurofilamentlike proteins, and membrane-associated cytoskeletal materials.[25,40,56]

2.1.2. Growth-Associated Proteins

Growth-associated proteins are cytoplasmic and membrane-associated polypeptides whose levels are correlated with growth during neuronal development and regeneration. The growth-associated proteins are hardly detectable in the mature intact neurons, but during regeneration they are expressed to a higher level in lower vertebrates (specifically in the visual system) and in mammalian PNS.[72]

No specific role has been assigned, so far, to any of the growth-associated proteins. However, the timing of appearance of individual proteins during regeneration implies that they play a distinct role in this process. Specifically, the acidic 43- to 49-kDa polypeptide[5] is synthesized on target disconnection (i.e., injury), but it is turned off independently of reconnection with the target. Distinctively, the 24- to 27-kDa polypeptides, although turned on by the disconnection from the target, return to their basal level only on reconnection.[4] Other regeneration-associated polypeptides are those whose levels transiently increase only if reconnection with the appropriate target organ is made. Their appearance may be associated with synaptogenesis and therefore with cessation of growth. This is further substantiated by the observation that in the absence of the primary target of the regenerating fibers, the regenerative response (manifested morphologically and biochemically) does not cease.[4,9,16,41] Similar changes in protein synthesis (putative growth-associated proteins) may appear in nonregenerative systems in response to artificially imposed external signals,[23,62] although they do not ordinarily appear in such systems after injury.

In both regenerative and nonregenerative systems, in addition to changes in protein synthesis, there are changes in translation products of mRNA derived from the tissues in which the cell bodies are located. This has been demonstrated so far in goldfish retinas with injured optic nerves[10,48,67] and in rabbit retinas having injured optic nerves supplied with exogenous factors.[67]

2.1.3. Lipids

The amounts of transported lipids,[13,19] especially gangliosides, are also increased after injury[61] in fish optic nerves. Gangliosides were shown to be involved in trophic interactions needed for axonal growth and maintenance.[18,65,66] Other lipids, such as cholesterol, may have a role in regeneration.[26] Exogenous application of phosphatidylcholine, phosphatidylserine, and cholesterol to regenerating retinas *in vitro* caused modulation of growth.[54] Other indications for the association between lipids and regeneration emerged from recent studies that identified a polypeptide (37 kDa) derived from nonneuronal cells of rat sciatic nerve as a form of apolipoprotein E (ApoE),[29,64] presumably involved in lipid degradation and metabolism.

2.2. NEURONAL–MICROENVIRONMENT RECIPROCAL RELATIONSHIP

2.2.1. RESPONSE TO AXONAL INJURY AND NERVE TRANSPLANTATION

The biochemical changes that occur in a regenerating neuron, described in the previous chapter, are associated with the establishment of a growth state and subsequent axonal elongation. The absence of these biochemical changes, including the obligatory ones, in nonregenerative nerves may stem from inappropriate behavior of the neuronal microenvironment in response to the injury.

In intact nerves there is a mutual relationship between the axon and the nonneuronal cells. This relationship is presumably required for the maintenance and functional activity of the axon and the fully differentiated nonneuronal cells. As a result of an injury, the neuron is deprived of target-derived substances, and the mutual relationship with the environment is disrupted, with a consequent transition of the environment to regeneration supportive or to regeneration inhibitory.

Axotomy induces changes in the state of growth of the surrounding nonneuronal cells,[44–47,70] which may lead to formation of an environment hostile to regeneration as a result of the appearance of either a glial scar tissue or axonal growth inhibitors.[39] In the last cited work, attempts were made to attribute the regenerative failure of axons in the adult mammalian CNS to the release of growth inhibitors from injured oligodendrocytes, from myelin sheath, or from both. Alternatively, the glial proliferation may lead to formation of a growth-supportive environment.[38,62,71,74] It appears that the formation of both hostile and supportive environments may occur at different time periods after injury.[47] It is the net outcome of these opposing contributions that may have an impact on the nature of the response to the injury, i.e, regeneration or degeneration.

Surgical manipulations were performed to determine whether a dense glial scar, which is formed by proliferating glial cells, interferes with outgrowth of neurites in regeneration. These studies showed that such a scar does not represent a major obstacle to axonal growth.[58,59] However, there is no conclusive information as to the contribution of scarring to the failure of regeneration in mammalian CNS.[8,35,43] It is possible that the lack of regeneration may stem not from hostile glial cells but from a deficiency in reactive glial cells.[54]

Nerve transplantation experiments demonstrated that the neuronal environment must be conducive for regeneration.[1,14,33,60] Injured spinal cord and brain axons regenerate readily through grafted columns of Schwann cells in peripheral

nerves but seldom enter grafted CNS nerve segments.[1,33,60] This indicates that
in contrast to glial cells, the nonneuronal cells of the peripheral nerves (e.g., the
Schwann cells) or components associated with them (e.g., diffusible or extracellular matrix) have the appropriate properties for regeneration.

2.2.2. ENVIRONMENT-DERIVED DIFFUSIBLE MOLECULES AND RESPONSE TO INJURY

Diffusible substances originating from nonneuronal cells may function as
trophic agents in the process of regeneration[38,71,74] and may affect glial proliferation and differentiation, neurite survival, and growth.

Axonal injury causes changes in the activity of diffusible substances originating from the nonneuronal environment and also from the target organ. Thus,
for example, the growth of the proximal stump of a transected PNS nerve is
facilitated by diffusible proteinaceous molecules possibly anchored in the basal
lamina and released from the distal stump of the transected nerve.[37] Similarly,
axonal injury induces increased neurite-promoting activity in extracts of the
target organ.[21,27,50,51] Furthermore, extracts prepared from denervated adult
skeletal muscle contain an increased amount of neurotrophic activity that promotes survival of dissociated motor neurons and outgrowth of neurites from
explants of spinal cord maintained in serum-free defined media.[51] This injury-
induced increase in activity has also been observed in the brain. For example, the
activity of a diffusible substance that is collected from the site of a brain lesion
and affects the survival of chick sensory neurons in culture is increased after a
lesion.[49] Injury-induced increased activity is also manifested by the better survival of brain grafts in wound cavities several days after the injury.[49,50]

Injury to optic nerves of fish[57] and peripheral nerves of mammals[63] (both
regenerative systems) causes changes in the type and amount of diffusible substances derived from surrounding nonneuronal cells. In the peripheral nervous
system, these changes were manifested by the selective accumulation of a 37-
kDa polypeptide that was identified as a form of apolipoprotein E.[29,64] In an
attempt to get an insight into how environment-derived factors affect regeneration competence, we have used visual systems of fish and rabbit, representing
regenerative and nonregenerative CNS, respectively. The results of our studies
are summarized below.

3. RESULTS OBTAINED IN THE VISUAL SYSTEM

Injury to the visual system of the lower vertebrate, which is endowed with a
high capacity for regeneration, causes alterations that are manifested by changes
in the appearance of polypeptides derived from nonneuronal cells. Among such
polypeptides are a 28-kDa polypeptide that is not detectable in the intact nerve[57]

and a 12-kDa polypeptide that appeared in the intact nerve but displays an increased synthesis during regeneration.[3] Other polypeptides expressed quantitative alterations in the course of regeneration. It is possible that among these there are polypeptides responsible, at least in part, for transforming the environment of the fish optic nerve from a "resting state" (needed for maintenance) into a "reactive state" (needed for growth support).

3.1. MODIFICATIONS OF NEURONAL ENVIRONMENT AND REGENERATION

3.1.1. SUBSTANCES DERIVED FROM REGENERATING FISH OPTIC NERVE ACTIVATE INJURED ADULT RABBIT OPTIC NERVE

To test the assumption, proposed above, that injury induces environmental changes needed for regeneration, a graft of regenerating fish optic nerve was inserted into an injured (but nonregenerative) optic nerve of adult rabbit.[62] The transplantation caused a regenerationlike response in the rabbit retina. However, immunologic rejection of the graft was noticed shortly after the surgery. To avoid the rejection, we used a "wrap around" implant as a substitute for the graft. The injured nerve of the rabbit was "wrapped around" with a silicone tube that was internally coated with collagen and incubated prior to implantation in diffusible substances (i.e., conditioned media) derived from regenerating optic nerves of fish (either carp or goldfish). The resulting response in the rabbit optic nerve included events that fulfilled the following criteria for regenerative response occurring spontaneously after injury in a regenerative system, and which were therefore chosen as parameters for a regeneration-associated response: (1) general alterations in protein synthesis in the retinas, (2) alterations in synthesis of specific polypeptides in the retinas, (3) *in vitro* sprouting activity, and (4) *in vivo* survival and sprouting.

Conditioned media derived from regenerating fish optic nerve caused a general increase in protein synthesis in retinas of crushed rabbit optic nerves. The right optic nerve (R) of each animal served as control. The ratio L/R provides an index for protein synthesis or for changes in protein synthesis determined by incorporation of [35S]methionine into TCA-precipitable molecules.[62] This increase was observed in 90% of the animals tested (L/R = 1.5, average of all the tested animals). Media conditioned by intact fish optic nerves caused only a slight increase in protein synthesis (L/R = 0.9) relative to retinas of injured but untreated nerves (L/R = 0.76).

Gel electrophoretic analysis of the [35S]methionine-labeled products in the rabbit retinas revealed a preferential increase in labeling of 130-, 110-, 74-, 64-, and 26-kDa polypeptides (Fig. 1). Polypeptides of similar molecular weights (74 and 65 kDa) were also observed by us in retinas of regenerating fish optic nerves. Two-dimensional gel electrophoretic analysis further revealed increased syn-

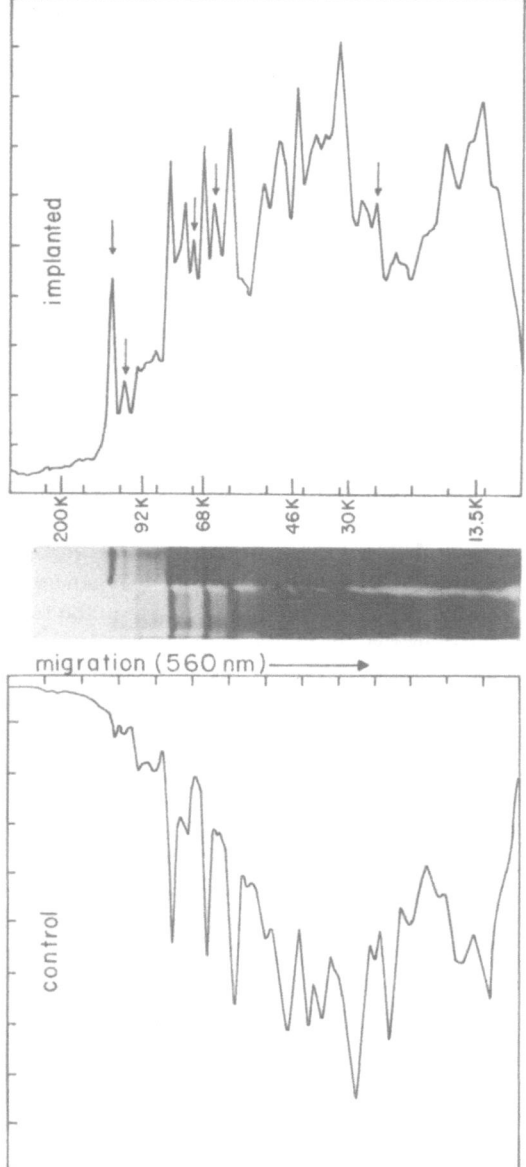

FIGURE 1. Gel analysis (SDS-PAGE, 7–20%) of rabbit retinal protein (100,000-g supernatant fraction) pulse labeled with [³⁵S]methionine. The retinal preparations were derived from untreated optic nerves (control) and optic nerves that were injured and implanted with substances originating from regenerating fish optic nerves (implanted). The figure illustrates both the fluorograms and their scans. Polypeptides that exhibited major changes (increase or newly appearing) are denoted by arrows. This pattern was found to be reproducible in ten tested preparations derived from distinct retinas. (From Schwartz et al.[62])

thesis of additional polypeptides. Some of these polypeptides are of similar molecular weights to the axonally transported proteins described in regenerating systems (including goldfish and toad optic nerves as well as mammalian sciatic nerves). It may be suggested that a few of these polypeptides function as specific growth-associated proteins and may be related to the GAPs defined by Willard and Skene.[72]

In vitro sprouting activity from the retinas was observed in culture. No sprouting could be detected in retinas of injured nerves that were implanted (as a control) with the silicone tubes that contained an irrelevant protein such as bovine serum albumin (Fig. 2).

Analysis of the rabbit optic nerve fibers using HRP labeling revealed the higher viability of fibers after conditioned medium implantation as opposed to fibers of nerves that were injured only. This higher viability was also manifested by the higher percentage of viable ganglion cells and nerve fibers in the treated nerves (Fig. 3). Along with this observation, electron microscopic analysis revealed the presence of growth cones in the injured nerves that were exposed to active conditioned medium derived from the regenerating fish optic nerves. Similarly, growth cones could not be detected in nerves that were injured and exposed to media free of active substances.

It should be noted that the observed growth cones in the implanted injured nerves seemed to be embedded in a tissue that appeared as the putative scar tissue (Fig. 4). This observation suggests that the proliferating glial cells do not necessarily impede growth and can even support it by forming a scaffold with a supportive surface for the growing fibers, provided that they acquire the appropriate properties at the appropriate time after the injury.

Thus, our study demonstrates that (1) an injured optic nerve of a non-regenerative system can be induced to express characteristics of regeneration provided that its environment is suitably modified, (2) an effective environmental modification can be achieved by diffusible substances derived from a regeneration-supportive environment, and (3) diffusible substances derived from regenerating optic nerves of fish have a significantly higher activity than those derived from intact optic nerves of fish. These results emphasize that changes in diffusible substances derived from the neuronal environment[57] are responsible for an increased activity of factors that can trigger a regenerative response. This higher activity may be the result of increased production of new or already existing substances. Alternatively, the higher activity may stem from activation of preexisting molecules, a reduced activity of inhibitors, or increased activity of materials that neutralize inhibitors.

Increased activity of media conditioned by regenerating fish optic nerve was also evident when the same conditioned media were examined for their effect on sprouting *in vitro*. This increase was shown to result, at least in part, from reduced levels of preexisting inhibitors.[57] It is not clear whether or not the same soluble substances are related to those that were found to be active *in situ* and, if

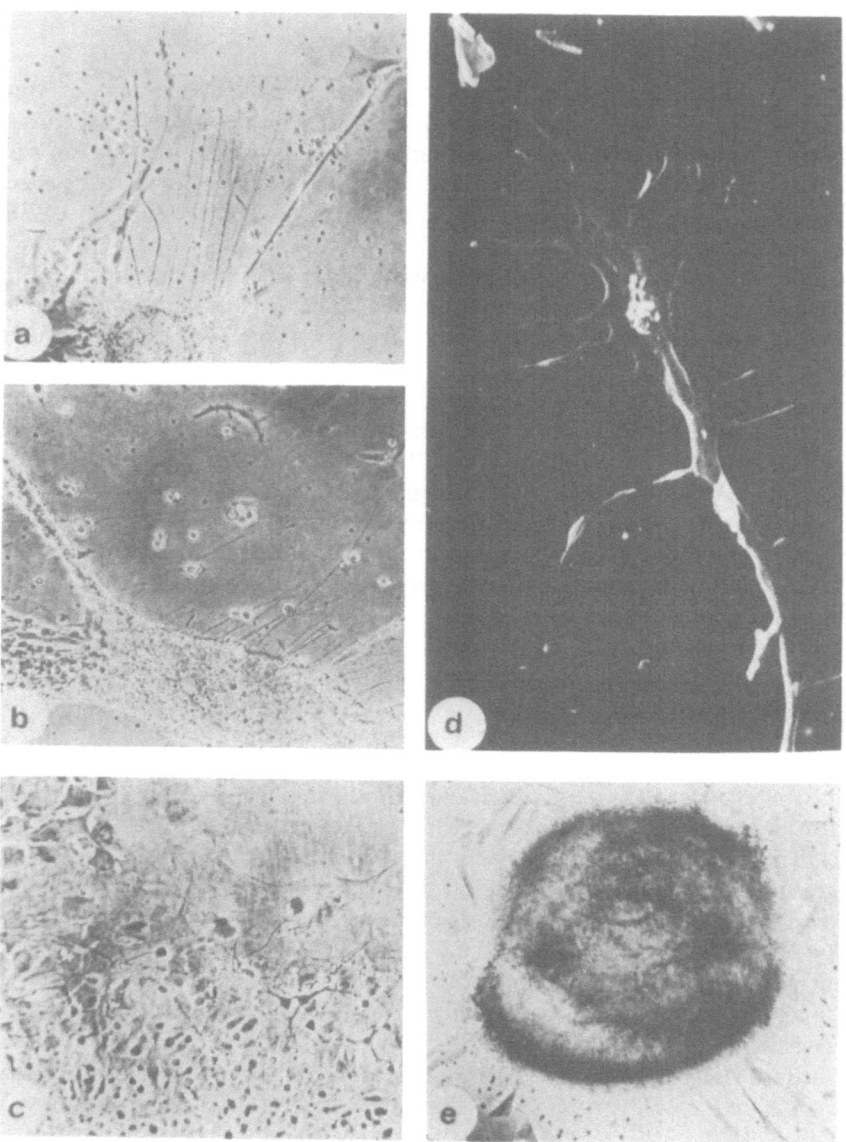

FIGURE 2. Neuritic outgrowth from rabbit retinas in culture. Rabbit retinas were excised 7 days following the surgery. The retinas were chopped into 400-μm squares and cultured on poly-L-lysine-coated dishes (0.1 mg/ml, Sigma) in DMEM supplemented with fetal calf serum (5%, Biolab), gentamycin sulfate (10 μg/ml, Sigma), HEPES (20 mM, Sigma), and glutamine (Biolab). Three retinas in each group were seperately examined. (a,b,d) Photomicrograph of cultured piece of rabbit retina of optic nerve that was injured and grafted with substances originating from regenerating optic nerve of fish; (a,b) ×70; (d) scanning electron micrograph of a growing fiber, ×9260. (c) Photomicrograph of a cultured retina of newborn rabbit optic nerve. (e) Micrograph of cultured rabbit retina of an injured optic nerve implanted with a silicone containing BSA. Note the lack of sprouts. ×140. (Three pictures in this composition were taken from Hadani *et al.*[23])

so, whether they are similarly regulated. This issue is currently under investigation.

Our study revealed that the observed activity is triggered by a non-NGF diffusible factor that is different from nerve growth factor (NGF), as an application of NGF in a silicone tube around the injured rabbit optic nerve did not cause any subsequent changes in the retinas (A. Harel, A. Solomon, M. Belkin, and M. Schwartz, unpublished data). Under the same experimental conditions, media conditioned by injured optic nerve of adult rabbit did not have any activity. In contrast, media conditioned by optic nerve of newborn rabbit displayed activity similar to that of media conditioned by the regenerating fish optic nerve, thus supporting our initial suggestion that the adult rabbit optic nerve can respond to exogenous factors but cannot provide them itself.[23] These results have led us to propose that the ability of a nerve to grow correlates with its ability to provide diffusible substances that can trigger a regenerationlike response in a non-regenerative system. For this reason, we named the active components growth-associated triggering factors (GATFs). It is possible that the observed effect induced by the conditioned medium is a result of several factors active consecutively or in concert. Purification of such a factor from media conditioned by regenerating fish optic nerve involved gel filtration and reverse-phase high-performance liquid chromatography. This procedure yielded a substance of about 500 daltons that caused a regenerationlike response in the retinas of the implanted injured nerves. Another factor, a protein of high molecular weight, caused an increase in laminin production. The latter is currently in the process of purification.

3.1.2. GATFs CAUSE ENVIRONMENTAL CHANGES

3.1.2a. THYMIDINE INCORPORATION AND PROTEIN PROFILE. The GATFs, when implanted around an injured optic nerve of an adult rabbit, may have a direct effect on the nonneuronal cells of the injured nerve. Alternatively, it is possible that the implanted triggering factors have a direct effect on the retinal cells (the ganglion cells or other neuronal or nonneuronal cells). To resolve this issue, several experiments were carried out in an attempt to find out whether the nonneuronal cells that surround the injured nerve displayed any changes after being exposed to these exogenous factors.

It appears that media conditioned by injured rabbit nerves that were implanted with neonatal-derived conditioned media and a week later dissected out and washed seemed to be able by themselves to provide active substances.[23] These changes in activity were accompanied by increased proliferation of perineural cells and changes in the profile of proteins derived from the GATF-treated nerves (Fig. 5). The major changes were in a 12-kDa polypeptide and in proteins having molecular weights similar to those of cytoskeletal elements. It is premature to attribute a role to the 12-kDa polypeptide. However, among other possibilities, it might be a secreted protein that comigrates with a polypeptide

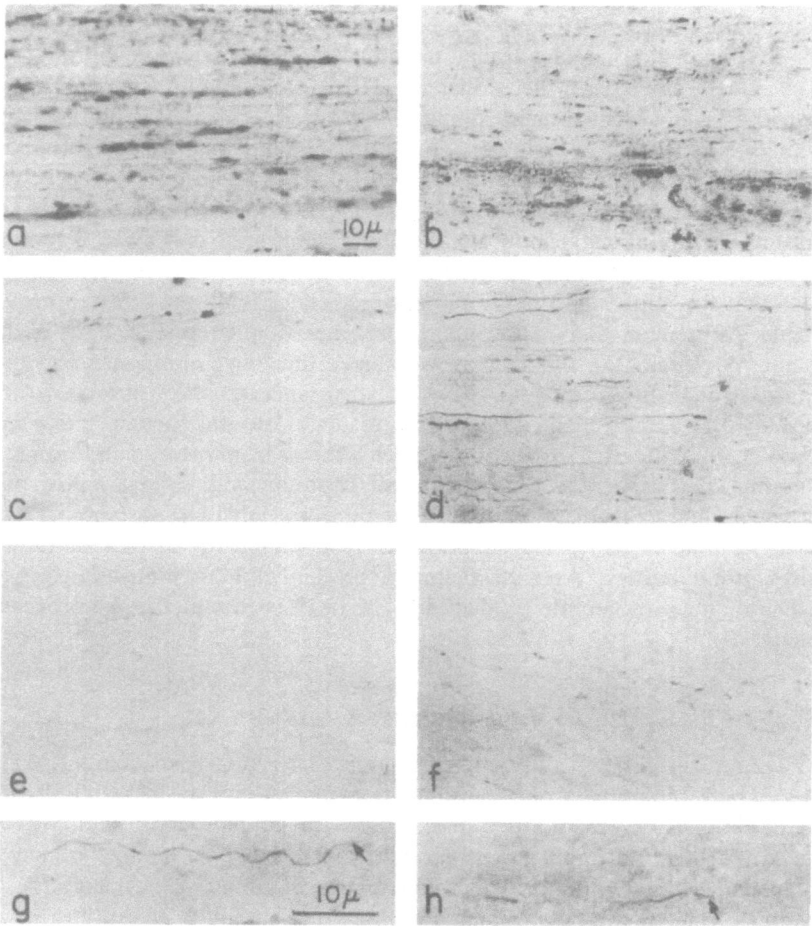

FIGURE 3. Horseradish-peroxidase-labeled optic nerves. Longitudinal cryosections were taken through the optic nerve, and labeled fibers were visualized with HRP using the Hanker–Yates method. (a,c,e) Nerve sections taken 1 week, 2 weeks, and 1 month, respectively, after the optic nerve crush. (b,d,f,g,h) Labeled nerves taken at the same time intervals as above, but after injury and implantation of silicone tube containing GATFs. Note the paucity of labeled fibers in the implanted injured nerve (f–h) and their absence in the control (e). The arrows point to structures that resemble growing fibers. (From Lavie *et al.*[36a])

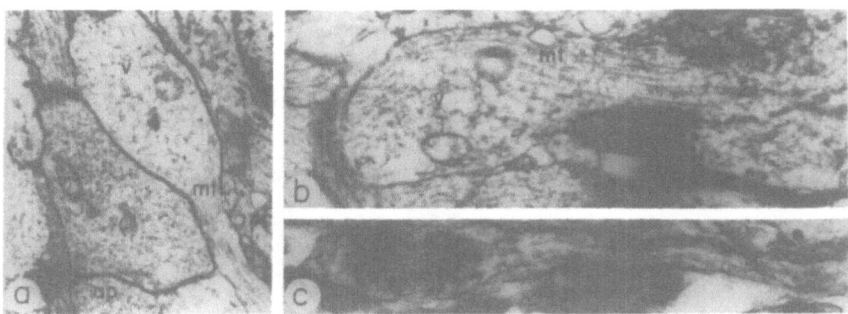

FIGURE 4. Growth cones in scaffold formed by glial processes after injury and implantation. Micrographs a and b represent sections taken from rabbit optic nerves that were injured and treated with GATF, whereas micrograph c represents a section taken from newborn rabbit optic nerve. In b, abundant glial cells with process (ap) are seen, among which a growth cone (gc) and nerve fibers are embedded. Typical growth cones of a newborn optic nerve of rabbit is seen in c.

originating from media conditioned by regenerating fish optic nerves (Fig. 5). Accordingly, the 12-kDa polypeptide might be a second mediator in the cascade of events that is induced by GATFs and leads to the neuronal regeneration response. This hypothesis can be tested by *in vitro* application of the isolated and purified 12-kDa polypeptide to nerves. (Isolation of the 12-kDa polypeptide is underway.) It is possible that GATFs cause additional alterations mainly in triggering growth-related events such as in the composition of the extracellular matrix, known to play a role in regeneration.[73] The technique used in Fig. 5 was not sufficiently sensitive to detect such components.

3.1.2b. LAMININ-IMMUNOREACTIVE SITES. To investigate possible GATF-induced alterations in the extracellular matrix, we decided to employ immunocytochemical tools. Specifically, we examined the presence of laminin-immunoreactive sites, since laminin is a matrix component that, in a regenerative system, contributes to the formation of a growth-supportive milieu.[15,28,73]

Our results revealed that in cryostat sections of intact adult rabbit optic nerve, laminin-immunoreactive sites appeared in the epineurium and around the sparsely distributed blood vessels. Following injury, laminin immunoreactivity could be detected in the epineurium, in connective tissue surrounding blood vessels, and in coarse bundles of scar tissue. However, after injury and application of GATF, the pattern of laminin immunoreactivity was changed, and additional laminin reactive sites could be detected. These appeared as a fine network coursing throughout the matrix of the nerve at the actual site of injury as well as at sites proximal, but not distal, to it. The more widespread distribution of laminin may be directly induced by the GATFs or may result from a cascade of events initiated by the GATFs. It could involve increased production or secretion of laminin or other metabolic changes that affect its accumulation.[75] Current

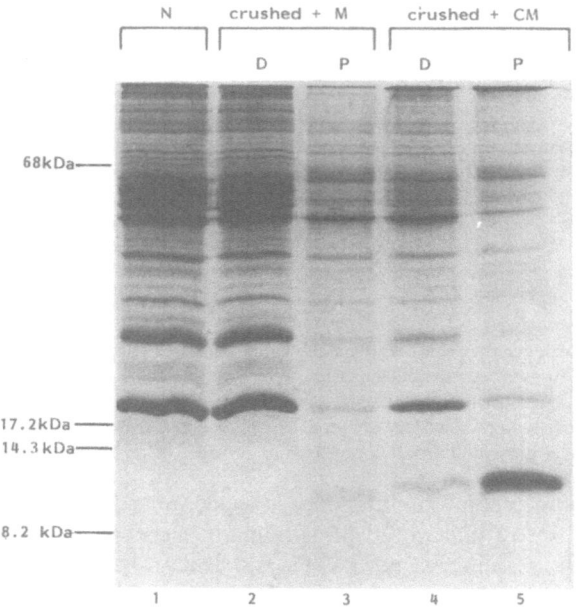

FIGURE 5. Exposure to GATFs induces the appearance of a 12-kDa polypeptide. Nerve homogenates (16 μ protein) of the various experimental groups were applied to SDS-polyacrylamide (15% acrylamide) gels. After electrophoresis, the gels were fixed and stained. The intensity of labeling of the 12-kDa polypeptide, as determined by densitometric scanning of the gel at 560 nm (Gilford), was approximately 30 times higher in the proximal segment of the GATF-treated nerve relative to the GATF-nontreated nerve. In nine of 13 GATF-treated rabbits, the 12-kDa polypeptide appeared as a prominent protein band. In none of the control rabbits (about 20 were tested) could such an increase be detected. (From Bawnik et al.[3])

studies are devoted to identifying the laminin-immunoreactive sites in fish and rabbit and to elucidating the mechanisms that regulate its accumulation in the adult fish optic nerve and its absence from the adult rabbit optic nerve.

3.2. MESSENGER RNA DERIVED FROM NONNEURONAL CELLS AND REGENERATION

We have shown that axonal injury in a system that is endowed with a high capacity for regeneration is accompanied by environmental changes. These changes are manifested by alterations in type, amount, and activity of diffusible molecules originating from such an environment. In order to get an insight into how these alterations are regulated and what might be the mechanism responsible for the changes in growth activity, several experiments were carried out in the fish visual system.

3.2.1. COMPARISON BETWEEN mRNA FROM REGENERATING AND NONREGENERATING FISH OPTIC NERVE

RNA extractions were achieved by the use of the guanidine isothiocyanate/CsCl protocol,[12] as it yielded the highest amount of translatable, nondegraded RNA. It appeared that regeneration is accompanied by changes in translated polypeptides from the RNA of nonneuronal cells surrounding a regenerating fish optic nerve as compared with RNA of an intact nerve analyzed by two-dimensional gel electrophoresis. The changes were mainly manifested in low-molecular-weight translated polypeptides.[68]

It is likely that the differences in translation of low-molecular-weight polypeptides in the regenerating preparation reflect true *in vivo* variability, yet they are not a direct result of variability in the average RNA size of the two preparations. Possibly the differences may stem from changes in the 5' ends of RNAs from the two preparations, making initiation of translation in one (the regenerating) more efficient than in the other (the normal). Indeed, much research is currently underway regarding the 5' terminus of the RNA and its effect on translation. In the regenerative CNS visual system of the fish, this may represent an efficient and finely tuned mechanism to control the proteins that the nonneuronal cells have available for themselves as well as for the axon under various physiological conditions.

3.2.2. NONNEURONAL CELLS IN REGENERATION AND ONCOGENES

Our results suggest that when the neuron regenerates, it initiates growth of fibers from the preexisting cell bodies while the perineural cells proliferate. The nonneuronal cell response may be typical of a growing tissue with a possible autonomous type of regulation that may be shifted back to a nonautonomous mode on termination of the axonal regeneration and growth. This might be a mechanism whereby a system transiently operates more efficiently to compensate for an increased need for growth factors. We therefore wanted to discover whether there is homology between the genes involved in the control of growth and proliferation of the nonneuronal cells in regeneration and cellular oncogenes. Oncogene products may function as growth factors, their membrane receptors, intracellular messengers, or other constituents in the growth response that leads ultimately to DNA synthesis, cell division, and regeneration. We therefore investigated whether, *in vivo*, the response to neuronal injury involves changes in the expression of any oncogene.

Our results suggest that RNA from cells surrounding optic nerves of fish contain sequences homologous to the oncogenes *fos* and *myc*. Hybridization with *fos* and *myc* was visible in mRNA derived from both noninjured nerves and regenerating nerves but was two to five times higher in the mRNA of regenerating nerve.[69]

Several *in vitro* studies have shown that expression of the *fos* gene is a transient and early response to mitogenic stimuli. It may be that in the visual system expression of *fos*, or *fos*-like activity, increases within hours or even days following the mitogenic stimulus of optic nerve injury. The observed increased expression in fish, measured 8 days after injury, may represent the peak or may already be a decline to base-line levels. The significance of *fos* and *myc* in the intact nerve, their increased level in regeneration, and their cellular origin among the nonneuronal cells warrant further study, as they may provide tools for understanding glial growth regulation in response to injury in regenerative and nonregenerative systems.

We have shown that after injury both the neurons and their surrounding nonneuronal cells are activated. The nonneuronal cells respond in a manner that might be similar to a reparative response of any other proliferative tissue. The lack of regeneration may stem from an inability of the glial cells of mammals to accomplish this response and thereby to acquire the appropriate properties at the right time. Perhaps the triggering factors provided by nonneuronal cells of growing (regenerating or developing) nerves can cause their activation.

Further characterization of the active components, analysis of their mode of action, determination of the extent of the anatomic regeneration that they induced, and establishment of other means of their application, possibly with other components known to be absent in mammalian CNS, may eventually contribute to alleviating the problem of the mammalian nonregenerative CNS.

REFERENCES

1. Aguayo, A., Samuel, D., Richardson, P., and Bray, G., 1978, Axonal elongation in peripheral and central nervous system transplantations, *Adv. Cell. Neurobiol.* 3:215–221.
2. Attardi, D. G., and Sperry, R. W., 1963, Preferential selection of central pathways by regenerating optic nerve, *Exp. Neurol.* 7:46–64.
3. Bawnik, Y., Harel, A., Stein-Izsak, C., and Schwartz, M., 1986, Environmental changes induced by growth associated triggering factors in injured optic nerve of adult rabbit, *Proc. Natl. Acad. Sci. U.S.A.* 84:2528–2531.
4. Benowitz, L. I., 1984, Target dependent and target independent changes in rapid axonal transport during regeneration of the goldfish retinotectal pathway, in: *Axonal Transport in Neuronal Growth and Regeneration* (J. S. Elam and P. Canalon, eds.), Plenum Press, New York, pp. 145–169.
5. Benowitz, L. I., and Lewis, E. R., 1983, Increased transport of 44,000 to 49,000 dalton acidic proteins during regeneration of the goldfish optic nerve, a two-dimensional gel analysis, *J. Neurosci.* 3:2153–2163.
6. Benowitz, L. I., Shashoua, V. E., and Yoon, M. G., 1981, Specific changes in rapidly transported proteins during regeneration of the goldfish optic nerve, *J. Neurosci.* 1981:300–307.
7. Benowitz, L. I., Yoon, M. G., and Lewis, E. R., 1983, Transported proteins in regenerating optic nerve regulation by interactions with optic tectum, *Science* 222:185–188.
8. Billingsley, M. L., and Mandel, H. G., 1982, Effect of DNA synthesis inhibitors on post-traumatic glial cell proliferation, *J. Pharmacol. Exp. Ther.* 222:765–770.

9. Burmeister, D. W., and Grafstein, B., 1984, Removal of optic tectum prolongs the cell body reaction to axotomy in goldfish retinal ganglion cell, *Brain Res.* **327**:45–51.

10. Burrel, H. R., Heacock, A. M., Water, R. D., and Agranoff, B W., 1979, Increased tubulin RNA in goldfish during optic nerve regeneration, *Brain Res.* **168**:628–632.

11. Cajal, S. Ramon y, 1928, *Degeneration and Regeneration of Nervous System,* Volume I (English translation by R. M. May), Hafner Publishing, New York, 1959.

12. Chirgwin, J. M., Przybyla, A. E., MacDonald, R. J., and Rutter, N. J., 1977, Isolation of biologically active ribonucleic acid from sources enriched in ribonuclease, *Biochemistry* **18**:5294–5299.

13. Currie, J. R., Grafstein, B., Whithall, M. H., and Alpert, R., 1978, Axonal transport of lipid in goldfish optic axons, *Neurochem. Res.* **3**:479–492.

14. David, S., and Aguayo, A. J., 1981, Axonal elongation into peripheral nervous system "bridges" after central nervous system injury in adult rats, *Science* **214**:931–933.

15. Davis, G. E., Varon, S., Engvall, E., and Manthorpe, M., 1985, Substratum-binding neurite promoting factors: relationships to laminin, *Trends Neurosci.* **8**:528–532.

16. Giulian, D., 1984, Target regulation of protein biosynthesis in retinal ganglion cells during regeneration of the goldfish visual system, *Brain. Res.* **296**:198–201.

17. Giulian, D., Des Ruisseaux, H., and Cowburn, D., 1980. Biosynthesis and intra-axonal transport of proteins during neuronal regeneration, *J. Biol. Chem.* **255**:6494–6501.

18. Gorio, A., Carnignoto, G., Facci, L., and Finesso, M., 1980, Motor nerve sprouting induced by ganglioside treatment, Possible implications for ganglioside on neuronal growth, *Brain Res.* **197**:236–241.

19. Grafstein, B., Miller, J. A., Ledeen, R. W., Haley, J., and Specht, S. C., 1975, Axonal transport of phospholipid in goldfish optic system, *Exp. Neurol.* **46**:261–278.

20. Grafstein, G., 1986, The retina as a regenerating organ, in: *The Retina as Model for Cell Biology Studies,* Part II (R. Adler and D. B. Farber, eds.), pp. 275–335.

21. Guilian, D., Allen, R. L., Baker, T. J., and Tomozawa, Y., 1986, Brain peptides and glial growth. I. Glial promoting factors as regulators of gliogenesis in the developing and injured central nervous system, *J. Cell Biol.* **102**:803–811.

22. Guth, L., and Windle, W., 1970, The enigma of central nervous system regeneration, *Exp. Neurol. [Suppl.]* **5**:1–43.

23. Hadani, M., Harel, A., Solomon, A., Belkin, M., Lavie, V., and Schwartz, M., 1984, Substances originating from the optic nerve of neonatal rabbit induce regeneration-associated response in the injured optic nerve of adult rabbit, *Proc. Natl. Acad. Sci. U.S.A.* **81**:7965–7969.

24. Heacock, A. M., and Agranoff, B. W., 1976, Enhanced labeling of retinal proteins during regeneration of the optic nerve in goldfish, *Proc. Natl. Acad. Sci. U.S.A.* **73**:828–832.

25. Heacock, A. M., and Agranoff, B. W., 1982, Protein synthesis and transport in the regenerating goldfish visual system, *Neurochem. Res.* **7**:771–778.

26. Heacock, A. M., Klinger, P. D., Deguin, E. B., and Agranoff, B. W., 1984, Cholesterol synthesis and nerve regeneration, *J. Neurochem.* **42**:987–993.

27. Henderson, C. E., Huchet, M., and Changeux, J.-P., 1983, Denervation increases a neurite-promoting activity in extracts of skeletal muscle, *Nature* **302**:609–611.

28. Hopkins, J. M., Ford-Holevinski, T. S., McCoy, J. P., and Agranoff, B. W., 1985, Laminin and optic nerve regeneration in the goldfish, *J. Neurosci.* **5**:3030–3038.

29. Ignatius, M. J., Gebicke-Harter, P. J., Skene, J. H. P., Schilling, J. W., Weisgraber, K. H., Mahley, R. W., and Shooter, E. M., 1986, Expression of apolipoprotein E during nerve degeneration and regeneration, *Proc. Natl. Acad. Sci. U.S.A.* **83**:1125–1129.

30. Ingolgia, N. A., and Tuliszewski, R., 1975, Transfer RNA may be axonally transported during regeneration of goldfish optic nerves, *Brain Res.* **112**:371–381.

31. Ingoglia, N. A., Sturman, J. A., and Eisner, R. A., 1977, Axonal transport of putrescine,

spermidine and spermine in normal and regenerating goldfish optic nerve, *Brain Res.* **130**:433–445.

32. Ingoglia, N. A., Sharma, S. C., Pilchman, J., Baranowski, K., and Sturman, J. A., 1982, Axonal transport and transcellular transfer of nucleosides and polyamines in intact and regenerating optic nerves of goldfish, speculation of the axonal regulation of periaxonal cell metabolism, *J. Neurosci.* **2**:1412–1423.

33. Kao, C. C., Chang, L. W., and Bloodworth, J. M. B., 1977, Axonal regeneration across transected mammalian spinal cords: An electron microscopic study of delayed microsurgical grafting, *Exp. Neurol.* **54**:591–615.

34. Kiernan, J. A., 1984, Hypotheses concerned with axonal regeneration in the mammalian nervous system, *Biol. Rev.* **54**:155–197.

35. Krikorian, J. G., Guth, L., and Donati, E. J., 1981, Origin of the connective tissue scar in transected rat spinal cord, *Exp. Neurol.* **72**:698–705.

36. Lasek, R. J., Dabrowski, C., and Norlander, R., 1977, Analysis of axoplasmic RNA from invertebrate giant axons, *Nature (New Biol.)* **244**:162–165.

36a. Lavie, V., Harel, A., Doron, A., Solomon, A., Lobel, D., Belkin, M., Benbasat, S., Sharma. S., and Schwartz, M., 1987, Morphological response of injured adult rabbit optic nerve to implants containing media conditioned by growing optic nerves, *Brain Res.* **419**:166–172

37. Longo, F. M., Skaper. S. D., Manthorpe, M., Williams, L. R., Lundborg, G., and Varon, S.. 1983, Temporal changes in neuronotrophic activities accumulating *in vivo* within nerve regeneration chambers. *Exp. Neurol.* **81**:756–769.

38. Manthorpe, M., Nieto-Sampedro, M., Skaper, S. D., Lewis, E. R., Longo, F. M., Cotman, C W., and Varon, S., 1983, Neurotrophic activity in brain wounds of the developing rat: Correlation with implants survival in the wound cavity, *Brain Res.* **267**:47–56.

39. McConnell, P., and Berry, M., 1982, Regeneration of ganglion cell axons in the adult mouse retina, *Brain. Res.* **241**:362–366.

40. McQuarrie, I. G., and Lasek, R. Y., 1981, Axonal transport of labeled neurofilaments proteins in goldfish optic axons, *J. Cell Biol.* **91**:234a.

41. Mizrachi, Y., Neuman, D., Sharma, S., and Schwartz, M., 1984, Target-dependent and independent stages in regeneration, *Brain Res.* **322**:115–118.

42. Mizrachi, Y., Rubinstein, M., Kimhi, Y., and Schwartz, M., 1986, A neurotrophic factor derived from goldfish brain: Characterization and purification, *J. Neurochem.* **46**:1675–1682.

43. Molander, H., Olsson, Y., Engkvist, O., Bowald, S., and Eriksson, I., 1982, Regeneration of peripheral nerve through a polyglactin tube, *Muscle Nerve* **5**:54–57.

44. Nathaniel, E. J. H., and Nathaniel, D. R., 1973, Regeneration of dorsal root fibers into the adult rat spinal cord, *Exp. Neurol.* **40**:333–350.

45. Nathaniel, E. J. H., and Nathaniel, D. R., 1981, The reactive astrocyte, *Adv. Cell. Neurobiol.* **2**:249–301.

46. Nathaniel, E. J. H., and Pease, D. R., 1963, Collagen and basement membrane formation by Schwann cells during nerve regeneration, *J. Ultrastruct. Res.* **9**:550–560.

47. Neumann, D., Yerushalmi, A., and Schwartz, M., 1983, Inhibition of nonneuronal cell proliferation in the goldfish visual pathway affects the regenerative capacity of the retina, *Brain Res.* **272**:237–245.

48. Neumann, D., Scherson, T., Ginzburg, I., Littauer, U. Z., and Schwartz, M., 1983, Regulation of mRNA levels for microtubule proteins during nerve regeneration, *FEBS Lett.* **162**:270–275.

49. Nieto-Sampedro, M., Manthorpe, M., Barbin, G., Varon, S., and Cotman, C. W., 1983, Injury-induced neuronotrophic activity in adult rat brain: Correlation with survival of delayed implants in the wound cavity, *J. Neurosci.* **3**:2219–2289.

50. Nieto-Sampedro, M., Whittemore, S. R., Needels, D. L., Larson, J., and Cotman, C. W., 1984, The survival of brain transplants is enhanced by extracts from injured brain, *Proc. Natl. Acad. Sci. U.S.A.* **81**:6250–6254.

51. Nurcombe, V., Hill, M. A., Eagleson, K. L., and Bennett, M. R., 1984, Motor neuron survival and neuritic extension from spinal cord explants induced by factors released from denervated muscle, *Brain Res.* **291**:19–28.

52. Perry, G. W., and Wilson, D. L., 1981, Protein synthesis and axonal transport during nerve regeneration, *J. Neurochem.* **37**:1203–1217.

53. Politis, M. J., 1985, Dynamics of induction of axonal regeneration in rat optic nerve, *Soc. Neurosci. Abstr.* **11**:1254.

54. Pollak-Rabinerson, N., Mizrachi, Y., Samuel, D., and Schwartz, M., 1985, The association between membrane fluidity and neuronal regeneration, *J. Neurochem.* **44**:525.

55. Quitschke, W., and Schechter, N., 1983, Specific optic nerve proteins during regeneration of the goldfish retinotectal pathway, *Brain. Res.* **258**:69–78.

56. Quitschke, W., and Schecter, N., 1984, 58,000 Dalton intermediate filament proteins of neuronal and nonneuronal origin in the goldfish visual pathway, *J. Neurochem.* **42**:569–576.

57. Rachailovich, I., and Schwartz, M., 1984, Molecular events associated with increased regenerative capacity of the goldfish retinal ganglion cells following x-irradiation: Decreased level of axonal growth inhibitors, *Brain Res.* **306**:149–155.

58. Reier, P. J., 1979, Penetration of grafted astrocytic scars by regenerating optic nerve axons in *Xenopus* tadpoles, *Brain Res.* **164**:61–68.

59. Reier, P. J., Stensaas, L. J., and Guth, L., 1983, The astrocytes scar as an impediment to regeneration in control nervous system, in: *Spinal Cord Reconstruction* (C. G. Kan, R. P. Bunge, and P. J. Reier, eds.), Raven Press, New York, pp. 163–195.

60. Richardson, P. M., Isaa, V. M. K., and Shemie, S., 1982, Regeneration and retrograde degeneration of axons in the rat optic nerve, *J. Neurocytol.* **11**:949–966.

61. Sbaschnig-Agler, M., Ledeen, R. W., Grafstein, B., and Alpert, R. M., 1984, Ganglioside changes in the regenerating goldfish optic system, comparison with glycoproteins and phospholipids in the regenerating goldfish optic system, *J. Neurosci. Res.* **12**:221–232.

62. Schwartz, M., Belkin, M., Harel, A., Solomon, A., Lavie, V., Hadani, M., Rachailovich, I., and Stein-Izsak, C., 1985, Regenerating fish optic nerves and regeneration-like response in injured optic nerve of adult rabbits, *Science* **228**:600–608.

63. Skene, J. H. P., and Shooter, E. M., 1983, Denervated sheath cells secrete a new protein after nerve injury, *Proc. Natl. Acad. Sci. U.S.A.* **80**:4173–4178.

64. Snipes, G. L., McGuire, C. B., Norden, J. J., and Freeman, J. A., 1986, Nerve injury stimulates the secretion of apolipoprotein E by non-neuronal cells, *Proc. Natl. Acad. Sci. U.S.A.* **83**:1130–1134.

65. Sparrow, J. R., McGuinness, C., Schwartz, M., and Grafstein, B., 1984, Antibodies to gangliosides inhibit goldfish optic nerve regeneration *in vivo*, *J. Neurosci. Res.* **12**:233–243.

66. Spirman, N., Sela, B. A., and Schwartz, M., 1982, Antiganglioside antibodies inhibit outgrowth from regenerating goldfish retinal explant, *J. Neurochem.* **39**:874–877.

67. Stein-Izsak, C., Harel, A., Solomon, A., Belkin, M., and Schwartz, M., 1985, Alterations in mRNA translation products are associated with regenerative response in the retina, *J. Neurochem.* **45**:1754–1760.

68. Stein-Izsak, C., Harel, A., Solomon, A., Neumann, D., Belkin, M., Rubinstein, M., and Schwartz, M., 1985, Molecular aspects of optic nerve regeneration in regenerative and non-regenerative systems, *Abstr. Neurosci.* **11**:1252.

69. Stein-Izsak, C., Breuer, O., and Schwartz, M., 1986, Expression of the proto-oncogenes *fos* and *myc* in optic nerve regeneration, *Abstr. Neurosci. Soc.* **12**:12.

70. Stevenson, J. A., and Yoon, M. G., 1978, Regeneration of optic nerve fibers enhances cell proliferation in the goldfish optic tectum, *Brain Res.* **153**:354–361.

71. Varon, S., Manthorpe, M., Longo, F. M., and Williams, L. R., 1983, Growth factors in regeneration of neural tissues, in: *Nerve, Organ and Tissue Regeneration, Research Perspectives* (F. Y. Seil, ed.), Academic Press, New York, p. 127.

72. Willard, M., and Skene, J. H., 1982, Molecular events in axonal regeneration, in: *Repair and Regeneration of the Nervous System* (J. G. Nicholls, ed.), Springer-Verlag, Berlin, Heidelberg, New York, pp. 71–81.

73. Williams, L. R., and Varon, S. S., 1985, Modification of fibrin matrix formation *in situ* enhances nerve regeneration in silicone chambers, *J. Comp. Neurol.* **213**:209–220.

74. Williams, L. R., Longo, F. M., Powell, H. C., Lundborg, G., and Varon, S., 1983, Spatial–temporal progress of peripheral nerve regeneration within a silicone chamber: Parameters for bioassay, *J. Comp. Neurol.* **218**:460–470.

75. Zak, N. B., Harel, A., Bawnik, Y., Benbasat, S., Vogel, Z., and Schwartz, M., 1986, Laminin immunoreactive sites are induced by growth-associated triggering factors in injured rabbit optic nerve, *Brain Res.* **408**:263–266.

15

Growth Factor Induction and Order of Events in CNS Repair

Manuel Nieto-Sampedro

ABSTRACT. In response to damage, the adult CNS exhibits capabilities, such as glial cell proliferation and differentiation and axonal sprouting and growth, typical of the developmental period. This "rejuvenation" of the CNS tissue arises as a consequence of the injury-induced increase in the activities of neurotrophic and sprouting factors and of glia, fibroblast, and endothelial cell mitogens and morphogens.

In the absence of neuronal division, true regeneration of the CNS is not possible. However, the knowledge of the biochemical events underlying the cellular response of the CNS to injury offers a way to intervene in the process and attempt functional repair.

Studies on the time course of induction of various growth activities after a lesion reveal that, contrary to what is observed during development, the process of injury repair does not follow a well-ordered temporal sequence. The increase in neurotrophic activity occurs simultaneously with that of axon-sprouting factors and at a time subsequent to most secondary neuronal death. The enhancement in the activity of nonneuronal mitogens (and the consequent proliferation of glial, fibroblast, and endothelial cells) precedes that of axon-sprouting factors. By giving priority to cell proliferation, the organism ensures the restitution of blood supply as well as that of the glia limitans and other CNS–body boundaries. But it compromises the regeneration of axons across the injury area.

This information, accumulated for the most part during the last 5 years, allows us to visualize various ways of intervention after CNS injury. One of the most obvious would be to supply purified neurotrophic factors to the affected area and thus save many neurons from secondary death. Another type of intervention that many of us have in mind is the replacement of lost neurons and their connections by means of transplants. Transplantation of donor CNS tissue at a time when production of neurotrophic and sprouting factors by the injured host is maximal would ensure optimal survival and integration of the donor neurons. Finally, the exogenous supply of purified neurite-sprouting and elongation factors, together with that of glial mitogen inhibitors (naturally present in the CNS), may facilitate the regeneration of interrupted pathways.

The purification and use of central growth factors and their inhibitors should eventually permit convergent multiple interventions to repair damaged CNS tissue. Correct timing and intertwining of the requirements of repair with the priorities of the organism seem essential.

MANUEL NIETO-SAMPEDRO • Department of Psychobiology, University of California at Irvine, Irvine, California 92717.

301

1. INTRODUCTION

Damage to the CNS breaks the physical and functional boundaries of the nervous tissue, disrupts the interactions between neural cells, and destroys both the neurons and the connections in which they are involved. Nerve cells do not proliferate, and damaged central nerve fibers regrow to a very limited degree. At the beginning of the century, Cajal showed that the damaged CNS, on its own, was unable to regenerate.[89] Subsequent morphological studies confirmed Cajal's observations while, at the same time, revealing that in response to injury the adult CNS "rejuvenates." Ironically, the damaged CNS exhibits most of the developmental capabilities required for regeneration. New capillary formation, glial proliferation and differentiation, axonal sprouting, and reactive synaptogenesis occur after mechanical trauma, stroke, and many degenerative diseases.[20,78] These responses seem appropriate to compensate for minor CNS lesions. However, the functional consequences of large CNS lesions are most frequently disastrous, and at present there are no treatments for CNS injury. In the absence of neuronal division, true regeneration, i.e., the restitution of the CNS to the preinjury state, is clearly impossible, and the best we can hope for is functional repair. This chapter describes the work carried out in our own and other laboratories, mostly in the last 6 years, attempting to find new ways to achieve such an objective.

2. CELLULAR EVENTS THAT FOLLOW CNS INJURY

The major events that follow severe CNS trauma are illustrated in Fig. 1. Immediately after severe CNS trauma, the blood–CNS barrier breaks down at the injury site. Local ischemia/hypoxia/hypoglycemia result from both vascular spasm and vascular disruption. Blood cells and serum proteins invade the injury area. Edema, resulting from both extracellular fluid accumulation and astrocyte swelling, is obvious 24 hr later.[43,49] Ultrastructural abnormalities in the axons in both gray and white matter can be observed immediately after a contusive injury, and uniform necrosis and myelin degeneration follow 8–24 hr later.[8] Many blood-derived macrophages accumulate 48 hr after an open wound and engulf degenerating myelin and other cell debris.[29]

Groups of neurons not killed immediately after injury begin to die 1–2 days later, and gradually enlarging cysts develop and coalesce to form cavities within the CNS parenchyma[45] that separate previously connected neurons. While phagocytosis is going on, astrocytes close to the lesion site begin to proliferate, and their enlarged fibrous processes form a web that isolates the surfaces of the injury from the surrounding tissue.[3,18] At about the same time, fibroblasts from the proximal connective tissue invade the injury site and overlay the injury surfaces with a layer of collagen,[51,111] completing the formation of a new boundary, the so-called "glial scar."

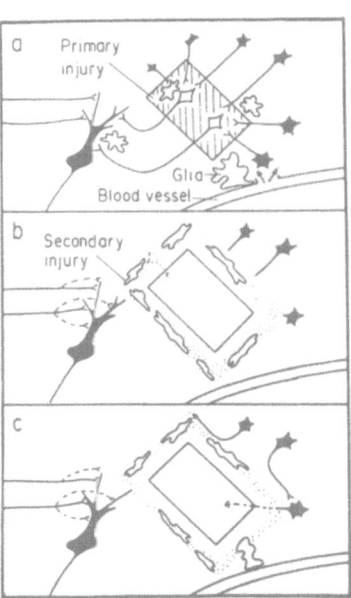

FIGURE 1. Sequence of events after CNS trauma. (a) Some neurons in the primary injury area die immediately. Other cells are axotomized or rendered ischemic by disruption of the local vasculature or vascular spasm. Injury triggers a cascade of events that results in (b) secondary neuronal death, that is, death of cells not directly affected by the injury. At the same time, debris is cleared, capillaries are repaired, and glial proliferation begins. A new CNS boundary is formed (so-called glial scar). Reactive and regenerative sprouts begin to grow. (c) However, regenerative sprouts are prevented from reaching their targets by a combination of the misguiding effects of the new glial boundary and reinnervation of their targets by reactive sprouts. Regenerative sprouts either die back or form inappropriate contacts near their site of origin. (Adapted from ref. 78.)

Complete clearing of degenerative debris may take many months, but in the adult, the bulk of it has been removed 4 or 5 days post-lesion, and sprouts from nearby undamaged neurons begin to appear at that time.[20] These fibers form new synapses that effectively repopulate vacated terminal fields. At about the same time, regenerating sprouts start to grow from axon stumps at the injury site. However, they have to grow a long distance before reaching their targets. Meanwhile, the glial scar (or neo-glia-limitans) has formed across the path of regenerating axons, which, deflected from their normal path, either die back or form new synapses with inappropriate proximal targets.[11a,89]

Unaided, the CNS cannot achieve complete functional repair. Intervention is necessary to prevent secondary neuronal death, to replace lost neurons, to control sprouting, and to guide the growth of regenerating sprouts across the glial boundary to their appropriate target. I consider each of these problems in turn and describe the progress achieved in dealing with them.

3. NEURONAL SURVIVAL AFTER CNS INJURY

Only a comparatively small number of neurons die acutely, i.e., in the first moments after a lesion. However, CNS injury does not terminate immediately after trauma. Many more neurons become necrotic within 24 hr post-lesion, and usually an even larger number die in the following 2–7 days in areas not directly affected by the injury (Fig. 1b). Cell death that is not acute is commonly denominated secondary death. Secondary neuronal death after CNS trauma arises from a combination of various injury-related causes, including axotomy, ischemia, formation of free radicals, alterations in the ionic balance,[25] and membrane phospholipid hydrolysis (P. Demediuk and A. I. Faden, Chapter 2).

Replacement of lost neurons by means of transplants is giving us invaluable understanding of the variables on which neuronal survival depends. Furthermore, transplants may become clinically important in the treatment of chronic injuries. However, when considering intervention after CNS lesions, preventing secondary neuronal death seems to be the obvious first approach. What are the mechanisms of secondary neuronal death? Can neuronal death be prevented or minimized? Would the same principles facilitate transplantation of neuronal replacements?

3.1. CENTRAL NEURONOTROPHIC FACTORS AND SECONDARY NEURONAL DEATH

The two major causes of secondary neuronal death in the CNS are probably axotomy and the sequels of disruption of the vasculature. A well-known feature of neurons subjected to axotomy is chromatolysis,[58] and a similar phenomenon has been described in the hippocampus after a brief ischemic episode.[48] Chromatolysis of sympathetic neurons is elicited by removal of their supply of nerve growth factor (NGF), and their health can be restored by providing exogenous NGF.[56] By analogy, we may expect that neurons that project into a CNS injury area and are deprived of their specific neuronotrophic factors will be affected much like peripheral neurons. Thus, deprivation of survival-promoting factors (also called neurotrophic or neuronotrophic factors, NTF) may be one of the mechanisms underlying secondary neuronal death in the CNS.

Do NTFs exist in the normal CNS, and, if so, how are they affected by injury? In order to answer these questions, rats were given a brain lesion and, at various times post-lesion, the animals were sacrificed, and extracts prepared from the tissue immediately surrounding the wound cavity.[79,80] The neuronotrophic activity of the extracts was then tested on cultures of dissociated neurons. Normal brain extracts contained low levels of neuronotrophic activity. However, after injury, these levels increased with time, reaching a maximum and decreasing thereafter (Fig. 2). The precise time at which maximal activity was reached depended on the age of the animal. The initial experiments were performed using neonatal animals,[68,79] and in this case maximal trophic activity accumulated after 3 days post-lesion. But the response was even more pronounced when the experiments were carried out with adult or aged animals, where maximal trophic titers were reached after 10 and 15 days post-lesion, respectively[75,80] (Fig. 2).

All types of injury examined, including chemical and ischemic insults and selective deafferentation, cause increases in NTF activity, generally proportional

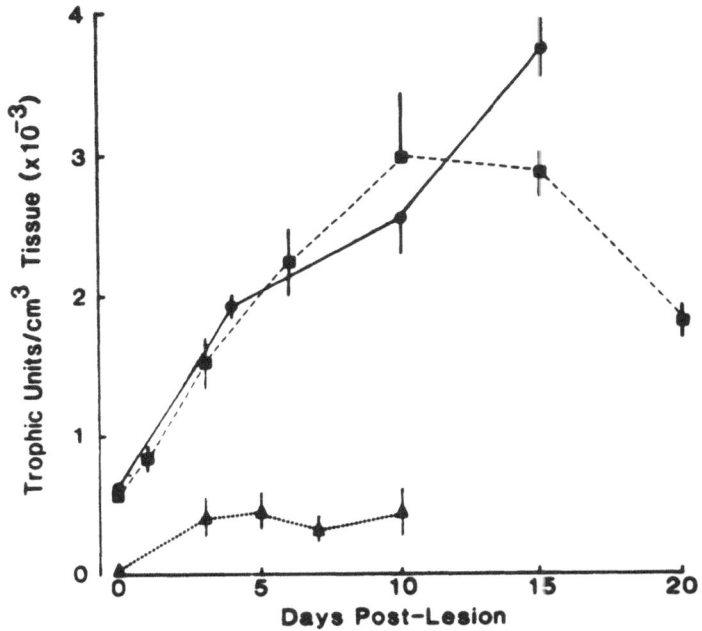

FIGURE 2. Postlesion increase in the neuronotrophic activity of Sprague–Dawley rats: (▲) 3 days old; (■) adult; (●) 24–26 months old. One trophic unit per milliliter supports 50% of the maximal neuron survival. Target cells were purified chick embryo (E8) ciliary ganglion neurons. Maximal neuron survival was 95 ± 8% of the cells seeded. The titer values (±S.E.M, $n = 3$–10) are expressed per milliliter of packed tissue (ca. per g tissue). (Adapted from ref. 75.)

to the extent of the lesion. The activity increased five to 50 times compared to normal brain, depending on the age of the animal and the neuronal type used as test cell in the assay.[68,75,80,108] The highest activity occurred in the tissue immediately surrounding the lesion at about the time when secondary neuronal death ceased. It seems that the increased supply of NTF prevented further neuronal death. If this were the case, an exogenous supply of such factors soon after injury might prevent most neuronal death arising from axotomy.

3.2. EXCITOTOXICITY AND SECONDARY NEURONAL DEATH

Of all the sequels of injury, disruption of the blood supply is perhaps the most traumatic. Recently, several lines of investigation have provided evidence that neuronal death subsequent to ischemia and the accompanying anoxia and hypoglycemia is mediated by excitatory amino acids (Fig. 3).[70,92,110] As a result of such trauma, excessive amounts of glutamate (up to eight times normal) are

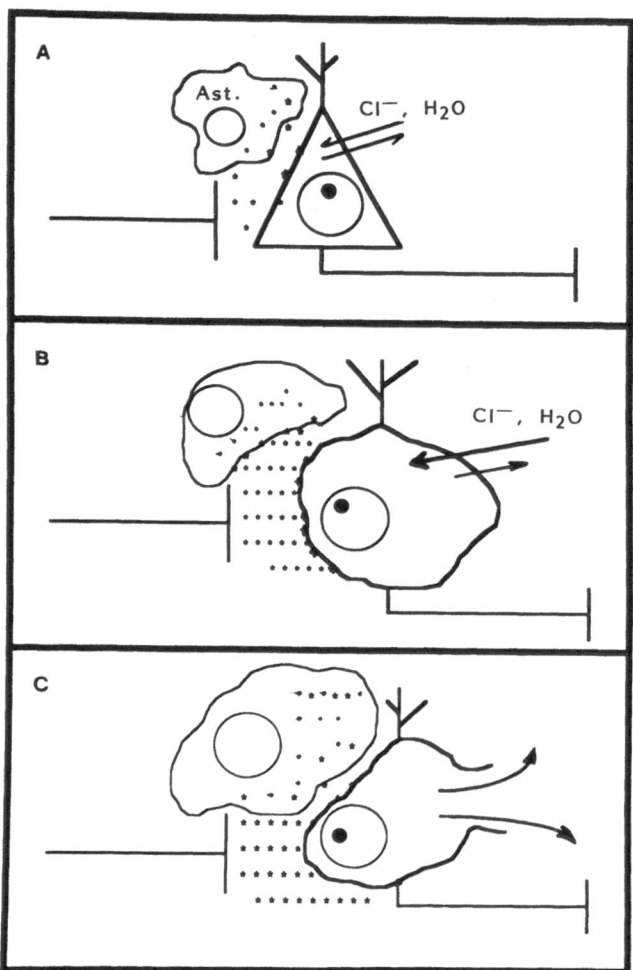

FIGURE 3. Excitotoxic neuronal death. (A) Under normal circumstances, the glutamate (∗) liberated at the synaptic cleft acts on the postsynaptic cell. Its excitatory action is terminated by removal into the astrocytic processes (Ast.) surrounding the synapse and amidation to glutamine (•), and repolarization is ensured. (B) Injury causes the liberation of a large excess of glutamate that overwhelms the capacity of the astrocyte to remove it from the synaptic region. The postsynaptic cell is permanently depolarized; large amounts of chloride (and the accompanying water) swell the cell, which finally (C) undergoes osmotic lysis.

released into the extracellular space.[11] If glutamate levels remain elevated for periods beyond several minutes, or if excitatory amino acids are injected directly into the CNS, cell death results.[92] Several glutamate antagonists, particularly those in the phosphonic acid series, can be protective if applied either immediately before or shortly after the insult.[70,102] The excitotoxic action of glutamate can be reproduced in cultured neurons or in brain slices, where the conditions can be precisely monitored.[93] Neuronal death results when cultures are maintained in a partially ischemic environment and exposed to glutamate (approximately 100 μm). Glutamate antagonists, particularly those of the N-methyl-D-aspartate (NMDA) class, protect against cell death in these systems.[28,93,94]

3.3. PREVENTING SECONDARY NEURONAL DEATH

Minimizing or preventing secondary neuronal death may greatly contribute to a favorable prognosis for recovery after CNS injury without further interventions to replace the lost cells. Several chapters in this volume deal with early postlesion deleterious events that may lead to neuronal loss and pharmacological treatments that may prevent it. From the work reported above, I propose two interventions: (1) treatment with glutamate antagonists specific for the NMDA receptor type; (2) treatment with neuronotrophic factors. A third intervention, astrocyte type 1 transplantation, is considered in Section 5.5.

A number of glutamate antagonists specifically inhibit binding to the NMDA receptor (Table I). Of these compounds, the best candidates for clinical use appear to be AP7, CPP, and compound MK-801. These compounds cross the blood–CNS barrier and, therefore, can be conveniently administered. Although CPP is the most potent glutamate antagonist at the NMDA receptor and MK-801

TABLE I. Excitatory Amino Acid Antagonists

Compound[a]	Receptor specificity	Reference
AP4	Presynaptic antagonist to AP4-type receptor	21
AP5	NMDA antagonist	22
AP6	Neuronodulator, acts at glial binding site	40
AP7	NMDA antagonist, crosses blood-brain barrier	70
CPP	Powerful NMDA antagonist; crosses blood-brain barrier	22
MK-801	Potent NMDA antagonist, active orally	28, 112
GDEE	Quisqualate receptor antagonist	94
Kynurenate[b]	General antagonist, occurs naturally in CNS	31
pBrBPzDa	Very powerful general antagonist	30

[a]Abbreviations: AP4, 4-aminophosphonobutanoic acid; AP5, 5-aminophosphonopentanoic acid; Ap6, 6-aminophosphonohexanoic acid; AP7, 7-aminophosphonoheptanoic acid; CPP, 3-([±]-2-carboxypiperazin-4-yl)-propyl-1-phosphonic acid; GDEE, glutamate diethyl ester; pBrBPzDA; p-bromobenzoylpiperazine dicarboxylic acid; MK-801, (+)-5-methyl-10,11-dihydro-5H-dibenzo[a,d]cyclohepten-5,10-imine maleate.
[b]Recent data from B. Meldrum (personal communication) indicate that kynurenic acid is useful in protecting the brain against ischemic damage.

is both potent and approved for clinical use as an anticonvulsant, other general antagonists may also prove useful. Kynurenate, in particular, has the advantage of being a naturally occurring CNS metabolite.

The therapeutic use of NTFs is far less advanced than, and may not be as convenient as, that of amino acid antagonists. However, NTF treatment of open CNS injuries may eventually prove very important. It has recently been shown that the best-known neuronotrophic factor, NGF, is present in brain and plays a key role in the survival of central cholinergic neurons.[50,100,107] The loss of septal cells following fimbria transection[109] could be almost completely prevented by infusion of NGF (F. H. Gage, personal communication; see also B. Will *et al.*, Chapter 16). Similar studies have not been carried out using other central NTFs. However, we have shown that an exogenous supply of a crude extract of injured brain tissue made possible the survival of fetal striatal tissue implanted immediately after an open injury.[82] These results clearly indicate that NTFs may be used as pharmacological agents in the treatment of CNS injury. Purification of injury-induced CNS neuronotrophic factors and cloning of the corresponding genes would make possible a clinical trial of these molecules.

3.4. REPLACING LOST NEURONS: INJURY-INDUCED NEURONOTROPHIC FACTORS AND TRANSPLANT SURVIVAL

Regardless of our success in preventing secondary neuronal death, a variable number of cells will be lost during the acute phase of injury. Furthermore, preventing neuronal loss is of little help to chronic CNS injury patients. In these cases, transplantation of fetal tissue into the injured CNS has been proposed as a means of replacing lost neurons. In order to be useful as therapeutic tools, transplants must survive in a wound cavity. Reliably successful survival of masses of neurons, that is, survival of tissue grafts, is therefore necessary.

However, the survival of solid fragments of embryonic CNS tissue in a wound cavity made in the host parenchyma is variable, depending not only on the age of the donor tissue but also on the type of neuron transplanted. Many cortical neurons survive well, septal or monoamine neurons less well, and striatal AChE-positive neurons survive poorly or not at all. The survival and growth of striatal neurons in a wound cavity were dramatically enhanced by placing the transplant in the host after neuronotrophic factor production had began to rise (Fig. 4a). There was a close correlation between NTF activity for striatal neurons in the tissue immediately adjacent to the cavity and survival of transplants of the same type of neurons.[68,79,80,108] Optimal survival coincided with maximal production of NTFs (Fig. 4b), and an exogenous supply of injured-brain extracts at the time of transplantation made the delay unnecessary.[82] Any donor tissue tested so far survives successfully when grafted using the delayed transplantation paradigm.

The delayed transplantation technique was introduced before information on

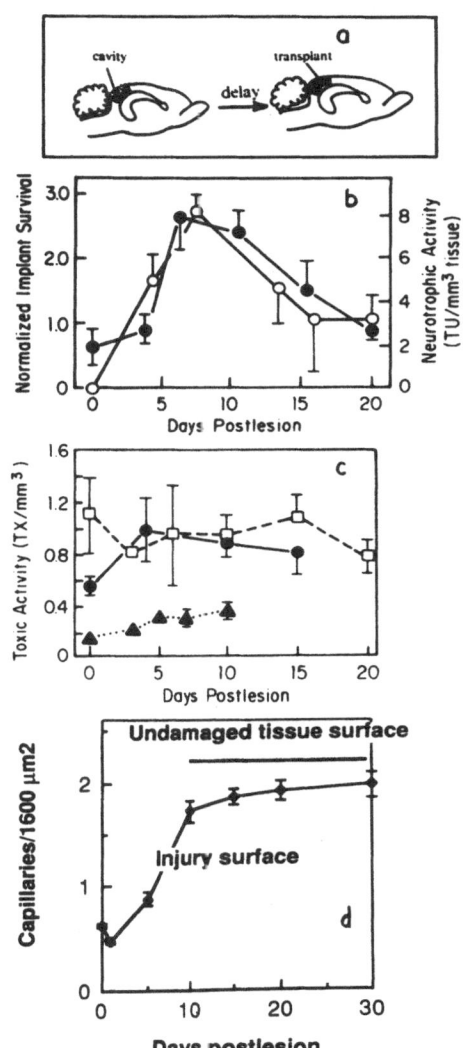

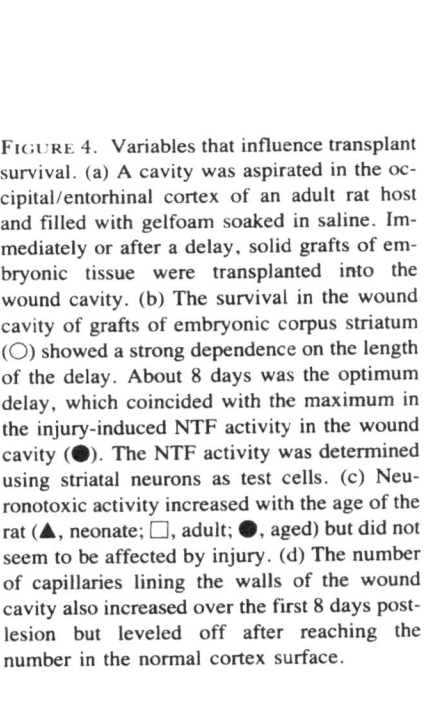

FIGURE 4. Variables that influence transplant survival. (a) A cavity was aspirated in the occipital/entorhinal cortex of an adult rat host and filled with gelfoam soaked in saline. Immediately or after a delay, solid grafts of embryonic tissue were transplanted into the wound cavity. (b) The survival in the wound cavity of grafts of embryonic corpus striatum (O) showed a strong dependence on the length of the delay. About 8 days was the optimum delay, which coincided with the maximum in the injury-induced NTF activity in the wound cavity (●). The NTF activity was determined using striatal neurons as test cells. (c) Neuronotoxic activity increased with the age of the rat (▲, neonate; □, adult; ●, aged) but did not seem to be affected by injury. (d) The number of capillaries lining the walls of the wound cavity also increased over the first 8 days postlesion but leveled off after reaching the number in the normal cortex surface.

injury-induced NTFs was available.[57,103] The delay was assumed to allow the formation of a vascular bed that facilitated transplant survival.[103] In adult rats, vascularization of a cortical wound surface occurs at the same time as the rise in NTF activity. However, whereas the number of capillaries in the new CNS surface levels off after 10 days post-lesion (Fig. 4d), both neuronotrophic activity and transplant survival reach a maximum at about 8–10 days post-lesion and decay thereafter (Fig. 4b). The decreased availability of NTFs explains why, with delays longer than 10 days, the transplants show diminished viability in spite of the presence of a well-established capillary bed in the host cavity.

Another variable that may be critical for transplant survival is the presence in the wound cavity of neuronotoxic factors, i.e., substances that cause neuronal death directly or that prevent the action of NTFs. Extracts of normal brain contain such substances. Their activity increases during development (Fig. 4c) and shows neuronal selectivity. Thus, brain neurotoxins kill central cells but less well or not at all peripheral ganglion neurons (see also G. Moonen *et al.*, Chapter 13). However, neurotoxic activity does not change after injury (Fig. 4c) and is therefore unlikely to be involved in the enhanced survival observed in the delayed implant paradigm.

In conclusion, establishing a blood supply is essential for long-term survival of the transplants.[88] But the major cause for the enhanced implant viability after a transplantation delay appears to be the presence of increased concentrations of neurotrophic factors in the host wound.

4. REACTIVE AND REGENERATIVE GROWTH AFTER CNS INJURY

Minor CNS injury is usually compensated by ongoing plasticity processes that, when required, can adapt to perform limited functional repair. At the neuronal level, the most general of these processes is called synapse turnover. Synapse turnover, i.e., synapse loss and replacement, is a maintenance process in the adult mammalian CNS that is elicited by a variety of normal stimuli[19,20] and is expressed massively in response to injury.[78] The first step of injury-induced synapse turnover, the degeneration of axon terminals separated from their parent bodies, results in partial denervation of undamaged cells. The undamaged and damaged axons remaining in the denervated area sprout, that is, differentiate new nerve endings that extend towards the vacated postsynaptic sites (Fig. 5A). New synapses replacing those lost by injury are then formed by these sprouts in the process called reactive synaptogenesis (Fig. 5B). The term reactive synaptogenesis denotes synapse formation triggered by stimuli that are not part of the developmental program.[20] If the new synapses arise from regenerative sprouts, the process is usually called regeneration or regenerative synaptogenesis. Regenerative synaptogenesis involves long-distance axonal extension and is not observed in the CNS except after transplantation. Reactive synaptogenesis has been extensively documented in many areas of the CNS, but the most extensive studies have been performed in the dentate gyrus of the hippocampal formation. I illustrate the essential features of reactive synaptogenesis by describing the effects of partial deafferentation of the dentate gyrus by unilateral entorhinal cortex ablation.

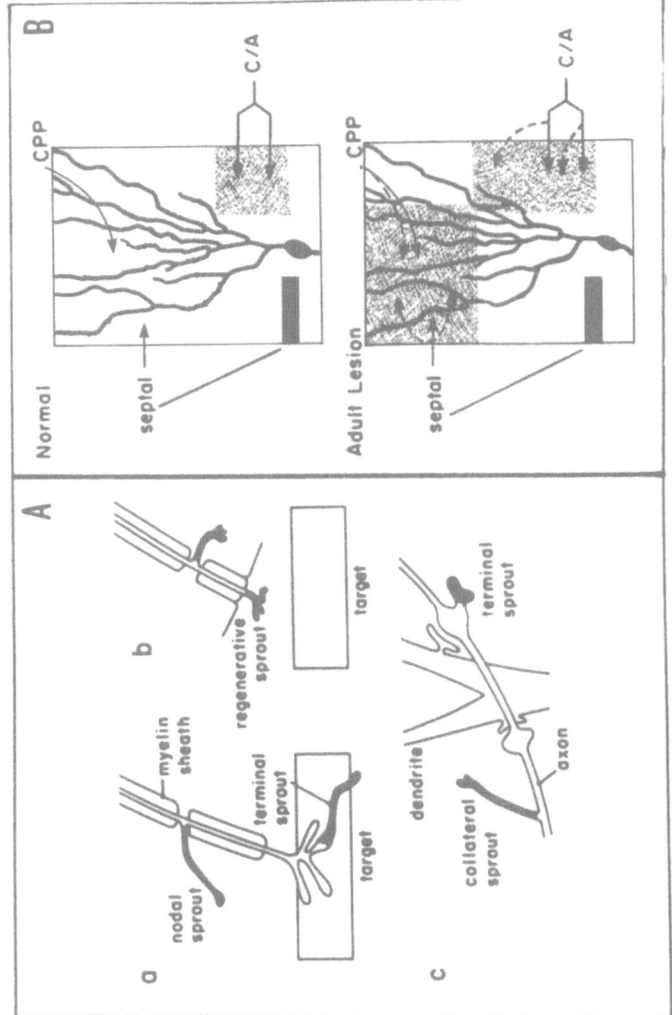

FIGURE 5. (A) After partial denervation, various types of sprouting are observed (a,b,c). Of these, only regenerative sprouts (b) have the potential to restore the initial circuitry. (B) Most frequently, the postsynaptic sites vacant after injury are filled by reactive sprouts from undamaged local fibers. In the dentate gyrus after ipsilateral entorhinal ablation, sprouts from undamaged septal, commisural/associational (C/A), and contralateral entorhinal (CPP) fiber systems occupy the postsynaptic sites that become available in the outer molecular layer. Broken lines indicate sprouting.

4.1. REACTIVE SYNAPTOGENESIS

The dentate gyrus is the only CNS structure where the response to deaf-ferentation of all known afferents has been monitored. In the adult rat, the sequence and timing of events after unilateral entorhinal ablation are stereotyped (for review, see ref. 78). One day after the lesion, 90% of the synapses in the outer two-thirds of the dentate molecular layer are lost, and fibers display exten-sive degeneration. Terminal degeneration proceeds rapidly for the first 10 days but continues at a lower rate therafter. The period of rapid degeneration coincides with the development of an impressive glial reaction. Astrocytes in the molecular layer hypertrophy within 48 hr post-lesion, orient their processes towards the denervated area, and actually migrate part way into this zone. At the same time, macrophages, probably originating from blood monocytes, reach three times their preoperative number by 4 days post-lesion.

At an early time post-lesion, degeneration and removal of degeneration products are the most prominent morphological features of the response to inju-ry. The processes of clearing the debris and initiation of axon sprouting appear closely related, both of them proceeding more rapidly in the zone invaded by commissural–associational fibers than in the rest of the molecular layer. In this initial period, and perhaps associated with astrocyte migration, a rearrangement of the vascular bed is observed in the outer dentate molecular layer. The capillar-ies change from a primarily vertical orientation with respect to the granule cell layer to one that is essentially horizontal.

The first clear signs of reactive sprouting by septal and commissural–asso-ciational fibers are observed 3–4 days post-lesion, and reactive synaptogenesis follows soon after. Maximal sprouting is achieved around 12–15 days post-lesion, but reactive synapse formation still continues 1 month later. Elec-trophysiological studies on the commissural afferents and temporodentate path show that new synapses first become functiol 9 days post-operation and that nearly all are functional after 15 days.[20]

4.2. FUNCTIONAL SIGNIFICANCE OF REACTIVE SYNAPTOGENESIS

The existence of reactive synaptogenesis proves that new synapses can indeed form in the mature CNS, replace those lost by injury, and mediate synaptic transmission.[20,78] Reactive synaptogenesis does not replace the original circuitry but results in a selective increase in the residual input that, in the case of small lesions, may have beneficial consequences. Thus, it has been argued that, in the hippocampus, reactive synaptogenesis facilitates recovery of performance on a reinforced alternation task after unilateral entorhinal ablation.[65] In addition, the reactive sprouts, by providing presynaptic input to deafferented neurons, may also help to prevent the dendritic atrophy associated with deafferentation.

On the negative side, reactive synaptogenesis may interfere with the process of functional recovery by introducing abnormal connections, some of which possibly compete with regenerative sprouts for available synaptic spaces. The finding that sprouting in the human hippocampus[17] appears to follow the same rules as those deduced from deafferented rodent models[33] emphasizes the need to understand the significance of this process.

4.3. NEURITE-PROMOTING FACTORS AND AXONAL SPROUTING

We have recently examined the effect of entorhinal ablation on the appearance in the cortex and the deafferented hippocampus of neurite-promoting factors, a class of growth factors capable of promoting neurite extension from cultured neurons.[74] Two types of lesion were performed with identical results. Electrolytic ablation selectively destroyed the entorhinal cortex without otherwise perturbing the hippocampus. Cortical ablation by vacuum aspiration transected the angular bundle but in addition also damaged the occipital cortex and deliberately nicked the dorsal hippocampus. In the case of electrolytic lesions, only the hippocampal tissue was sampled, whereas with aspiration lesions, both the hippocampus and the tissue surrounding the lesion were examined.

The animals were sacrificed at various times post-lesion, and extracts of tissue were prepared and tested for neurite-promoting factor (NPF) activity. Test cells were primary cultures of embryonic ciliary ganglion neurons that were freed on nonneuronal elements and plated at low density to avoid indirect interfering effects.[75] In addition, the survival and initiation of neurite outgrowth by the cells are totally insensitive to NGF. These neurons can be maintained alive with neuronotrophic factors that lack neurite-promoting activity or by increasing the K^+ concentration of the culture medium. Under these conditions, the neurons assume a rounded morphology, which they maintain for prolonged periods (up to 2 weeks). However, addition of brain extract, either fresh or freeze-thawed in the presence of sulfhydryl agents, causes extensive neurite outgrowth from these cells[74] (Fig. 6).

Uninjured brain had a basal NPF activity of 1300 units/g tissue that increased fourfold 10 to 15 days after a lesion (Fig. 6). Both basal and injury-induced brain NPF activities had the properties of proteins, i.e., were nondiffusible and temperature and protease sensitive. The injury-induced increase in activity originated, at least in part, from the appearance of new molecules. The molecular weight of most of the basal activity was 9000–17,000. Injured brain had additional activities with molecular masses of 30, 70, and ≥200 kDa. Injury-induced NPF activities further differed from the basal NPF in their greater sensitivity to oxidation, although both activities were abolished by treatment with N-ethylmaleimide.

The time course of appearance of injury-induced NPF activity closely correlated with the sprouting of commissural–associational or septal fibers after entorhinal ablation (Fig. 6), lending support to the hypothesis that brain NPF activity

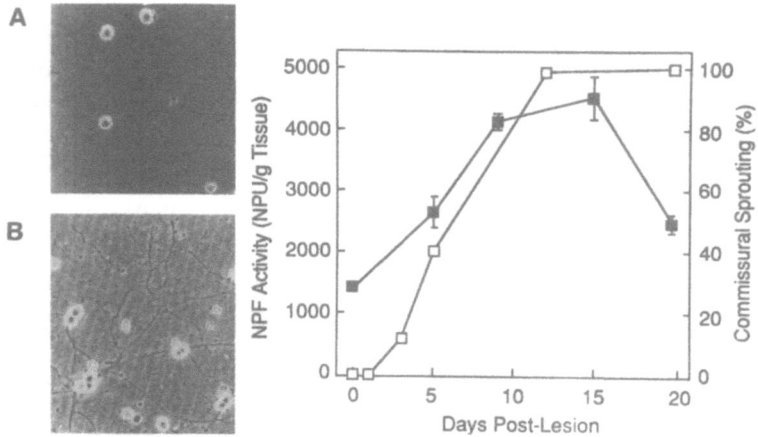

FIGURE 6. Effect of brain neurite-promoting factors. (A) Purified ciliary ganglion neurons can be maintained in culture as healthy, spherical cells with no neurites. (B) Addition of brain extracts causes profuse neurite outgrowth. (C) In the dentate gyrus, the postlesion increase in neurite-promoting activity after entorhinal lesion closely correlates with the sprouting of C/A fibers. (Adapted from ref. 74.)

is responsible for the sprouting response observed histologically after partial denervation. The hippocampal sprouting response was considerably delayed in aged animals[97]; correspondingly, hippocampal NPF activity showed no increase after entorhinal ablation in 24 to 26-month-old rats, although neuronotrophic activity increased after the lesion as much as in young adults. Furthermore, in initial experiments in my laboratory, injections of injured-brain extract into the hippocampi of rats that had received an entorhinal lesion accelerated sprouting in the dentate gyrus. After extract injection, sprouting of septohippocampal and commissural fibers was evident 2 days after entorhinal ablation compared to 4–5 days in controls injected comparable amounts of serum albumin (unpublished observations). These results open the way to the study of the molecules responsible for injury-induced sprouting in the CNS.

From the point of view of interventive CNS repair, an important open question is whether or not the same molecules that cause reactive sprouting will also mediate regenerative sprouting. It would be a great advantage if the molecules that mediate the two phenomena were different. In any case, naturally occurring NPF inhibitors or antibodies against NPFs could, in principle, be used clinically to control maladaptive sprout formation after CNS injury. The sensitivity of NPF to oxidants could explain one of the deleterious effects of peroxides on regeneration.[25] It also opens an independent pharmacological approach to controlling sprouting.

4.4. REGENERATIVE SYNAPTOGENESIS AND TRANSPLANT–HOST INTEGRATION

Axonal extension during reactive synaptogenesis is limited to a few tens of micrometers. The greatest expansion of a terminal field so far reported is that of hippocampal CA4 fibers, which sprout 40 to 60 μm in the dentate molecular layer after entorhinal ablation.[78] On the other hand, the reconstruction of a disrupted CNS pathway generally requires extension of renerative sprouts over much longer distances, a process usually called regeneration. Unaided, CNS axons fail to regenerate, but such failure is not because of lack of ability of transected central axons to sprout new growth cones or lack of growth capacity of these sprouts. Central fibers can be induced to grow many times their normal length (up to several centimeters) into a segment of the sheath of a myelinated peripheral nerve. Such peripheral nerve implants have been used to join the stumps of transected spinal cord, to bridge two widely separated levels of the brain and spinal cord, to guide the growth of CNS axons into other tissues, and, more recently, to guide the growth of transected retinal axons to the superior colliculus.[4,5] The central axons that emerge from the peripheral nerve grow into the CNS tissue for a short distance, conduct normal nerve impulses, and seem to form functional synapses.[5]

Thus, the success or failure of axonal regeneration seems to depend on signals that the regenerating neurons exchange with their immediate environment. It is possible that the CNS extracellular territory is inappropriate for axons to navigate over long distances once connections are established during development. The use of transplants of embryonic CNS tissue into adult hosts provides a way to test that hypothesis. A transplant of embryonic CNS tissue homologous to that lost by injury would function as a relay station, receiving the original input from the host and sending to the original target projections similar to those interrupted by the lesion. This arrangement permits the examination of long-distance navigation in the adult CNS by both developing and adult fibers.

4.4.1. PROJECTIONS FROM TRANSPLANT TO HOST: SPECIFICITY

In general, embryonic fibers are remarkably successful in forming the appropriate synapses with the adult target after growing over long distances in the adult CNS. Implants of embryonic locus coeruleus,[12] septum,[13] raphe,[6,14] and entorhinal cortex[34] form their own distinctive pattern of connections in the rat dentate gyrus, identical to that of the original synapses. The positioning of the implants in very abnormal locations, i.e., occipital cortex, does not prevent the fibers from reaching their correct target.[57,80] Furthermore, it appears that the specificity of the connections formed by a given type of afferent is determined by the neurotransmitter used by that type of fiber. For example, after fimbria–fornix transection in the adult rat, transplants of cholinergic cells from embryonic corpus striatum[80] or habenula[35] form similar termination fields as those of septal transplants or the original septal fibers.

Thus, the specificity of synapse formation resides in both the afferent originating in the transplant and the host target cells. The embryonic axons reach their target independently of whether they will eventually be myelinated (such as the perforant path) or unmyelinated (i.e., septal fibers). In summary, the adult CNS environment does not seem to offer obstacles to the progress of embryonic axons. However, adult growth cones seem to find greater difficulties.

4.4.2. PROJECTIONS FROM HOST TO TRANSPLANT: AN UNSOLVED PROBLEM

Most CNS circuits seem to require accurate point-to-point connectivity for correct function. Therefore, if transplants are to have therapeutic value in repairing this type of circuit, it is not sufficient that the projections from the transplant reach the correct host target. The converse must also occur, i.e., host axons must be able to innervate the appropriate cells in the transplant.

Can adult axons grow, reach embryonic transplants, and there form appropriate contacts? A preliminary answer is possible, with the caveat that only a few studies dealing with this question have appeared. Thus, nonmyelinated host septal or dorsal raphe fibers are capable of entering the transplants and correctly innervating the hippocampal[53,105] or cortical[34] cells. This is even more remarkable because the cellular organization of embryonic transplants tends to be more disarranged than that of the normal tissue.[34,52,84,105]

In contrast, damaged myelinated fiber systems are rarely able to penetrate into the transplant. Thus, transplanted entorhinal neurons usually do not receive innervation from the thalamus, contralateral entorhinal cortex, presubiculum, or subiculum (Fig. 7). Typically, these fibers grow around the transplant but do not enter it. However, in one case, contralateral entorhinal and subicular fibers entered the implant.[34] The zone of the implant where the host fibers were seen entering was that where the layer of glial cells usually surrounding transplants[7,64,66] was either very sparse or absent (R. Gibbs, personal communication). It appears that the layer of glia in the surface of the implant and/or the surface of the host injury cannot be crossed by these axons.

Thus, in general, CNS transplants are incomplete relay stations. They send acurate output but receive only a minor proportion of input. In order to achieve effective transplant—host integration, the problem of the glial boundary has to be solved. At this time, it appears essential to define the various roles that astroglia can play and search for the mechanisms that control the number and type of these cells.

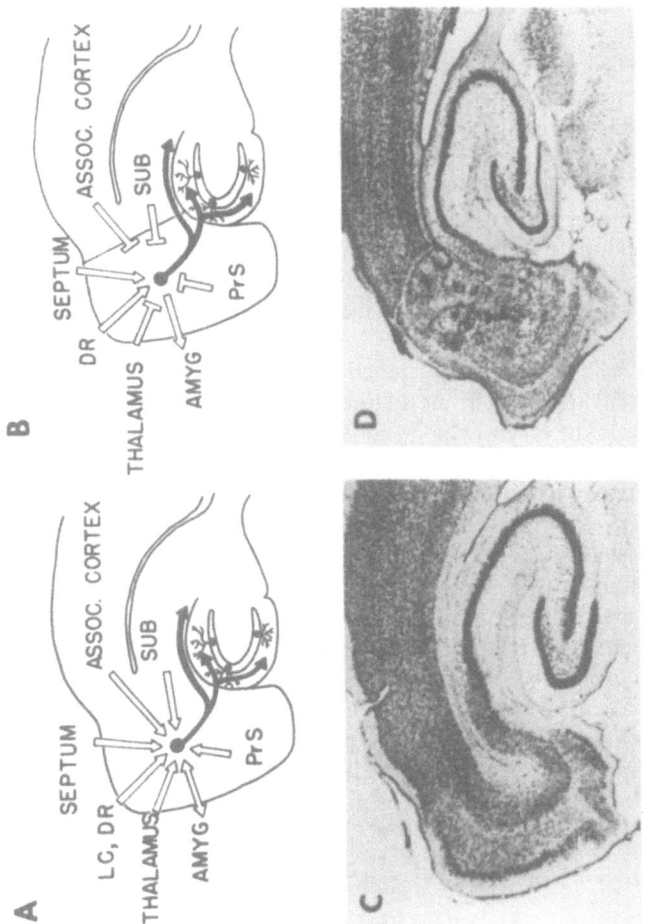

FIGURE 7. Transplant–host integration. (B,D) Embryonic entorhinal cortex transplanted into an entorhinal wound in an adult host 8 days post-lesion grows about ten times its initial size and innervates the host hippocampus. However, the transplant received only three of the normal eight inputs in controls (A,C).

5. MULTIPLE ROLES OF ASTROGLIA

Increased interest in the study of astrocyte development and physiology has revealed an almost bewildering number of roles for these cells. Such variety of functions has led us to investigate the possibility that astrocytes may in fact be a number of morphologically similar but functionally (and phenotypically) different classes of cells. Although this work is only in its beginning, the initial results are very exciting.

In vivo, two types of astrocytes, traditionally denominated protoplasmic and fibrous and more recently type 1 and type 2, can be observed. These two types of glial cell differ in immunophenotype and appear to be developmentally distinct.[72,87] Type 1 astrocytes usually show a flat, fibroblastlike morphology, whereas type 2 cells exhibit a more fibrous, stellate shape. However, morphology alone is not a good criterion to distinguish between the two glial types. *In vivo,* after a lesion or in culture in the absence of serum or in the presence of various substances with morphogenic activity, type 1 astrocytes may assume type 2 morphology but not immunophenotype; intermediate morphologies are not uncommon.

After injury, astrocytes become reactive, a condition typically characterized by enlargement and increase in the number of GFAP filaments. It is not clear whether both astrocyte types respond independently to injury or even if injury may trigger the interconversion of one type into the other. Type 1 astrocytes respond more actively to mitogens and seem responsible for the majority of the cell division observed after a lesion. The morphologically fibrous astrocytes that form the ''glial scar'' are predominantly type 1,[71] as are those forming the original glia limitans.

Most of the astrocytes grown in culture in the experiments that are described below were cortical type 1 astrocytes. These are the astrocytes associated with synapses and are probably concerned with maintaining local ionic balance, neurotransmitter removal and inactivation, and growth factor secretion. It is suspected that astroglial cells associated with particular neuronal or synaptic populations may be unique in ways specific to that synaptic population.[38,39,98,99] The fundamental role of astrocytes in neural function is described at the end of this section in terms of a model, the unit of function neuron–glia.

5.1. THE "GLIAL SCAR" OR NEO-GLIA LIMITANS

The ''glial scar'' is a layer of glial cells that forms at the surface of a CNS injury or, indeed, at any new CNS surface. In the case of an occipital cortex lesion, a loose layer of nonneuronal cells, predominantly astrocytes and blood monocytes (the latter frequently confused with microglia), is apparent 4–5 days after injury. This layer is penetrated by new blood vessels and becomes more compact, reaching a stable structure in the following 15 days (M. Nieto-Sampedro, unpublished observations). At this point, astroglia are the major cellular component in contact with the CNS, but fibroblast layers are laid over the glial cells. The final glial layer, frequently called "glial scar," closely resembles the glia limitans and probably fulfills the same functions, an idea also advanced by Reier et al.[90] Both, glial scar and glia limitans are formed by type 1 astrocytes.[72]

A more or less obvious neo-glia limitans also surrounds solid embryonic transplants[7,64,66] and probably contributes in preventing or making difficult the ingrowth of fibers from the host. The glial scar is widely regarded as an obstacle to regeneration and transplant–host integration. Regenerating axons usually fail to grow across an injury zone or the host–transplant boundary. Most frequently, they turn around and either die back or make inappropriate synaptic contact on available sites proximal to their place of origin. Reactive glia are traditionally held responsible for this behavior. Astrocytes in an injury area become reactive less than 1 day after the lesion. In the following days they both migrate and proliferate, and their enlarged fibrous processes form a web that isolates the new surface of the brain from nonneural tissue.[2,18]

The glial scar does not act as a simple mechanical barrier. Axons do not cross a transection zone even when the scar is very thin or virtually absent[32,37] but can cross collagen barriers[24] or dense implanted scar tissue.[90] The neo-glia limitans functions in much the same way as the normal glia limitans. Although we do not know why, axons do not cross either the glia limitans or the glial scar. It is possible that, because astrocytes prefer growing guided by astrocytic processes, they are actually misguided by the glial scar.

Another view, initially proposed by Ramón y Cajal,[89] is that astrocytes actively inhibit axonal growth. However, this view is contradicted by two facts: (1) some axons can in fact penetrate the glial web; (2) there is evidence from multiple sources (see Section 5.4) that astrocytes secrete substances that promote the survival, attachment, and sprouting of neurons.

This paradox ceases when we consider that astrocytes may not be a homogeneous population. The age of astrocytes seems to determine their morphology[27] and their behavior with respect to axon growth. Using a preparation consisting of transected sciatic nerve regenerating in a silicone chamber, Kalderon[44] showed that immature blastlike astrocytes (15-day-old cells) facilitate peripheral nerve regeneration, whereas older, mature cells (45 days old) prevent it. The transition from young astrocytes to mature, reactive astrocytes correlated with the disappearance in the latter of plasminogen activator molecules.[44]

All these observations place the glia in the center stage of the regeneration problem and emphasize the importance of the cellular and molecular processes that control the number and type of the various glial populations.

5.2. THE CONTROL OF GLIAL POPULATIONS IN ADULT CNS:
MITOGENS, MORPHOGENS, AND INHIBITORS

How are CNS glial populations controlled, and how do these controls respond to injury? Type 1 astrocytes can be easily prepared from embryonic or neonatal rat cortex and maintained in greater than 95% pure cultures.[69] With the help of these cultures, it is possible to study the activity of molecules that *in vitro* promote astrocyte proliferation (mitogens) and morphological transformation from protoplasmic into fibrous (morphogens). Thus, we can correlate the proliferation of glia following CNS injury and the changes in the injured tissue of mitogenic and morphogenic activities.

Astrocytes rarely, if ever, divide in the normal CNS. The number of CNS glial cells reaches a maximum soon after birth and then remains practically constant throughout adulthood. Although glial cells retain their ability to proliferate,[104] and the normal CNS contains molecules capable of causing division and differentiation of cultured astrocytes,[55,62,86,106] glial cell division in a healthy adult is a potentiality rather than a normal event. After injury, however, astrocytes become reactive (i.e., enlarge and become more fibrous-looking) and multiply.

Do mitogenic and morphogenic activities increase after CNS injury? Do glial proliferation and fibrous appearance follow the increase in mitogens and morphogens? Recently, we have studied the effect of extracts of injured brain tissue on the proliferation and differentiation of purified astrocytes in culture.[81] A cavity was aspirated in the occipital cortex of adult rats; at intervals ranging from 1 hr to 60 days post-lesion, the animals were sacrificed, and the mitogenic and morphogenic activities were determined. Parallel groups of injured animals were perfused, and the number of glial cells/unit area counted in thin sections.

The mitogenic activity in the tissue surrounding the wound increased rapidly, reaching maximum values after 6 days post-lesion (Fig. 8a). Tissue morphogenic activity began to increase at a later time (6 days post-lesion) and remained high 60 days later (Fig. 8c). Glial cell number in the injury area also increased rapidly, closely following the rise in mitogenic activity (Fig. 8b).

The injury-induced increase in mitogenic activity seems to be largely caused by the postlesion loss of mitogen inhibitory activity. Two lines of evidence support this statement. The first is the shape of the dose–response curves for the mitogenic activity of extracts from uninjured versus injured brain (Fig. 9). The bell shape of the dose–response curve for uninjured tissue is diagnostic of the presence of inhibitory activity. The second line of evidence was the recovery, after filtration of the extracts through an Amicon membrane of considerably greater than 100% of the mitogenic activity.[81] As a simplistic first approach, it appears that astrocytes do not divide in the CNS under normal circumstances because inhibitory molecules prevent the action of the mitogens. The nature and site of action of these

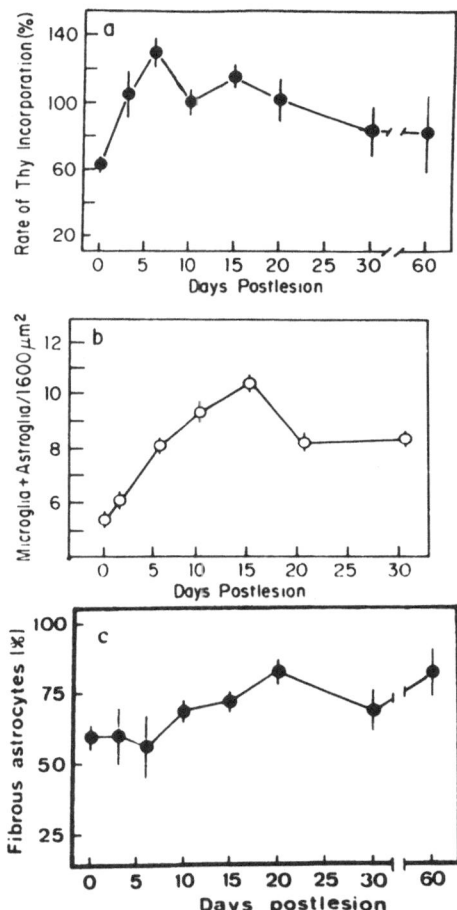

FIGURE 8. Glial response to injury. (a) The mitogenic activity in the rat brain tissue adjacent to an injury increased rapidly, and (b) nonneuronal cell proliferation in the tissue at the edge of the injury followed the increase in mitogenic activity. (c) Morphogenic activity experienced a much slower increase.

mitogen inhibitors are subjects of active research (see G. Moonen *et al.*, Chapter 13).

5.3. ASTROCYTES ACCUMULATE AND DETOXIFY GLUTAMATE

Glial proliferation after injury, by contributing to the closing of the boundaries that separate the CNS from the rest of the organism, has a definite survival value. However, the increase in glial number has several additional beneficial effects, one of which is control of extracellular excitotoxin concentration.

The great majority of the CNS synapses are excitatory, and most of these

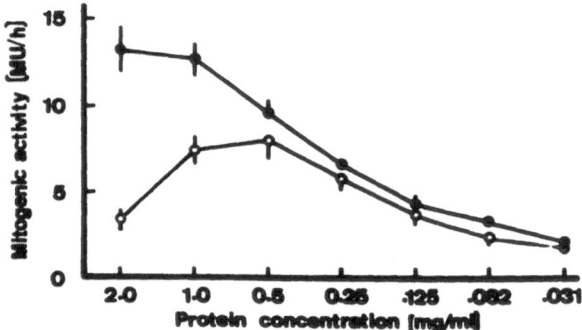

FIGURE 9. A decrease in the activity of mitogen inhibitors was probably responsible for the increase in brain mitogenic activity after injury: (○) normal adult brain extract; (●) extract of tissue adjacent to an injury 10 days post-lesion.

use glutamate or related compounds as neurotransmitters. It has been hypothesized that, under normal circumstances, the excitatory action of glutamate is terminated by its uptake into the astrocytes surrounding the synapses; it is inactivated by amidation and, in this inactive form, shuttled back to the neurons.[77] Although definitive evidence for this cycle is not yet available, we have shown that one of its key elements, a chloride-dependent high-affinity glutamate receptor with a K_D of 0.5 μM, is present in astrocytes.[16]

The glutamate receptor of astrocytes has unique binding and pharmacological properties that distinguish it from the five Glu binding sites present in neurons (Table II). Highly excitotoxic compounds such as kainate or N-methyl-D-aspar-

TABLE II. Ligand Specificity of Glutamate Binding
to Astrocyte Membranes

Displacer	Glutamate bound (%)
None	100
L-Aspartate	4 ± 3
Quisqualate	49 ± 2
D-Aspartate	76 ± 6
N-Methyl-D-aspartate	106 ± 26
2-Amino-5-phosphonopentanoate	84 ± 6
Kainate	86 ± 11
L-2-Amino-4-phosphonobutyrate	95 ± 15
AMPA[a]	106 ± 26

[a]AMPA, α-amino-3-hydroxy-5-methyl-4-isoxazole propionate. Specific binding of [³H]Glu (100nM) to astrocyte membranes was determined in 50 mM Tris-HCl, 1 mM CaCl₂, at 30°C, 60 min, in the presence of the compounds indicated (100μM).[16]

tate are unable to bind to the astrocyte receptor. They are toxic because they cannot be removed by astrocytes. Glutamate and aspartate are able to use the astrocyte binding site and are neurotoxic only when they are in large excess with respect to their physiological concentration, as is the case following CNS trauma.[11]

Astrocytes, by their ability to bind excitatory amino acids, constitute a natural protective system against excitotoxic lesions. Their rapid proliferation after injury may help to arrest secondary neuronal death.

5.4. ASTROCYTES PRODUCE FACTORS THAT PROMOTE NEURONAL SURVIVAL, SPROUTING, AND SUBSTRATE ATTACHMENT

Central neurons show no long-term survival in culture in the absence of astrocytes or their secretion products. Astrocytes seem to be a major source of NGF and non-NGF neuronotrophic and neurite-promoting factors,[9,63,73,95] particularly laminin.[59] Furthermore, astrocytes are an excellent substrate for neuron attachment and neurite extension both in culture[26,83,85] and *in vivo*,[90,101] perhaps because of their ability to produce laminin.[59−61,67,91] Following injury to the adult CNS, the conditions and time course of production of neuronotrophic and neurite-promoting factors *in vivo* parallel those of astrocytosis and astrogliosis[78,80] (Fig. 10). Suppression of glial proliferation causes suppression of injury-induced factor production.[42] In summary, both *in vitro* and *in vivo*, astrocytes provide neurons with trophic support, growth signals, and substrate attachment. Astrocytes could be responsible for the enhanced postlesion plasticity of the CNS. From this point of view, astrocyte proliferation following injury also appears beneficial, i.e., adaptive.

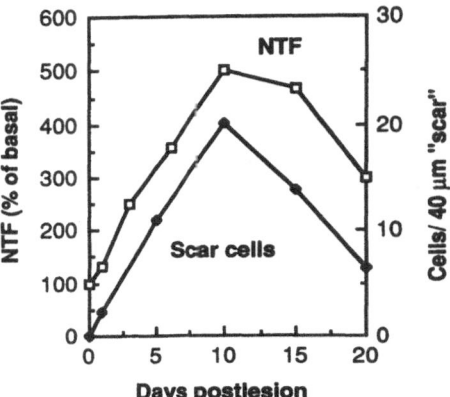

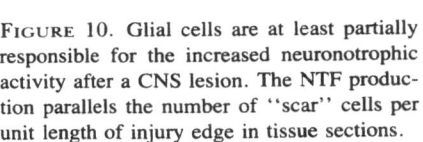

FIGURE 10. Glial cells are at least partially responsible for the increased neuronotrophic activity after a CNS lesion. The NTF production parallels the number of "scar" cells per unit length of injury edge in tissue sections.

5.5. TRANSPLANTS OF PURIFIED ASTROCYTES PROMOTE FUNCTIONAL RECOVERY

Astrocytes bind excitotoxins, secrete neuronotrophic and neurite-promoting factors, and are a preferred substrate for axonal growth. From these properties it could be expected that astrocytes transplanted into an injury area immediately after a lesion may help recovery of function in two ways: (1) by preventing secondary neuronal death and (2) by stimulating neuronal plasticity. We have recently shown that after a cortical lesion this prediction is correct.[46]

Bilateral ablation of the mediofrontal cortex of adult rats causes severe deficits in the learning of spatial tasks. Typically, cortically damaged animals require at least twice as many trials as normal controls to learn a simple reinforced alternation task in a T-maze. Stein and collaborators showed that recovery from this deficit could be accelerated by transplantation of embryonic frontal cortex and that the T-maze performance of those injured animals that subsequently received transplants was indistingishable from that of controls.[54] A puzzling observation in these experiments was that formation of transplant–host connections did not appear to be involved. The authors suggested that trophic mechanisms could be responsible for the recovery, an idea suceptible to experimental test.

We operated on a set of neonatal rats, placed a gelfoam fragment in the injury cavity, and, when the neuronotrophic activity in the gelfoam reached maximal levels, transferred the gelfoam (called "injury gelfoam") from the neonates to a group of adult test animals that had received a medial frontal cortex ablation immediately before. The T-maze performance of the injury gelfoam recipients was indistinguishable from that of either sham-operated controls or controls that received a delayed transplant of embryonic frontal cortex. However, if the gelfoam fragments were extracted and the extract applied to the lesions soaked in a fresh gelfoam fragment, the improvement in performance did not occur (Fig. 11).

The only difference between the gelfoam fragments transferred directly to the test animals and those that were first extracted and the extract then supplied absorbed in a new gelfoam fragment was the presence in the former of glial cells. Accordingly, we tested the ability of glial cells to mediate functional recovery. Purified astrocytes were cultured in gelfoam fragments, and the fragments implanted immediately after frontal cortex ablation, as for injury gelfoam. The performance in the T-maze alternation task of this group of rats was indistiguishable from that of sham-operated controls. Astrocyte transplants accelerated recovery to the same extent as did transplants of either injury gelfoam or embryonic frontal cortex[46] (Fig. 11). On the other hand, when astrocyte transplants were performed 8 days after the lesion, no recovery of function was observed.

These results indicate that astrocytes, when transplanted immediately after

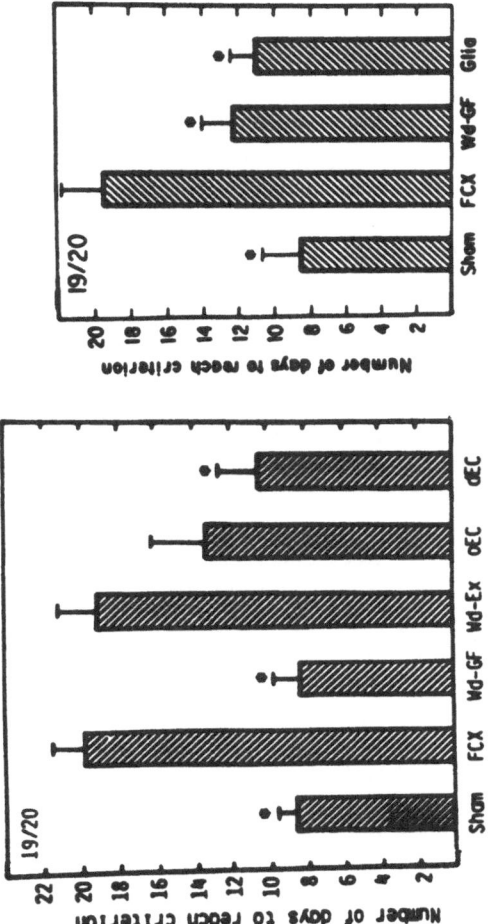

FIGURE 11. Astrocyte transplants promote behavioral recovery. Number of days that adult rats require to reach criterion performance (19 out of 20 correct alternations in two consecutive days) after the following treatments: Sham, sham-operated control; FCX, bilateral medial frontal cortex ablation control. All animals in the remaining groups received bilateral ablations followed by the indicated implants: Wd-Gf, implanted wound gelfoam; Wd-Ex, implanted gelfoam soaked in wound gelfoam extract; oEC, no-delay embryonic tissue transplant; dEC, delayed (8 days) embryonic tissue transplants; Glia, purified astrocyte transplant. There were no significant differences in performance among the groups marked with an asterisk. (Adapted from ref. 46.)

injury, may act in two independent ways: (1) removing and inactivating excitotoxins, thus preventing secondary neuronal death; (2) producing neuronotrophic and neurite-promoting factors that stimulate the plasticity response of the surviving neurons.

5.6. CONTROL OF THE NEURAL ENVIRONMENT BY ASTROCYTES: A NEURON–ASTROCYTE UNIT OF FUNCTION

Many CNS responses are best understood in terms of dynamic units of function, neuron–glia. Astrocytes are intimately associated with neurons and, because of their sensitivity to ions and their ability to bind and transport neurotransmitters, are able continuously to monitor and modify their microenvironment. Furthermore, astrocytes can be depolarized by excitatory neurotransmitters,[15,47] show specialized regions of high conductance,[76] and are able to conduct action potentials.[1] These properties make astrocytes able to monitor (receive, interpret, and act according to) continuously the information signaled by neurons. They seem to function as "environment stats" that maintain the environmental composition appropriate for a normal pattern of neuronal activity. Any deviation from that composition triggers a glial response, for example, by removing excess excitatory molecules before they reach excitotoxic levels or by producing levels of neuronotrophic and sprouting factor activities adequate to ongoing neuronal requirements. In summary, astrocytes seem to be the primary controllers of the CNS environment as regards ionic composition, neurotransmitter concentration, and supply of neuronal growth factors.

Under normal circumstances, astrocytes are able to fulfill a large variety of unrelated roles. After injury, glial cells are subject to greatly increased demands. The number of cells available attempts to meet the new demands by various types of reaction, including hypertrophy and, if necessary, cell division. However, large injuries appear to overwhelm the astrocyte capabilities. A general and immediate consequence of CNS injury is astrocyte swelling at the injury site. Swollen cells may be impaired in their ability to carry out their functions. Neurons near an injury may die from the combination of excitotoxicity, a decrease in the availability of trophic factors, and/or an increase in neuronotrophic requirements. Transplantation of purified astrocytes could have great therapeutic usefulness in CNS repair by helping the indigenous cells to carry the additional load imposed by the lesion. Implanted astrocytes would help to restore the neuronal environment to a composition that falls within the buffering capacity of the available glial cells.

6. CELLULAR SOURCES OF TROPHIC FACTORS

Central nervous system injury begins with the initial traumatic event but does not end with it. Trauma triggers a cascade of events, some independent of each other and some causally related, that continue in time far after the initial trauma. Some of these events, particularly those leading to secondary cell death, are clearly deleterious and increase the extent of the initial injury. Others, like glial scar formation, are apparently deleterious in that they may prevent recovery of function; however, they fulfill an adaptive function because they are keyed to protect the survival of the whole organism.

What are the cells that produce glial mitogens, morphogens, and inhibitors and neuron survival and sprouting factors? When, after injury, do they begin to produce these substances? Do these cells proliferate, and, if so, when? We have enough data to propose reasonable answers to several of these questions.

Two working hypotheses, by no means mutually exclusive, propose that neuron survival and neurite-promoting factors are (1) produced by the neuronal target—in this case, it is common to assume that sprouting factor production is inhibited in the fully innervated state and rises after denervation[20] and (2) produced by nonneuronal cells and regulated by neuron–glia interactions.[78] A number of solid experimental observations (see refs. 20 and 78) support both hypotheses, and it is unlikely that either may be totally incorrect. A hypothetical model for the increase in NTF and NPF production after a lesion is summarized in Fig. 12. Under normal conditions, neurons and glia exchange signals about their mutual metabolic state; astrocytes maintain appropriate levels of extracellular growth factors, ions, and neurotransmitters. Neurons produce mitogen

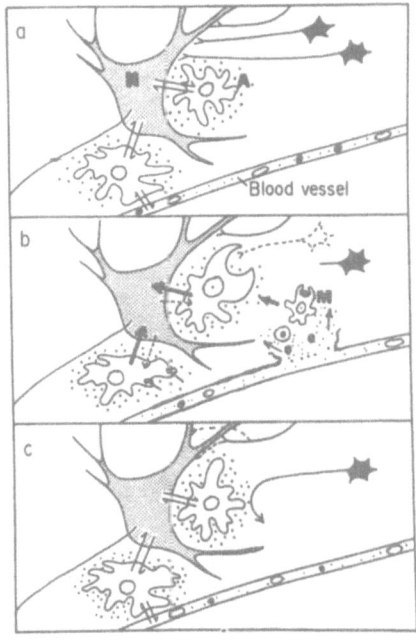

FIGURE 12. Cellular sources of trophic signals. (a) Normally, astrocytes (A) and neurons (N) exchange signals on their mutual metabolic state. Neuronal mitogen inhibitors maintain the normal glial population stationary. (b) Injury disrupts both the blood–CNS barrier and the neuronal circuitry. Blood components invade the CNS. Neurons cease to produce mitogen inhibitors. Mitogenic signals from monocytes (M) help trigger astrocyte proliferation and perhaps enhance growth factor secretion. (c) These growth factors help axotomized and ischemic neurons to survive and initiate sprouting. Repair of the capillaries, restitution of the glial boundary, and reinnervation of neurons by sprouts shut the sources of initiating signals, and a new steady state is achieved.

inhibitors that maintain glial populations stationary (Fig. 12a). Denervation (Fig. 12b) may directly cause an increase in factor secretion by the deafferented target or indirectly through the glia. Astrocytes could detect CNS damage, for example, as an elevation in the levels of K^+ or of excitatory amino acids. These or other signals may trigger the additional production of trophic factors. Alternatively, each astrocyte may continue to produce its usual amount of trophic factors, but the total output will increase through local astrocyte proliferation.

Signals to initiate astrocyte proliferation may come from activated blood monocytes (Fig. 12b; "ameboid microglia"[37]). Blood monocytes may become activated by cell debris in the injury area. Alternatively, astrocyte proliferation may be directly initiated by activation of astrocyte voltage-gated K^+ channels.[23] At the same time, damaged neurons may decrease or cease their output of mitogen inhibitors.[41] The process thus initiated will lead to astrocyte proliferation. The new cells, in turn, will reform the glia limitans and secrete survival and sprouting factors. Closing of the blood–CNS barrier and reinnervation of deafferented neurons by reactive sprouts will shut the sources of the initiating signals, and the CNS will return to a new steady state (Fig. 12c).

7. Timing of the Intervention in CNS Repair

Extensive CNS trauma has a major impact on the survival of the whole organism. Has any priority system evolved for the response of the CNS to such an emergency? Indications may be obtained by comparing the order of events during development (Fig. 13A) with that following injury (Fig. 13B).

During development, the two earliest events observed concomitantly with the appearance of the CNS as a distinct organ are the development of a primitive vasculature and the appearance of a boundary, a basal lamina. This points to two major CNS priorities: first, to ensure the supply of oxygen and nutrients and the removal of catabolites; second, to develop structures that protect the CNS from indiscriminate influences from the rest of the organism. The second priority is emphasized by the subsequent rapid formation of an incipient blood–CNS barrier, a layer of glia limitans and a pia–arachnoid system. These events occur in the early days of development and affect the CNS as a whole. Most neuronal and glial proliferation, axonal and dendritic growth, and synapse formation occur subsequently, over a period that in rats is measured in weeks rather than days. They are local events that have their own pace in each individual CNS locus, although in each case the sequence of events is highly coordinated and reproducible.

The same priorities seem to be maintained throughout the lifetime of the organism and are expressed in the spontaneous response to injury. The CNS is critically dependent on blood supply. At the same time, the blood–CNS barrier has to be strictly maintained so that concentrations of metabolites that would be normal in other organs, such as glutamate or aspartate, cannot cause havoc in the

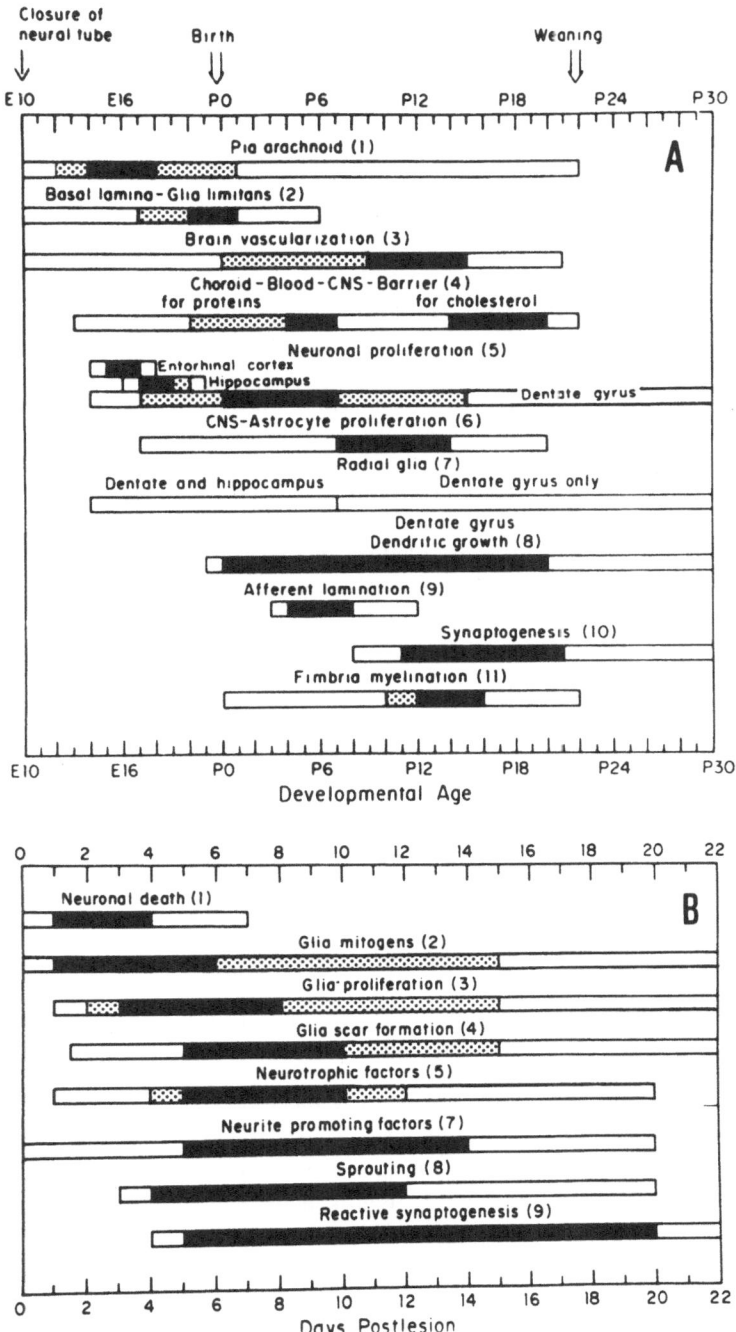

FIGURE 13. Order of events in the CNS: (A) During development. (B) After injury. (Adapted from ref. 78.)

CNS by indiscriminately flooding all excitatory synapses. Therefore, re-vascularization and glia proliferation leading to the formation of the neo-glia limitans begin very rapidly after a CNS lesion (Fig. 13B). A vascularized glial boundary is observed 5 days after mechanical damage to the rat cortex. Mean-while, secondary neuronal death is in progress, reaching a maximum around 4 days post-lesion. Maximal production of neuronotrophic factors that could arrest neuronal death is only reached around 8–10 days post-lesion. In development, sprouting and synaptogenesis occur within a system enclosed by the glia lim-itans, and most astrocyte proliferation follows sprouting. After injury, the con-verse is true: sprouting follows astrocyte proliferation and glial scar formation (Fig. 13B). Consequently, regenerating axon sprouts find between themselves and their target the new glial boundary, which they cannot cross.

The spontaneous repair response of the mammalian CNS seems only ade-quate to cope with minor injury. When faced with major lesions, the overall time course of events seems to be directed to CNS survival but not to restoration of function. It appears that, during the evolution of mammals, functional repair of the CNS after a major injury provided no selective advantage.

The priorities of the neurologist are the same as those of the tissue—to a certain point. Preserving the organism is essential, but functional recovery also has major importance. Our increasing understanding of the biochemical and cellular events after CNS injury permits a new optimism concerning the pos-sibility of functional CNS repair. From the work carried out thus far, we may derive a few general principles. I believe that in order to achieve functional repair: (1) we should try to use as far as possible the natural repair response of the CNS; (2) interventions should be directed to manipulate, when necessary, the temporal expression of this natural response; (3) therefore, timing of the inter-ventions will be critical; (4) multiple interventions, intertwining our priorities and those of the CNS, will most likely be necessary; (5) we should try to use, as far as possible, the same compounds and cells that the injured CNS does.

Treatment of CNS injury in animal models, using a global approach based on the conceptual advances made in recent years, has not yet been performed. The sequence of treatments of an open CNS injury proposed below is certain to be very simplistic and incomplete, but it gives an idea of the type of multiple interventions that I have in mind.

As soon after injury as possible, we want to "engineer" the neuronal environment in order to prevent secondary neuronal death. This may be possible by treatment with glutamate antagonists and infusion of neuronotrophic factors. It seems reasonable to continue this treatment for about 4–6 days post-lesion. Treatment with other substances, such as antiinflammatory drugs, sulfhydryl reagents, and inhibitors of lipolysis, may be added, keeping in mind that it may be as important to avoid treatments that are deleterious as to provide the correct ones. In this respect, high levels of glucocorticoids seem to potentiate excitotoxic neuronal death[96] and should perhaps be avoided. Finally, implantation of cultured astrocytes, also performed as soon after trauma as possible, would help to normalize the neuronal environment and promote neuronal survival and sprouting.

Treatment with neurite-promoting factors may help to initiate sprouting, thus stimulating process regeneration. There are no data indicating the optimal time to initiate treatment with NPFs. Here, we face the contradiction that we want to initiate regenerative growth as soon as possible, yet we do not want to encourage reactive sprouting. Treatment with neurite-promoting factors is questionable until we have data on their specificity. Research is essential to investigate whether regenerative sprouting and reactive sprouting are both promoted by the same factors. Also, the possibility of isolating substances that accelerate neurite elongation is critical to intervention in axonal regeneration. Virtually no studies are available in this area.

Ideally, one should use purified injury-induced factors from the same species as that of the injured animal. However, these factors have not yet been purified. Other factors such as NGF, acidic and basic FGF, EGF, plasminogen activator, and its inhibitors are available in pure form. Their general neuronotrophic and/or neurite-promoting activity has not yet been fully evaluated.

Following the early treatment, large injuries would receive, 8–10 days postlesion, a transplant of homologous embryonic tissue. Local injections of mitogen and/or morphogen inhibitors may facilitate innervation of the implant by host fibers and make possible functional transplant–host integration. However, a major problem remains in that the CNS needs a glial boundary, whereas the neurologist needs regenerative growth across this glial layer. Glial inhibition has to be local, and axon growth directed to that particular area. More intense research into the molecules and processes that contribute to the guidance of axonal growth is essential.

Sprouts from nondamaged local axons are close to the deafferented neurons and will occupy all available postsynaptic sites before regenerating fibers are able to reach them. After neurons are fully innervated, the competition between reactive and regenerative fibers would be limited to that allowed by ongoing synapse turnover. This is a problem that may require additional surgery to provide postsynaptic space or the application of molecules that accelerate synapse renewal. The reports that monoamines and acetylcholine[10] increase synapse turnover deserve to be examined in this context.

8. CONCLUSION

Learning about glial cells and about the various types of sprouting response is a key problem in CNS repair. Neuronotrophic and neurite-promoting activities may be a byproduct of glial proliferation. In general, astroglia play a peculiar dichotomous role—they are both beneficial and detrimental. Functional repair of the CNS will probably require the development of methods that permit the control of glial proliferation and differentiation at precise anatomic loci. It may also require selective stimulation of the initiation and growth of regenerative sprouts. Much of the work outlined in this chapter was performed within the last 5 years. The basic findings permit the visualization of new conceptual approaches to CNS repair. The clinical crystallization of these concepts has not yet occurred but is likely to follow soon.

REFERENCES

1. Abbot, N. J., 1985. Are glial cells excitable after all? *Trends Neurosci.* **8**:141–142.
2. Adrian, E. K., 1963, Cell division in injured spinal cord, *Am. J. Anat.* **123**:501–520.
3. Adrian, E. K., and Williams, M. G., 1973, Cell proliferation in injured spinal cord. An electron microscopic study, *J. Comp. Neurol.* **151**:1–24.
4. Aguayo, A., 1985, Axonal regeneration from injured neurons in the adult mammalian nervous system. In: *Synaptic Plasticity* (C. W. Cotman, ed.), The Guilford Press, New York, pp. 457–484.
5. Aguayo, A., Vidal-Sanz, M., and Bray, G. M., 1986, PNS transplants into the CNS: A tool for the study of axonal regeneration and connectivity in the mammalian brain, *Proceedings of the Symposium on Neural Grafts*, UCLA, Los Angeles, pp. 33–34.
6. Azmitia, E. C., Perlow, M. J., Brennan, M. J., and Lauder, J. M., 1981, Fetal raphe and hippocampal transplants into adult and aged C57 BL/6N mice: A preliminary immunocytochemical study, *Brain Res. Bull.* **7**:703–710.
7. Azmitia, E. C., and Whittaker, P. M., 1983, Formation of a glial scar following microinjection of fetal neurons into the hippocampus or midbrain of adult rat: An immunocytocchemical study, *Neurosci. Lett.* **38**:145–150.
8. Balentine, J. D., 1978, Pathology of experimental spinal cord trauma. II. Ultrastructure of axons and myelin, *Lab. Invest.* **39**:254–266.
9. Banker, G. A., 1980, Trophic interactions between astroglial cells and hippocampal neurons in culture, *Science* **209**:809–810.
10. Bear, M. F., and Singer, W., 1986, Modulation of visual cortical plasticity by acetylcholine and noradrenaline, *Nature* **320**:172–176.
11. Beneviste, H., Drejer, J., Schousboe, A., and Diemer, N. H., 1984, Elevation of the extracellular concentrations of glutamate and aspartate in rat hippocampus during transient cerebral ischemia monitored by intracerebral microdialysis, *J. Neurochem.* **43**:1369–1374.
11a. Bernstein, J. J., and Bernstein, M. E., 1971, Axonal regeneration and formation of synapses proximal to the site of lesion following hemisection of the rat spinal cord, *Exp. Neurol.* **19**:25–32.
12. Bjorklund, A., Segal, M., and Stenevi, U., 1979, Functional reinnervation of rat hippocampus by locus coeruleus implants *Brain Res.* **170**:409–426.
13. Bjorklund, A., and Stenevi, U., 1977, Reformation of the severed septohippocampal cholinergic pathway in the adult rat by transplanted septal neurons, *Cell Tissue Res.* **185**:289–302.
14. Bjorklund, A., Stenevi, U., and Svengaard, N.-A., 1976, Growth of transplanted monoaminergic neurons into the adult hippocampus along the perforant path, *Nature* **262**:787–790.
15. Bowman, C. L., and Kimelberg, H. K., 1984, Excitatory amino acids directly depolarize rat brain astrocytes in primary culture, *Nature* **311**:656–659.
16. Bridges, R. J., Nieto-Sampedro, M., and Cotman, C. W., 1985, Stereospecific binding of L-glutamate to astrocyte membranes, *Soc. Neurosci. Abstr.* **11**:110.

17. Cassell, M. D., and Brown, M. W., 1984, The distribution of Timm's stain in the non-sulphide perfused human hippocampal formation *J. Comp. Neural.* **222**:461–471.
18. Clemente, C. D., 1955, Structural regeneration in the mammalian CNS and the role of neuroglia and connective tissue, in: *Regeneration in the Central Nervous System* (W. F. Windle, ed.), Charles C. Thomas, Springfield, IL, pp. 147–161.
19. Cotman, C. W., and Nieto-Sampedro, M., 1984, Cell biology of synaptic plasticity, *Science* **225**:1287–1294.
20. Cotman, C. W., Nieto-Sampedro, M., and Harris, E. W., 1981, Synapse replacement in the nervous system of adult vertebrates, *Physiol. Rev.* **61**:684–784
21. Cotman, C. W., Flatman, J. A., Ganong, A. H., and Perkins, M. N., 1986, Effects of excitatory amino acid antagonists on evoked and spontaneous excitatory potentials in guinea pig hippocampus, *J. Physiol. (Lond.)* **378**:403–415.
22. Davies, J., Evans, R. H., Herrling, P. L., Jones, A. W., Olverman, H. J., Pook, P., and Watkins, J. C., 1986, CPP, a new potent and selective NMDA antagonist. Depression of central neuron responses, affinity for ^{3}H-D-AP5 binding sites on brain membranes and anticonvulsant activity, *Brain Res.* **382**:169–173.
23. De Coursey, T. E., Chandy, K. G., Gupta, S., and Cahalan, M. D., 1984, Voltage-gated K $^+$ channels in human T lymphocytes: A role in mitogenesis? *Nature* **307**:465–468.
24. de la Torre, J. C., 1982, Catecholamine fiber regeneration accross a collagen bio-implant after spinal cord transection, *Brain Res. Bull.* **9**:545–552.
25. Faden, A. I., 1983, Recent pharmacological advances in experimental spinal injury, *Trends Neurosci.* **6**:375–377.
26. Fallon, J., 1985, Neurite guidance by non-neuronal cells in culture: Preferential outgrowth of peripheral neurites on glial as compared to nonglial cell surfaces, *J. Neurosci.* **5**:3169–3177.
27. Fedoroff, S., and Doering, L., 1987, Transplantation of mouse astrocyte precursor cells cultured in vitro into neonatal cerebellum, *Ann. N.Y. Acad. Sci.* **495**:24–34.
28. Foster, A. C., Gill, R., Iverson, L. L., and Woodruff, G. N., 1987, Systems administration of MK-801 protects against ischemia-induced hippocampal neurodegeneration in the gerbil, *Br. J. Pharmacol* **90**:9P.
29. Fujita, S., and Kitamura, T., 1976, Origin of the brain macrophages and the origin of the microglia, *Prog. Neuropathol.* **3**:1–50.
30. Ganong, A. H., Jones, A. W., Watkins, J. C., and Cotman, C. W., 1986, Parallel antagonism of synaptic transmission and kainate/quisqualate responses in the hippocampus by piperazine-2,3-dicarboxylic acid analogs, *J. Neurosci.* **6**:930–937.
31. Ganong, A. H., Lanthorn, T. H., and Cotman, C. W., 1983, Kynurenic acid inhibits synaptic and acidic amino acid-induced responses in the rat hippocampus and spinal cord, *Brain Res.* **273**:170–174.
32. Gearhart, J., Oster-Granite. M. L., and Guth, L., 1979, Histological changes after transection of the spinal cord of fetal and neonatal mice, *Exp. Neurol.* **66**:1–15.
33. Geddes, J. W., Monaghan, D. T., Cotman, C. W., Lott, I. T., Kim, R. C., and Chui, H. C., 1985, Plasticity of hippocampal circuitry in Alzheimer's disease, *Science* **230**:1179–1181.
34. Gibbs, R. B., Harris, E. W., and Cotman, C. W., 1985, Replacement of damaged cortical projections by homotypic transplants of entorhinal cortex, *J. Comp. Neurol.* **237**:47–64.
35. Gibbs, R. B., Anderson, K., and Cotman, C. W., 1987, Factors affecting innervation in the CNS: Comparison of three cholinergic cell types transplanted to the hippocampus of adult rats, *Brain Res.* **383**: 362–366.
36. Giulian, D., and Baker, T. J., 1985, Peptides released by ameboid microglia regulate astroglial proliferation, *J. Cell Biol.* **101**:2411–2415.
37. Guth, L., Barrett, C. P., Donati, E. J., Dashpande, S. S., and Albuquerque, E., 1981, Histopathological reactions and axonal regeneration in the transected spinal cord of hibernating squirrels, *J. Comp. Neurol.* **203**:297–308.

38. Hansson, E., Rönnbäck, L., Lowenthal. A., and Noppe, M., 1985, Primary cultures from defined brain areas: Effects of seeding time on cell growth, astroglial content and protein synthesis, *Dev. Brain Res.* **21:**175–185.

39. Hansson, E., 1985, Primary cultures from defined brain areas; effects of seeding time on the development of β-adrenergic- and dopamine-stimulated cAMP-activity during cultivation, *Dev. Brain Res.* **21:**187–192.

40. Harris, E. W., Ganong, A. H., Monaghan, D. T., Watkins, J. C., and Cotman, C. W., 1986, Action of CPP: A new and highly potent antagonist of NMDA receptors in the hippocampus, *Brain Res.* **382:** 174–177.

41. Hatten, M. E., 1985, Neuronal regulation of astroglial morphology and proliferation *in vitro, J. Cell Biol.* **100:**384–396.

42. Heacock, A. M., Schonfeld, A. R., and Katzman, R., 1986, Hippocampal neurotrophic factor: Characterization and response to denervation, *Brain Res.* **363:**299–306.

43. Hirano, A., 1969, The fine structure of brain in edema, in: *The Structure and Function of the Nervous Tissue* (G. H. Bourne, ed.), Academic Press, New York, pp. 69–135.

44. Kalderon, N., 1987, The astrocyte and the failure of CNS neural regeneration: A study of innoculated astrocytes in a PNS regenerating model system, *Ann. N.Y. Acad. Sci.* **495:**722–725.

45. Kao, C. C., and Chang, L. W., 1977, The mechanism of spinal cord cavitation following spinal cord transection. Part 1: A correlative histochemical study, *J. Neurosurg.* **46:**197–206.

46. Kesslak, J. P., Nieto-Sampedro, M., Globus, J., and Cotman, C. W., 1986, Transplants of purified astrocytes promote behavioral recovery after frontal cortex ablation, *Exp. Neurol.* **92:**377–390.

47. Kettenmann, H., and Schachner, M., 1985, Pharmacological properties of γ-aminobutyric acid-, glutamate- and aspartate-induced depolarizations in cultured astrocytes, *J. Neurosci.* **5:**3295–3301.

48. Kirino, T., 1982, Delayed neuronal death in the gerbil hippocampus following ischemia, *Brain Res.* **239:**57–69.

49. Klatzo, I., 1967, Neuropathological aspects of brain edema, *J. Neuropathol. Ept. Neurol.* **26:**1–14.

50. Korschig, S., Auburger, G., Heumann, R., Scott, J., and Thoenen, H., 1985, Levels of nerve growth factor and its mRNA in the central nervous system of the rat correlate with cholinergic innervation, *EMBO J.* **4:**1389–1393.

51. Krikorian, J. G., Guth, L., and Donati, E., 1981, The origin of connective tissue scar in the transected rat spinal cord, *Exp. Neurol.* **72:**698–707.

52. Kromer, L. F., Bjorklund, A., and Stenevi, U., 1984, Intracephalic embryonic implants in the adult brain. I. Growth and mature organization of brainstem, cerebellar and hippocampal implants, *J. Comp. Neurol.* **218:**433–459.

53. Kromer, L. F., Bjorklund, A., and Stenevi, U., 1980, Innervation of embryonic hippocampal implants by regenerating axons of cholinergic septal neurons in the adult brain, *Brain Res.* **210:**153–171.

54. Labbe, R., Firl, E. F., Jr., Mufson, E. J., and Stein, D. G., 1983, Fetal brain transplants: Reduction of cognitive deficits in rats with frontal cortex lesions, *Science* **221:**470–472.

55. Lemke, G. E., and Brockes, J. P., 1984, Identification and purification of glial growth factor, *J. Neurosci.* **4:**75–83.

56. Levi-Montalcini, R., and Angeletti, P. U., 1968, Nerve growth factor, *Physiol. Rev.* **48:**534–569.

57. Lewis, E. R., and Cotman, C. W., 1983, Neurotransmitter characteristics of brain grafts: Striatal and septal tissues form the same laminated input to hippocampus, *Neuroscience* **8:**57–66.

58. Lieberman, A. R., 1971, The axon reaction: A review of the principal features of perikaryal responses to axonal injury, *Int. Rev. Neurobiol.* **14:**49–124.

59. Liesi, P., Dahl, D., and Vaheri, A., 1983, Laminin is produced by early rat astrocytes in primary culture, *J. Cell Biol.* **96:**920–924.
60. Liesi, P., Dahl, D., and Vaheri, A., 1984, Neurons cultured from developing rat brain attach and spread preferentially to laminin, *J. Neurosci. Res.* **11:**241–251.
61. Liesi, P., Kaakkola, S., Dahl, D., and Vaheri, A., 1984, Laminin is induced in astrocytes of adult brain by injury, *EMBO J.* **3:**683–686.
62. Lim, R., 1985, Glia maturation factor and other factors acting on glia, in: *Growth and Maturation Factors,* Volume 3 (G. Guroff, ed.), John Wiley & Sons, New York, pp. 119–147.
63. Lindsay, R. M., 1979, Adult rat brain astrocytes support the survival of both NGF-dependent and NGF-insensitive neurons, *Nature* **282:**80–82.
64. Lindsay, R. M., and Raisman, G., 1983, An autoradiographic study of neuronal development, vascularization and neuronal cell migration from hippocampal transplants labelled in intermediate explant culture, *J. Neurosci.* **12:**513–530.
65. Loesche, J., and Steward, O., 1977, Behavioral correlates of denervation and reinnervation of the hippocampal formation of the rat: recovery of alternation performance following unilateral entorhinal cortex lesions, *Brain Res. Bull.* **2:**31–39.
66. Lundberg, J. J., and Møllgard, K., 1979, Mitotic activity in adult rat brain induced by implantation of pieces of fetal rat braen and liver, *Neurosci. Lett.* **13:**265–270.
67. Manthorpe, M., Envall, E., Ruoslahti, E., Longo, F. M., Davis, G. E., and Varon, S., 1983, Laminin promotes neurite regeneration from cultured peripheral and central neurons, *J. Cell Biol.* **97:**1882–1890.
68. Manthorpe, M., Nieto-Sampedro, M., Skaper, S. D., Lewis, E. R., Barbin, G., Longo, F. M., Cotman, C. W., and Varon, S., 1983, Neuronotrophic activity in wounds of the developing rat. Correlation with implant survival in the wound cavity, *Brain Res* **267:**47–56.
69. McCarthy, K. D., and de Vellis, J., 1980, Preparation of separate astroglial and oligodendroglial cell cultures from rat cerebral tissue, *J. Cell Biol.* **85:**890–902.
70. Meldrum, B., 1985, Possible applications of antagonists of excitatory amino acid neurotransmitter, *Clin. Sci.* **68:**113–122.
71. Miller, R. H., Abney, E. R., David, S., ffrench-Constant, C., Lindsay, R., Patel, R., Stone, J., and Raff, M. C., 1986, Is reactive gliosis a property of a distinct subpopulation of astrocytes? *J. Neurosci.* **6:**22–29.
72. Miller, R., and Raff, M. C., 1984, Fibrous and protoplasmic astrocytes are biochemically and developmentally distinct, *J. Neurosci.* **4:**585–592.
73. Müller, H. W., and Seifert, W., 1982, A neurotrophic factor (NTF) released from primary glial cultures supports survival and fiber outgrowth of cultured hippocampal neurons, *J. Neurosci. Res.* **8:**195–204.
74. Needels, D. L., Nieto-Sampedro, M., and Cotman, C. W., 1986, Induction of a neurite-promoting factor in rat brain following injury or deafferentation, *Neuroscience* **18:**517–526.
75. Needels, D. L., Nieto-Sampedro, M., Whittemore, S. R., and Cotman, C. W., 1985, Neuronotrophic activity for ciliary ganglion neurons. Induction following injury to the brain of neonatal, adult and aged rats, *Dev. Brain Res.* **18:**275–284.
76. Newman, E. A., 1986, High potassium conductance in astrocyte end feet, *Science* **233:**453–454.
77. Nicklas, W. J., 1986, Glia–neuronal interrelationships in the metabolism of excitatory amino acids, in: *Excitatory Amino Acids* (P. J. Roberts, J. Storm-Mathisen, and H. F. Bradford, eds.), Macmillan, London, pp. 57–66.
78. Nieto-Sampedro, M., and Cotman, C. W., 1985, Growth factor induction and temporal order in CNS repair, in: *Synaptic Plasticity* (C. W. Cotman, ed.), Guilford Press, New York, pp. 407–455.
79. Nieto-Sampedro, M., Lewis, E. R., Cotman, C. W., Manthorpe, M., Skaper, S. D., Barbin, G., Longo, F. M., and Varon, S., 1982, Brain injury causes a time-dependent increase in neuronotrophic activity at the lesion site, *Science* **221:**860–861.

80. Nieto-Sampedro, M., Manthorpe, M., Barbin, G., Varon, S., and Cotman, C. W., 1983, Injury-induced neuronotrophic activity in adult rat brain: Correlation with survival of delayed implants in the wound cavity, *J. Neurosci.* **3**:2219–2229.
81. Nieto-Sampedro, M., Saneto, R. P., de Vellis, J., and Cotman, C. W., 1985, The control of glial populations in brain: Changes in astrocyte mitogenic and morphogenic factors in response to injury, *Brain Res.* **343**:320–328.
82. Nieto-Sampedro, M., Whittemore, S. R., Needels, D. L., Larson, J., and Cotman, C. W., 1984, The survival of brain transplants is enhanced by extracts from injured brain, *Proc. Natl. Acad. Sci. U.S.A.* **81**:6250–6254.
83. Noble, M., Fok-Seang, J., and Cohen, J., 1984, Glia are a unique substrate for the *in vitro* growth of central nervous system neurons, *J. Neurosci.* **4**:1892–1903.
84. Oblinger, M. M., and Das, G. D., 1982, Connectivity of neural transplants in adult rats: Analysis of afferents and efferents of neocortical transplants in the cerebellar hemisphere, *Brain Res.* **249**:31–49.
85. Peacock, J. H., Rush, D. E., and Mathers, L. H., 1979, Morphology of dissociated hippocampal cultures from fetal mice, *Brain Res.* **169**:231–246.
86. Pettmann, B., Weibel, M., Sensenbrenner, M., and Labourdette, G., 1985, Purification of two astroglial growth factors from bovine brain, *FEBS Lett.* **189**:102–108.
87. Raff, M. C., Abney, E. R., Cohen, J., Lindsay, R., and Noble, M., 1983, Two types of astrocytes in cultures of developing rat white matter: Differences in morphology, surface gangliosides, and growth characteristics, *J. Neurosci.* **6**:1289–1300.
88. Raisman, G., Lawrence, J. M., Zhou, C.-F., and Lindsay, R. M., 1985, Some neuronal, glial and vascular interactions which occur when developing hippocampal primordia are incorporated into adult host hippocampi, in: *Neural Grafting in the Mammalian CNS* (A. Bjorklund and U. Stenevi, eds.), Elsevier, New York.
89. Ramon y Cajal, S., 1928, *Degeneration and Regeneration in the Nervous System*, Hoffner, New York.
90. Reier, P. J., Stensaas, L. J., and Guth, L., 1983, The astrocytic scar as an impediment to regeneration in the central nervous system, in: *Spinal Cord Reconstruction* (C. C. Kao, R. P. Bunge, and P. J. Reier, eds.), Raven Press, New York, pp. 163–195.
91. Rogers, S. L., Letourneau, P. C., Palm, S. L., Mc Carthy, J., and Furcht, L. T., 1983, Neurite extension by peripheral and central nervous system neurons in response to substratum-bound fibronectin and laminin, *Dev. Biol.* **98**:212–220.
92. Rothman, S. M., and Olney, J. W., 1986, Glutamate and the pathology of hypoxic/ischemic brain damage, *Ann. Neurol.* **19**:105–111.
93. Rothman, S. M., 1984, Synaptic release of excitatory amino acid neurotransmitter mediates anoxic neuronal death, *J. Neurosci.* **4**:1884–1891.
94. Rothman, S. M., 1985, The neurotoxicity of excitatory amino acids is produced by passive chloride influx, *J. Neurosci.* **5**:1483–1489.
95. Rudge, J. S., Manthorpe, M., and Varon, S., 1985, The output of neuronotrophic and neurite-promoting agents from rat brain astroglial cells: A microculture method for screening potential regulatory molecules, *Dev. Brain Res.* **19**:161–172.
96. Sapolsky, R. M., and Pulsinelli, W. A., 1985, Glucocorticoid toxicity in the hippocampus: Temporal aspects of neuronal vulnerability, *Science* **229**:1397–1400.
97. Scheff, S. W., Benardo, L., and Cotman, C. W., 1980, Decline in reactive fiber growth in the dentate gyrus of aged rats compared to young adult rats following entorhinal cortex removal, *Brain Res.* **199**:21–38.
98. Schousboe, A., and Divac, I., 1979, Differences in glutamate uptake in astrocytes cultured from different brain regions, *Brain Res.* **177**:407–409.
99. Schousboe, A., Drejer, J., and Divac, I., 1980, Regional heterogeneity in astroglial cells. Implications of neuron–glia interactions, *Trends Neurosci.* **3**:XIII–XIV.

100. Shelton, D. L., and Reichardt, L. F., 1986, Studies on the expression of the β nerve growth factor (NGF) gene in the central nervous system: Level and regional distribution of NGF mRNA suggest that NGF functions as a trophic factor for several distinct populations of neurons, *Proc. Natl. Acad. Sci. U.S.A.* **83:**2714–2718.

101. Silver, J., 1986, Use of transplanted astroglial cells to direct callosal fibers in the adult brain, *Ann. N.Y. Acad. Sci.* **495:**185–206.

102. Simon, R. P., Swan, J. H., Griffiths, T., and Meldrum, B. S., 1984, Blockage of N-methyl-D-aspartate receptors may protect against ischemic damage in the brain, *Science* **226:**850–852.

103. Stenevi, U., Bjorklund, A., and Svendgaard, N.-A., 1976, Transplantation of central and peripheral monoamine neurons to the adult rat brain: Techniques and conditions for survival, *Brain Res.* **114:**1–20.

104. Sturrock, R. R., 1982, Cell division in the normal central nervous system, *Adv. Cell Neurobiol.* **3:**3–33.

105. Sunde, N., and Zimmer, J., 1983, Cellular, histochemical and connective organization of the hippocampus and fascia dentata transplanted to different regions of immature and adult rat brain, *Dev. Brain Res.* **8:**165–191.

106. Thomas, K. A., and Giménez-Gallego, G., 1986, Fibroblast growth factors: Broad spectrum mitogens with potent angiogenic activity, *Trends Biochem. Sci.* **11:**81–84.

107. Whittemore, S. R., Ebendal, T., Lärkfors, L., Olson, L., Seiger, A., Strömberg, I., and Persson, H., 1986, Developmental and regional expression of β nerve growth factor mRNA and protein in the rat central nervous system, *Proc. Natl. Acad. Sci. U.S.A.* **83:**817–821.

108. Whittemore, S. R., Nieto-Sampedro, M., Needels, D., and Cotman, C. W., 1985, Neuronotrophic factors for mammalian brain neurons: Injury induction in neonatal, adult and aged rat brain, *Dev. Brain Res.* **20:**169–178.

109. Wictorin, K., Fischer, W., Williams, L. R., Varon, S., Bjorklund, A., and Gage, F. H., 1985, Loss of acetylcholine esterase positive cells and choline acetyl transferase activity in the septal area and diagonal band of Broca following fimbria–fornix transection, *Neurosci. Abstr.* **11:**257.

110. Wieloch, T., 1986, Endogenous excitotoxins as possible mediators of ischemic and hypoglycemic brain damage, *Prog. Brain Res.* **63:**69–85.

111. Windle, W. F., 1956, Regeneration of axons in the vertebrate central nervous system, *Physiol. Rev.* **36:**427–440.

112. Wong, E. H. F., Kemp, J. A., Priestley, T., Knight, A. R., Woodruff, G. N., and Iversen, L. L., 1986, The novel anticonvulsant MK-801 is a potent NMDA antagonist, *Proc. Natl. Acad. Sci. U.S.A.* **83:**7104–7108.

16

NERVE GROWTH FACTOR
EFFECTS ON CNS NEURONS AND ON BEHAVIORAL RECOVERY FROM BRAIN DAMAGE

BRUNO WILL, FRANZ HEFTI, VIVIANE PALLAGE, AND GUY TONIOLO

ABSTRACT. Nerve growth factor (NGF) is a well-characterized protein that acts as a neurotrophic factor for catecholaminergic neurons of the peripheral sympathetic nervous system and for a subpopulation of peripheral sensory neurons. In the central nervous system, catecholaminergic neurons are not affected, but evidence obtained in recent years indicates that NGF acts as a neurotrophic factor for cholinergic neurons of the basal forebrain innervating cortex and hippocampus. Nerve growth factor affects survival, fiber growth, and expression of transmitter-specific enzymes by these cholinergic neurons. Intracerebral administration of NGF has been found in several studies to modify the behavioral recovery of animals from experimentally induced brain damage. Such effects were observed after lesions in target areas and areas of origin of forebrain cholinergic neurons (septum, fimbria–fornix, hippocampus, cortex) and also after lesions in hypothalamus, striatum, and nucleus accumbens, i.e., in areas not innervated by forebrain cholinergic neurons. The mechanisms mediating the behavioral effects of NGF and the possible involvement of central cholinergic and peripheral sympathetic neurons are discussed.

1. INTRODUCTION

In recent years, evidence has accumulated that neuronal maintenance and survival as well as developmental, adaptive, and restorative neuroplasticity (e.g., ref. 76) depend on the humoral and cellular microenvironment of the neurons. The dependence of neuronal "behavior" on specific sets of microenvironmental

BRUNO WILL, VIVIANE PALLAGE, AND GUY TONIOLO • Department of Neurophysiology and Biology of Behavior, Center of Neurochemistry, C.N.R.S., 67084 Strasbourg, France. FRANZ HEFTI • Department of Neurology, University of Miami School of Medicine, Miami, Florida 33101.

influences was demonstrated mainly by *in vitro* techniques of neural tissue and cell cultures (e.g., ref. 71). For instance, it has been extensively documented that peripheral nervous system (PNS) terrain favors, whereas central nervous system (CNS) terrain prevents, the regeneration of both PNS and CNS injured axons. The humoral, surface-associated, or architectural factors responsible for the competence or incompetence of a terrain were often shown to be not only source specific but also target specific. These factors are mostly proteins and act as local mediators rather than as hormones and show (1) trophic effects (neuronotrophic, i.e., supporting neuronal growth and survival, and/or neurite-promoting, i.e., stimulating specifically neurite extension), (2) antitrophic effects (inhibiting growth and facilitating cell death), and/or (3) tropic or tactic effects (inducing directional guidance by attraction or by restriction, respectively).

In this chapter, only one of these factors is considered, namely, the nerve growth factor (NGF), because it has recently been demonstrated that, in addition to its already well-known action on PNS neurons, NGF also plays a role in CNS. The latter observation suggests that this compound (or similar compounds) may be used for pharmacological symptomatic and perhaps even etiologic management of some patients suffering from brain injury or neural degeneration.

2. THE NERVE GROWTH FACTOR AND ITS EFFECTS ON PNS NEURONS

The prototype macromolecular factor showing trophic, tactic, and tropic effects is the NGF discovered by Levi-Montalcini and Hamburger more than 30 years ago.[39,40] First identified in sarcoma-180 tumors, NGF was also fortuitously found in snake venom that was being used for degrading the nucleic acids of the active fraction extracted from sarcoma-180 cells. Many other sources of NGF were found later, the richest being the convoluted tubules of adult male mouse submaxillary glands, which are similar in certain respects to the venom glands of snakes.[18]

Nerve growth factor was first isolated from mouse submaxillary glands and biochemically characterized. Submaxillary gland NGF is a protein multimer (the 7 S NGF complex) with a molecular weight of 131,500 that can be subdivided into two α subunits, two γ subunits, and one β subunit. The neurotrophic and neurotropic activity of NGF resides in the β subunit, a basic polypeptide with an isoelectric point of 9.3 (2.5 S NGF being a partial degradation product of β-NGF). The β subunit of NGF is a dimer, i.e., a complex of two identical polypeptide chains, each of which has a molecular weight of 13,250. The gene coding for β-NGF has recently been sequenced and cloned, and its organization has been elucidated.[12,58,70] Another recent study revealed that in the iris, one of the target areas of peripheral sympathetic neurons, NGF exists in the form of the β-NGF, since the α and γ subunits were not found.[48] It therefore seems possible that the 7 S complex of NGF represents a special storage form synthesized by secretory organs. In the present chapter, NGF is used synonymously with β-NGF.

Nerve growth factor has been extensively characterized in its role as neurotrophic and neurotropic factor for peripheral sympathetic neurons and was shown to be a selective neurotrophic factor for a subpopulation of peptidergic sensory neurons also (for reviews see refs. 15, 67, 68). Nerve growth factor is necessary for the normal development, maintenance, and survival of these sympathetic and sensory cells. It is synthesized by target tissues of NGF-sensitive neurons and acts on specific receptors located on their plasma membranes. Following internalization and retrograde transport to the cell body, NGF stimulates the biosynthesis of RNA, of neurotubule proteins, and of key enzymes (tyrosine hydroxylase, TH, and dopamine β-hydroxylase, DBH) necessary for norepinephrine production. Treatment with NGF results in a marked hypertrophy of embryonic dorsal root ganglia and sympathetic ganglia.[37] Administration of antibodies to rodent embryos results in atrophy and irreversible degeneration of the sympathetic nervous system.[35,36,38] In animals subjected to experimental axotomy of peripheral neurons, which frequently results in their retrograde degeneration, NGF-sensitive neurons can be rescued by direct administration of NGF.[1,16,26,49] This observation suggests that the primary injury signal in these neurons is the absence of target-derived NGF.

3. Effects of NGF on CNS Neurons

After peripheral sympathetic (noradrenergic) neurons were shown to be highly sensitive to NGF, several studies were carried out in order to characterize the influence of NGF on central catecholaminergic neurons. The findings clearly demonstrated that NGF fails to affect central catecholaminergic neurons. However, recent investigations have accumulated evidence showing, surprisingly, that NGF acts as a neurotrophic factor for central cholinergic neurons in a similar way to that by which it influences peripheral sympathetic neurons.

First, with enzyme-linked immunoassays for quantification of endogenous NGF and cDNA or cRNA probes for quantification of the messenger RNA coding for NGF (mRNA-NGF), it was recently demonstrated that NGF and the mRNA-NGF are present in the rat brain.[29,34,59,72,73] The distribution of NGF and mRNA-NGF correlates well with that of central cholinergic neurons. The NGF levels are highest in hippocampus, cortex, septum, and nucleus basalis, whereas mRNA-NGF localization remains restricted to hippocampus and cortex, suggesting that, in CNS as in PNS, NGF is produced by target cells and retrogradely transported to cell bodies of NGF-sensitive neurons.

A second group of findings indicates that central cholinergic neurons contain receptors for NGF. Indirect evidence for such localization of NGF receptors is provided by experiments showing that exogenous $[^{125}I]$NGF injected into target areas of forebrain cholinergic neurons (i.e., hippocampus and cortex), is taken up by nerve terminals and retrogradely transported to the cell bodies of cholinergic neurons located in the basal forebrain but not to other cell bodies projecting to the same target areas.[57] More recently, NGF receptors were directly demonstrated in the rat forebrain by immunoprecipitation with a monoclonal antibody to the NGF receptor protein.[64,65] By autoradiographic techniques, NGF receptors have been found in the septum and nucleus basalis of the rat brain.[53] Furthermore, NGF receptors were visualized on cholinergic neurons of the rat and human forebrain using immunohistochemical procedures and monoclonal antibodies to NGF receptors[21] (Fig. 1).

A third group of findings provides evidence that the stimulation of NGF receptors on forebrain cholinergic neurons mediates trophic effects on these cells. Nerve growth factor has been found to elevate the activity of choline acetyltransferase (ChAT) in central cholinergic neurons and in aggregate cultures of fetal telencephalic neurons of rats, especially after continued treatment[31] and when added together with triiodothyronine, which plays an important role in normal brain development.[30] In cultures of dissociated neurons of the fetal rat septum, both murine and bovine NGF increased ChAT activity, and the effect of NGF was blocked by antiserum to NGF.[23] In these *in vitro* studies performed on fetal rat cells, NGF was shown to evoke only a slight increase in acetylcholinesterase (AChE) activity. Initial studies failed to reveal effects of NGF on survival and fiber outgrowth of cholinergic neurons.[23] However, in slice cultures of brain tissue from neonatal rats grown for several weeks, the presence of NGF stimulated the growth of septal cholinergic neurons towards target cells in the hippocampus.[13] Several *in vivo* studies showed that NGF selectively stimulates ChAT activity of forebrain cholinergic neurons. In neonatal rats, repeated intracerebroventricular (i.c.v.) injections of murine or bovine NGF elevated ChAT activity measured a few days after the last injection in those brain regions that are rich in cholinergic perikarya (septum, diagonal band of Broca, nucleus basalis) or nerve terminals (cortex, hippocampus). No effect of NGF treatment on AChE, TH, and glutamate decarboxylase (GAD) was observed.[14,47] Finally, in adult rats with partial transection of the fimbria, i.c.v. injections of NGF for 4 weeks also increased ChAT activity in the hippocampus and in the septum when measured 3 days after the last NGF injection.[22]

However, the NGF-induced ChAT activation was not observed in the hippocampus of adult rats when this structure received its normal cholinergic input,[22] nor when it was virtually devoid of septal afferents.[69] In this last study we made unilateral fimbria–fornix lesions by aspiration through the overlying cingulate cortex and found that acetylcholine-rich fetal forebrain tissue grafted in the severely denervated hippocampus of adult rats partially restored hippocampal ChAT activity and that repeated intrahippocampal NGF injection further enhanced ChAT activity in cholinergic neurons grafted in the deafferented hippocampus yet had no effect on cells grafted in the intact hippocampus (Fig. 2).

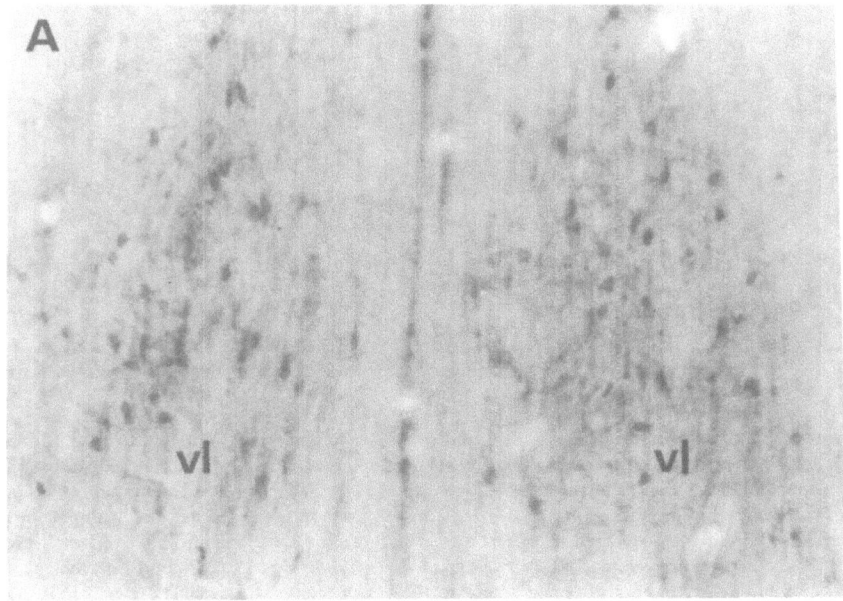

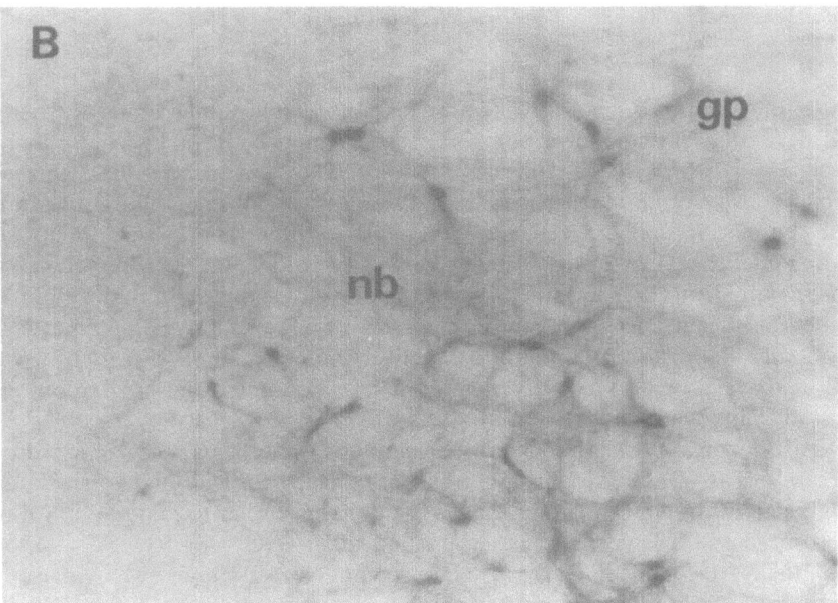

FIGURE 1. Visualization of NGF receptors in rat brain with an immunohistochemical procedure using a monoclonal antibody recognizing this receptor. This procedure located the receptors in the medial septal nucleus, the nucleus of the diagonal band of Broca, and the nucleus basalis. The localization corresponds to that of cholinergic neurons in the basal forebrain. A: NGF receptor staining in the diagonal band of Broca. B: In the nucleus basalis. gp, globus pallidus; nb, nucleus basalis; vl, vertical limb of the nucleus of the diagonal band of Broca.

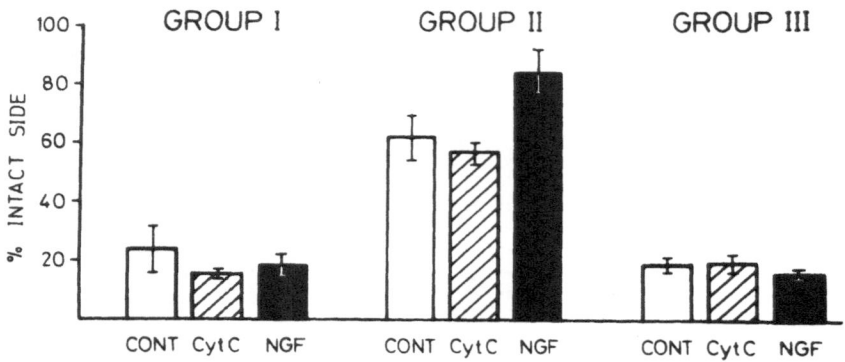

FIGURE 2. Choline acetyltransferase activity in the right hippocampus on the side of the fimbria–fornix lesions, grafts, and treatments as a percentage of activity in the left (intact) hippocampus. The three groups of rats received either lesion alone (group I), ACh-rich ventral forebrain grafts placed into the lesioned hippocampus (group II), or ACh-rich grafts placed into the intact hippocampus, which was subsequently lesioned just prior to sacrifice (group III). Separate rats from each group received six treatments of either NGF or cytochrome c (Cyt C, a control protein) injected into the hippocampus at 4-day intervals or no injections at all (CONT, control). Vertical bars indicate S.E.M. Group II differs significantly from groups I and III ($P < 0.001$), and within group II the NGF treatment differs significantly from the two control treatments ($P < 0.05$).

In the absence of cholinergic terminals, locally injected NGF may be unable to affect cholinergic function merely because it cannot be taken up by cholinergic terminals on which NGF receptors are located, or, in the case of a virtually normal density of cholinergic terminals (with or without the addition of grafted fetal cholinergic cells), NGF may be unable to affect cholinergic function in adult animals because these cells are supplied by endogenous NGF, which ascertains maximal survival and function. A role of endogenous NGF in development of cholinergic neurons has recently been established by Otten et al.[50] In 6-week-old rats treated in utero (at embryonic day E15.5) by a single injection of anti-NGF antibodies, ChAT activity was reduced in the nucleus basalis region, septum, and hippocampus.

In the partially deafferented hippocampus of adult rats, the NGF-induced increase of ChAT activity was only transitory (lasting for less than 10 weeks), as ChAT activity in NGF-treated rats was found to be similar to that of control rats when measured 10 weeks after termination of the NGF injections.[75] Furthermore, the NGF-mediated increase in hippocampal ChAT activity was not accompanied by increased AChE activity or by an increased density of cholinergic fibers in this area.[22] Based on these findings, it was concluded that NGF transitorily stimulates ChAT activity in spared or grafted cholinergic neurons without affecting their regenerative or sprouting capacity. However, in these experiments, NGF also increased ChAT activity in the septum, and this increase was not transitory but was still observed 10 weeks after completion of NGF treatment.[22,75]

To account for these findings, it was hypothesized that NGF might affect survival of septal cholinergic neurons and that 10 weeks was probably too short a period for observing any regenerated processes from septal fibers into the hippocampus. Indeed, Hefti[21] reported that NGF is able to enhance survival of septal cholinergic neurons after axonal transection in adult rats. Using Nissl and AChE (with diisopropylfluorophosphate pretreatment) staining, Hefti found that fimbrial transections resulted in retrograde degeneration of cholinergic septohippocampal neurons and that repeated i.c.v. NGF treatment strongly attenuated this lesion-induced degeneration. In control rats with lesions, the total number of AChE-positive cells contained in the medial septal nucleus and in the vertical limb of the diagonal band of Broca on the lesion side was reduced by 50% as compared to the number on the intact side. In rats treated with NGF, the number of cholinergic cells on the lesion side was reduced by only 12%. Similar findings were recently presented by Williams and co-workers,[76] showing that continuous intraventricular infusion of NGF ipsilateral to a fimbria–fornix transection resulted in substantial protection of cholinergic and other neurons in the medial septum and diagonal band against their otherwise expected death. The findings of these studies indicate that NGF is able to rescue rat forebrain cholinergic (and perhaps even other) neurons from degeneration after transection of their processes; they broaden the role of NGF in the function of these neurons and provide a further line of evidence demonstrating that NGF acts as a neurotrophic factor.

Finally, a fifth group of findings suggests that central cholinergic neurons and peripheral sympathetic neurons react to the same neurotrophic factor, NGF. Indeed, when cholinergic neurons innervating the hippocampus are destroyed, endogenous and exogenous (i.e., transplanted) sympathetic fibers grow to and occupy the same anatomic target sites that were previously occupied by cholinergic fibers.[5,6,42,43,63]

Taken together, the five groups of findings presented in the preceeding paragraphs (see Table I) strongly support the hypothesis that NGF acts as a neurotrophic factor for central cholinergic neurons. All cholinergic neurons of the forebrain seem to react to NGF. These neurons include the ascending cholinergic neurons of the basal forebrain, which have their cell bodies in medial septal nucleus, nucleus of the diagonal band of Broca, substantia innominata, and nucleus basalis and project to hippocampus, cortex, olfactory tubercle, and amygdala (for review of the anatomy of central cholinergic systems, see Mesulam et al.[46]).

The ascending cholinergic projections of the basal forebrain are topographically organized. Cell bodies located in the medial septal nucleus project primarily to the hippocampus and give rise to the cholinergic septohippocampal projection. The cortical input is derived from cell bodies of substantia innominata and nucleus basalis (cholinergic basalocortical projection). Besides

TABLE I. Effects of NGF on Central Cholinergic Neurons[a]

	Subjects	Lesion	NGF	Method	Results
Schwab et al.[57]	Adult rats	No	M	Intracerebral injections	Transport to cell bodies af ACh neurons (septum + DBB)
Korsching et al.[34] Shelton and Reichardt[60] Whittemore et al.[73]	Adult rats	No		Measurement of NGF levels and of mRNA(NGF)	mRNA(NGF) in target areas of forebrain ACh neurons NGF distribution correlated with that of forebrain ACh neurons
Riopelle et al.[53] Hefti et al.[24]	Adult rats	No		Immunohistochemistry with antibody to NGF receptors [^{125}I]NGF autoradio	NGF receptors located on ACh neurons
Honegger and Lenoir[31] Honegger[30] Hefti et al.[23] Martinez et al.[44]	Cultured fetal telencephalic neurons	No	M and bovine NGF (+/−T3)	Biochemistry	Increased ChAT activity, especially after continued treatment; effect blocked by anti-NGF antiserum
Gnahn et al.[14] Mobley et al.[47] Johnston et al.[32a]	Neonatal rats	No	M and bovine (i.c.v.) and repeated	Biochemistry a few days after last injection	Increased ChAT activity in septum, hippocampus, s.innominata, neostriatum No effect on AChE, TH, GAD
Otten et al.[50]	Rat fetuses (ED 19.5)		Anti-NGF	Biochemistry 7 weeks later	Decreased ChAT activity in n.basalis, septum, hippocampus
Hefti et al.[22] Will and Hefti[74] Toniolo et al.[69]	Adult rats	Fimbria or fornix + fimbria	M (i.c.v. or intrahipp.) repeated	Biochemistry a few days after last injection	Increased ChAT activity in hippocampus + septum
Hefti[21] Williams et al.[76]	Adult rats	Fimbria or fornix + fimbria	M (i.c.v. repeated or continuous)	Immunohistochemistry	Increased survival of ACh cells in septum and DBB Increased cholinergic sprouting in septum

[a]Abbreviations: AChE, acetylcholinesterase; ChAT, choline acetyltransferase; DBB, diagonal band of Broca; ED, embryonic day; GAD, glutamic acid decarboxylase; i.c.v., intracerebroventricular; M, mouse 2.5 S NGF; TH, tyrosine hydroxylase.

these ascending projection neurons, cholinergic interneurons of the striatum also respond to NGF.[44,47] As judged by immunohistochemical visualization, none of the noncholinergic neurons in the forebrain express receptors for NGF.[24] In the forebrain, the ability to respond to NGF seems to be a selective capability of cholinergic neurons. It would be valuable to complement the studies performed on the cholinergic forebrain neurons (sectors Ch1 to Ch4 according to the classification by Mesulam *et al.*[46]) with similar studies on the cholinergic neurons located within the pontomesencephalic reticular formation and the tegmental gray of the periventricular area (neurons of sectors Ch5 and Ch6), areas that provide the major cholinergic innervation of the thalamus. Cholinergic motoneurons were already shown not to respond to NGF.[9]

4. Effects of NGF on Behavior

As shown in Table II, NGF treatment of adult animals with brain lesions was reported several times to enhance and/or accelerate recovery from behavioral deficits produced by the lesions. However, some "negative" reports (no NGF effect or even NGF-induced behavioral impairments) must also be taken into account in order to evaluate the processes underlying the NGF-induced modulation of behavioral recovery.

The first behavioral experiments carried out in the 1970s were all implicitly based on the assumption that NGF might trophically affect catecholaminergic neurons in the CNS as it does in the PNS. Indeed, this assumption had actually received some support from an experiment that tended to demonstrate that NGF is able to stimulate regenerative processes in central catecholaminergic neurons.[4] Berger *et al.*[2] reported that a single i.c.v. injection of NGF given at the time of brain damage facilitated recovery from feeding deficits associated with lateral hypothalamic lesions, enhanced the feeding response to exogenous norepinephrine (i.c.v.) administration, and conferred a lasting protection against reinstatement of the lateral hypothalamic syndrome by 6-hydroxydopamine. Berger *et al.* considered that NGF may stimulate the regeneration of reversibly damaged neurons in the noradrenergic feeding system or may promote supersensitivity to norepinephrine.

Similar assumptions stimulated the work by Tarpy and co-workers,[66] who reported that NGF antiserum, administered either centrally at adult age or systematically at birth (producing immunosympathectomy), decreased subsequent self-stimulation under variable-ratio schedules of reinforcement with the stimulation electrodes implanted in the posterior hypothalamus. The authors interpreted their results as an antiserum-induced reduction in central catecholamine levels.

Later studies that were still based on the assumption of catecholaminergically mediated behavioral effects of NGF were conducted by Donald Stein and his group. Rats with bilateral lesions of the caudate nucleus that were given intracau-

TABLE II. Behavioral Effects of NGF in Brain-Damaged Animals

	Subjects[a]	Lesion[b]	NGF[c]	Dose[d]	Delay[e]	Behavior	Results[f]
Berger et al.[2]	$	LH (Elec)	M* (i.c.v.)	4	*	Food intake	(+) and increased resistance to 6-OHDA
Hart et al.[20]	$	Caudate (RF)	M* (caudate)	4	* **	Spatial reversal	(+) (0)
Lewis et al.[41]	$	Accumbens (6-OHDA)	M* (s. nigra)	2.5	*	Activity; response to d-amphetamine	(+)
Kimble et al.[33]	$	Hippocampus (Asp.)	7 S* (hippocampus)	20	**	Maze learning	(0)
Stein et al.[61]	$	LH (RF)	M* (i.v.c.)	4 or 2	*	Water intake, reactivity discrimination	(+) (0) (−) increased freezing
Yip and Grafstein[77]	Goldfish	Optic nerve (Crush)	M + 7 S + β * + continued (intraocular) (optic nerve)	900 to 1790 BU	* *	Startle reaction	(+) similar effects for acute and repeated treatment
Stein and Will[62]	$	Entorhinal cortex (Elec)	M* (hippocampus)	4	* **	Maze learning	(+) (0)
Eclancher et al.[10]	Female rats (7 days)	Septum (Elec) VMH (Elec)	M* (i.c.v.) M* (i.c.v.)	30	*,** *,**	Two-way active avoidance	(+) in septal rats (i.e., decreased performance)
Will and Hefti[74]	$	Fimbria (section)	M (i.c.v.) repeated	8 × 10	* **	Maze learning	(+) (0)
Pallage et al.[51]	Female rats	Medial septum (Elec)	M* (hippocampus)	8	** ***	Spont. alternation Maze learning	(−) (−)

[a]Subjects: $, male juvenile or adult rats.
[b]Lesion: Asp, aspiration; Elec, electrolytic; LH, lateral hypothalamus; RF, radiofrequency; VMH, ventromedial hypothalamus.
[c]NGF: M, mouse 2.5 NGF; *acute; i.c.v., intracerebroventricular.
[d]Dose: micrograms/animal or biological units (BU).
[e]Delay between last NGF injection and start of behavioral testing: *, less than 3 weeks; **, between 3 weeks and 2.5 months; ***, more than 2.5 months.
[f]Results: (+) facilitation of recovery; (0) no effect on recovery; (−) deleterious effects.

date injections of NGF were found to show faster recovery of normal appetitive behavior and perseverated less than their buffer-treated counterparts on a spatial reversal task.[20] However, NGF had no ameliorating effect on some other behavioral deficits that accompany bilateral caudate–putamen damage, nor had NGF any effect on steady-state caudate dopamine levels. In another study, Lewis and collaborators[41] found that following 6-hydroxydopamine-induced depletion of dopamine in the nucleus accumbens, NGF administration in the vicinity of the substantia nigra promoted recovery of the locomotor response to d-amphetamine. However, this apparent behavioral recovery could not be related to increased dopaminergic neuronal reinnervation of the nucleus accumbens.

In a further study, Stein and his collaborators found that in intact rats, NGF disrupted behavioral performance in visual discrimination learning, whereas in rats with lateral hypothalamic lesions they did not find any difference between NGF-treated and control rats.[61] They suggested that this failure to replicate the findings of Berger et al.[2] may be associated with the lesion size, which might have been larger in their study than in that of Berger et al.[2] Finally, in the late 1970s, Kimble and collaborators published a report that further increased the complexity of the situation concerning behavioral NGF effects.[33] They examined the effect of NGF on maze-learning behavior of rats with hippocampal lesions and on the development of lesion-induced anomalous noradrenergic innervation of the hippocampus by peripheral sympathetic fibers. Neither behavior nor sympathetic sprouting was found to be affected by the single administration of NGF, which was made directly into the damaged brain tissue. Thus, near the end of the 1970s, NGF seemed to have beneficial consequences in some experimental conditions, whereas in others it was found to be completely ineffective. The reasons for the discrepant findings were not clear, perhaps partly because knowledge of neurotrophic effects of NGF on CNS neurons was still scarce at that time.

The situation changed noticeably in the early 1980s. In 1982, Yip and Grafstein[77] reported that various forms of NGF (β, 2.5 S, and 7 S), administered by intraocular injection or by local application to the lesion site on the goldfish optic nerve, increased axonal outgrowth and decreased the time required for recovery of the startle reaction to a bright light. The effect produced by a single intraocular injection given at the time of surgery was not further increased by subsequent injections. Thus, in the lower vertebrate CNS, NGF was shown for the first time not only to facilitate behavioral recovery following CNS injury but also to enhance axonal regeneration.

However, there are many examples demonstrating that generalization from lower vertebrate CNS to mammalian CNS should be done with great caution because of the large evolutionary separation of the two classes.

These data, as well as the discovery of the neurotrophic effects of NGF on central cholinergic neurons of mammalians, prompted us to start a series of experiments based on an assumption that focuses not on the neurotrophic role of

NGF in catecholaminergic systems but rather on its role in cholinergic systems. In three separate experiments we studied the effects of NGF on behavioral recovery from various lesions to the hippocampal system. In our first study,[62] mature rats with entorhinal cortex lesions received a single bilateral injection of NGF into the dorsal hippocampus because we assumed that NGF might affect the lesion-induced fiber sprouting from the remaining, particularly cholinergic, intact neurons. In our second study (D. G. Stein, F. Deluzarche, and B. Will, unpublished data), mature rats with dorsal hippocampal lesions received a single bilateral injection of NGF into the dorsal hippocampus. Here, the assumption was that NGF might affect the regeneration and/or survival of the cholinergic septohippocampal neurons. In both studies we found that NGF produced a facilitation of behavioral recovery in maze learning but that this facilitation was no longer detectable 8 weeks after NGF treatment. Because it was possible that chronic or repeated administration of NGF may have promoted a more persistent functional recovery, we used the repeated-i.c.v.-injection paradigm, which was shown by Hefti and collaborators[22] to enhance hippocampal and septal ChAT activity in adult rats with partial fimbria lesions. Again, we found that NGF produced only an acceleration of maze learning (after an initial impairment) in rats with such lesions[74] (Fig. 3). We also found that the NGF-induced increase of ChAT activity was observable at the end of behavioral testing only in the septum and not in the hippocampus.

In contrast, the data recently reported by Eclancher and her co-workers[10] tend to demonstrate that NGF can have lasting effects on functional recovery from brain damage. In rats with lesions of either the ventromedial hypothalamus or septal nucleus, they found that a single i.c.v. injection of NGF given at the time of surgery can facilitate recovery of function by attenuating lesion-induced symptoms in each case: NGF treatment increased two-way active avoidance performance in rats with hypothalamic lesions and decreased performance in rats with septal lesions. This study by Eclancher and collaborators, showing some more persistent behavioral effects of NGF than in most previously mentioned reports, also differs from them in that CNS lesions and NGF administration were performed in infant rats (7-day-old rats), whereas in the other studies rats were operated on at a much later developmental stage.

Finally, in a study aimed at investigating the interaction between NGF and intrahippocampal septal grafts on the behavior of rats after a medial septal lesion, we followed up the behavioral alterations over a much longer postoperative period than in the preceeding studies because of the late behavioral expression of transplant effects.[51] We were surprised not only to find very long-lasting behavioral effects of NGF in female rats that were given surgery and NGF injections at young adult age but also to find that these effects were "negative," i.e., that the deleterious lesion and NGF effects were additive (Fig. 4). Specifically, in a radial maze task, both immediate and delayed grafts reduced the lesion-induced deficit several months after surgery, whereas the single intrahippocampal NGF

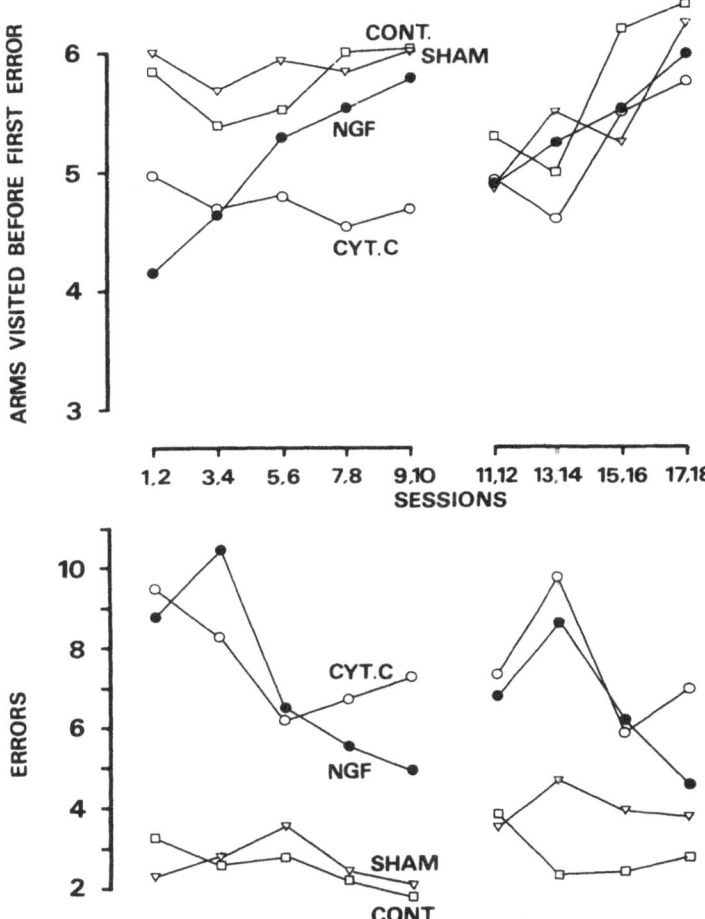

FIGURE 3. Number of arms visited before first error (top figure; means and S.E.M.) and number of errors (bottom figure; means and S.E.M.) shown by the rats of the four treatment groups (CYT.C, cytochrome *c* injected; NGF, nerve growth factor injected; CONT., nonoperated control rats; SHAM, "cortical" control rats) in an eight-arm radial maze. Only the NGF-treated rats improved their performance significantly over time during the first test period (trials 1–10). During the second test period (trials 11–16), 6 weeks later, the performance of the NGF- and cytochrome-*c*-treated rats did not differ.

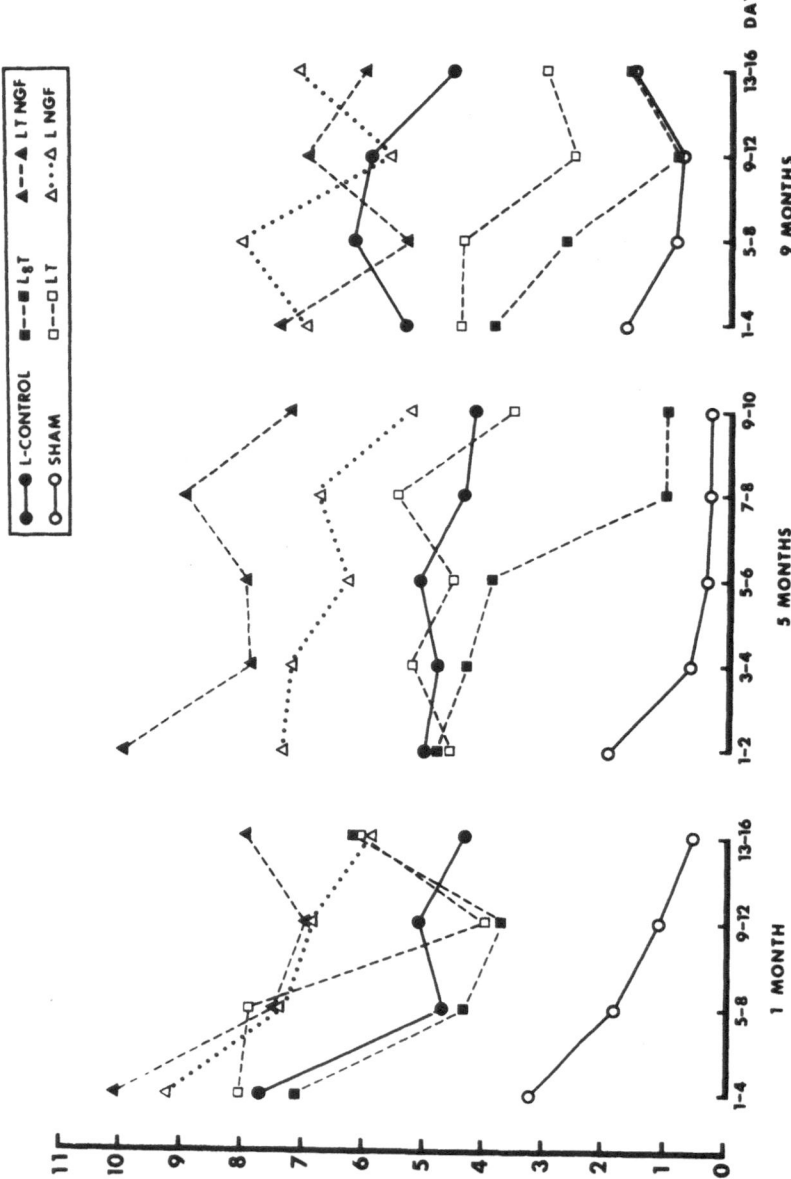

FIGURE 4. Mean performance in an eight-arm radial maze shown 1 month (blocks of four trials), 5 months (blocks of two trials), and 9 months (blocks of four trials) after treatment. SHAM, sham-operated rats; L-CONTROL, lesion-control rats; L8T, delayed grafted rats; LT, immediately grafted rats; LTNGF, grafted rats that received an NGF injection; LNGF, NGF-treated rats.

injection (whether given without or in conjunction with grafted dissociated cells) increased this deficit, especially 5 months postoperatively.

In order to explain the long-term detrimental effects of NGF observed in that study, several possibilities can be considered. One of these possibilities is based on the already mentioned fact that destruction of the cholinergic input to the hippocampus results in an ingrowth of peripheral sympathetic fibers originating from the superior cervical ganglia into the CA3 and dentate gyrus. In fact, this ingrowth of peripheral sympathetic fibers is presumably the most readily apparent effect of intracerebrally administered NGF. Because peripheral sympathetic neurons are responsive to NGF, we have speculated that the detrimental effects produced by NGF might result from an enhanced sympathetic sprouting into the deafferented hippocampus, preventing cholinergic (endogenous and/or grafted) septal fibers to reinnervate their hippocampal targets.

5. Discussion

Although NGF has been characterized primarily by its effects on the development, maintenance, and survival of peripheral sympathetic and sensory neurons, there is now a strong body of evidence demonstrating that this protein plays also a role in the function of central cholinergic neurons. Does this recent demonstration of a NGF-mediated modulation of CNS function give us any help in understanding the NGF-mediated behavioral effects reported above?

Lesions of the ascending cholinergic projections of the basal forebrain result in learning and memory deficits in rats.[11,27,28,52,56] However, no lesion technique exists permitting the specific and exclusive destruction of cholinergic neurons. Therefore, we also need to take into consideration a host of pharmacological experiments that all tend to confirm the notion that cholinergic systems are involved, to a major degree, in cognitive functions necessary for mastering the behavioral tasks (maze learning and retention, spontaneous and reinforced alternation, acquisition of active and passive avoidance conditioned responses, etc.) used in most reported experiments for testing NGF efficiency.[3,8,17,32,45,54] Thus, some of the findings reported above suggest the possibility that the behavioral improvements observed in NGF-treated animals reflect its promotion of ChAT activity and/or survival of cholinergic neurons. The long-term behavioral impairments observed in the NGF-treated rats with lesions of the medial septum may be caused by a functional antagonism between the abnormal sympathetic and normal cholinergic innervation of the hippocampus. If sympathetic neurons show a competitive advantage over cholinergic neurons for occupying the deafferented cholinergic sites in the hippocampus, NGF may thwart behavioral recovery as measured by learning and memory tests by enhancing sympathetic sprouting. However, these interpretations remain highly speculative until we know much more about the causal link between behavioral events and modulation of cholinergic as well as sympathetic function in the various brain areas considered. In any case, the early behavioral experiments reported during the 1970s need to be reconsidered in the light of the recent findings on NGF-mediated effects on central cholinergic neurons.

Several other features may help us to approach a more synthetic view of the varied behavioral data reviewed. One of these features may be the time course of behavioral modifications after NGF administration (or after last administration when NGF was given repetitively). Indeed, all the studies that reported "positive" effects of NGF treatment on behavioral recovery in adult animals have found that these effects are detectable only during the second and third weeks after the last NGF injection, or they have used too short a period of testing to allow an appreciation of the persistence of such behavioral effects. "Negative" effects of NGF treatment[51] have been observed after much longer delays (5 months), at which time the NGF-mediated ChAT activation is no longer found in the hippocampus,[74] and the sprouting of sympathetic fibers (possibly enhanced by NGF treatment) has had enough time to produce reinnervation of the hippocampal sites vacated by degenerated septohippocampal fibers. The absence of NGF effects reported by Kimble and co-workers[33] could be explained either (1) by the fact that they conducted behavioral testing at about 50 days after surgery, i.e., between periods at which "positive" and "negative" effects had been observed, respectively, or (2) by one of several other possibilities, one of which is the small number of animals used (five hippocampal saline- and six hippocampal NGF-treated rats).

A second feature that may help us to understand the variability found in the reported behavioral data is the age of the subjects at surgery (and NGF treatment). Indeed, in infant rats, as compared to adult rats, Eclancher et al.[10] found similar time courses in behavioral results after septal lesions but not after ventromedial hypothalamic lesions. With the latter lesions, the NGF effects appeared only after a longer delay, and the differences between NGF- and saline-treated rats were persistent (at least for 7 weeks after surgery). However, the discrepancies between these and other results may also reflect differences in lesion locus and in the locus of NGF administration.

Although these few indications for a tentative synthesis of the available behavioral data remain unsatisfactory, some important clues for a more comprehensive view of NGF-induced behavioral effects have already appeared. First, although Honegger and Lenoir[31] have shown that in vitro continued NGF treatment is more effective for stimulating ChAT activity than a more acute treatment, most behavioral experiments have demonstrated that chronic (or repeated) treatment by NGF seems to be no more efficient than a single administration given at the time of surgery (e.g., ref. 77); however, no behavioral testing has been performed during continued NGF treatment.

Second, the possibility that the small amounts of renin that contaminate most mouse salivary gland NGF preparations might act on central cholinergic neurons seems unlikely, as it has been shown that bovine NGF, which is renin-free, and mouse NGF, which is renin-contaminated, have similar biological activities[19] and similar effects on central cholinergic neurons.[23] Renin itself actually impaired performance of intact and brain-damaged rats in a spatial reversal task[55] and seems, therefore, not to be a good candidate for explaining the transient "positive" NGF effects observed in several experiments. Renin, however, might explain the detrimental long-term effects of NGF treatment found by Pallage *et al.*,[51] and this possibility should be considered in association with the explanation of these detrimental NGF-induced effects in terms of the action of this protein on sympathetic sprouting.

Third, at least in infant rats, NGF was shown to promote genuine recovery of behavioral function and did not merely increase performance.[10] Nerve growth factor attenuated symptoms by improving performance in rats that showed lesion-induced impairment of performance (ventromedial hypothalamus lesions) and by reducing performance in rats that showed a lesion-induced increase of performance (septal nucleus lesions). Similar studies need to be conducted using adult animals.

Fourth, although it is certainly unjustified to claim that a substance must have an endogenous physiological role because it has an effect when administered to an organism, evidence is now accumulating for an endogenous function of NGF in the CNS. Endogenous NGF and mRNA coding for NGF have recently been localized in the brain, and it seems highly probable that this endogenous NGF is able to affect the function of central cholinergic neurons as does exogenous intracerebrally injected NGF. Since NGF is able to affect neurons of the CNS trophically, one should consider the use of NGF as a therapeutic tool for the treatment of nervous system injury. A degenerative disease, such as Alzheimer's disease, associated with degeneration of forebrain cholinergic neurons has been speculatively explained by a lack of endogenous NGF.[25] It can thus be assumed that compounds mimicking the action of NGF by trophic influences on central cholinergic neurons might be beneficial in the treatment of Alzheimer's and similar diseases. Beneficial effects of NGF can also be anticipated even with causative factors other than NGF itself. Increasing the availability of NGF to cholinergic neurons is likely to stimulate many synthetic processes in these cells. This may result in strengthening of their morphological structures and in a higher capability for transmitter synthesis. Such neurons might be less vulnerable to primary disease processes and have an augmented probability of survival. The possible application of NGF in Alzheimer's disease is discussed in detail in a recent review.[25]

Nerve growth factor is a protein that does not cross the blood–brain barrier. For human application it is therefore necessary to develop a carrier system with which NGF can be delivered to the brain. Alternatively, drugs might be developed that mimic the actions of NGF on its central receptors. Very little is known about the structural requirements by which NGF stimulates its receptor(s), and its receptor domain has not been characterized. It is therefore not possible at the present time to outline a rational strategy for the development of orally active agonists of NGF.

A further note of caution is suggested by our findings indicating that NGF administration in rats can produce "negative" effects after certain experimental lesions. It is likely that, besides destroying NGF-responsive cells, experimental lesions also sever other, nonresponsive neurons. Application of NGF might therefore stimulate survival or regrowth of one cellular population only, resulting in a functional imbalance that produces behavioral effects more detrimental than the original lesion itself. A similar situation might arise in the human brain when a disease process affects several neuronal populations. Enhanced survival of a given neuronal population might not be sufficient to improve the general behavioral status of patients.

At the present time, NGF represents the only isolated neurotrophic factor that affects central neurons. With the knowledge obtained in recent years about neurotrophic factors in the PNS,[68] it seems likely that many more trophic factors with selective and different specificities exist in the mammalian brain. The isolation and characterization of such neurotrophic factors remains one of the major goals of modern neurobiology. The knowledge gained on NGF's role in the brain will serve in a paradigmatic way to characterize the actions of these new factors. We can speculate that a combination of neurotrophic factors promoting survival and functions of affected populations of neurons might represent a future treatment for neurodegenerative diseases.

ACKNOWLEDGMENTS. This work was supported in part by grants to B. Will from the Fondation pour la Recherche Médicale and from I.N.S.E.R.M. (ATP 866.019) and to F. Hefti from the Alzheimer's Disease and Related Disorders Association, Chicago, and the National Parkinson Foundation, Miami.

REFERENCES

1. Banks, B. E. C., and Walter, S. J., 1977, The effects of post-ganglionic axotomy and nerve growth factor on superior cervical ganglia of developing mice, *J. Neurocytol.* **6**:287–297.
2. Berger, B. D., Wise, C. D., and Stein, L., 1973, Nerve growth factor: Enhanced recovery of feeding after hypothalamic damage, *Science* **185**:506–508.
3. Biedermann, G. B., 1975, The search for the chemistry of memory; recent trends and the logic of investigation in the role of cholinergic and adrenergic transmitters, in: *Progress in Neurobiology*, Volume 2 (G. A. Kerkut and J. W. Phyllis, eds.), Pergamon Press, New York, pp. 49–123.
4. Björklund, A., and Stenevi, U., 1972, Nerve growth factor: Stimulation of regenerative growth of central noradrenergic neurons, *Science* **175**:1251–1253.
5. Björklund, A., and Stenevi, U., 1977, Experimental reinnervation of the rat hippocampus by grafted sympathetic ganglia: I. Axonal regeneration along the hippocampal fimbria, *Brain Res.* **138**:259–270.

6. Crutcher, K. A., Brothers, L., and Davis, J. N., 1979, Sprouting of sympathetic nerves in the absence of afferent input, *Exp. Neurol.* **66**:778–783.
7. Crutcher, K. A., Brothers, L., and Davis, J. N., 1981, Sympathetic noradrenergic sprouting in response to central cholinergic denervation: A histochemical study of neuronal sprouting in the rat hippocampal formation, *Brain Res.* **210**:115–128.
8. Deutsch, J. A., 1971, The cholinergic synapse and the site of memory, *Science* **174**:788–794.
9. Dribin, L. E., and Barrett, J. N., 1985, Conditioned medium enhances neuritic outgrowth from rat spinal cord explants, *Dev. Biol.* **74**:184–195.
10. Eclancher, F., Ramirez, J. J., and Stein, D. G., 1985, Neonatal brain damage and recovery: Intraventricular injection of NGF at time of injury alters performance of active avoidance, *Dev. Brain Res.* **19**:227–235.
11. Flicker, C., Dean, R. L., Watkins, D. L., Fisher, S. K., and Bartus, R. T., 1983, Behavioral and neurochemical effects following neurotoxic lesions of a major cholinergic input to the cerebral cortex in the rat, *Pharmacol. Biochem. Behav.* **18**:973–981.
12. Francke, U., DeMartinville, B., Coussens, L., and Ullrich, A., 1983, The human gene for the beta-subunit of nerve growth factor is located on the proximal short arm of chromosome 1, *Science* **222**:1248–1250.
13. Gähwiller, B. H., and Hefti, F., 1987, Nerve growth factor is involved in establishment of septo-hippocampal cholinergic projection, *Neurosci. Lett.* **75**:6.
14. Gnahn, H., Hefti, F., Heuman, R., Schwab, M. E., and Thoenen, H., 1983, NGF-mediated increase in choline acetyltransferase (ChAT) in the neonatal rat forebrain; evidence for a physiological role of NGF in the brain? *Dev. Brain Res.* **9**:45–52.
15. Greene, L. A., and Shooter, E. M., 1980, The nerve growth factor: Biochemistry, synthesis and mechanism of action, *Annu. Rev. Neurosci.* **3**:353–402.
16. Hamburger, V., Brunsobechtold, J. K., and Yip, J. W., 1981, Neuronal death in the spinal ganglia of the chick embryo and its reduction by nerve growth factor, *J. Neurosci.* **1**:60–71.
17. Harountunian, V., Barnes, E., and Davis, K. L., 1985, Cholinergic modulation of memory, *Psychopharmacology* **87**:266–271.
18. Harper, G. P., and Thoenen, H., 1980, Nerve growth factor: Biological significance, measurement, and distribution, *J. Neurochem.* **34**:5–16.
19. Harper, G. P., Barde, Y. A., Edgar, D., Ganten, D., Hefti, F., Heuman, R., Naujoks, K. W., Rohrer, H., Turner, J. E., and Thoenen, H., 1983, Biological and immunological properties of nerve growth factor from bovine seminal plasma: Comparison with the properties of mouse nerve growth factor, *Neuroscience* **8**:375–387.
20. Hart, T., Chaimas, N. B., Moore, R. Y., and Stein, D. G., 1978, Effects of nerve growth factor on behavioral recovery following caudate nucleus lesions in rats, *Brain Res. Bull.* **3**:245–251.
21. Hefti, F., 1986, Nerve growth factor (NGF) promotes survival of septal cholinergic neurons after fimbrial transections, *J. Neurosci.* **6**:2155–2162.
22. Hefti, F., Dravid, A., and Hartikka, J., 1984, Chronic intraventricular injections of nerve growth factor elevate hippocampal choline acetyltransferase activity in adult rats with partial septo-hippocampal lesions, *Brain Res.* **293**:305–311.
23. Hefti, F., Hartikka, J., Eckenstein, F., Gnahn, H., Heumann, R., Schwab, M., and Thoenen, H., 1985, Nerve growth factor (NGF) induces choline acetyltransferase but fails to affect survival of fiber outgrowth of cholinergic neurons in cultures of dissociated septal neurons of fetal rat brain, *Neuroscience* **14**:55–68.
24. Hefti, F., Hartika, J., Salvatierra, A., Weiner, W. J., and Mash, D. C., 1986, Localization of nerve growth factor receptors in cholinergic neurons of the human basal forebrain, *Neurosci. Lett.* **69**:37–41.
25. Hefti, F., and Weiner, W. J., 1986, Nerve growth factor and Alzheimer's disease, *Ann. Neurol.* **20**:275–281.

26. Hendry, I. A., 1975, The response of adrenergic neurons to axotomy and nerve growth factor, *Brain Res.* **94:**87–97.
27. Hepler, D. G., Olton, D. S., Wenk, G. L., and Coyle, J. T., 1985, Lesions in nucleus basalis magnocellularis and medial septal area of rats produce qualitatively similar memory impairments, *J. Neurosci.* **5:**866–873.
28. Hepler, D. G., Wenk, G. L., Cribbs, B. L., Olton, D. S., and Coyle, J. T., 1985, Memory impairments following basal forebrain lesions, *Brain Res.* **346:**8–14.
29. Heumann, R., Korsching, S., and Thoenen, H., 1985, Regulation of nerve growth factor (NGF) specific messenger RNA in the peripheral and the central nervous system, *Soc. Neurosci. Abstr.* **11:**939.
30. Honegger, P., 1983, Nerve growth factor-sensitive brain neurons in culture, *Monogr. Neurol. Sci.* **9:**36–42.
31. Honegger, P., and Lenoir, D., 1982, Nerve growth factor (NGF) stimulation of cholinergic telencephalic neurons in aggregating cell cultures, *Dev. Brain Res.* **3:**229–238.
32. Jaffard, R., Galey, D., Micheau, J., and Durkin, T. P., 1985, The cholinergic septo-hippocampal pathway, learning and memory, in: *Brain Plasticity, Learning and Memory* (B. Will, P. Schmitt, and J. Dalrymple-Alford, eds.), Plenum Press, New York, pp. 167–181.
32a. Johnson, M. V., Buchanan, K., Rutkowski, J. L., and Mobley, W. C., 1985, Nerve growth factor effects on developing central cholinergic neurons: Temporal response characteristics in septum, hippocampus and striatum, *Soc. Neurosci. Abstr.* **11:**661.
33. Kimble, P. D., Bremiller, R., and Perez-Polo, J. R., 1979, Nerve growth factor applications fail to alter behavior of hippocampal-lesioned rats, *Physiol. Behav.* **23:**653–657.
34. Korsching, B., Auburger, G., Heumann, R., Scott, J.. and Thoenen, H., 1985, Levels of nerve growth factor and its mRNA in the central nervous system of the rat correlate with cholinergic innervation, *EMBO J.* **4:**1389–1393.
35. Levi-Montalcini, R., 1966, The nerve growth factor: Its mode of action on sensory and sympathetic nerve cells, *Harvey Lect.* **60:**217–259.
36. Levi-Montalcini, R., and Angeletti, P. U., 1966, Immunosympathectomy, *Pharmacol. Rev.* **18:**619–628.
37. Levi-Montalcini, R., and Booker, B., 1960, Excessive growth of sympathetic ganglia evoked by a protein isolated from mouse salivary gland, *Proc. Natl. Acad. Sci. U.S.A.* **46:**373–384.
38. Levi-Montalcini, R., and Booker, B., 1960, Destruction of the sympathetic ganglia in mammals by an antiserum to the nerve-growth promoting factor, *Proc. Natl. Acad. Sci. U.S.A.* **46:**384–391.
39. Levi-Montalcini, R., and Hamburger, V., 1951, Selective growth-stimulating effects of mouse sarcoma on the sensory and sympathetic nervous system of the chick embryo, *J. Exp. Zool.* **116:**321–362.
40. Levi-Montalcini, R., and Hamburger, V., 1953, A diffusible agent of mouse sarcoma producing hyperplasia of sympathetic ganglia and hyperneurotization of viscera in the chick embryo, *J. Exp. Zool.* **123:**233–278.
41. Lewis, M. E., Brown, R. M., Brownstein, M. J., Hart, T., and Stein, D. A., 1979, NGF: Effects on D-amphetamine induced activity and brain monoamines, *Brain Res.* **176:**297–310.
42. Loy, R., Milner, T. A., and Moore, R. Y., 1980, Sprouting of sympathetic axons in the hippocampal formation: Conditions necessary to elicit ingrowth, *Exp. Neurol.* **67:**399–411.
43. Loy, R., and Moore, R. Y., 1977, Anomalous innervation of the hippocampal formation by peripheral sympathetic axons following mechanical injury, *Exp. Neurol.* **57:**645–650.
44. Martinez, H. J., Dreyfus, C. F., Jonakait, D. G., and Black, I. B., 1985, Nerve growth factor promotes cholinergic development in brain striatal cultures, *Proc. Natl. Acad. Sci. U.S.A.* **82:**777–7781.
45. Matthies, H., 1974, The biochemical basis of learning and memory, *Life Sci.* **15:**2017–2031.
46. Mesulam, M. M., Mufson, E. J., Wainer, B. H., and Levey, A. I., 1983, Central cholinergic

pathways in the rat: An overview based on an alternative nomenclature (Ch1–Ch6), *Neuroscience* **10**:1185–1201.

47. Mobley, W. C., Rutowski, J. L., Tennekoon, G. I., Buchanan, K. and Johnston, M. V., 1985, Choline acetyltransferase activity in striatum of neonatal rats increased by nerve growth factor, *Science* **229**:284–286.

48. Murphy, R. A., Landis, S. C., Bernanke, J., and Siminoski, K., 1986, Absence of the alpha and gamma subunits of 7S nerve growth factor in denervated rodent iris: Immunocytochemical studies, *Dev. Biol.* **114**:369–380.

49. Nja, A., and Purves, D., 1978, Effects of nerve growth factor and its antiserum on synapses in the superior cervical ganglion of the guinea pig, *J. Physiol. (Lond.)* **277**:53–75.

50. Otten, U., Weskamp, G., Schlumpf, M., Lichtensteiger, W., and Mobley, W. C., 1985, Effects of antibodies against nerve growth factor on developing cholinergic forebrain neurons in rats, *Soc. Neurosci. Abstr.* **11**:661.

51. Pallage, V., Toniolo, G., Will, B., and Hefti, F., 1986. Long-term effects of nerve growth factor and neural transplants on behavior of rats with medial septal lesions, *Brain Res.* **386**:197–208.

52. Pepeu, G., 1983, Brain acetylcholine: An inventory of our knowledge on the 50th anniversary of its discovery, *Trends Pharmacol. Sci.* **4**:416–418.

53. Riopelle, R. J., Richardson, P. M., and Verge, V. M. K., 1985, Receptors for nerve growth factor in the rat central nervous system, *Soc. Neurosci. Abstr.* **11**:1056.

54. Russell, R. W., 1982, Cholinergic system in behavior: The search for mechanisms of action, *Annu. Rev. Pharmacol.* **22**:435–463.

55. Sabel, B. A., Kardon, G. B., and Stein, D. G., 1983, Behavioral effects of intracerebral injections of renin and captopril in intact and brain-damaged rats, *Brain Res. Bull.* **11**:637–642.

56. Salamone, J. D., Beart, P. M., Alpert, J. E., and Iversen, S. D., 1984, Impairment in T-maze reinforced alternation performance following nucleus basalis magnocellularis lesions in rats, *Behav. Brain Res.* **13**:63–70.

57. Schwab, M., Otten, U., Agid, Y., and Thoenen, H., 1979, Nerve growth factor (NGF) in the rat CNS: Absence of specific retrograde axonal transport and tyrosine hydroxylase induction in locus coeruleus and substantia nigra, *Brain Res.* **168**:473–483.

58. Scott, J., Selby, M., Urdea, M., Quiroga, M., Bell, G. I., and Rutter, W. J., 1983, Isolation and nucleotide sequence of cDNA encoding the precursor of mouse nerve growth factor, *Nature* **302**:538–540.

59. Shelton, D. L., and Reichardt, L. F., 1984, Expression of the nerve growth factor gene correlates with the density of sympathetic innervation in effector organs, *Proc. Natl. Acad. Sci. U.S.A.* **81**:7951–7955.

60. Shelton, D. L., and Reichardt, L. F., 1986, Studies on the expression of the beta nerve growth factor (NGF) gene in the central nervous system: Level and regional distribution of NGF mRNA suggest that NGF functions as a trophic factor for several distinct populations of neurons, *Proc. Natl. Acad. Sci. U.S.A.* **83**:2714–2718.

61. Stein, D. G., Blake, C. A., and Weiner, H. W., 1980, Nerve growth factor disrupts metabolism and behavioral performance of intact rats but does not affect recovery from hypothalamic lesions, *Brain Res.* **190**:278–284.

62. Stein, D. G., and Will, B. E., 1983, Nerve growth factor produces a temporary facilitation of recovery from entorhinal cortex lesions, *Brain Res.* **261**:127–131.

63. Stenevi, U., and Björklund, A., 1978, Growth of vascular sympathetic axons into the hippocampus after lesions of the septo-hippocampal pathway: A pitfall in brain lesions studies, *Neurosci. Lett.* **7**:219–224.

64. Taniuchi, M., and Johnson, E. M., 1985, Characterization of the binding properties and retrograde axonal transport of a monoclonal antibody directed against the rat nerve growth factor receptor, *J. Cell. Biol.* **101**:1100–1106.

65. Taniuchi, M., Schweizer, J. B., and Johnson, E. M., 1986, Nerve growth factor receptor molecules in rat brain, *Proc. Natl. Acad. Sci. U.S.A.* **83:**1950–1954.
66. Tarpy, R. M., Augenbraun, C. B., and Holman, W. L., 1975, Hypothalamic self-stimulation in rats following immunosympathectomy or central nerve growth factor antiserum injection, *Comp. Physiol. Psychol.* **88:**528–533.
67. Thoenen, H., and Barde, Y. A., 1980, Physiology of nerve growth factor, *Physiol. Rev.* **60:**1284–1335.
68. Thoenen, H., and Edgar, D., 1985, Neurotrophic factors, *Science* **229:**238–242.
69. Toniolo, G., Dunnett, S. B., Hefti, F., and Will, B., 1985, Acetylcholine-rich transplants in the hippocampus: Influence of intrinsic growth factors and application of nerve growth factor on choline acetyltransferase activity, *Brain Res.* **345:**141–146.
70. Ullrich, A., Gray, A., Berman, C., and Dull, T. J., 1983, Human beta-nerve growth factor gene sequence highly homologous to that of mouse, *Nature* **303:**821–825.
71. Varon, S., and Manthorpe, M., 1985, *In vitro* models for neuroplasticity and repair, in: *Central Nervous System Plasticity and Repair* (A. Bignami, F. E. Bloom, C. L. Bolis, and A. Adeloye, eds.), Raven Press, New York, pp. 13–23.
72. Weskamp, G., Lorez, H. P., and Otten, U., 1985, Development of a highly sensitive immunoassay for measurement of endogenous NGF in peripheral and central nervous system of the adult rat, *Soc. Neurosci. Abstr.* **11:**940.
73. Whittemore, S. R., Ebendal, T., Läkfors, L., Olson, L., Seiger, A., Strömberg, I., and Persson, H., 1985, Developmental, regional and post-lesion expression of nerve growth factor (NGF) and NGF mRNA in rat brain, *Soc. Neurosci. Abstr.* **11:**660.
74. Will, B., and Hefti, F., 1985, Behavioural and neurochemical effects of chronic intraventricular injections of nerve growth factor in adult rats with fimbria lesions, *Behav. Brain Res.* **17:**17–24.
75. Will, B. E., Schmitt, P., and Dalrymple-Alford, J. (eds.), 1985, *Brain Plasticity, Learning and Memory*, Plenum Press, New York.
76. Williams, L. R., Varon, S., Petersen, J. M., Victoreen K., Fischer, W., Björklund, A., and Gage, F. H., 1986, Continuous infusion of nerve growth factor prevents basal forebrain neuronal death after fimbria–fornix transection, *Proc. Natl. Acad. Sci. U.S.A.* **83:**9231–9235.
77. Yip, H. K., and Grafstein, B., 1982, Effect of nerve growth factor on regeneration of goldfish optic axons, *Brain Res.* **238:**329–339.

17

Recovery from Stroke

Andrew Kertesz

ABSTRACT. The pharmacological approach to first-stage recovery in acute stroke is aimed at controlling edema and improving microcirculation and cellular protection in the ischemic penumbra. Limiting lesion size with these early measures may influence outcome significantly. Careful methodology is necessary to measure recovery rates and outcome. The extent of recovery is influenced by initial severity. Lesion size in a stroke population correlates significantly with outcome measures. Recovery in the initial period, the first 3 months, is significantly greater in all groups and in all functional deficits. Evidence appears to indicate that both homologous contralateral and ipsilateral functionally connected hemispheric structures play a role in recovery. Comprehension and semantic processing may have more widespread cerebral compensation than motor and assembly functions of language, which are more left hemisphere dependent. Pharmacological studies in recovery must consider these factors and utilize more precise methodology to define functional deficits.

1. Introduction

Human brain injury from stroke or trauma produces deficits that recover to a variable extent. Human ischemic deficit and recovery from it have a special neurobiology. In order to investigate the effect of any form of therapy on recovery, first- and second-stage recovery should be distinguished. Some of the recovery studies have concentrated on preventing ischemic damage or increasing the resistance of the brain to ischemia. Recent developments in describing various patterns of cerebral perfusion, electrical activity, and ionic pump failure in ischemia have provided a conceptual basis for pharmacological intervention.[1] Much of the change in the acute phase is related to the recovery from the acute effects of hemorrhage, edema, electrolyte disturbances, and cellular reaction, which subside in a matter of days and weeks.

In addition, the concept of "ischemic penumbra," which is a zone of viable but metabolically lethargic cells surrounding an area of focal infarction, is also

ANDREW KERTESZ • Research Institute, St. Joseph's Hospital, University of Western Ontario, London, Ontario N6A 4V2, Canada.

important in first-stage recovery. It is the reversibility of electrical activity and ionic changes in this area that provides the impetus for pharmacological research. The ischemic threshold of cerebral perfusion for membrane failure is around 8 ml/100 g per min. Therefore, damage can be reversed if blood flow can be elevated. The rapid recovery from neurological deficit after a stroke is often attributed to the recovery of function of the cells in this ischemic penumbra.

There are many experimental models for cerebral ischemia. Most studies of pharmacological agents deal with these models, which widely differ in their reliability and relevance to clinical stroke. The literature in first-stage intervention is very extensive and is reviewed only selectively.

The interest in our laboratory has focused on second-stage recovery, beyond the acute effects of ischemia, hemorrhage, cellular reaction, and chemical alterations. Recovery of human cognitive function, especially recovery of language, can provide an important behavioral model for the biological determinants of second-stage recovery. The study of recovery from brain damage is more than just a practical prognostic exercise for the clinician or a baseline for therapy. It also provides an important theoretical framework for cerebral reorganization.

Monakow[43] realized the changing nature of aphasic and cognitive deficits, and his explanation for second-stage recovery, which he called "diaschisis," is still a valid concept in neurobiology. He thought that in acute injury, the damaged brain deprives the surrounding, mostly functionally connected areas from a trophic influence of innervation. The denervation would then cause the initial deficit to be larger than would have been expected from a mere loss of function. Monakow suggested that these areas recover by acquiring innervation from somewhere else or becoming autonomously functional.

Much of what we know about the reorganization of brain function in man comes from the functional analysis of deficits and their relationship to brain lesions. After stroke, trauma, or infection, human cognition is affected in a complex fashion, and its measurement and analysis are difficult. The reproducibility of observations is influenced by many biological and psychological factors. The main areas investigated are language, nonverbal cognition, visuomotor performance. and memory. The complexity of deficit analysis in cognition and in aphasia has been recognized, and some quantitation has been achieved by several advances in methodology. Aphasia tests became better standardized and more specific for a language-disordered population, and the methods of follow-up and the statistical evaluation of change have become more sophisticated.[17,25,26] Also, advances in cognitive psychology and linguistics have contributed to deficit analysis. Developments in neuroimaging, such as computerized tomography (CT) and magnetic resonance imaging (MRI), allow us to localize and quantitate lesions in patients who can be examined in detail with neuropsychological tests at the same time.

In this chapter, the pharmacological aspects of first- and second-stage recovery and the methodological advances in measuring recovery from aphasia as an example of human second-stage recovery are discussed.

2. PHARMACOLOGICAL INTERVENTION AND FIRST-STAGE RECOVERY

The pharmacological treatment of stroke patients is usually aimed at first-stage recovery. Since many of these drugs have vasodilating as well as cellular protective effects, and some are platelet antiaggregants that decrease the viscosity of the blood, the classifications of these antiischemic medications are overlapping (Table I). In the first few days after stroke, there is often progressive deterioration. In fact, a recent survey indicated that about a third of stroke patients show worsening that may interfere with their ultimate recovery.[19] Most of this initial deterioration is related to cerebral edema, occasionally to secondary hemorrhage into a dry infarct and at times recurrent embolism or what is often

TABLE I. Drugs in Acute Stroke

Edema control
    Hyperosmolar agents: mannitol, glycerol
    Corticosteroids: dexamethasone
    Barbiturates
Oxygen enhancers
    Hyperbaric oxygen
    Fluorocarbons
Cerebral vasodilators
    Papaverine
    Aminophylline
    CO_2 inhalation
    β-Blockers
    Prostacyclin and thromboxane inhibitors
    Calcium channel blockers: nimopidine
    Serotonin inhibitors
Microcirculation enhancers
    Low-molecular-weight dextran
    Prostacyclin and thromboxane inhibitors
    Platelet antiaggregants: ASA, dipyridamole
    Anticoagulants: coumadin, heparin
Fibrinolytics: streptokinase, urokinase, viper venom
Cellular protection
    Barbiturates
    Calcium antagonists: flurazine
    Opiate antagonists: naloxone
    Prostacyclin

called "stroke in evolution." At times drug effects, metabolic complications, most often generalized anoxia, or diabetes contribute to a negative change. Most of the time the physician is restricted to controlling the nonspecific complications.

Some of the pharmacological treatment of first-stage deterioration is an attempt to control cerebral edema. Hyperosmolar agents such as mannitol and glycerol reduce brain volume and increase cerebral blood flow, but most of the acutely effective drugs unfortunately have only a temporary effect, and some even produce a rebound edema. The hypervolemia after repeated administration leads to renal or cardiac failure and electrolyte disturbance. Mannitol and glycerol are used extensively in head injury, but their efficacy has not been proven in stroke. Similarly, the use of corticosteroids is controversial, to say the least. Most neurologists do not use it because a recent study suggested that not only is it not effective even in very high doses,[44] but it actually increases mortality[11] by increasing the risk of infections and worsening diabetes. There is evidence that high glucose levels produce high lactate, which is cytotoxic, rather than acting to increase available substrate for metabolism.[48]

Acute oxygen therapy of hyperbaric oxygen has been tried, but the hyperbaric effect seems to last only a few hours, and prolonged use of high concentrations of oxygen may be toxic.[42] Fluorocarbons apparently have some protective effect in acute ischemic models.[45] Subsequent studies showed only moderate modification on pathology.[46]

Cerebral vasodilators have obvious therapeutic potential, but the problem is the loss of autoregulation of the arteries in ischemic areas. Therefore, vasodilators, such as papaverine and carbon dioxide, tend to dilate normal cerebral blood vessels, stealing blood from ischemic areas.[33] Theophylline and papaverine were also found to be ineffective in influencing the outcome of cerebral infarction.[5,41] Attempts to exploit this paradoxical failure of autoregulation use the opposite effect of vasoconstrictors. These drugs should shunt blood into ischemic areas, because only normal cerebral vessels will vasoconstrict. Vasoconstrictors would also have the added effect of increasing systemic blood pressure and improving cerebral circulation by the proportionate increase of blood delivered to the brain. However, vasoconstrictors may contribute further to ischemia, and increased blood pressure may produce hemorrhages. Therefore, vasoconstrictors have not been used extensively in acute stroke except to support hypotension and failure of circulation. Hyperventilation and alkalosis are also potential vasoconstrictors of the cerebral circulation. The treatment of stroke with hyperventilation has failed to be effective and caused several complications.[7] Drug-induced metabolic alkalosis using aminomethane was also ineffective.[40]

Other drugs that would increase microcirculation and possibly reverse ischemia have been tried in great numbers in animal models as well as in clinical experiments. Low-molecular-weight dextran decreased platelet aggregation and blood viscosity and improved cerebral blood flow.[20] In a double-blind study in patients, fewer deaths after treatment were seen in severe stroke, but survivors were equally disabled at 6 months.[38] Platelet antiaggregants have been used after stroke not only to prevent recurrence but also to improve microcirculation.[4] Recent studies of hemodilution showed a moderate but definite effect.[55] Fibrinogen contributes to blood viscosity, and viper venom, which is fibrinolytic, was used successfully in ischemic stroke to decrease viscosity.[22]

Prostacyclin causes vasodilation and inhibition of platelet aggregation, reduces the size of myocardial infarction, decreases the oxygen demand of tissue, and counteracts the effect of endotoxins. However, the efficacy of prostacyclin in stroke has not been confirmed by controlled trials, even though some stroke patients appear to have benefited.[18] Other studies showed that prostacyclin reduced blood–brain barrier leakage.[2] A double-blind study showed some neurological improvement in the first 3 days, but no significant effect was observed by 2 weeks after the initial stroke.[23] Thromboxane synthesis inhibitors have been tried in order to alter cerebral blood flow and perfusion of ischemic areas. Indomethacin is thought to inhibit all the products of cyclooxygenase that accumulate in cerebral ischemia and contribute to thromboxane synthesis inhibition.

One of the important electrolyte changes in acute ischemia is the increase of intracellular calcium (Ca), which inhibits mitochondrial respiration. Impaired membrane permeability increases Ca influx, which seriously interferes with neuronal functioning. Calcium channel antagonists not only inhibit Ca influx but also prevent the postischemic reduction of cerebral blood flow and reduce mortality in various animals.[57] Different calcium blockers have different organ specificity: some like bepridil and verapamil have mostly cardiac effects and are antiarrhythmic and antianginal; others like nifedipine exert a therapeutic effect mainly by vasodilation. However, protection from calcium at the cellular level also contributes to the antiischemic effect.[15] Calcium antagonists seem to have a potentially useful effect in first-stage recovery, but this is still insufficiently documented.[12]

Barbiturates have been tried for their effect of decreasing cerebral metabolism and lowering intracranial pressure. Recent studies also demonstrated that barbiturates may protect the brain by scavenging free radicals released by ischemia.[13] Although barbiturate anesthesia reduced the neurological disability and the severity of cerebral infarction in the stroke model using carotid artery occlusion in dogs, the use of barbiturates in severe stroke or deteriorating stroke has not been proven.[52] Most neurologists avoid inducing barbiturate coma in stroke because of the difficulty in monitoring patients and the problems of overloading intensive care unit capacity.

Dramatic response to naloxone, an opiate antagonist, has been reported for focal cerebral ischemia.[24] Improvement, however, tends to be temporary and may be related to cerebral arousal rather than to a specific vasogenic protective effect. Amphetamines have also been used for their protective effect in cerebral

ischemia (see D. M. Feeney and R. L. Sutton, Chapter 7). Reports of intracerebral hemorrhage related to amphetamine use discouraged the clinical trial of
this drug.[54] Studies of circulating catecholamines after stroke provided the rationale for treatment with serotonin and dopamine inhibitors. Seratonin antagonists (cephaloridine) have shown to protect the CNS from experimental ischemia.[50] Tradozone appears to have an ischemic effect through the selective
inhibition of serotonin reuptake. Currently, a clinical trial is underway to determine its effectiveness in acute stroke.[12]

Fibronolytic agents have been initially rejected because of the danger of
hemorrhage. Some of these early studies demonstrated the thrombi were dissolved with greater frequency with streptokinase, but no clinical improvement
was evident, and a small risk of hemorrhage was noted.[39] Urokinase injections
later than 24 hr after the onset of symptoms of completed strokes was not
effective.[14] Recent large-scale studies on cardiac uses of fibrinolysis did not
show any increase in the incidence of intracranial hemorrhage.[56] Limited clinical
experience indicated that improvement can occur in some patients in acute stroke
even with intravenous injection.[9] The experience in myocardial ischemia indicates that the best results are obtained when the treatment begins within 6 hr of
the onset of ischemia. This would maximize functional tissue recovery by limiting the duration of parenchymal injury. More recent studies used a local intraarterial infusion of streptokinase or urokinase, and although recanalization occurred in most patients, the recovery rate was modest, and 17% of patients had
some hemorrhage.[9]

3. PHARMACOLOGICAL TREATMENT IN SECOND-STAGE RECOVERY

The range of pharmacological agents used to promote second-stage recovery in established stroke is much smaller than in the acute period. However, the
extent of recovery is considerable, and the potential for drugs to promote this
stage of compensation has not been explored extensively. The common foci of
treatment in second-stage stroke are physio-, speech, and occupational therapy
aimed at functional restoration. Physiatrists and rehabilitation specialists have
traditionally relied on physical and psychological means of restoration rather
than drugs. Nevertheless, there are a few commonly used drugs and a few
experimental ones. The role of baclofen or dantrolene sodium or centrally active
muscle relaxants in controlling muscle spasm is controversial. Most physicians
only use these drugs with severe, incapacitating spasticity, because many am-
bulating stroke patients need a little spasticity, in fact, to stand up, and if this is
taken away, one can hinder rehabilitation and actually increase weakness.

Anecdotal reports of the use of L-dopa and dopa decarboxylase inhibitor in a
few aphasic patients have been presented, but there has been no reliably con-

trolled study. Sodium amobarbital and amphetamines have also been tried with no significant success. Barbiturates only increase the dysarthric component of speech but do not release the severe word-finding problem, which has all the appearance of a blockage that should respond to a drug that releases inhibitors in the central nervous system.

The process of structural reorganization may be promoted by brain gangliosides, which are natural components of cellular membranes.[49] Stroke patients 2 weeks post-onset who were treated with monosialogangliosides for 6 weeks showed a moderate but significant benefit.[3]

Finally, the judicious use of antidepressants is well accepted, but the diagnosis of depression is difficult at times because of the communication problem in left-hemispheric stroke and because of the effect of disturbed emotional expression and processing in right-hemisphere stroke. The peculiar forced crying and laughter that are often part of the so-called "pseudobulbar palsy" seen in bilateral or more caudally (often in the brainstem) located strokes is not caused by depression, although it is often mistaken for it, leading to unnecessary medication.

4. FACTORS IN SECOND-STAGE RECOVERY

Second-stage recovery is a complex and largely unexplained phenomenon.[53] A study of any therapeutic modality has to account for a variety of important factors influencing outcome. Some of the methodological issues discussed below are valid also for first-stage recovery. It is essential to control some of these second-stage recovery factors in order to study drug effects in humans for acute-stage studies as well.

Among the factors important in recovery is initial severity. Early investigators considered initial severity to have a highly predictive value in aphasia.[16,29] The severity of deficit at onset has a considerable effect on recovery rates because mildly affected aphasics do not have much room for recovery (a "ceiling effect") and severe aphasics often have more potential. The lack of consideration of initial severity is a major error in design in some treatment studies. Treated patients tend to be selected from the less severe groups and bias the results. Unless initial severity is controlled, studies of treatment should not be considered reliable. There are various methods of controlling for initial severity, such as analysis of covariance or using outcome measures instead of recovery rates or expressing the change as a percentage of the initial severity or comparing patient groups with equal severity.

The methodology of patient selection is also an important issue. Often patients are included in recovery studies at various stages on the recovery curve. In our studies, we took care to start our evaluation within the acute period, usually between 10 and 45 days after a stroke. Since most of our patients were examined at exactly 14 days after onset, this population is rather homogeneous. Only the more severely affected patients, who could not be examined at that time because of intercurrent medical illness or obtundation, were kept until the upper limit of the time period.

Various etiologies were grouped together in many early studies, but this seems a significant disadvantage. Traumatic aphasia, for instance, improves quickly if it is related to closed head injury. Dysarthria, however, tends to be persistent in severe trauma, and this often disrupts communication to such a degree that the extent of posttraumatic aphasia is difficult to determine. Penetrating head injury affects a different age group and behaves differently because of the variation in the speed and path of the missile and the associated concussion. Therefore, posttraumatic aphasia is biologically different from the vascular type. There are many similarities, however, indicating that the recurring patterns of aphasic types are not necessarily related to the distribution of vascular lesions. A recent study by Ludlow et al.[37] on Vietnam veterans showed that the lesions that produce persisting asyntactic or Broca's aphasia are large and involve subcortical and parietal structures in addition to Broca's area, very similar to recovery after stroke.

Age or sex does not seem to be a significant factor as long as an adult population with strokes is studied. Prepubertal children recover quite well from injury, and even infantile hemispherectomies develop normal speech with only slight limitation on verbal intelligence.[10] Etiology compounds the age factor, since young individuals are much less likely to suffer from stroke. When only similar etiologies are studied, the differences between childhood and adult recovery rates tend to decrease significantly.[58] Other pathological variables, such as repeated stroke insults, cerebral atrophy, or intercurrent latent dementia, remain factors to be considered or even studied directly, although they can be controlled by exclusion such as was done in our studies.

5. THE MEASUREMENTS OF DEFICIT

Various recovery studies used different language examinations. Extremely detailed testing of function does not allow a practical number of follow-up studies. We used the Western Aphasia Battery (WAB) because it covers language functions comprehensively yet is practical to administer to most patients.[26] The interrater, test–retest, and reliability content, intratest validity, and rationale of the test have been described.[25] The WAB provides a summary of the language subscores as a measure of overall severity called the aphasia quotient (AQ). Among the subtests, the information content provides a measure of functional communication, and it can also be used separately as a measure of recovery. Comprehension is tested with yes/no questions, a pointing task of auditory word recognition, and a syntactically complex sentence task. Naming of visually presented common objects, sentence completion, and responsive speech are measures of lexical access. Repetition is tested with words and sentences of increasing difficulty. The test includes reading, writing, and an assessment of praxis, calculation, and a section of nonverbal performance such as block design, Raven's Colored Progressive Matrices, drawing, and line bisection. The tests are done at 10–45 days, 3 months, 6 months, and 12 months after stroke.

6. Recovery Rates and Time Intervals

Second-stage recovery is most marked in the first 3 months, and recovery curves are initially steeper in all aphasic groups and also for the total group. More severely affected aphasics continue to recover at a later stage if they are followed for a sufficient length of time. Some investigators, such as Broida[6] suggested that recovery continues beyond 1 year, although this was based on only a few selected cases. In our previous study,[29] we found no significant recovery beyond 1 year when a larger population was looked at.

7. Lesion Size and Recovery

Lesion size and location have also been recognized as relevant but complex factors. Until recently, clinicians relied on autopsy correlations, but modern neuroimaging has provided an opportunity to study lesion characteristics *in vivo*. We presented our first study of lesion size measured on CT and recovery from aphasia in 1979.[28] We found that the larger the lesion the poorer the outcome with one unexpected exception: the recovery rate of comprehension was found to increase with lesion size! Why this occurred can be best understood if another study of ours is considered in which the best-recovered modality was found to be comprehension.[36] Patients with large lesions having global or severe Broca's aphasia often show greater improvement in comprehension than patients with smaller lesions, such as anomics, who already have good comprehension and therefore have less room for recovery (ceiling effect). The large lesions with more recovery and small lesions with little change give rise to a consistently positive correlation between lesion size and recovery unless the initial severity is covaried, as was done in our subsequent studies.

Since then, various other authors dealt with localization of the lesions in a somewhat different, symptom-oriented approach.[32,50] Knopman et al.[32] looked at fluency, lesion size, and location and found that in the language area about 60 cm^3 was a critical size; a larger lesion results in relatively less recovery. Motor speech has less redundancy, and if the areas surrounding Broca's area and the precentral gyrus are involved, less recovery will take place. Semantic access is severely impaired in Wernicke's aphasics, and after large lesions there is less recovery. The symptom-orientation approach generally leads to less focal localization of functional deficits, as some of these functions are widely distributed in the brain and can be affected from several sites.

Improvement in imaging techniques and in measuring the lesion parameters increased the accuracy beyond that of CT studies. The recent magnetic resonance imager (MRI) utilizes greater white and gray matter contrast and allows visualization of the brain in quasianatomic sections in any desired plane *in vivo,* while the patients are being examined.

Lesion tracing should be performed blindly without knowledge of the patient's clinical features to avoid bias in locating the anatomic structures that are involved. The issue of direct tracing of lesions or using templates onto which the lesions are drawn cannot be resolved easily. Direct tracing is more reproducible between observers, but because of the variability of head positioning, different scanning techniques, and different skull shapes of individuals, tracing on standard templates by a human observer allows mental adjustment for angulation of the head and various differences in the size and shape of the scans of different patients. The digitization of the lesion areas is a fairly standard process, and modern scanners have algorithms that provide for an automated pixel count. Even in this case, the human observer has to draw the edges or limits of the lesion. When a lesion is digitized for each slice, the areas can be multiplied by the slice thickness, and a volumetric measurement can be obtained.

8. LESION LOCATION AND RECOVERY

Lesion location is often determined by a checklist of regions of interest that has been worked out in several laboratories[37,50] including ours (see below). The actual involvement in each structure may be scored as a percentage of involvement, but this is difficult to reproduce and may create a spurious source of variability. A simplified scoring system of less than half, more than half, or total involvement is more realistic.

The CT scan evaluation of lesion locations, using a three-point rating of the extent of involvement of each anatomic structure was carried out in 22 Broca's aphasics divided by the median for poor and good recovery. The structures with significant involvement (more than 50%) were the inferior frontal gyrus, especially the pars opercularis and triangularis, and the insula in both groups. There were only two patients in whom the posterior inferior frontal gyrus was not involved, and both of these patients had significant involvement of the putamen or the caudate nucleus or both. The difference between the persisting and recovered cases of Broca's aphasia was most prominent in the involvement of the precentral, postcentral, and supramarginal gyri in the cases of poor recovery. In those cases in which recovery was good, supramarginal and inferior parietal gyri were not involved. The subcortical regions showed significant differences in the involvement of the putamen and the caudate, which was twice as frequent in the persistent cases.

Specific structural correlates of recovery were also examined for Wernicke's aphasia. Those who have better recovery rates have clearly smaller mean lesion volumes, and certain structures are less frequently involved than others. The most consistently involved structure was the superior temporal gyrus. In cases of poor recovery, the middle temporal gyrus and the supramarginal gyrus are significantly more frequently involved in addition to the postcentral gyrus and the insula, which is twice as frequently involved in unrecovered cases.

9. CEREBRAL ASYMMETRY

The possible interaction of cerebral asymmetry or atypically distributed language in the two hemispheres and recovery was explored in Broca's and Wernicke's aphasics by measurings the frontal and occipital "petalias" (prominence of one side or the other) and width on CT scans according to the methodology of LeMay and Kido.[34] It has been suggested that more bilaterally distributed language capacity could result in better recovery in unilateral brain damage.[47] We divided the "petalias" and width measurements into groups of right larger than left, equal, or left larger than right.[27] Broca's aphasics were then grouped according to their recovery. Those who remained Broca's aphasics were compared to those who changed into other categories such as anomics, conduction or transcortical motor aphasia, or recovered completely. Those patients with better recovery were in the majority ($n = 16$). Although there were some trends for the better-recovered patients to have less typical cerebral asymmetry with cerebral petalia and width measures, the differences between the two groups were not significant. A similar lack of significance for asymmetries was found in Wernicke's aphasics.

Certain aspects of hemispheric specialization may vary according to individuals even though anatomic asymmetries do not seem to play a role in recovery as was suggested. It could be that anatomic asymmetries relate more to handedness than to language distribution, as suggested by some of our studies in normals,[27] and this may be the reason why we are not seeing an effect on language recovery. The individual variations in the intra- and interhemispheric distribution of various functional components may contribute to an important extent to the ability of the mature brain to compensate after a single nonprogressive lesion.

10. FUNCTIONAL REORGANIZATION

Rather than anatomic reorganization through axonal regrowth or collateral sprouting, which can be demonstrated in the peripheral nervous system and to a lesser extent in the CNS of rodents, it is probably "functional reorganization" that underlies recovery in the human brain. Parts of the intact and functionally connected brain substitute for others, and the homologous portion of the contralateral hemisphere may do this to some extent. Right hemisphere compensation has been suggested by Wernicke and subsequently by Henschen.[21] This principle was based largely on anecdotal evidence of large left hemisphere lesions with good recovery.

In some patients who became aphasic with a single left-hemisphere stroke and subsequently recovered, a second right-hemisphere stroke may produce language deficit.[35] These cases are rarely documented and may represent bilateral language organization to begin with rather than a common mechanism of functional transfer to the contralateral hemisphere after destruction of a certain amount of language-related structure in the left hemisphere. One of the most dramatic demonstrations of the residual capacity of the right hemisphere to compensate for the loss of language resulting from left hemisphere lesions is given by the hemispherectomy studies[51] that indicated that symptoms resembling global aphasia occur after a left hemispherectomy. Some comprehension recovers, but the patient continues to remain nonfluent. When written or verbal input was separated to each of the hemispheres, converging evidence from callosal-sectioned patients demonstrated that the right hemisphere is capable of processing single words, usually concrete nouns.[59]

The idea that compensation after partial left hemisphere damage occurs through right hemisphere functions was supported to some extent by studies of sodium amobarbital given to aphasics who have recovered.[8,30] The studies indicated that even though the aphasic disturbance occurred from a left-hemisphere lesion it was the right hemispheric injection that increased the language disturbance, indicating that the right hemisphere compensated for the previous deficit. Recent studies of cerebral blood flow with xenon 133 also indicated right hemisphere participation in recovery to a variable degree.[31]

Our studies, nevertheless, demonstrated the importance of structures that surround the lesion areas in the recovery process. Those left hemispheric structures that are connected sequentially with the opercular and anterior insular regions play a crucial role in recovery from Broca's aphasia. Patients who have adjacent involvement, especially the inferior portion of the precentral gyrus and the anterior parietal region, show less recovery than those in whom these areas are spared, thus indicating their role in compensation. Phonemic output mechanisms are processed by a cortical–subcortical network that can be damaged partially with good recovery. However, if both cortical and subcortical components of the network are impaired, recovery is much less likely.

A complex integration of structures also takes place for the processing of language comprehension, although interhemispheric connections may play a larger role in comprehension than in motor output. It seems that a restricted deficit in the dominant hemisphere auditory association area, the posterior superior temporal gyrus and the planum temporale, can be compensated for by the opposite, homologous hemispheric structures or by surrounding structures in the temporal and inferior parietal regions and in the insula. However, when either of these compensating structures is affected, or when the lesion is large, precluding right hemisphere access, recovery is not as likely.

11. IMPLICATIONS FOR PHARMACOLOGICAL TRIALS IN PATIENTS

Language recovery following stroke provides a potential measure of the efficacy of pharmacological intervention in stroke patients. The variables that have been carefully analyzed could serve as a baseline, and the methodology of sequential follow-up utilized in comparing treated and untreated groups. Regardless of whether the drug treatment is in the acute or in the second stages of recovery, the final outcome is influenced by certain variables that need to be considered in order to match experimental groups. The major ones are etiology, initial severity, lesion size, and lesion location. These are interdependent variables, and considering one will account for some of the others, but each contributes additional variability and is worth examining separately.

The functional analysis should be as detailed as possible, considering not only the overall deficit but all the separate cognitive and language processes whenever practicable. Even if early assessment at the time of administration is impossible in detail, subsequent testing may still serve as a base line for longitudinal follow-up.

Group comparisons of repeated measure with ANOVA, multiple regression analysis, and contingency tables can be used to determine the efficacy of treatment. Covariance of initial severity is important for recovery rates to avoid a ceiling effect. Sample size estimation can be based on the above-quoted studies of rates of recovery for various stroke groups. Careful attention should be given to choosing outcome measures or recovery rates, because the two often differ. Correlation analysis using recovery rates can give results opposite to those obtained from outcome measures. Neglecting the complexity of second-stage recovery may result in negative drug trials or even in false claims of efficacy.

REFERENCES

1. Astrup, J., Siesjo, B. K., and Symon, L., 1981, Thresholds in cerebral ischemia—the ischemic penumbra, *Stroke* **12**:723–725.
2. Awad, I., Little, J. R., Lucas, F., Skrinska, V., Slugg, R., and Lesser, R. P., 1983, Treatment of acute focal cerebral ischemia with prostacyclin, *Stroke* **14**:203–209.
3. Bassi, S., Albizzati, M. G., Sbacchi, M., Frattola, L., and Massarotti, M., 1985, Monosialo-ganglioside therapy in stroke, *Stroke* **16**:899–900.
4. Bousser, M. G., Eschwege, E., Haguenau, M., Lefaucconnier, J. M., Thibult, N., and Touboul, D., 1983, "AICLA" controlled trial of aspirin and dipyridamole in the secondary prevention of athero-thrombotic cerebral ischemia, *Stroke* **14**:5–14.

5. Britton, M., de Faire, U., Helmers, C., Miah, K., and Rane, A., 1980, Lack of effect of theophylline on the outcome of acute cerebral infarction, *Acta Neurol. Scand.* **62:**116–123.
6. Broida, H., 1977, Language therapy effects in long term aphasia, *Arch. Phys. Med. Rehabil.* **58:**248–253.
7. Christensen, M. S., Paulson, O. B., Olesen, J., Alexander, S. C., Skinhoj, E., Dom, W. H., and Lassen, N. A., 1973, Cerebral apoplexy (stroke) treated with or without prolonged artificial hyperventilation. 1. Cerebral circulation, clinical course, and cause of death, *Stroke* **4:**568–631.
8. Czopf, J., 1972, Role of the non-dominant hemisphere in the restitution of speech in aphasia, *Arch. Psychiatr. Nervenkr.* **216:**162–171.
9. Del Zoppo, G. J., Zeumer, H.. and Harker, L. A., 1986, Thrombolytic therapy in stroke: Possibilities and hazards, *Stroke* **17:**595–607.
10. Dennis, M., and Kohn, B., 1975, Comprehension of syntax in infantile hemiplegics after cerebral hemidecortication: Left hemisphere superiority, *Brain Lang.* **2:**472–482.
11. Dyken, M., and White, P. T., 1956, Evaluation of cortisone in the treatment of cerebral infarction, *J.A.M.A.* **132:**1531–1956.
12. Fieschi, C., Lenzi, G. L., and Rasura, M., 1986, Role of calcium entry blockers in neurological diseases, *Eur. Neurol.* **25**(Suppl. 1):68–71.
13. Flamm, E. S., Demopoilos, H. B., Seligman, M. L., *et al.*, 1977, Possible molecular mechanisms of barbiturate-mediated protection in regional cerebral ischemia, *Acta Neurol. Scand.* **56**(64):150–151.
14. Fletcher, A. P., Alkjaersig, M., Lewis, M., Tulevski, V., Davies, A., Brooks, J. E., Mardin, W. B., Landau, W. M., and Raichle, M. E., 1976, A pilot study of urokinase therapy in cerebral infarction, *Stroke* **7:**135–142.
15. Gelners, H. J., 1984, The effects of nimopidine on the clinical course of patients with acute ischemic stroke, *Acta Neurol. Scand.* **69:**232–239.
16. Godfrey, C. M., and Douglass, E., 1959, The recovery process in aphasia, *Can. Med. Assoc. J.* **80:**618–624.
17. Goodglass, H., and Kaplan, E., 1983, *Boston Naming Test,* Lea & Febiger, Philadelphia.
18. Gryglewski, R. J., Nowak, S., Kostka-Trabka, E., Kusmiderski, J., Dembinska-Kiec, A.. Bieron, K., Basista, M., and Blaszczyk, B., 1983, Treatment of ischemic stroke with prostacyclin, *Stroke* **14:**197–202.
19. Hachinski, V., and Norris, J. W., 1985, *The Acute Stroke,* F. A. Davis, Philadelphia.
20. Hass, W. K., 1979, Drug effects in regional cerebral blood flow in focal cerebrovascular disease, *J. Neurol. Sci.* **19:**461.
21. Henschen, S. E., 1920–1922, *Klinische und anatomische Beitrage zur Pathologie des Gehirns.* Volumes 5–7, Nordiska Bokhandel, Stockholm.
22. Hossman, V., Heiss, W., Bewermeyer, H., and Wiedemann, G., 1983, Controlled trial of ancrod in ischemic stroke, *Stroke* **40:**803–808.
23. Huczynski, J., Kostka-Trabka, E., Sotowska, K., Bieron, L., Grodzinska, L., Dembinska-Kiec, A., Pykosz-Mazur, E., Peczak, E., and Gryglewski, R. J., 1985, Double-blind controlled trial of the therapeutic effects of prostacyclin in patients with completed ischemic stroke, *Stroke* **16:**810–813.
24. Jabally, J., and Davis, J. N., 1984, Naloxone administration to patients with acute stroke, *Stroke* **15:**36–39.
25. Kertesz, A., 1979, *Aphasia and Associated Disorders,* Grune & Stratton, New York.
26. Kertesz, A., 1982, *The Western Aphasia Battery,* Grune & Stratton, New York.
27. Kertesz, A., Black, S. E., Polk, M., and Howell, J., 1986, Cerebral asymmetries on magnetic resonance imaging, *Crotex* **22:**117–127.
28. Kertesz, A., Harlock, W., and Coates, R., 1979, Computer tomographic localization, lesion size and prognosis in aphasia, *Brain Lang.* **8:**34–50.

29. Kertesz, A., and McCabe, P., 1977, Recovery patterns and prognosis in aphasia, *Brain* **100**:1–18.
30. Kinsbourne, M., 1971, The minor cerebral hemisphere as a source of aphasic speech, *Arch. Neurol.* **25**:302–306.
31. Knopman, D. S., Rubens, A. B., Selnes, O. A., Klassen, A. C., and Meyer, M. W., 1984, Mechanisms of recovery from aphasia: Evidence from serial xenon 133 cerebral blood flow studies, *Ann. Neurol.* **15**(6):530–535.
32. Knopman, D. S., Selnes, O. A., Niccum, N., and Rubens, A. B., 1983, A longitudinal study of speech fluency in aphasia: CT scan correlates of recovery and persistent nonfluency, *Neurology (N.Y.)* **33**:1170–1178.
33. Lassen, N. A., and Palvolgyi, R., 1968, Cerebral steal during hypercapnia and the inverse reaction during hypocapnia observed by the 133-xenon technique in man, *Scand. J. Clin. Lab. Invest.* **22**:13D.
34. Lemay, M., and Kido, D. K., 1978, Asymmetries of the cerebral hemispheres on computed tomograms, *J. Comput. Assist. Tomogr.* **2**:471–476.
35. Levine, D. M., and Mohr, J. P., 1979, Language after bilateral cerebral infarctions: Role of the minor hemisphere, *Neurology (Minneap.)* **29**:927–938.
36. Lomas, J., and Kertesz, A., 1978, Patterns of spontaneous recovery in aphasic groups: A study of adult stroke patients, *Brain Lang.* **5**:388–401.
37. Ludlow, C., Rosenberg, J., Fair, C., Buck, D., Schesselman, S., and Salazar, A., 1986, Brain lesions associated with nonfluent aphasia fifteen years following penetrating head injury, *Brain* **109**:55–80.
38. Matthews, W. B., Oxbury, J. M., Grainger, M. R., and Greenhall, R. C. D., 1976, A blind controlled trial of Dextran 40 in the treatment of ischemic stroke. *Brain* **99**:193–206.
39. Meyer, J. S., *et al.*, 1965, Therapeutic thrombolysis in cerebral thrombus–embolism. Randomized evaluation of intravenous streptokinase, in: *Cerebral Vascular Diseases* (C. H. Millikan, R. G. Siekert, and J. Whisnant, eds.), Grune & Stratton, New York, pp. 200–213.
40. Meyer, J. S., Fukuuchi, Y., Shimazu, K., Ohuchi, T., and Ericsson, A. D., 1972, Abnormal hemispheric blood flow and metabolism in cerebrovascular disease, ii. Therapeutic trials with 5% CO_2 inhalation, hyperventilation and intravenous infusion of THAM and mannitol, *Stroke* **3**:157–167.
41. Meyer, J. S., Gotoh, F., Gilroy, J., 1965, Improvement in brain oxygenation and clinical improvement in patients with stroke treated with papaverine hydrochloride. *JAMA* **194**:957–961.
42. Meyer, J. S., and Mathew, N. T., 1974, Medical management in cerebral ischemia, in: *Controversy in Internal Medicine, Volume 2* (F. Ingelfinger, ed.), W. B. Saunders, Philadelphia, p. 771.
43. Monakow, C. von, 1914, *Die Lokalisation im Grosshirn und der Abbau der Funktionen durch corticale Herde*, Bergmann, Wiesbaden.
44. Norris, J. W., and Hachinski, V. C., 1985, Megadose steroid therapy in ischemic stroke, *Stroke* **16**:150.
45. Peerless, S. J., Ishikawa, R., Hunter, I. G., and Peerless, M. J., 1981, Protective effect of Fluosol-DA in acute cerebral ischemia, *Stroke* **12**:558–563.
46. Peerless, S. J., Nakamura, R., Rodriguez-Salazar, A., and Hunter, I. G., 1985, Modification of cerebral ischemia with Fluosol, *Stroke* **16**:38–43.
47. Pieniadz, J. M., Naeser, M. A., Koff, E., and Levine, H. L., 1983, CT scan cerebral hemispheric asymmetry measurements in stroke cases with global aphasia: Atypical asymmetries associated with improved recovery, *Cortex* **19**:371–393.
48. Plum, F., 1983, What causes infarction in ischemic brain? *Neurology (N.Y.)* **33**:222–233.

49. Sabel, B. A., Slavin, M. D., and Stein, D. G., 1984, GM₁ ganglioside treatment facilitates behavioral recovery from bilateral brain damage, *Science* **225**:340–342.

50. Selnes, O. A., Knopman, D. S., Niccum, N., and Rubens, A. B., (1983), CT scan correlates of auditory comprehension deficits in aphasia: A prospective recovery study, *Ann. Neurol.* **13**:558–566.

51. Smith, A., 1966, Speech and other functions after left (dominant) hemispherectomy, *J. Neurol. Neurosurg. Psychiatry* **29**:467–471.

52. Smith, A. L., Hoff, J. T., and Nielsen, S. L., 1974, Barbiturate protection in acute focal cerebral ischemia, *Stroke* **5**:1–7.

53. Stein, H. D., Rosen, J. J., and Butters, N., 1974, *Plasticity and Recovery of Function in the Central Nervous System*, Academic Press, New York.

54. Stoessl, A. J., Young, G. B., and Feasby, T. E., 1985, Intracerebral hemorrhage and angiographic beading following ingestion of catecholaminergics, *Stroke* **16**:734–736.

55. Strand, T., Asplund, K., Eriksson, S., Hagg, E., Lithner, F., and Wester, P., 1984, A randomized controlled trial of hemodilution therapy in acute ischemic stroke, *Stroke* **15**:980–989.

56. TIMI Study Group, 1985, Special report: The thrombolysis in myocardial infarction (TIMI) trial, *N. Engl. J. Med.* **312**:932–936.

57. Wauquier, A., 1984, Effect of calcium entry blockers in models of brain hypoxia, in: *Calcium Entry Blockers in Cardiovascular and Cerebral Dysfunctions* (Godfraind, Herman, and Wellens, eds.), Martinus Nijhoff, The Hague, pp. 241–254.

58. Woods, B. T., and Teuber, H. L., 1978, Changing patterns of childhood aphasia, *Ann. Neurol.* **3**:273–280.

59. Zaidel, E., 1976, Auditory vocabulary in the right hemisphere following brain bisection or hemidecortication, *Cortex* **12**:191–211.

60. Zivin, J. A., and Venditto, J. A., 1984, Experimental CNS ischemia: Serotonin antagonists reduce or prevent damage, *Neurology (N.Y.)* **34**:469–474.

INDEX

Acetylcholinesterase (AChE), 172, 182, 342, 344–346
  staining, 197
ACTH, 234, 235
  $ACTH_{4-10}$, 234–237, 243
Adenylate cyclase, 105, 114
Adrenal medulla, 135
Age-dependent event, 185
AGF2, 195, 206, 207, 209–211, 226, 227
  ganglioside inner ester, 204, 227
Allopurinol, 9
Alpha$_2$ adrenoceptors, 133
Alpha-glycerophosphate dehydrogenase, 129
Alpha-methyltyrosine, 106
Alternation
  reinforced, 353
  spontaneous, 348, 353
Alzheimer's disease, 103, 355
Aminomethane, 364
Amphetamine (AMP), 54, 55, 67, 121–129, 131–139, 201, 204, 206, 207, 209, 210, 348, 365, 366
Amygdala, 105, 106
Anastomosis
  preganglionic, 171
  postganglionic, 171
Anoxia, 305, 364
Anticoagulant, 363
  coumadin, 363
  heparin, 363
Anticoagulation, 11
Antidepressants, 367
Antihypertensives, 138
Antioxidants, 32, 54, 63, 65
Aphasia, 138, 362, 367–369, 371
  Broca's, 368–372
  Wernicke's, 369, 371
  Western Aphasia Battery (WAB), 368
Apomorphine, 115, 129, 201
  apomorphine-induced rotations, 201, 202
Arachidonate, 54
  arachidonic acid, 6, 9, 23, 24, 28–30, 33–36

Aromatic amino acid decarboxylase (AAAD), 105, 107, 110
Aspirations, 185
Astrocytes, 5, 259, 262, 270–273, 318–328
  astroglia, 144, 316, 318, 319
  transplants of purified astrocytes, 324–326
  type 1 astrocytes, 318–320
  type 2 astrocytes, 318
Asymmetry, 203, 222
Atrophy, 168, 185
Atropine, 127, 128
Autoreceptors, 108, 114
Avoidance behaviors, 197
  active avoidance, 182, 198, 210
  avoidance learning, 348, 350, 353
  passive avoidance, 198, 200, 210, 211
Axons, 169, 270
  axonal connections, integrity of, 184
  axonal growth, 170, 283, 285
    growing axonal membranes, 171
  axonal transport, 168, 180, 283
    anterograde axonal transport techniques, 180
    reestablishment of axonal transport, 176
  axon branches, 179
  axon terminals, 179
  injured axon, 282
  spared axons, 173
  surviving axons, 175
Axoplasmic flow, 169
Axotomy, 169, 191, 285

Basal lamina, 4
Behavior
  behavioral deficits, 183
  behavioral sparing, 173, 181
  behavioral substitution, 127
  open-field, 196
Beta-blockers, 363
Beta-endorphin, 89
Bicuculline, 67
Binding sites, 148
Binocular vision, 12, 125

377

Biomechanics, 58
Biorheologic factors, 11
Biotransduction of membrane-mediated information, 146
Blood–brain barrier, 4, 14, 83, 173, 207, 227, 365
Blood flow
    cerebral (CBF), 5, 126–128, 138, 200, 372
    regional, 79–81
    spinal cord, 82, 85
Brain damage, 168
Brain gray matter, 148
Brain repair, 167, 181
    mechanisms of, 169
Broca, diagonal band of, 342, 343, 345, 346
Bromlysergic acid diethylamide (BOL), 83–86
Bufotenine, 84–85

Cajal, Ramon y, 168, 191, 274
Calcium, 53, 54, 61–65, 365
    Ca²⁺, 61, 65, 149, 270
    calcium cascade, 6, 7, 11
Calcium channel antagonists, 363, 365
    calcium channel blockers, 9, 53, 63, 65, 363, 365
        flunarizine, 9, 363
        nifedipine, 9, 365
        nimodipine, 9, 53, 63, 64, 363
        verapamil, 9, 365
Carotid artery, 76, 81
    ligation, 76, 77
    occlusion, 77
Cat, 121, 122, 124–127, 134, 135, 171
Catecholamines (CA), 121–123, 127, 128, 132, 134, 135, 138, 139, 366
    catecholaminergic fibers, 180
    catecholaminergic fluorescence, 171
    cathecholaminergic neurons, 339, 341, 347
    cathechol-O-methyltransferase (COMT), 105
Caudate nucleus (CN), 105, 109, 113, 173, 175, 184, 190, 195, 207, 347–349
Cell adhesion molecules (CAMs), 4, 5, 263, 264
    neural cell adhesion molecules (nCAMs), 263
Cell counts, 202
Cell death, 185
    retrograde, 187, 190
Cell shrinkage, 198
Cell surface, 171
Cell survival, 183
    enhanced, 183
Cellular differentiation, 153
Cellular distribution, 145
Cellular membrane, 168
Cerebellum, 123, 132–134, 260
    Bergman fibers, 263
Cerebral asymmetry, 371
Cerebral perfusion, 362
Cerebral vascular occlusion, 76

Cerebrovascular accidents, 200
Chemical features, 145
Cholera toxin, 148, 149, 272
Choline acetyltransferase (ChAT), 145, 172, 173, 181, 182, 197, 198, 342, 344, 347, 350, 353, 354
    activity, 198
    levels, 198
Cholinergic afferents, 172
Cholinergic cell line, 173
Cholinergic connections, 182
Cholinergic deafferentation, 182
Cholinergic enzymes, 182
Cholinergic forebrain nuclei, 198, 211
Cholinergic neurons, 181, 198, 308, 339, 341–349, 353–355
    firing activity of residual cholinergic neurons, 181, 182
    metabolic activity of residual cholinergic neurons, 181, 182
Cholinergic terminal degeneration, 181
Chromaffin cell grafts, 135
Chromatolysis, 3, 185
Cinanserin, 84
Clinical trials, 3, 12
Clonidine, 54
Cognitive function, 362
Compensation, 187, 188
Computer-controlled injury, 56
Computerized tomography (CT), 200, 362, 369–371
Conditioned avoidance response (CAR), 54
Conditions medium, 287, 291
Consummatory behavior, 204
Contusion, 43
Corpus striatum, 105, 106, 110, 112, 114
Cortex, 17, 171, 339, 341, 342, 345
    cerebral, 174, 195, 196, 201, 210
    entorhinal (EC), 196, 220, 221, 315, 348, 350
    frontal, 181
    mediofrontal, 200
    motor, 14, 122, 123
    neo, 176, 185
        rat neocortex, 174
    sensorimotor, 122, 124, 125, 128, 132–135, 138
    visual, 122, 187, 198, 200, 211, 214
Cortical ACh, 182
Cortical blindness, 198, 211, 214
Cortical contusion, 135
Cortical metabolism, 129
Cortical slices, 173
Corticosteroids, 47, 54, 61, 363, 364
    dexamethasone, 363
Critical window, 211
Cyclic nucleotides, 8
Cyclooxygenase, 23, 30, 31, 33, 34, 36
    cyclooxygenase cascade inhibitors, 33
    cyclooxygenase inhibitors, 65

Cyproheptadine, 84–86
Cytochrome oxidase (CYO), 132

Deafferentation, 169
  hippocampal deafferentation, 171
Decortication, 176
Degeneration, 51, 174, 181
  in adulthood, 181
  anterograde, 181, 184
  prevention of, 185
    prevention of terminal, 182
  retardation of degeneration processes, 172
  retrograde, 169, 186
  secondary, 169, 181, 187, 189, 202
    reduction of, 182
  transsynaptic degeneration, 185
Dendritic loss, 182
Denervated postsynaptic cells, 169
Denervation, 51
  supersensitivity, 47, 51, 169, 187, 190
    prevention of, 187
Dentate gyrus, 172
[^{14}C]2-deoxyglucose (2-DG), 129, 131
Deoxyribonucleic acid (DNA), 295
Depression
  functional, 169
  temporary, 170
Depth perception, 121, 125, 126
Development, 170, 171, 185
  postnatal development, 176
Diacylglycerol (DG) (DAG), 8, 23–28
Diaschisis, 126, 128, 129, 131, 362
  crossed cerebellar diaschisis, 131
3,4-dihydroxyphenylacetic acid (DOPAC), 105, 107,
    108, 110, 112, 113, 176
Discrimination
  brightness, 54, 198, 211
  pattern, 198, 211
Dopamine (DA), 104–110, 113–116, 121–123, 138,
    176, 183, 202, 366
  beta-hydroxylase, 341
  levels, striatal, 202
  release, 107–110, 112–114
  supersensitivity, 201
  synthesis, 107–114, 183
  [^{3}H]DA uptake, 174, 185
Dopaminergic, 15, 103–109, 112–114, 225
  agonists, 173
  receptors, 115
Drug contraindications, 138
Drug therapy, 3
Dynorphin, 10, 53, 89, 95–97
Dysarthria, 368

Edema, 45, 181, 223, 228, 229, 302, 361
  antiedema agents, 11

Edema (cont.)
  cerebral edema, 363, 364
  reduction in, 223
EDTA, 9
Electron microscopy, 180, 289
Electrophysiological activity, spontaneous, 183
Electrophysiological evidence, 176
Emboli, 80, 86
Emotionality, 197
Environment-derived factors, 283
Enzyme recovery, 172
Epilepsy, 17, 18
EPSPs, 176–177
Excitotoxicity, 305
  excitotoxins, 5, 268
Exogenous factors, 144

Factors promoting neuronal survival, 323
Factors promoting sprouting, 323
Factors promoting substrate attachment, 323
Fetal mesencephalic tissue, 179
Fiber outgrowth, 173
Fibrinolytics, 363, 366
  streptokinase, 363, 366
  urokinase, 363, 366
  viper venom, 363, 365
Fibroblast growth factor (FGF), 271
Fimbria, 342, 344, 345, 348, 350, 399
Fink–Heimer procedure, 178, 184
Fish, 287
Fluorescence histochemistry, 174
Fluorocarbons, 363, 364
Forepaw dexterity, 135, 136, 138
Fornix, 342, 344
Free fatty acids (FFA), 23–28, 35
Free radicals, 8, 365
Function, restoration of, 169
Functional connectivity, 168
Functional reorganization, 371, 372

GABA, 1, 3, 14–18, 270
Gamma butyrolactone (GBL), 110, 111
Ganglion cells, 289, 291
Gangliosides, 66, 146–154, 156, 157, 167, 168,
    181, 195–207, 209–211, 219–222, 224,
    227, 228, 284, 367
  acute effects of, 203, 219, 220
  antibodies, 157
    antiganglioside antibodies, 156
  in biological membranes, 149
  cellular localization of, 146, 148
  and cellular response, 150, 151
  chemical characteristics of, 146
  chemical diversity of, 146
  distribution of, 148
  effects, 210

Gangliosides (*cont.*)
  exogenous gangliosides, 150, 153, 154
    effects of, 151
    exogenously supplemented single ganglioside
      species, 156
    ganglioside-induced facilitation of NA$^+$, K$^+$-AT-
      Pase activity, 203
  membrane organization of, 146, 149
  mixture, 177
  patterns, 151
  stable insertion of, 156
  storage diseases, 152
  tissue distribution of, 148
  treatments, 202, 204, 205, 210, 211, 214, 219–
    222, 224–228
Gel electrophoresis, 295
Gerbil, 77
  Mongolian, 226, 227
GM1 (monosialoganglioside), 143, 145–159, 172–
    180, 182–190, 367
  affinity-purified antibodies to GM1, 157
    anti-GM1 antibodies, 152
  derivative, 185
  effects *in vivo*, 158
    relationship of GM1 effects *in vivo* with neu-
      ronotrophic factors, 158
  gangliosidosis, 171
  -plus-amphetamine, 207
  systemic administration of GM1, 158
  versus other gangliosides, 156
Glia, 4, 285
  neo-glia limitans, 318
  radial, 262, 264
  glial cells, 282
    proliferation, 285
  glial inhibitors, 320, 321, 327
  glial mitogens, 320, 327, 329
  glial morphogens, 320, 327
  glial reaction, 312
  glial scar, 302, 303, 318, 319, 329
  gliosis, 271, 272
Glutamate, 8
  glutamate antagonists, 307
  glutamate decarboxylase (GAD), 342, 346
  glutaminergic input, 172
Glycerol, 363, 364
Grafts, 180, 287, 342, 344, 350, 352, 353
Grid-walking task, 58, 60
Growth, abnormal, 178
Growth-associated proteins (GAPs), 234, 284, 289
  B-50, 234–240
  GAP43, 239, 240
Growth-associated triggering factors (GATFs), 291
Growth cones, 289, 293
Growth factors, 270, 292–295
  growth factor receptors, 149

Haloperidol (HAL), 15, 112, 121, 123, 124, 126,
    131, 138
Hamster, 176, 177
Handedness, 371
Hemiplegia, 14, 121–125, 127, 129, 131, 133–135
  hemiplegic syndrome, 15
Hemispherectomy, 372
Hemitransections, 173, 201, 222, 224
  unilateral, 201, 203, 224, 225
High-affinity choline uptake (HACU), 181, 182
Hippocampal AChE, 197
Hippocampal slices, 188
Hippocampus, 105, 113, 135, 144, 145, 172, 174,
    182, 197, 210, 228, 312, 317, 339, 341,
    342, 344–350, 353, 354
Homovanillic acid (HVA), 105, 107–110, 112, 113,
    173, 174, 201
Horseradish peroxidase (HRP), 46, 174–176, 203,
    207
Hot plate test, 52
5-HT, 176
Huntington's disease, 5, 104
Hydroperoxyeicosatetraenoic acids (HPETEs), 29,
    30, 33
6-hydroxydopamine (6-OHDA), 106–111, 115, 173,
    174
Hydroxyeicosatetraenoic acids (HETEs), 29, 30, 33
5-hydroxyindoleacetic acid (5-HIAA), 77, 82, 83,
    85, 86
  5-HIAA concentrations, 86
Hydroxyl radicals (OH), 9
Hyperactivity, 172, 196, 210, 221
Hyperbaric oxygen, 363, 364
Hyperglycemia, 6
Hyperreflexia, 51
Hypervolemia, 364
Hypocalcia, 63
Hypoglycemia, 268, 305
Hypothalamus, 339, 347–350, 354, 355

Idazoxan, 132, 133
Immune response, 5
Immunocytochemical material, 183
Immunofluorescence, 173, 201
Immunoreactivity, 183
Impact injuries, 44, 46, 47, 49
  impaction device, 43, 56
  impactor, 56
  impact trauma, 66
Inclined plane, 52
  inclined-plane test, 57, 60
Indomethacin, 9
Infarcts, 76
  infarction, 82, 86
Inflammatory response, 5
Initial deficit, 181

Injury model, 173
Inositol, 8
Insulin, 261, 271
Interleukin, 5
Internal capsule, 105
Intracranial pressure, 77
Intramuscular, 171
Intraperitoneal, 171
Iodoantipyrine, 79, 80
Ion equilibrium, 181
Ion permeability, 151
Ischemia, 1, 3, 5–10, 45, 47, 63, 75–77, 79, 82–
        85, 92, 93, 200, 219, 226, 228, 268, 302,
        304, 305, 361, 362, 365, 366
    cerebral, 77, 365, 366
        transient cerebral, 200
    CNS, 77–80, 82, 83, 86
        therapies, 80
    duration of, 79, 80, 84
    global, 77
    ischemic damage, 75
    ischemic penumbra, 6, 11, 361, 362
    rabbit spinal cord ischemia model (RSCIM), 78–
        81, 83, 86
    reversible, 80
        irreversible, 80

K^+ concentration, extracellular, 268
Kainic acid, 8, 270
κ-receptor, 89

Laminin immunoreactivity, 293, 294
Lateral geniculate body, 200
L-dopa, 115, 127
Lesions
    bilateral, 172
    caudate nucleus, 202, 204, 209
    electrocoagulation, 172
    entorhinal cortex, 172
    intermediate, 56
    location, 370
    medical complications of, 3, 10
    mediofrontal cortex, 198, 199
    neurological complications of, 3, 10
    nigrostriatal, 173
    paradigm, 186
    partial, 46, 49, 107–113, 188
    placement, 183
    primary, 169
    septal, 197
    size, 369, 370
    suppression of eating and drinking, 204
    tectal, 186
    untreated, 207
    volume, 58
Leucine-enkephalin, 89, 97, 98

Leukotrienes (LTs), 23, 24, 29, 30, 31, 34, 35, 99
Levallorphan, 10
Lipase inhibitors, 32
Lipids, 284, 285
    cholesterol, 284
    peroxidation of, 29, 54, 65, 181
    phosphatidylcholine, 284
    phosphatidylserine, 284
Lipoxygenases, 20, 23, 31, 33, 34, 36, 46
    lipoxygenase inhibition, 34
Localization, 171
Locomotor ability, 57, 127
    locomotor function, 49, 52
    locomotor performance, 54
Locus coeruleus (LC), 129, 132, 133, 134
    fetal locus coeruleus tissue, 180
Long-term potentiation (LTP), 8
Low-molecular-weight dextran, 363, 364
Lysergic acid diethylamide (LSD), 83–85
Lysosomes, 171

Macrophage, 49, 302, 312
Magnetic resonance imaging, 362, 370
Mammalian nonregenerative CNS, 296
Mannitol, 363, 364
Matrix components, extracellular, 263
    collagen, 263, 264
    laminin, 264
Maze learning, 348, 349, 350, 351, 352, 353
Medial forebrain bundle, 105
Mediofrontal aspirations, 198
Melanocortins
    administration, 243, 249–251
    clinical trials, 251–253
    development, 235
    dose–response relations, 241
    electrophysiology, 243–246
    eye opening, 235
    histology, 246, 247
    motor function, 242, 243
    neural injury, 233
    pathophysiological mechanism, 247–249
    sensory function, 240–242
    tissue culture, 236
Membrane
    failure, 223
    fluidity, 150
    function, 150
    lipids, 23, 25, 27, 35
    organization, 145
    protection, 228
Membrane Na^+, K^+-ATPase, 219, 223–225, 227,
        228
Mesolimbic, 105
Messengers, second, 168
Metabolic activity, 170

Metabolic depression, 131
Methionine, 287, 288
1-methyl-4-phenyl-1,2,3,6-tetrahydropyridine
    (MPTP), 106
Methylsergide, 84
Microcirculation, 11
Microscope, light, 179
Microspheres, 81, 82
    radiolabeled, 81
Migration, radial, 262
Molecular cascade, 168
Molecular mechanisms, 168
Molecules, diffusible, 286
Monoamine oxidase (MAO), 105
Monoclonal antibody A2B5, 157
Monocular deprivation, 187
Morphine, 89, 110
Morphogens, 275
    morphogenesis, inborn errors of, 262
Mortality, 220
    decrease in, 228
    reduced, 227
Motor deficits, 15
    severe, 206
MSH, 234, 235
    administration, 243, 249–251
    clinical trials, 251–253

Nerve growth factor (NGF), 144, 145, 154–159,
    259, 265, 291, 304, 308, 313, 323, 331,
    339–360
    and cell survival, 345, 355
    and ChAT, 342, 343, 344
    mRNA coding for, 341, 355
    receptors, 341–344, 346, 347, 355, 356
    transport, 341
    and triiodothyronine, 342
Nerve transplantation, 285
Neural environment, control of, 326
Neuraminidase, 188
Neurites, 171
    meganeurites, 152, 171
    neurite outgrowth, 153, 154, 156, 157
    neurite promoting factors (NPF), 313, 314, 324,
        326, 327, 329, 331
    neurite repair, 151
    neurite sprouting, 179
    neuritogenesis, 151
Neurobiology, developmental, 259
Neuroblastoma cells, 153, 154, 155
Neurofilament protein, 156
Neuroimaging, 362
Neuron(s), 145
    ghost neurons, 189
    cell survival of, 144, 158, 259
    connections, 183

Neuron(s)(cont.)
    death of, 169, 265
        in development, 185
        secondary, 268, 304, 305, 307, 330
            prevention of, 307, 324, 326, 330
    development of, 152
    membrane-mediated transfer of information, 145
    migration of, 262
    networks of, 168
    primary fetal (E8) chick neurons, 156, 158
        chick sensory neurons, 286
    primary PNS neurons, 154
    primary sensory neurons, 154
    proliferation of, 260, 261
    regeneration of, 282
    residual neurons, 182
        undamaged, 202
    shrinkage of, 185
    spared neurons, 202
    stabilization of, 260, 261, 265, 267
    survival of, 174, 175, 183, 196, 270, 303, 327
Neuronotoxic factors, 268, 310
    astrocytic neuronotoxic factor, 268
Neuronotrophic activity after injury, 144
Neuronotrophic effects, 197, 267
Neuronotrophic factors (NTF), 143–146, 151, 158,
        260, 265–267, 270, 275, 304, 305, 308–
        310, 313, 323, 324, 326, 327
    ciliary neuronotrophic factor (CNTF), 158
    neuronal cell responsiveness to, 151
        modulation of neuronal cell responsiveness to,
            146
Neuronotrophic substances, 180
Neuroontogenesis, 259, 260
Neurotoxin, 176
Neurotransmission, 173
    neurotransmitter, 8, 14
Neurotrophic factors, 304, 310, 329, 339, 360
    activity, 286
Neurotropic factors, 339–360
Neurotubule proteins, 341
Nicotine, 112, 114
Nictitating membrane, 171
    supersensitivity of, 187
Nigrostriatal system, 105–116, 171, 173, 195, 196
    axons, 201
    pathway, 184, 201, 203, 205, 210, 211, 222, 224,
        225
    transections, 204
Nissal-stain, 202
N-methyl-D-aspartate (NMDA), 8
Nonneuronal cells, 286, 291, 294–296
Norepinephrine (NE), 121–125, 132–134, 176
    degeneration of, 174
Nuclei
    dorsal lateral geniculate nuclei of the thalamus
        (LGd), 179, 185

Nuclei (*cont.*)
magnocellular nuclei (MFN), 181
pretectal nuclei (PT), 179
ventral lateral geniculate nuclei of the thalamus
(LGv), 179
Nucleus accumbens, 105, 106, 348, 349
Nucleus, basal, 182
Nucleus basalis, 342–343, 345
magnocellularis, 198
Nucleus, red, 176, 180

Occlusion, 200
Ocular dominance, 187
shift, 187
Olfactory tubercle, 105
Oligodendrocytes, 4, 5, 259, 271
Oncogenes, 295
fos, 295, 296
myc, 295, 296
Opiate antagonists, 47, 53, 54, 363, 365
naloxone, 10, 11, 47, 53, 54, 61, 63, 67, 90–95,
98, 363, 365
Opiate receptors, 91, 95
opiate-receptor antagonists, 90, 93, 95, 98
Opioids, 10
endogenous opioid peptides, 89
opioid receptor, 53
Optic nerve, 286, 292, 296, 348, 349
fish, 287–291, 295
rabbit, 287, 289–291, 293
optic tract axons, 185
obtic tract sprouting, 185
Org.2766, 234
clinical trials, 251–253
development, 235
electrophysiology, 243–246
histology, 246, 247
motor function, 242, 243
sensory function, 242, 243
Osmotic minipump, 174

Paralysis, 171
Parkinson's disease, 5, 103, 104, 106–109, 113–115
Pathophysiology, 6
Peripheral nerve regeneration, 170
Peripheral nervous system (PNS), 148, 154, 170
Peroneal nerve, 174
Perturbation, subcellular, 181
Petalias, 371
Pharmacodynamic parameters, 13
Pharmacokinetic parameters, 13
Pharmacological agents, 181
Pharmacological intervention, 2, 44, 52, 65, 363
Pharmacological protection, 9, 11
barbiturates, 9–11, 363, 365, 366
Pharmacological treatment, 3, 366, 367
Phase of injury, acute, 200

Phenothiazines, 9
Phenotypic expression, 168
Phenoxybenzamine, 124
Phentermine, 134
Phenylpropanolamine (PPA), 134
Phenytoin, 15
Pheochromocytoma, PC_{12}, 154, 155, 156
Phorbol ester, 8
Phosphoglycerides, 25
Phospholipases, 25–28, 32, 54
Phospholipid degradation, 65
Photosensitivity, 18
Physical therapy, 125, 137
Placebo, 12, 13, 137
placebo injections, 200
Placing responses, 54
Planum temporale, 372
Plasma half-life, 206, 207
Plasma membrane 156, 228
Plasminogen activators, 262, 264, 272
tissue type, 263, 272
urokinase type, 263, 272, 273
Platelet antiaggregants, 363, 365
ASA, 363
dipyridamole, 363
platelet antiaggregation drugs, 11
Polyamine, 283
Polypeptides, 282–289, 291, 293–295
Postepileptic paralysis, 17
Postoperative day, 206
Postsynaptic cells, response of, 170
sensitivity alterations of postsynaptic receptors,
187
slow-rising postsynaptic potentials, 176
up-regulation of postsynaptic receptors, 170
Presynaptic markers, 189
presynaptic nerve terminals, 172
presynaptic transmitter release, 170
presynaptic transmitter synthesis, 170
Primary insult, 181
Projections from host to transplant, 316
projections from transplant to host, specificity, 315
Proopiomelanocortins, 234
Propranolol, 124
Prostacyclin (PGI_2), 9, 29–31, 34, 363, 365
Prostaglandins (PGs), 23, 24, 29–31
Protective action, 185
Protein kinase, 6
protein kinase C (PKC), 6, 8
Proteins, 284
structural proteins, 283
tubulin, 283
synthesis, 287
Pruning, 180
Pupil, 171
Putamen, 105, 370
Pyramidal layer, 188

Quipazine, 85

Rabbit, 78, 79, 81, 82, 84, 287
Raven's Colored Progressive Matrices, 369
Reactivation, 169
Receptors, 114–116
  affinity, 187
  expression, 116
  sensitivity, 168
Recovery, 171, 173
  behavioral, 168, 207
  of function, 127, 168, 181, 220–222, 226, 324
  spontaneous recovery, 210
Reducing agents, 9
Regeneration, 44, 47, 49, 66, 67, 168–170, 174,
      176, 201, 282–285, 302
  injury-induced regeneration, 283
  true regeneration, 180
Regrowth, 169, 174
Rehabilitation, 14, 17
Reinnervation, 172, 180, 196, 197, 201, 202, 220
Reinstatement of benefits, 124
Rejection, immunologic, 287
Remote functional depression (RFD), 126, 128, 131,
      132, 134, 139
Renin, 354, 355
Repair processes, 144
  functional repair, 168
  structural repair, 168
Residual capacities, 55
Retina, 287–290
Retinofugal fibers, 177
Retrograde cell atrophy, 181
Retrograde cell labeling, 180
Retrograde soma shrinkage, 182
Retrograde transport, 174, 175
Ribonucleic acid (RNA), 282–284, 295
  biosynthesis, 341
  messenger (mRNA), 294–296
Rotation, 173, 202, 204
  rotational asymmetry, 201, 203, 210, 222–225
    amphetamine-induced rotational asymmetry, 203
  rotational behavior, 115, 202, 205
  stereotyped rotation, 201

Saline injections, 206
  saline-injected controls, 187
Sarcoma-180 tumors, 340
Scar formation, 5
Schaffer collateral–commissural fibers, 188
Schwann cells, 4, 49, 264, 269, 272, 274, 285
Segregation, 178
Septohippocampal system, 182, 195, 196
Septum, 105, 106, 145, 182, 315, 339, 341–346,
      348, 350, 353–355

Septum (cont.)
  dorsal septum, 172
  medioventral septum, 172
Serotonin, 75–77, 82, 83, 85
  agonists, 83, 84
  antagonists, 83, 85, 86
  inhibitors, 85, 363, 366
    competitive inhibitor, 84
  intravenously administered, 85
  serotinergic enzymes, 182
Serum-free defined media, 286
Serum glucose, 6
Sham control, 207
Shrinkage, 187
Signaling, transmembrane, 151
Signal recognition, 151
Signal transduction, 151
Silver grains, 179
Smoking, 114
Snare ligature, 78
Somatosensory evoked potentials (SEPs), 46, 51, 52
Spared fibers in recovery process of partially
      damaged system, 180
Spasticity, 51
Spatial alternation task, 196, 198, 199
  spatial alternation deficits, 202
    learning deficits, 207
Spinal cord, 171, 174, 176
  grafts, 66
  injury, 43, 44, 53, 55, 63, 68, 92, 93, 98
    acute phase of, 43, 45, 46, 52, 53, 61, 65
    chronic phase of, 43, 45, 52, 54, 55, 66, 67
    compression injuries of the spinal cord, 45
    experimental spinal cord injury, 53
  spinal transections, 54, 55, 66, 67
Spines, 171
Spontaneous outgrowth, 180
Sprouting, 67, 168–171, 174, 178, 188, 196, 197,
      202, 220, 221, 289, 329, 344, 346, 350,
      353–355
  axonal, 188, 312, 313
    collateral axonal, 51
  collateral, 47, 180, 182, 196, 198, 202, 371
  enhancement of, 172
  intrasystem, 172
  neuronal, 195, 197, 201, 210, 220
  nigrostriatal fiber, 204
  potentiate, 179
  promote central, 180
  regenerative, 2, 201
  suppression of, 172
  time course of, 189, 190
Statistical tests, 12
Status epilepticus, 268, 270
Steroids, 11, 53
Striatal Na^+, K^+-ATPase activity, 203

Striatum, 174, 346, 347
Stroke, 1, 3, 6, 11, 76, 78, 80, 121, 134, 138, 139, 200, 214, 226, 302, 361, 362, 365–369, 372, 373
  acute stroke, 363, 364, 366
  embolic stroke model, 80
    microsphere embolic stroke model, 78, 80, 86
  stroke patients, 137, 363, 367, 373
Structural–functional paradox, 189
Subcellular mechanisms, 168
Substantia innominata, 345, 346
Substantia nigra (SN), 104, 107, 109, 110, 114, 115, 174, 175, 183, 190, 222
  substantia nigra pars compacta (SNc), 202, 207
  substantia nigra pars reticulata (SNr), 174, 184
Substrate adhesion molecules (SAM), 4
Superior cervical ganglion, 171
Superior colliculus (rSC), 176, 177, 179, 185, 186
Supersensitivity, 115
Sympathetic neurons, 339, 340, 341, 345, 349, 353–355
Synapse turnover, 310
Synaptic efficiency, 169, 187, 188
Synaptic mechanisms, 172
Synaptic response, potentiated, 188
Synaptogenesis
  reactive, 2, 310, 312, 329
  regenerative, 315
Synaptosomes, 174
  striatal, 185

Tactile placing, 122
Target field, 185
Terminals, 174
  terminal fields, 178
    abnormally formed, 178
    diencephalic, 179
Termination density, 179
Thalamus
  lateral posterior nucleus of (LP), 179
  medial dorsal nucleus of, 199
Theories, 2
Thiazides, 138
Thromboxane, 363, 365
  thromboxane A_2 (TXA$_2$), 29–31, 34, 35
Thymidine, 291
Thyrotropin-releasing hormone (TRH), 53, 54, 65, 98, 99

Tissue culture, 274
T-maze performance, 324
Todd's phenomenon: see Postepileptic paralysis,
Transections, 176
  unilateral, 201
    unilateral nigrostriatal, 203, 222
Transmitter
  biosynthesis, 168, 188
    up-regulation of, 173
  release, 107–109, 168
  synthesis, 107–109, 114, 169
    compensatory up-regulation of transmitter synthesis, 183
Transplants, 135
Trauma, 368
Treadmill locomotion, 54, 55
Treatment modalities, 53
Trophic factors, 185, 260
  sources of trophic factors, 326, 327
  trophic availability, 144
  trophic deficit, 144
  trophic effects, 144, 145
  trophic substances, 185, 189
  trophic support, 185
Tyrosine hydroxylase (TH), 105–108, 173, 198, 202, 206, 341, 342, 346
  activity, 174

Underlying mechanisms, 156

Vasoconstrictors, 364
  vasoconstrictive properties, 76
Vasodilators, 364
  carbon dioxide, 364
    CO_2 inhalation, 363
  papaverine, 363, 364
  theophylline, 364
Vasospasm, 77
Ventral tegmental area, 105
Vestibular free-fall responses, 52
Vicariation, 126, 127
Visual cliff, 122, 126
Visual system, 177, 180, 286, 295

Wallerian degeneration, 4, 47, 50
Weight loss, 204
Withdrawal, 18